Herbs and Herbalism

nova
Medicine & Health
New York

Herbs and Herbalism

Indian Medicinal Plants of Ladakh Himalaya Used in Sowa Rigpa
Mayaram Uniyal, Deepak Kumar Semwal,
Ruchi Badoni Semwal and Ankit Kumar
2022 ISBN: 979-8-88697-210-8 (Softcover)
2022 ISBN: 979-8-88697-427-0 (eBook)

***Alpinia nigra* (Gaertn) Burtt: Prospects in Controlling Diabetes**
Biman Bhuyan, Angkita Baruah, M Pharm.
and Prakash Rajak, PhD
2022 ISBN: 979-8-88697-225-2 (Softcover)
2022 ISBN: 979-8-88697-300-6 (eBook)

Healing Medicinal Plants (Ajwain, Asafoetida, Barberry, Fenugreek and Fig) and Sustainable Human Health
Mohamad Hesam Shahrajabian, PhD and Wenli Sun, PhD
2022 ISBN: 978-1-68507-496-8 (eBook)

An Introduction to Medicinal Herbs
Mila Emerald, PhD, Dr. Sc. (Editor)
2021 ISBN: 978-1-68507-147-9 (Hardcover)
2021 ISBN: 978-1-68507-287-2 (eBook)

Ginger's Antimicrobial, Anti-Nausea and Anti-Osteoarthritic Activities
Diana R. Cundell, PhD (Editor)
2021 ISBN: 978-1-68507-117-2 (Hardcover)
2021 ISBN: 978-1-68507-165-3 (eBook)

More information about this series can be found at https://novapublishers.com/product-category/series/herbs-and-herbalism/

Sun-Chong Wang

Herbal Prescriptions for Signs and Symptoms:

GMP Herbal Formulations for Treating Clinical Manifestations of Diseases

nova
Medicine & Health
New York

DOI: https://doi.org/10.52305/PNQX5883.

Library of Congress Cataloging-in-Publication Data

ISBN: 979-8-88697-835-3

Published by Nova Science Publishers, Inc. † New York

This book is dedicated to Gao Yue Wang.

Contents

Preface

Herbal Prescriptions for Signs and Symptoms: GMP Herbal Formulations for Treating Clinical Manifestations of Diseases serves those who, by the use of cGMP herbal products, treat suboptimal health, practice preventive healthcare, and exercise personalized medicine.

According to a worldwide survey by the World Health Organization, only 5% and 20% of the population are respectively healthy and diseased. The rest, i.e., 75%, of the world population are subhealthy, a condition that, albeit suboptimal, does not reach the diagnostic criteria of a disease by the standard methods of modern Western medicine. In contrast to the few options offered by modern Western medicine, such as vitamins and minerals, various cGMP-certified herbal products are available over the counter for the subhealthy in the Asia-Pacific region including Japan, Taiwan, Hong Kong, and Singapore. The book's first aim is to benefit the vast majority of people in the world who are overlooked or underserved by conventional medicine.

As signs and symptoms are observed or experienced before diagnosis, if signs and symptoms can be treated early in disease progression, diseases could be prevented, saving a lot of cost of the society and individuals. The same idea was proposed 1400 years ago by Sūn Sīmiǎo, a famous Taoist physician and pharmacist in the Tang dynasty and author of Essential Prescriptions Worth a Thousand in Gold for Every Emergency (Bèi jí qiānjīn yào fang). Sūn Sīmiǎo was also the first who combined herbal formulas to enhance the effectiveness of the treatment, a practice that has since been followed by later herbalists. Throughout the book, we will also see prescriptions consisting of multiple formulas and herbs for the subhealthy conditions.

A disease can manifest a constellation of signs and symptoms. However, the specific combination of signs and symptoms varies from patient to patient. For example, high blood glucose levels can damage the retinas in some patients while the peripheral nerves in the foot in other patients with diabetes. Instead of the 'one size fits all' paradigm of conventional medicine, different herbs are combined into a prescription for patients with the same disease but different signs and symptoms. To this aim, the book lists herbal prescriptions for not only signs and symptoms but also for diseases given signs and symptoms. Note that as genes underlie one's predispositions to signs and symptoms, the personalized herbal prescriptions work best for the patients.

The herbs that make up the prescriptions in this book are, in granular form, made by PIC/S GMP-compliant pharmaceutic manufacturers. This level of government-industry enforcement helps ensure the safety and quality of the herbal products, paving the way toward modernization and globalization of traditional herbal medicine. The terms that we use for the signs and symptoms in the book are from the MeSH (Medical Subject Headings) thesaurus which is a controlled and hierarchically organized vocabulary generated and maintained by the National Library of Medicine of the National Institute of Health, the U.S. The MeSH hierarchy helps the reader capture the relatedness and grouping among the signs and symptoms.

This book contains 300 such signs and symptoms and their associated herbal prescriptions. Likewise, the diseases appearing in the book are in ICD-9 and ICD-10 (the 9th and 10th revision of the International Classification of Diseases issued by the WHO), which are what patients receive from their modern Western medical doctors' diagnoses in most countries across the world. Adoption of the MeSH symptom and ICD disease terms in the book helps bridge the gap between modern Western medicine and traditional herbal medicine.

Finally, the herbal prescriptions in this book result from the multilingual neural machine translation method with state-of-the-art Transformer model on a large dataset consisting of a decade's worth of reimbursement records from the National Health Insurance Program, Taiwan. The current wave of artificial intelligence advances in natural language processing makes possible the book with the aforementioned features.

Sun-Chong Wang
New Taipei, Taiwan
January 2023

Acknowledgments

The author is indebted to Gao Yue Wang, Lanying Huang, Jessie J.Y. Liu, and Peggy P.C. Chu for their support and assistance.

Part I. Signs and Symptoms to Herbs

Chapter 1

Pain

Pain is a sensation initiated by a stimulus which harms one's body. Because the stimulus is damaging, the sensation is unpleasant, causing one to become averse to the stimulus or the situation which could cause harm for one's own benefit in the future. Sensation is a nervous system physiological phenomenon. Pain is a manifestation of neurology or a pathological condition of the nervous system. Since the nerves of the nervous system innervate all parts of the body, pain can be expressed in various areas. In this chapter, we present herbal prescriptions for pains on the head (including the eye, ear, tooth and tongue), neck, shoulder, chest, breast, abdomen, flank, back, low back, pelvis, hip, buttock, leg, and foot. Other pains and their classifications are shown in Figure 1.1.

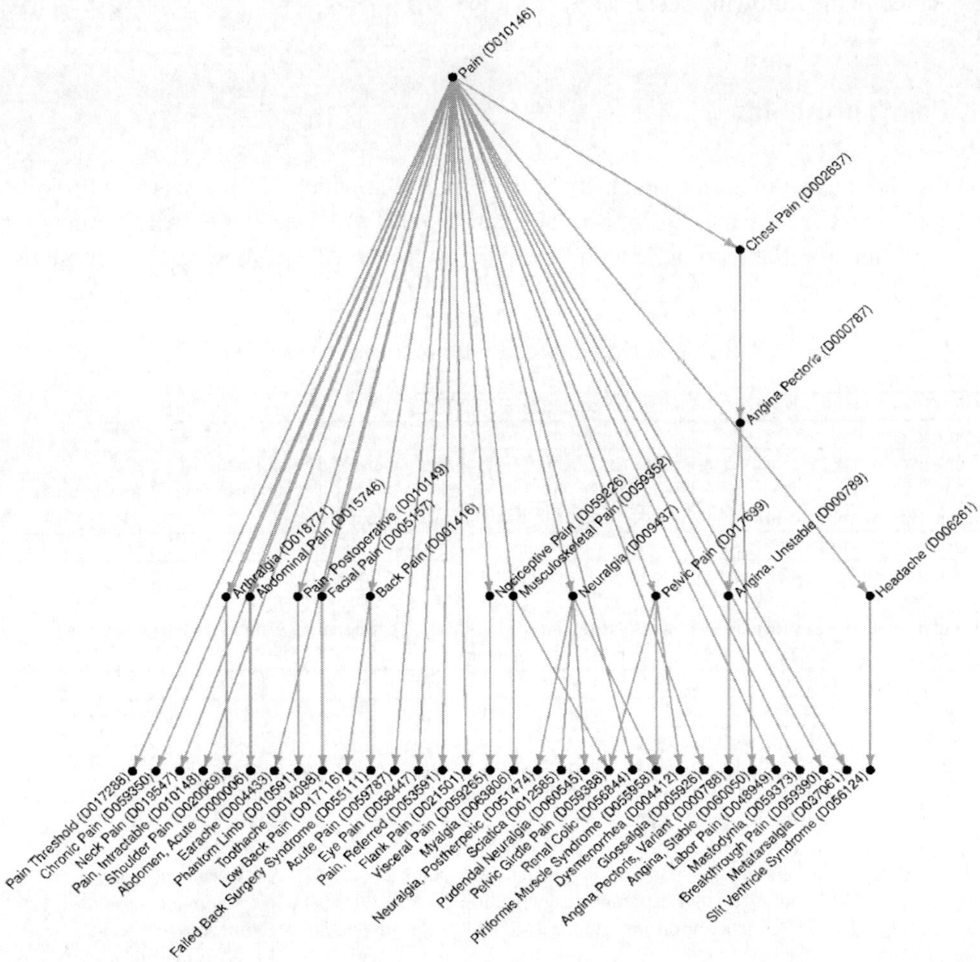

Figure 1.1. Pain sensation, a nervous system physiological phenomenon, occurs in different ways and regions of the body.

Note that because mind and body connect, physical pain can induce emotional reactions such as anxiety, fear and depression. A better pain management program should therefore also attend to patient's psychological state.

As the painful sensation is so unwelcome, natural products that kill pain have been vigorously sought throughout the history of human existence. Indeed, many herbs have been found to relieve pain including Yánhúsuǒ, Sāngzhī, Jiānghuáng, Yùjīn, Niúxī, Mòyào and Rǔxiāng, many of which are now known to be anti-inflammatory. The diseases appearing in this chapter that can cause the described signs and symptoms include disorders of nervous system, cardiovascular diseases, myoneural disorders, disorders of metabolism, conditions of brain, myopathy, heart diseases, disorders of joint, and so on. In modern herbology, individual herbs have been combined into herbal formulas to treat the complexity of a disease which can have multiple signs and symptoms. The multi-herb formulas commonly used to manage pain in this chapter include Shūjīnghuóxuètāng, Sháoyàogāncǎotāng, Guìzhītāng, Dāngguīniāntòngtāng, Sìnìtāng, Xuèfǔzhúyūtāng, Huángqíwǔwùtāng, Jiāwèixiāoyáosǎn, Èrshùtāng, Dúhuójìshēngtāng, and so on. Finally, we observe that acupuncture is used along with herbal prescriptions in most of the pain prescriptions in this chapter. Specific regimens are detailed in the following sections.

1.1. Pain Threshold

Pain threshold is the minimum intensity of the stimulus at which one begins to feel pain. Pain threshold varies from person to person and can change with one's age or health conditions such as systemic inflammation and chronic pain. In Table 1.1 we show the prescriptions for pain threshold.

Table 1.1. Herbal prescriptions for pain threshold

Pain Threshold: https://meshb.nlm.nih.gov/record/ui?ui=D017288.
Common prescriptions:
Huángqíwǔwùtāng 5g chuānxiōng 1g dānshēn 1g zhúrú 1g sāngzhī 1g dāngguī 1g jiānghuáng 1g Huángqíwǔwùtāng 5g chuānxiōng 1g dānshēn 1g zhúrú 1g sāngzhī 1g dāngguī 1g jiānghuáng 1g + acupuncture Huángqíwǔwùtāng 5g dānshēn 1g zhúrú 1g sāngzhī 1g jiānghuáng 1g + acupuncture
Alternative prescriptions:
Huángqíwǔwùtāng 5g dānshēn 1g zhúrú 1g sāngzhī 1g jiānghuáng 1g jīxuèténg 1g Guìzhītāng 5g báizhú 2g fùzǐ 2g báisháo 2g fúlíng 2g dǎngshēn 1g shēngjiāng 1g Huángqíwǔwùtāng 5g chuānxiōng 1g dānshēn 1g zhúrú 1g yánhúsuǒ 1g sāngzhī 1g dāngguī 1g jiānghuáng 1g + acupuncture Guìzhītāng 5g báizhú 1g fúlíng 1g + acupuncture
Indicated diseases:
Myopathy, unspecified 359.9 (Myopathy, unspecified G729); Myoneural disorders 358; Unspecified disorders of nervous system 349.9 (Disorder of central nervous system, unspecified G969); Cardiovascular disease, unspecified 429.2 (Atherosclerotic heart disease of native coronary artery without angina pectoris I2510); Other dermatoses 702; Polyneuropathy in diabetes 357.2 (Diabetes mellitus due to underlying condition with diabetic polyneuropathy E0842, Drug or chemical induced diabetes mellitus with neurological complications with diabetic polyneuropathy E0942, Type 1 diabetes mellitus with diabetic polyneuropathy E1042, Type 2 diabetes mellitus with diabetic polyneuropathy E1142, Other specified diabetes mellitus with diabetic polyneuropathy E1342); Diabetes with neurological manifestations 250.6; Diabetes with peripheral circulatory disorders 250.7; Diabetes mellitus 250; Unspecified endocrine disorder 259.9 (Endocrine disorder, unspecified E349); Unspecified disorder of metabolism 277.9 (Metabolic disorder, unspecified E889); Unspecified disorder of joint, site unspecified 719.90 (Joint disorder, unspecified M259)

Pain Threshold: https://meshb.nlm.nih.gov/record/ui?ui=D017288.	
Myopathy, unspecified 359.9/G729 with pain threshold D017288:	
Huángqíwǔwùtāng 5g juānbìtāng 5g dānshēn 1g zhúrú 1g sāngzhī 1g jiānghuáng 1g to ♀	Huángqíwǔwùtāng 5g dānshēn 1g zhúrú 1g sāngzhī 1g jiānghuáng 1g to ♂
Cardiovascular disease, unspecified 429.2/I2510 with pain threshold D017288:	
Yùzhú 5g sìnìtāng 5g mǔdānpí 1g zhīzǐ 1g huánglián 0g to ♀	Sìnìtāng 5g gānlùyǐn 5g lóngdǎnxiègāntāng 5g to ♂

The dominant component in both the common and alternative prescriptions for pain threshold is Huángqíwǔwùtāng, which tonifies Qi, the vital energy or life force in any living organism according to many medical traditions. The nervous system enables us to not only sense stimuli through our sense organs but also respond to changes in the environment via skeletal muscles. Muscle cells and neurons function together as the neuromuscular system, and any pathological condition in one can impact the other. Myopathy and myoneural disorders are therefore indicated by the symptom in the table. Herbal prescriptions can be sex specific, as shown in the table. Note that a prescription is typically served three time a day (after meals) for three, five, six or seven days till the pain is relieved. In the prescription package, one spoonful of medicinal granules weighs one gram. If the weight of the medicinal granules is 0.4 grams or less, it is indicated as 0g in the table.

1.2. Chronic Pain

When pain lasts for longer than three months, the pain becomes chronic. Examples of chronic pain are low back pain and headache. Chronic pain can accompany chronic diseases such as osteoarthritis, shingles, diabetes and cancer. Table 1.2 lists the herbal treatments for chronic pain.

Table 1.2. Herbal prescriptions for chronic pain

Chronic Pain: https://meshb.nlm.nih.gov/record/ui?ui=D059350.
Common prescriptions:
Xiǎohuóluòdān 5g shūjīnghuóxuètāng 5g dāngguīniāntòngtāng 5g + acupuncture Shūjīnghuóxuètāng 5g dāngguīniāntòngtāng 5g + acupuncture Xiǎohuóluòdān 5g shūjīnghuóxuètāng 5g + acupuncture
Alternative prescriptions:
Shūjīnghuóxuètāng 5g guìzhī 0g Táohóngsìwùtāng 5g Xuèfǔzhúyūtāng 5g shēntòngzhúyūtāng 5g dāngguīniāntòngtāng 5g huángbò 1g cāngzhú 1g + acupuncture Juānbìtāng 5g shūjīnghuóxuètāng 4g dāngguīniāntòngtāng 4g yǐtiáogēn 1g chuānqī 1g mùguā 1g sāngzhī 1g jīxuèténg 1g xùduàn 1g + acupuncture Shūjīnghuóxuètāng 5g guìzhī 0g huángqín 0g + acupuncture
Indicated diseases:
Myopathy, unspecified 359.9 (Myopathy, unspecified G729); Myoneural disorders 358; Unspecified disorders of nervous system 349.9 (Disorder of central nervous system, unspecified G969); Unspecified disorder of joint, site unspecified 719.90 (Joint disorder, unspecified M259); Cardiovascular disease, unspecified 429.2 (Atherosclerotic heart disease of native coronary artery without angina pectoris I2510); Other dermatoses 702; Polyneuropathy in diabetes 357.2 (Diabetes mellitus due to underlying condition with diabetic polyneuropathy E0842, Drug or chemical induced diabetes mellitus with neurological complications with diabetic polyneuropathy E0942, Type 1 diabetes mellitus with diabetic polyneuropathy E1042, Type 2 diabetes mellitus with diabetic polyneuropathy E1142, Other specified diabetes mellitus with diabetic polyneuropathy E1342); Diabetes with neurological manifestations 250.6; Diabetes with peripheral circulatory disorders 250.7; Diabetes mellitus 250; Unspecified endocrine disorder 259.9 (Endocrine disorder, unspecified E349); Unspecified disorder of metabolism 277.9 (Metabolic disorder, unspecified E889)

Table 1.2. (Continued)

Chronic Pain: https://meshb.nlm.nih.gov/record/ui?ui=D059350.	
Myopathy, unspecified 359.9/G729 with chronic pain D059350:	
Huángqíwǔwùtāng 5g juānbìtāng 5g dānshēn 1g zhúrú 1g sāngzhī 1g jiānghuáng 1g to ♀	Huángqíwǔwùtāng 5g dāngguīsìnìtāng 5g dānshēn 1g zhúrú 1g sāngzhī 1g jiānghuáng 1g to ♂
Cardiovascular disease, unspecified 429.2/I2510 with chronic pain D059350:	
Yùzhú 5g sìnìtāng 5g mǔdānpí 1g zhīzǐ 1g to ♀	Sìnìtāng 5g gānlùyǐn 5g lóngdǎnxiègāntāng 5g to ♂

Shūjīnghuóxuètāng has traditionally been used for soreness of the musculoskeletal system that includes the muscles, joints and nerves. It 'dredges meridians, activates Blood and eliminates Wind.' The words enclosed in single quotation marks represent the author's translation of the expression from Chinese medical classics. In addition, the author may capitalize the first letter of certain traditional terms, such as "Blood," because in traditional Chinese medicine, the concept of Blood encompasses more than what is understood as blood in modern Western medicine. Finally, we note that since Blood activating medicines can quicken blood circulation, they are contraindicated in patients taking anticoagulants such as heparin and warfarin.

1.3. Neck Pain

Many people in modern days suffer from neck pain because longtime use of smartphones and computers strains the muscles and tendons around the neck and upper back. Most neck pain resolves in days, however others become chronic depending on the cause. Table 1.3 shows that problems with the spinal cord can also cause neck pain.

Table 1.3. Herbal prescriptions for neck pain

Neck Pain: https://meshb.nlm.nih.gov/record/ui?ui=D019547.
Common prescriptions:
Guìzhītāng 5g báizhú 1g fùzǐ 1g Guìzhītāng 5g chuānwū 1g yánhúsuǒ 1g Guìzhītāng 5g báizhú 1g fùzǐ 1g fúlíng 1g Guìzhītāng 5g chuānwū 1g
Alternative prescriptions:
Guìzhītāng 5g shēngjiāng 1g guìzhī 1g Guìzhītāng 5g gégēn 1g dàhuáng 0g Guìzhītāng 5g chuānwū 1g dàhuáng 0g Guìzhītāng 5g chuānwū 1g dàhuáng 0g + acupuncture Huángqíwǔwùtāng 5g dānshēn 1g zhúrú 1g sāngzhī 1g jiānghuáng 1g
Indicated diseases:
Myopathy, unspecified 359.9 (Myopathy, unspecified G729); Myoneural disorders 358; Unspecified disorders of nervous system 349.9 (Disorder of central nervous system, unspecified G969); Unspecified disease of spinal cord 336.9 (Disease of spinal cord, unspecified G959); Malignant neoplasm of spinal cord 192.2 (Malignant neoplasm of spinal cord C720, Malignant neoplasm of cauda equina C721); Neuroendocrine tumors 209; Malignant neoplasm of nervous system, part unspecified 192.9 (Malignant neoplasm of central nervous system, unspecified C729); Unspecified disorder of joint, site unspecified 719.90 (Joint disorder, unspecified M259)

Neck Pain: https://meshb.nlm.nih.gov/record/ui?ui=D019547.	
Myopathy, unspecified 359.9/G729 with neck pain D019547:	
Shēntòngzhúyūtāng 5g shūjīnghuóxuètāng 5g to ♀	Huángqíwǔwùtāng 5g dāngguīsìnìtāng 5g dānshēn 1g zhúrú 1g sāngzhī 1g jiānghuáng 1g to ♂
Unspecified disease of spinal cord 336.9/G959 with neck pain D019547:	
Shūjīnghuóxuètāng 5g dúhuójìshēngtāng 5g + acupuncture to ♀	Shūjīnghuóxuètāng 5g dúhuójìshēngtāng 5g + acupuncture to ♂

Guìzhītāng was originally composed for patients with headache, neck pain and fever due to the common cold or influenza. Because the viral infection can cause vomiting and diarrhea in some patients, Guìzhītāng also 'harmonizes digestion and defence,' in addition to its effect of 'muscle releasing and Wind expelling' on the respiratory symptoms. Chuānwū 'expels Wind, eliminates Dampness,' 'disperses chills, stops pain,' and has mainly been used as a rheumatic pain killer. Its modern uses are for other and unspecified disorders of back and joint (Wang, 2019). Note that raw Chuānwū, i.e., aconite root, is toxic to the central nervous system, so is Fùzǐ. One should never ingest unprocessed Chuānwū and Fùzǐ.

1.4. Intractable Pain

Intractable pain refers to persistent pain that is resistant to standard pain treatment. It is a severe form of chronic pain and can lead to patient's disability and eventual death if the pain is not relieved. Intractable pain can be the result of such diseases as migraine and degenerative disc disease. Table 1.4 shows herbal prescriptions for intractable pain and also for diseases presenting intractable pain.

Xiǎohuóluòdān is a formula consisting of Chuānwū and Rǔxiāng, which are single herbs known for their pain relieving. We see from the table that cancer or cancer treatment can cause intractable pain.

Table 1.4. Herbal prescriptions for intractable pain

Intractable Pain: https://meshb.nlm.nih.gov/record/ui?ui=D010148.
Common prescriptions:
Guìzhītāng 5g yánhúsuǒ 1g + acupuncture Guìzhītāng 5g chuānwū 1g Guìzhītāng 5g chuānwū 1g yánhúsuǒ 1g Guìzhītāng 5g yánhúsuǒ 1g Guìzhītāng 5g gégēn 1g
Alternative prescriptions:
Guìzhītāng 5g shēngjiāng 1g guìzhī 1g Sìnìtāng 5g shēngjiāng 1g guìzhī 1g dàhuáng 0g Huángqíwǔwùtāng 5g dānshēn 1g zhúrú 1g sāngzhī 1g dāngguī 1g jiānghuáng 1g Guìzhītāng 5g báizhú 1g fùzǐ 1g Huángqíwǔwùtāng 5g chuānxiōng 1g sāngzhī 1g dāngguī 1g jiānghuáng 1g
Indicated diseases:
Myopathy, unspecified 359.9 (Myopathy, unspecified G729); Myoneural disorders 358; Unspecified disorders of nervous system 349.9 (Disorder of central nervous system, unspecified G969); Unspecified disorder of intestine 569.9 (Disease of intestine, unspecified K639); Malignant neoplasm of rectum 154.1 (Malignant neoplasm of rectum C20); Diseases of the jaws 526; Unspecified disease of spinal cord 336.9 (Disease of spinal cord, unspecified G959);

Table 1.4. (Continued)

Intractable Pain: https://meshb.nlm.nih.gov/record/ui?ui=D010148.	
Malignant neoplasm of spinal cord 192.2 (Malignant neoplasm of spinal cord C720, Malignant neoplasm of cauda equina C721); Malignant neoplasm of nervous system, part unspecified 192.9 (Malignant neoplasm of central nervous system, unspecified C729)	
Myopathy, unspecified 359.9/G729 with pain, intractable D010148:	
Huángqíwǔwùtāng 5g juānbìtāng 5g dānshēn 1g zhúrú 1g sāngzhī 1g jiānghuáng 1g to ♀	Huángqíwǔwùtāng 5g dānshēn 1g zhúrú 1g sāngzhī 1g jiānghuáng 1g to ♂
Unspecified disorder of intestine 569.9/K639 with pain, intractable D010148:	
Máziřénwán 5g to ♀	Lǐzhōngtāng 5g fùzǐ 1g to ♂
Unspecified disease of spinal cord 336.9/G959 with pain, intractable D010148:	
Xiǎohuóluòdān 5g shūjīnghuóxuètāng 5g dāngguīniāntòngtāng 5g jìshēngshènqìwán 5g to ♀	Shūjīnghuóxuètāng 5g dāngguīniāntòngtāng 5g dúhuójìshēngtāng 5g + acupuncture to ♂

1.5. Arthralgia

Arthralgia is pain or soreness of the joint. Joint pain can be caused by damage to the ligaments, tendons and bursas surrounding the joint, resulting from injury (such as strain, sprain or dislocation) or infection.

Dāngguīniāntòngtāng is today used for unspecified gout, and rheumatoid arthritis (Wang, 2019). Note that arthropathies such as rheumatoid arthritis have their articular features and associated dermatological manifestations (Jagadeesan and Shenoy, 2017).

Table 1.5. Herbal prescriptions for arthralgia

Arthralgia: https://meshb.nlm.nih.gov/record/ui?ui=D018771.	
Common prescriptions:	
Dāngguīniāntòngtāng 5g niúxī 1g huángbò 1g cāngzhú 1g yìyǐrén 1g Dāngguīniāntòngtāng 5g niúxī 1g huángbò 1g cāngzhú 1g yìyǐrén 1g + acupuncture Dāngguīniāntòngtāng 5g niúxī 1g huángbò 1g cāngzhú 1g + acupuncture Dāngguīniāntòngtāng 5g niúxī 1g huángbò 1g cāngzhú 1g	
Alternative prescriptions:	
Shàngzhōngxiàtōngyòngtòngfēngwán 5g niúxī 1g huángbò 1g cāngzhú 1g yìyǐrén 1g + acupuncture Zhènggǔzǐjīndān 5g shēntòngzhúyūtāng 5g dāngguīniāntòngtāng 5g huángbò 1g cāngzhú 1g + acupuncture Shàngzhōngxiàtōngyòngtòngfēngwán 5g shūjīnghuóxuètāng 5g dāngguīniāntòngtāng 5g + acupuncture Dāngguīniāntòngtāng 5g shūjīnghuóxuètāng 4g niúxī 1g huángbò 1g cāngzhú 1g yìyǐrén 1g + acupuncture	
Indicated and associated diseases:	
Cardiovascular disease, unspecified 429.2 (Atherosclerotic heart disease of native coronary artery without angina pectoris I2510); Vascular disorders of skin 709.1 (Vasculitis limited to the skin, unspecified L959); Panuveitis 360.12 (Panuveitis, unspecified eye H44119); Behcet's syndrome 136.1 (Behcet's disease M352); Other dermatoses 702; Disorder of eye, unspecified 379.90 (Unspecified disorder of eye and adnexa H579); Unspecified disorder of joint, site unspecified 719.90 (Joint disorder, unspecified M259); Deformity and disproportion of reconstructed breast 612; Other disorders of breast 611; Benign mammary dysplasias 610; Amyloidosis 277.3; Unspecified disorder of metabolism 277.9 (Metabolic disorder, unspecified E889); Myopathy, unspecified 359.9 (Myopathy, unspecified G729); Myoneural disorders 358; Unspecified disorders of nervous system 349.9 (Disorder of central nervous system, unspecified G969)	
Cardiovascular disease, unspecified 429.2/I2510 with arthralgia D018771:	
Yùzhú 5g sìnìtāng 5g mǔdānpí 1g zhīzǐ 1g huánglián 1g to ♀	Sìnìtāng 5g gānlùyǐn 5g lóngdǎnxiègāntāng 5g to ♂

Arthralgia: https://meshb.nlm.nih.gov/record/ui?ui=D018771.	
Other dermatoses 702 with arthralgia D018771:	
Dāngguīniāntòngtāng 5g tǔfúlíng 1g báixiānpí 1g dìfūzǐ 1g to ♀	Bàidúsǎn 5g zhēnrénhuómìngyǐnqùchuānshānjiǎ 4g huángliánjiědútāng 4g to ♂
Unspecified disorder of joint, site unspecified 719.90/M259 with arthralgia D018771:	
Zhènggǔzǐjīndān 5g yánhúsuǒ 1g pǔjìxiāodúyǐn 1g to ♀	Zhènggǔzǐjīndān 5g yánhúsuǒ 1g pǔjìxiāodúyǐn 1g to ♂
Myopathy, unspecified 359.9/G729 with arthralgia D018771:	
Guìzhīsháoyàozhīmǔtāng 5g dāngguīniāntòngtāng 5g niúxī 1g huángbò 1g cāngzhú 1g yìyǐrén 1g to ♀	Guìzhīsháoyàozhīmǔtāng 5g dāngguīniāntòngtāng 5g niúxī 1g huángbò 1g cāngzhú 1g yìyǐrén 1g to ♂

1.6. Shoulder Pain

The muscles and tendons that stabilize the head of the upper arm bone within the shoulder socket can be injured due to overuse in sports. The connective tissues in the shoulder can become stiff due to underuse of the joint or the natural aging process. Either can cause shoulder pain, which is a type of arthralgia, as shown in Figure 1.1.

Table 1.6. Herbal prescriptions for shoulder pain

Shoulder Pain: https://meshb.nlm.nih.gov/record/ui?ui=D020069.	
Common prescriptions:	
Èrshùtāng 5g sháoyàogāncǎotāng 5g shūjīnghuóxuètāng 5g + acupuncture Èrshùtāng 5g shūjīnghuóxuètāng 5g + acupuncture	
Alternative prescriptions:	
Èrshùtāng 5g gégēntāng 5g Èrshùtāng 5g shūjīnghuóxuètāng 5g Èrshùtāng 5g guìzhīsháoyàozhīmǔtāng 5g yánhúsuǒ 1g jiānghuáng 1g + acupuncture Èrshùtāng 5g juānbìtāng 5g yánhúsuǒ 1g wēilíngxiān 1g Èrshùtāng 5g sháoyàogāncǎotāng 5g shūjīnghuóxuètāng 5g	
Indicated diseases:	
Unspecified disorder of joint, site unspecified 719.90 (Joint disorder, unspecified M259); Deformity and disproportion of reconstructed breast 612; Other disorders of breast 611; Benign mammary dysplasias 610; Myopathy, unspecified 359.9 (Myopathy, unspecified G729); Myoneural disorders 358; Unspecified disorders of nervous system 349.9 (Disorder of central nervous system, unspecified G969); Polymyalgia rheumatica 725 (Polymyalgia rheumatica M353); Malignant neoplasm of thorax 195.1 (Malignant neoplasm of thorax C761)	
Myopathy, unspecified 359.9/G729 with shoulder pain D020069:	
Èrshùtāng 5g sháoyàogāncǎotāng 5g shūjīnghuóxuètāng 5g + acupuncture to ♀	Èrshùtāng 5g juānbìtāng 5g to ♂
Myoneural disorders 358 with shoulder pain D020069:	
Èrshùtāng 5g juānbìtāng 5g + acupuncture to ♀	Èrshùtāng 5g juānbìtāng 5g + acupuncture to ♂
Unspecified disorder of joint, site unspecified 719.90/M259 with shoulder pain D020069:	
Zhènggǔzǐjīndān 5g yánhúsuǒ 1g pǔjìxiāodúyǐn 1g to ♀	Zhènggǔzǐjīndān 5g yánhúsuǒ 1g pǔjìxiāodúyǐn 1g to ♂

The modern use of Èrshùtāng is for adhesive capsulitis of shoulder (Wang, 2019). We also note from the table that shoulder pain can occur after treatment of breast conditions.

1.7. Acute Abdomen

A common type of acute abdominal pain is acute appendicitis which is caused by blockage to the appendix. Different localizations from the spleen, stomach, gallbladder, pancreas, kidney, to small and large intestines give rise to different diagnoses. Acute abdomen is a common medical emergency that accounts for many hospitalizations, with some cases requiring immediate surgical intervention.

Table 1.7. Herbal prescriptions for acute abdomen

<table>
<tr><td colspan="2">Acute Abdomen: https://meshb.nlm.nih.gov/record/ui?ui=D000006.</td></tr>
<tr><td colspan="2">Common prescriptions:</td></tr>
<tr><td colspan="2">Mùxiāngbīnglángwán 5g mázǐrénwán 5g
Mázǐrénwán 5g rùnchángwán 5g dàhuáng 1g
Mùxiāngbīnglángwán 5g mázǐrénwán 5g rùnchángwán 5g
Mùxiāngbīnglángwán 5g mázǐrénwán 5g rùnchángwán 5g dàhuáng 1g</td></tr>
<tr><td colspan="2">Alternative prescriptions:</td></tr>
<tr><td colspan="2">Mázǐrénwán 5g rùnchángwán 5g dàhuáng 1g hòupò 1g zhǐshí 1g
Dàchéngqìtāng 5g dǐdāngtāng 2g
Xiǎochéngqìtāng 5g mázǐrénwán 5g xuánshēn 2g dìhuáng 2g màiméndōng 2g
Tiáowèichéngqìtāng 5g dàhuáng 1g
Tiáowèichéngqìtāng 5g dàhuáng 2g</td></tr>
<tr><td colspan="2">Indicated and associated diseases:</td></tr>
<tr><td colspan="2">Cholecystitis, unspecified 575.10 (Cholecystitis, unspecified K819); Unspecified disorder of gallbladder 575.9 (Disease of gallbladder, unspecified K829); Unspecified disorder of biliary tract 576.9 (Disease of biliary tract, unspecified K839); Unspecified disorder of intestine 569.9 (Disease of intestine, unspecified K639); Malignant neoplasm of appendix vermiformis 153.5 (Malignant neoplasm of appendix C181); Diseases of the jaws 526; Cardiovascular disease, unspecified 429.2 (Atherosclerotic heart disease of native coronary artery without angina pectoris I2510); Perforation of intestine 569.83 (Perforation of intestine (nontraumatic) K631); Other diseases of appendix 543; Unspecified disorder of metabolism 277.9 (Metabolic disorder, unspecified E889)</td></tr>
<tr><td colspan="2">Cholecystitis, unspecified 575.10/K819 with abdomen, acute D000006:</td></tr>
<tr><td>Dàcháihútāng 5g chìsháo 1g jīnqiáncǎo 1g yùjīn 1g huǒmárén 0g to ♀</td><td>Dàcháihútāng 5g chìsháo 1g jīnqiáncǎo 1g yùjīn 1g huǒmárén 0g to ♂</td></tr>
<tr><td colspan="2">Unspecified disorder of intestine 569.9/K639 with abdomen, acute D000006:</td></tr>
<tr><td>Lǐzhōngtāng 5g mázǐrénwán 2g báisháo 1g dàhuáng 0g to ♀</td><td>Lǐzhōngtāng 5g báisháo 1g guìzhī 1g to ♂</td></tr>
<tr><td colspan="2">Cardiovascular disease, unspecified 429.2/I2510 with abdomen, acute D000006:</td></tr>
<tr><td>Sìnìtāng 5g gānlùyǐn 5g mǔdānpí 1g zhīzǐ 1g huánglián 0g to ♀</td><td>Sìnìtāng 5g gānlùyǐn 5g mǔdānpí 1g zhīzǐ 1g huánglián 1g to ♂</td></tr>
</table>

Mùxiāngbīnglángwán has traditionally been used for the treatment of indigestion through its effect of 'moving Qi and guiding stagnation' through the digestive tract. It is of note that heart problems can manifest pain in the upper abdomen and jaw.

1.8. Earache

Inflamed epithelium of the ear canal by microbial infection after such aquatic activities as swimming can cause ear pain. Most earache resolves in a couple of days. Table 1.8 shows the possible conditions causing the pain and the associated herbal treatments.

Table 1.8. Herbal prescriptions for earache

Earache: https://meshb.nlm.nih.gov/record/ui?ui=D004433.	
Common prescriptions:	
Xiǎocháihútāng 5g língguìshùgāntāng 5g shíchāngpú 1g yuǎnzhì 1g Xiǎocháihútāng 5g língguìshùgāntāng 5g shíchāngpú 1g jiégěng 1g yuǎnzhì 1g Xiǎocháihútāng 5g língguìshùgāntāng 5g shíchāngpú 1g jiégěng 1g jīngjiè 1g yuǎnzhì 1g Xiǎocháihútāng 5g língguìshùgāntāng 5g shíchāngpú 1g jiégěng 1g jīngjiè 1g liánqiáo 1g yuǎnzhì 1g Xiǎocháihútāng 5g língguìshùgāntāng 5g chuānxiōng 1g shíchāngpú 1g jiégěng 1g jīngjiè 1g yuǎnzhì 1g	
Alternative prescriptions:	
Xiǎocháihútāng 5g língguìshùgāntāng 5g shíchāngpú 2g qīnghāo 2g jiégěng 2g jīngjiè 2g liánqiáo 2g yuǎnzhì 2g Yìqìcōngmíngtāng 5g shíchāngpú 0g yuǎnzhì 0g Xiǎocháihútāng 5g língguìshùgāntāng 5g niúxī 1g chēqiánzǐ 1g liánqiáo 1g yuǎnzhì 1g Xiǎocháihútāng 5g língguìshùgāntāng 5g niúxī 2g chēqiánzǐ 2g jiégěng 2g yuǎnzhì 2g Yìqìcōngmíngtāng 5g xiǎocháihútāng 2g shíchāngpú 1g yuǎnzhì 1g	
Indicated diseases:	
Other dermatoses 702; Cholesteatoma of middle ear 385.32 (Cholesteatoma of tympanum, bilateral H7113, Polyp of middle ear, unspecified ear H7440); Cholesteatoma, unspecified 385.30 (Unspecified cholesteatoma, bilateral H7193); Unspecified disorder of ear 388.9 (Unspecified disorder of ear, bilateral H9393); Unspecified disease of pharynx 478.20 (Other diseases of pharynx J392); Malignant neoplasm of anterior wall of nasopharynx 147.3 (Malignant neoplasm of anterior wall of nasopharynx C113); Unspecified otitis media 382.9 (Otitis media, unspecified, unspecified ear H6690)	
Other dermatoses 702 with earache D004433:	
Xiāofēngsǎn 5g jīngjièliánqiáotāng 5g zhēnrénhuómìngyǐnqùchuānshānjiǎ 4g huángliánjiědútāng 4g to ♀	Xiāofēngsǎn 5g bàidúsǎn 5g zhēnrénhuómìngyǐnqùchuānshānjiǎ 4g huángliánjiědútāng 4g to ♂
Unspecified disease of pharynx 478.20/J392 with earache D004433:	
Xiǎocháihútāng 5g bànxiàhòupòtāng 5g xuánshēn 1g jiégěng 1g to ♀	Xiǎocháihútāng 5g língguìshùgāntāng 5g xuánshēn 2g jiégěng 2g jīngjiè 2g liánqiáo 2g yuǎnzhì 2g to ♂
Unspecified otitis media 382.9/H6690 with earache D004433:	
Xiǎocháihútāng 5g língguìshùgāntāng 5g shíchāngpú 2g qīnghāo 2g jiégěng 2g liánqiáo 2g yuǎnzhì 2g to ♀	Xiǎocháihútāng 5g língguìshùgāntāng 5g shíchāngpú 2g qīnghāo 2g jiégěng 2g liánqiáo 2g yuǎnzhì 2g to ♂

Xiǎocháihútāng was initially designed for improving Liver health. As the Gallbladder meridian goes through the liver and ear, Xiǎocháihútāng has also been used for hearing problems. The formula is now believed to be anti-inflammatory as its modern uses are for chronic hepatitis and chronic bronchitis (Wang, 2019). Note that tonsillitis can cause earache.

1.9. Toothache

Dental caries, also known as tooth decay, is the breakdown of the enamel covering a tooth due to the acidic by-products produced by bacteria in the mouth when they metabolize sugars. When the enamel is eroded, the nerves surrounding of the tooth can become irritated, causing pain. Dental caries is the most prevalent chronic disease in not only children but also adults, although it can be prevented by practicing proper oral hygiene and using fluoride-containing toothpaste. Other dental problems such as pulpitis can cause toothache as seen in Table 1.9.

Yùnǚjiān 'clears the Stomach and quenches Fire.' Traditional Chinese medicine believes that inflammation of oral tissues is caused by baking of the oral cavity by the Fire from the stomach. Yùnǚjiān has therefore been used for problems with the mouth.

The same thinking explains why Qīngwèisǎn, which literally means 'clearing the Stomach,' is combined with Yùnǚjiān into the prescription in the end of the table for dental caries with toothache. We notice from the table that, in addition to heart disease, multiple myeloma, also known as plasma cell myeloma, can cause toothache (Wehrhahn et al., 2018).

Table 1.9. Herbal prescriptions for toothache

Toothache: https://meshb.nlm.nih.gov/record/ui?ui=D014098.	
Common prescriptions:	
Chuānxiōngchádiàosǎn 5g gégēntāng 5g + acupuncture Yùnǚjiān 5g gānlùyǐn 5g qīngwèisǎn 5g	
Alternative prescriptions:	
Sháoyàogāncǎotāng 5g gégēntāng 5g + acupuncture Qīngwèisǎn 5g yùnǚjiān 2g Gégēntāng 5g báizhǐ 1g xìxīn 1g dàhuáng 0g + acupuncture Chuānxiōngchádiàosǎn 5g shūjīnghuóxuètāng 2g gānlùyǐn 1g xìngsūyǐn 1g shēngmàiyǐn 0g gāncǎo 0g Gégēntāng 5g báizhǐ 1g xīnyí 1g + acupuncture	
Indicated diseases:	
Cardiovascular disease, unspecified 429.2 (Atherosclerotic heart disease of native coronary artery without angina pectoris I2510); Multiple myeloma 203.0; Unspecified hemorrhagic conditions 287.9 (Hemorrhagic condition, unspecified D699); Unspecified diseases of blood and blood-forming organs 289.9 (Disease of blood and blood-forming organs, unspecified D759); Pulpitis 522.0 (Reversible pulpitis K0401, Irreversible pulpitis K0402); Geniculate ganglionitis 351.1 (Geniculate ganglionitis G511); Facial nerve disorders 351; Unspecified disorder of cranial nerves 352.9 (Cranial nerve disorder, unspecified G529); Unspecified disorders of nervous system 349.9 (Disorder of central nervous system, unspecified G969); Dental caries of smooth surface 521.07 (Dental caries on smooth surface limited to enamel K0261, Dental caries on smooth surface penetrating into dentin K0262, Dental caries on smooth surface penetrating into pulp K0263)	
Cardiovascular disease, unspecified 429.2/I2510 with toothache D014098:	
Yùzhú 5g sìnìtāng 5g mǔdānpí 1g zhīzǐ 1g huánglián 1g to ♀	Sìnìtāng 5g gānlùyǐn 5g mǔdānpí 1g zhīzǐ 1g huánglián 1g to ♂
Pulpitis 522.0/K0401,K0402 with toothache D014098:	
Qīngwèisǎn 5g dǎodìwúgōng 1g zhīzǐ 1g liánqiáo 1g gégēn 1g mùxiāng 1g xuánshēn 1g báizhǐ 1g huángbò 1g to ♀	Qīngwèisǎn 5g dǎodìwúgōng 1g zhīzǐ 1g liánqiáo 1g gégēn 1g mùxiāng 1g xuánshēn 1g báizhǐ 1g huángbò 1g to ♂
Geniculate ganglionitis 351.1/G511 with toothache D014098:	
Gégēntāng 5g báizhǐ 1g báijiāngcán 1g fángfēng 1g qínjiāo 1g chántuì 1g gōuténg 1g + acupuncture to ♀	Wūyàoshùnqìsǎn 5g bǔyánghuánwǔtāng 5g báizhǐ 1g báijiāngcán 1g dìlóng 1g + acupuncture to ♂
Dental caries of smooth surface 521.07/K0261,K0262,K0263 with toothache D014098:	
Yùnǚjiān 5g gānlùyǐn 5g qīngwèisǎn 5g to ♀	Yùnǚjiān 5g qīngwèisǎn 5g to ♂

1.10. Facial Pain

Facial pain is pain anywhere in the face. Facial pain can be caused by trigeminal neuralgia, sinusitis, shingles, migraine, skin abscess, and mouth cancer.

Sháoyàogāncǎotāng 'regulates and harmonizes Qi-Blood,' 'quells convulsion, stops pain,' and is today used for unspecified myalgia and myositis, and neuralgia, neuritis and radiculitis (Wang, 2019).

Table 1.10. Herbal prescriptions for facial pain

Facial Pain: https://meshb.nlm.nih.gov/record/ui?ui=D005157.	
Common prescriptions:	
Sháoyàogāncǎotāng 5g shūjīnghuóxuètāng 5g + acupuncture Shūjīnghuóxuètāng 5g + acupuncture Shūjīnghuóxuètāng 5g huángqíwǔwùtāng 5g + acupuncture	
Alternative prescriptions:	
Huángqíwǔwùtāng 5g dānshēn 1g zhúrú 1g sāngzhī 1g dāngguī 1g jiānghuáng 1g + acupuncture Huángqíwǔwùtāng 5g chuānxiōng 1g dānshēn 1g zhúrú 1g sāngzhī 1g dāngguī 1g jiānghuáng 1g + acupuncture Shūjīnghuóxuètāng 5g sháoyàogāncǎotāng 3g mòyào 1g rǔxiāng 1g jiānghuáng 1g jīxuèténg 1g + acupuncture Shēntòngzhúyūtāng 5g sháoyàogāncǎotāng 2g yánhúsuǒ 1g + acupuncture Huángqíwǔwùtāng 5g chuānxiōng 1g dānshēn 1g zhúrú 1g sāngzhī 1g jiānghuáng 1g + acupuncture	
Indicated diseases:	
Trigeminal neuralgia 350.1 (Trigeminal neuralgia G500); Geniculate ganglionitis 351.1 (Geniculate ganglionitis G511); Facial nerve disorders 351; Unspecified disorder of cranial nerves 352.9 (Cranial nerve disorder, unspecified G529); Unspecified disorders of nervous system 349.9 (Disorder of central nervous system, unspecified G969); Malignant neoplasm of cranial nerves 192.0 (Malignant neoplasm of unspecified cranial nerve C7250); Neuroendocrine tumors 209; Malignant neoplasm of nervous system, part unspecified 192.9 (Malignant neoplasm of central nervous system, unspecified C729); Myopathy, unspecified 359.9 (Myopathy, unspecified G729); Unspecified disorder of joint, site unspecified 719.90 (Joint disorder, unspecified M259); Somatization disorder 300.81 (Somatization disorder F450); Myoneural disorders 358	
Trigeminal neuralgia 350.1/G500 with facial pain D005157:	
Gégēntāng 5g báizhǐ 1g báijiāngcán 1g qínjiāo 1g chántuì 1g gōuténg 1g + acupuncture to ♀	Gégēntāng 5g báizhǐ 1g báijiāngcán 1g fángfēng 1g qínjiāo 1g gōuténg 1g + acupuncture to ♂
Geniculate ganglionitis 351.1/G511 with facial pain D005157:	
Wūyàoshùnqìsǎn 5g huángqíwǔwùtāng 5g + acupuncture to ♀	Wūyàoshùnqìsǎn 5g bǔyánghuánwǔtāng 5g + acupuncture to ♂
Myopathy, unspecified 359.9/G729 with facial pain D005157:	
Huángqíwǔwùtāng 5g juānbìtāng 5g dānshēn 1g zhúrú 1g sāngzhī 1g jiānghuáng 1g to ♀	Huángqíwǔwùtāng 5g juānbìtāng 5g + acupuncture to ♂

1.11. Phantom Limb

A limb is still being felt even though it is no longer there is called phantom limb. Most amputees would experience phantom limb soon after the amputation, with the sensation going away gradually. The mechanism of phantom limb is poorly understood.

As phantom limb is about limb sensations, it is treated here by herbal therapists using Sìnìtāng which, containing Fùzǐ, has traditionally been used to warm up the patients who, due to the loss of 'Yang Qi', feel cold in their four limbs. Yang Qi is believed to be responsible for every aspect of proactivity in life.

Because of the effect of reversing the dwindling of Yang, extensive use of Sìnìtāng for various conditions throughout the book is not surprising. From the prescriptions in the beginning of the table, we learn that a common practice of cGMP herbal prescription composition is to add single herbs, e.g., Fùzǐ and Gānjiāng, to formulas, e.g., Sìnìtāng, which already contain the single herbs, in order to enhance the effect of the formulas.

Table 1.11. Herbal prescriptions for phantom limb

Phantom Limb: https://meshb.nlm.nih.gov/record/ui?ui=D010591.	
Common prescriptions:	
Sìnìtāng 5g dāngguīsìnìtāng 5g wúzhūyú 1g gānjiāng 1g Sìnìtāng 5g dāngguīsìnìtāng 5g wúzhūyú 1g fùzǐ 1g gānjiāng 1g Sìnìtāng 5g lǐzhōngtāng 5g ròuguì 1g yánhúsuǒ 1g zhìgāncǎotāng 1g Sìnìtāng 5g dāngguīsìnìtāng 5g wúzhūyú 1g Sìnìtāng 5g lǐzhōngtāng 5g ròuguì 1g yánhúsuǒ 1g zhìgāncǎotāng 1g + acupuncture	
Alternative prescriptions:	
Sìnìtāng 5g guìzhī 1g máhuáng 1g xìxīn 1g Sìnìtāng 5g lǐzhōngtāng 5g Sìnìtāng 5g guìzhī 1g shēngjiāng 1g Máhuángfùzǐxìxīntāng 5g shēngjiāng 2g zhìgāncǎo 2g guìzhī 2g dàzǎo 1g	
Indicated or associated diseases:	
Unspecified disorders of nervous system 349.9 (Disorder of central nervous system, unspecified G969); Malignant neoplasm of nervous system, part unspecified 192.9 (Malignant neoplasm of central nervous system, unspecified C729); Somatization disorder 300.81 (Somatization disorder F450); Cardiovascular disease, unspecified 429.2 (Atherosclerotic heart disease of native coronary artery without angina pectoris I2510); Myoneural disorders 358; Phobia, unspecified 300.20 (Phobic anxiety disorder, unspecified F409)	
Unspecified disorders of nervous system 349.9/G969 with phantom limb D010591:	
Huángqíwǔwùtāng 5g chuānxiōng 1g dānshēn 1g zhúrú 1g sāngzhī 1g dāngguī 1g jiānghuáng 1g to ♀	Huángqíwǔwùtāng 5g chuānxiōng 1g dānshēn 1g zhúrú 1g sāngzhī 1g dāngguī 1g jiānghuáng 1g to ♂
Cardiovascular disease, unspecified 429.2/I2510 with phantom limb D010591:	
Yùzhú 5g sìnìtāng 5g mǔdānpí 1g zhīzǐ 1g huánglián 0g to ♀	Sìnìtāng 5g gānlùyǐn 5g mǔdānpí 1g zhīzǐ 1g huánglián 0g to ♂
Myoneural disorders 358 with phantom limb D010591:	
Huángqíwǔwùtāng 5g juānbìtāng 5g dānshēn 1g zhúrú 1g sāngzhī 1g jiānghuáng 1g to ♀	Huángqíwǔwùtāng 5g dānshēn 1g zhúrú 1g sāngzhī 1g jiānghuáng 1g + acupuncture to ♂

1.12. Low Back Pain

Overstretch of the muscles and ligaments supporting the back can cause acute low back pain. Damage to the spinal joints or intervertebral discs can lead to chronic low back pain.

Table 1.12. Herbal prescriptions for low back pain

Low Back Pain https://meshb.nlm.nih.gov/record/ui?ui=D017116
Common prescriptions:
Dúhuójìshēngtāng 5g shūjīnghuóxuètāng 3g Dúhuójìshēngtāng 5g shūjīnghuóxuètāng 4g Dúhuójìshēngtāng 5g Dúhuójìshēngtāng 5g + acupuncture
Alternative prescriptions:
Dúhuójìshēngtāng 5g sháoyàogāncǎotāng 4g dāngguīniāntòngtāng 4g shūjīnghuóxuètāng 2g gégēntāng 2g niúxī 1g Dúhuójìshēngtāng 5g niúxī 1g mòyào 1g rǔxiāng 1g yánhúsuǒ 1g fùzǐ 1g guìzhī 1g jīxuèténg 1g xùduàn 1g + acupuncture Dāngguīniāntòngtāng 5g dúhuójìshēngtāng 5g sháoyàogāncǎotāng 4g guīlùèrxiānjiāo 4g cháigéjiějītāng 2g shūjīnghuóxuètāng 2g niúxī 1g gǔsuìbǔ 1g Dúhuójìshēngtāng 5g dùzhòng 2g xùduàn 2g + acupuncture Dúhuójìshēngtāng 5g shūjīnghuóxuètāng 4g niúxī 1g mòyào 1g rǔxiāng 1g fùzǐ 1g guìzhī 1g jīxuèténg 1g + acupuncture

Low Back Pain https://meshb.nlm.nih.gov/record/ui?ui=D017116	
Indicated diseases:	
Cardiovascular disease, unspecified 429.2 (Atherosclerotic heart disease of native coronary artery without angina pectoris I2510); Multiple myeloma 203.0; Unspecified hemorrhagic conditions 287.9 (Hemorrhagic condition, unspecified D699); Unspecified diseases of blood and blood-forming organs 289.9 (Disease of blood and blood-forming organs, unspecified D759); Unspecified disease of spinal cord 336.9 (Disease of spinal cord, unspecified G959); Malignant neoplasm of spinal cord 192.2 (Malignant neoplasm of spinal cord C720, Malignant neoplasm of cauda equina C721); Unspecified disorders of nervous system 349.9 (Disorder of central nervous system, unspecified G969); Myopathy, unspecified 359.9 (Myopathy, unspecified G729); Unspecified disorder of joint, site unspecified 719.90 (Joint disorder, unspecified M259); Myoneural disorders 358; Malignant neoplasm of nervous system, part unspecified 192.9 (Malignant neoplasm of central nervous system, unspecified C729); Neuroendocrine tumors 209	
Cardiovascular disease, unspecified 429.2/I2510 with low back pain D017116:	
Yùzhú 5g sìnìtāng 5g mǔdānpí 1g zhīzǐ 1g huánglián 0g to ♀	Yùzhú 5g sìnìtāng 5g zhìgāncǎotāng 5g to ♂
Unspecified disease of spinal cord 336.9/G959 with low back pain D017116:	
Shūjīnghuóxuètāng 5g dúhuójìshēngtāng 5g + acupuncture to ♀	Shūjīnghuóxuètāng 5g dúhuójìshēngtāng 5g xiǎohuóluòdān 2g xiāngshālìujūnzǐtāng 2g to ♂
Myopathy, unspecified 359.9/G729 with low back pain D017116:	
Huángqíwǔwùtāng 5g dāngguīsìnìtāng 5g dānshēn 1g zhúrú 1g sāngzhī 1g jiānghuáng 1g to ♀	Huángqíwǔwùtāng 5g dāngguīsìnìtāng 5g dānshēn 1g zhúrú 1g sāngzhī 1g jiānghuáng 1g to ♂
Myoneural disorders 358 with low back pain D017116:	
Huángqíwǔwùtāng 5g dānshēn 1g zhúrú 1g sāngzhī 1g jiānghuáng 1g + acupuncture to ♀	Huángqíwǔwùtāng 5g dānshēn 1g zhúrú 1g sāngzhī 1g jiānghuáng 1g + acupuncture to ♂

According to classical Chinese medical literature, Dúhuójìshēngtāng was designed for the treatment of weakened Liver, Kidney, Qi and Blood which cause prolonged paralysis, pain of the body, and in particular soreness of the waist and knees. Indeed, its modern uses include lumbago, sciatica, and rheumatoid arthritis (Wang, 2019). There is evidence that cardiovascular morbidities are associated with chronic low back pain (Fernandez et al., 2016).

1.13. Back Pain

Back pain is commonly caused by sudden awkward movements that strain and sprain the muscle or ligament in the back. Physical therapies such as back massage and back exercise are believed to ease back pain.

Table 1.13. Herbal prescriptions for back pain

Back Pain: https://meshb.nlm.nih.gov/record/ui?ui=D001416.
Common prescriptions:
Dúhuójìshēngtāng 5g + acupuncture Dúhuójìshēngtāng 5g Dúhuójìshēngtāng 5g shūjīnghuóxuètāng 3g Dúhuójìshēngtāng 5g shūjīnghuóxuètāng 4g
Alternative prescriptions:
Dúhuójìshēngtāng 5g dùzhòng 1g gǔsuìbǔ 1g xùduàn 1g Sānbìtāng 5g dúhuójìshēngtāng 5g Dúhuójìshēngtāng 5g dùzhòng 1g xùduàn 1g Dúhuójìshēngtāng 5g sháoyàogāncǎotāng 2g + acupuncture Dúhuójìshēngtāng 5g dùzhòng 1g jīxuèténg 1g mòyào 0g rǔxiāng 0g + acupuncture

Table 1.13. (Continued)

Back Pain: https://meshb.nlm.nih.gov/record/ui?ui=D001416.	
Indicated diseases:	
Cardiovascular disease, unspecified 429.2 (Atherosclerotic heart disease of native coronary artery without angina pectoris I2510); Multiple myeloma 203.0; Unspecified hemorrhagic conditions 287.9 (Hemorrhagic condition, unspecified D699); Unspecified diseases of blood and blood-forming organs 289.9 (Disease of blood and blood-forming organs, unspecified D759); Unspecified disease of spinal cord 336.9 (Disease of spinal cord, unspecified G959); Malignant neoplasm of spinal cord 192.2 (Malignant neoplasm of spinal cord C720, Malignant neoplasm of cauda equina C721); Unspecified disorders of nervous system 349.9 (Disorder of central nervous system, unspecified G969); Neuroendocrine tumors 209; Malignant neoplasm of nervous system, part unspecified 192.9 (Malignant neoplasm of central nervous system, unspecified C729); Myoneural disorders 358	
Cardiovascular disease, unspecified 429.2/I2510 with back pain D001416:	
Yùzhú 5g sìnìtāng 5g mǔdānpí 1g zhīzǐ 1g huánglián 0g to ♀	Yùzhú 5g sìnìtāng 5g zhìgāncǎotāng 2g to ♂
Unspecified disease of spinal cord 336.9/G959 with back pain D001416:	
Guīlùèrxiānjiāo 5g shūjīnghuóxuètāng 2g dāngguīniāntòngtāng 2g xiǎohuóluòdān 1g xiāngshāliùjūnzǐtāng 1g to ♀	Shūjīnghuóxuètāng 5g dúhuójìshēngtāng 5g xiǎohuóluòdān 2g xiāngshāliùjūnzǐtāng 2g to ♂

Sānbìtāng in traditional Chinese medicine treats pain and numbness resulting from Wind, Dampness and chills. One of its modern uses is for lumbago (Wang, 2019).

1.14. Failed Back Surgery Syndrome

When pain in the back and leg continues after lumbar spine surgery, it is called failed back surgery syndrome. The factors contributing to failed back surgery syndrome are complex and can involve patient's mental conditions and lifestyle behaviors such as smoking. The reported prevalence of failed back surgery syndrome varies from country to country.

Sháoyàogāncǎotāng has traditionally been used for the treatment of muscle spasms and muscle cramps. We will therefore see its use for other pains later in the chapter.

Table 1.14. Herbal prescriptions for failed back surgery syndrome

Failed Back Surgery Syndrome: https://meshb.nlm.nih.gov/record/ui?ui=D055111.
Common prescriptions:
Sháoyàogāncǎotāng 5g shūjīnghuóxuètāng 5g dāngguīniāntòngtāng 5g + acupuncture Sháoyàogāncǎotāng 5g shūjīnghuóxuètāng 5g + acupuncture
Alternative prescriptions:
Sháoyàogāncǎotāng 5g shūjīnghuóxuètāng 5g dúhuójìshēngtāng 5g + acupuncture Sháoyàogāncǎotāng 5g shēntòngzhúyūtāng 5g mòyào 1g rǔxiāng 1g + acupuncture Shūjīnghuóxuètāng 5g sháoyàogāncǎotāng 2g yánhúsuǒ 1g jīxuèténg 1g + acupuncture Shūjīnghuóxuètāng 5g niúxī 0g mòyào 0g rǔxiāng 0g fùzǐ 0g guìzhī 0g jīxuèténg 0g + acupuncture Jiāwèixiāoyáosǎn 5g gāncǎoxiǎomàidàzǎotāng 5g + acupuncture
Indicated diseases:
Unspecified condition of brain 348.9 (Disorder of brain, unspecified G939); Unspecified diseases of blood and blood-forming organs 289.9 (Disease of blood and blood-forming organs, unspecified D759); Unspecified disorders of nervous system 349.9 (Disorder of central nervous system, unspecified G969); Unspecified disorder of metabolism 277.9 (Metabolic disorder, unspecified E889); Alcohol abuse 305.0; Cardiovascular disease, unspecified 429.2 (Atherosclerotic heart disease of native coronary artery without angina pectoris I2510); Multiple myeloma 203.0; Unspecified hemorrhagic conditions 287.9 (Hemorrhagic condition, unspecified D699); Alexia 315.01 (Dyslexia and alexia R480)

Failed Back Surgery Syndrome: https://meshb.nlm.nih.gov/record/ui?ui=D055111.	
Unspecified condition of brain 348.9/G939 with failed back surgery syndrome D055111:	
Bǔyánghuánwǔtāng 5g dānshēn 1g tiānmá 1g shíchāngpú 1g yuǎnzhì 1g + acupuncture to ♀	Bǔyánghuánwǔtāng 5g dānshēn 1g tiānmá 1g shíchāngpú 1g yuǎnzhì 1g + acupuncture to ♂
Unspecified disorders of nervous system 349.9/G969 with failed back surgery syndrome D055111:	
Shūjīnghuóxuètāng 5g píngwèisǎn 2g mùguā 1g sāngzhī 1g jīxuèténg 1g to ♀	Shūjīnghuóxuètāng 5g píngwèisǎn 2g mùguā 1g sāngzhī 1g jīxuèténg 1g to ♂
Cardiovascular disease, unspecified 429.2/I2510 with failed back surgery syndrome D055111:	
Sìnìtāng 5g gānlùyǐn 5g mǔdānpí 1g zhīzǐ 1g huánglián 0g to ♀	Shēngmàiyǐn 5g zhìgāncǎotāng 5g dānshēn 1g to ♂

1.15. Acute Pain

Acute pain is a sudden, sharp pain resulting from, for example, a cut, sting, pinch, burn, sprained ligament, strained muscle or broken bone. The pain typically stops when the wound heals.

Guìzhītāng is used for neck pain and intractable pain in previous sections. Here it is enhanced with Shēngjiāng to treat acute pain. Shēngjiāng, i.e., fresh ginger root, is a food flavoring. Addition of ginger into the prescription is considered to aid patient's digestion and sleep, which in turn help patient's recovery from the wound.

Table 1.15. Herbal prescriptions for acute pain

Acute Pain: https://meshb.nlm.nih.gov/record/ui?ui=D059787.	
Common prescriptions:	
Guìzhītāng 5g shēngjiāng 1g báisháo 1g dàhuáng 0g Guìzhītāng 5g shēngjiāng 1g guìzhī 1g Guìzhītāng 5g shēngjiāng 1g guìzhī 1g dàhuáng 0g Guìzhītāng 5g shēngjiāng 1g báisháo 1g guìzhī 1g Guìzhītāng 5g shēngjiāng 1g báisháo 1g	
Alternative prescriptions:	
Guìzhītāng 5g chuānwū 1g Guìzhītāng 5g báizhú 1g fúlíng 1g dàhuáng 0g Guìzhītāng 5g fùzǐ 1g dàhuáng 0g	
Indicated diseases:	
Cardiovascular disease, unspecified 429.2 (Atherosclerotic heart disease of native coronary artery without angina pectoris I2510); Myopathy, unspecified 359.9 (Myopathy, unspecified G729); Compartment syndrome, unspecified 958.90 (Compartment syndrome, unspecified, initial encounter T79A0XA); Heart disease, unspecified 429.9 (Heart disease, unspecified I519); Myoneural disorders 358; Unspecified disorders of nervous system 349.9 (Disorder of central nervous system, unspecified G969); Unspecified disorder of joint, site unspecified 719.90 (Joint disorder, unspecified M259)	
Cardiovascular disease, unspecified 429.2/I2510 with acute pain D059787:	
Sìnìtāng 5g gānlùyǐn 5g mǔdānpí 1g zhīzǐ 1g huánglián 0g to ♀	Sìnìtāng 5g gānlùyǐn 5g mǔdānpí 1g zhīzǐ 1g huánglián 1g to ♂
Heart disease, unspecified 429.9/I519 with acute pain D059787:	
Sìnìtāng 5g gānlùyǐn 5g mǔdānpí 1g zhīzǐ 1g huánglián 0g to ♀	Sìnìtāng 5g gānlùyǐn 5g mǔdānpí 1g zhīzǐ 1g huánglián 0g to ♂
Myopathy, unspecified 359.9/G729 with acute pain D059787:	
Huángqíwǔwùtāng 5g juānbìtāng 5g + acupuncture to ♀	Guīlùèrxiānjiāo 5g to ♂
Unspecified disorder of joint, site unspecified 719.90/M259 with acute pain D059787:	
Zhènggǔzǐjīndān 5g to ♀	Zhènggǔzǐjīndān 5g yánhúsuǒ 1g pǔjìxiāodúyǐn 1g to ♂

1.16. Eye Pain

When one in the work focuses his or her eyes on a near object, such as a computer monitor, for a long time, the ciliary muscles in the eyes, which normally relax when one focuses on distant objects, can spasm, causing an ache. Eye strain can be prevented by periodically shifting the focus away from the digital devices. Other eye conditions such as glaucoma can cause eye pain.

Table 1.16. Herbal prescriptions for eye pain

Eye Pain: https://meshb.nlm.nih.gov/record/ui?ui=D058447.	
Common prescriptions:	
Sháoyàogāncǎotāng 5g shūjīnghuóxuètāng 5g dāngguīniāntòngtāng 5g + acupuncture Xǐgānmíngmùtāng 5g zīshènmíngmùtāng 5g Sháoyàogāncǎotāng 5g shūjīnghuóxuètāng 5g + acupuncture	
Alternative prescriptions:	
Dāngguīsìnìtāng 5g shēngjiāng 1g wúzhūyú 1g fùzǐ 1g Sháoyàogāncǎotāng 5g dāngguīniāntòngtāng 5g dúhuójìshēngtāng 5g guīlùèrxiānjiāo 5g shūjīnghuóxuètāng 3g gégēntāng 3g niúxī 2g Sháoyàogāncǎotāng 5g gǒuqǐzǐ 2g júhuā 2g + acupuncture Xǐgānmíngmùtāng 5g zīshènmíngmùtāng 5g mùzéicǎo 1g cǎojuémíng 1g	
Indicated diseases:	
Disorder of eye, unspecified 379.90 (Unspecified disorder of eye and adnexa H579); Malignant neoplasm of other specified sites of eye 190.8 (Malignant neoplasm of overlapping sites of unspecified eye and adnexa C6980); Neuroendocrine tumors 209; Malignant neoplasm of nervous system, part unspecified 192.9 (Malignant neoplasm of central nervous system, unspecified C729); Primary open angle glaucoma 365.11 (Primary open-angle glaucoma, right eye, stage unspecified H401110, Primary open-angle glaucoma, right eye, mild stage H401111, Primary open-angle glaucoma, right eye, moderate stage H401112, Primary open-angle glaucoma, right eye, severe stage H401113, Primary open-angle glaucoma, right eye, indeterminate stage H401114, Primary open-angle glaucoma, left eye, stage unspecified H401120, Primary open-angle glaucoma, left eye, mild stage H401121, Primary open-angle glaucoma, left eye, moderate stage H401122, Primary open-angle glaucoma, left eye, severe stage H401123, Primary open-angle glaucoma, left eye, indeterminate stage H401124, Primary open-angle glaucoma, bilateral, stage unspecified H401130, Primary open-angle glaucoma, bilateral, mild stage H401131, Primary open-angle glaucoma, bilateral, moderate stage H401132, Primary open-angle glaucoma, bilateral, severe stage H401133, Primary open-angle glaucoma, bilateral, indeterminate stage H401134, Primary open-angle glaucoma, unspecified eye, stage unspecified H401190, Primary open-angle glaucoma, unspecified eye, mild stage H401191, Primary open-angle glaucoma, unspecified eye, moderate stage H401192, Primary open-angle glaucoma, unspecified eye, severe stage H401193, Primary open-angle glaucoma, unspecified eye, indeterminate stage H401194); Open-angle glaucoma 365.1; Glaucoma 365; Ocular hypertension 365.04 (Ocular hypertension, unspecified eye H40059); Cardiovascular disease, unspecified 429.2 (Atherosclerotic heart disease of native coronary artery without angina pectoris I2510); Diabetic retinopathy 362.0; Diabetes with peripheral circulatory disorders 250.7; Unspecified retinal disorder 362.9 (Unspecified retinal disorder H359); Diabetes mellitus 250; Unspecified endocrine disorder 259.9 (Endocrine disorder, unspecified E349); Unspecified disorder of metabolism 277.9 (Metabolic disorder, unspecified E889)	
Disorder of eye, unspecified 379.90/H579 with eye pain D058447:	
Qǐjúdìhuángwán 5g xǐgānmíngmùtāng 5g zīshènmíngmùtāng 5g to ♀	Qǐjúdìhuángwán 5g xǐgānmíngmùtāng 5g zīshènmíngmùtāng 5g to ♂
Primary open angle glaucoma 365.11/H401110,H401111,H401112,H401113,H401114,H401120,H401121,H401122,H401123, H401124,H401130,H401131,H401132,H401133,H401134,H401190,H401191,H401192, H401193,H401194 with Eye pain D058447:	
Qǐjúdìhuángwán 5g xǐgānmíngmùtāng 5g zīshènmíngmùtāng 5g to ♀	Qǐjúdìhuángwán 5g xǐgānmíngmùtāng 5g zīshènmíngmùtāng 5g to ♂
Cardiovascular disease, unspecified 429.2/I2510 with eye pain D058447:	
Yùzhú 5g sìnìtāng 5g mǔdānpí 1g zhīzǐ 1g huánglián 1g to ♀	Sìnìtāng 5g gānlùyǐn 5g lóngdǎnxiègāntāng 5g to ♂

We learn in previous sections that Sháoyàogāncǎotāng relieves muscle spasms and that Shūjīnghuóxuètāng promotes blood circulation. Combination of the two here is believed to relieve ocular muscle strain, easing the pain. Both Xǐgānmíngmùtāng and Zīshènmíngmùtāng contain the term míngmù, which is literally translated as 'clear the eyes.' Because of the similarity in the vasculature between the heart and eye, cardiovascular diseases and eye diseases are highly associated (Flammer et al., 2013), as we also notice in the table.

1.17. Referred Pain

When location of the perceived pain is away from that of the damaged organ, the pain is called referred pain. Examples of referred pain are pains in the teeth, jaw or left shoulder triggered by a heart attack. Numerous hypotheses have been proposed to explain the phenomenon, many of them involving convergence of multiple afferent sensory information to the same dorsal horn neurons in the spine and then loss or mislocalization of the original information by the thalamic neurons in the brain. Treatment for referred pain should target the damaged organ instead of the site in pain. Table 1.17 shows herbal prescriptions and conditions causing referred pain.

Phantom limb can be considered an example of referred pain. We therefore see that Sìnìtāng, which is used for phantom limb in Section 1.11, is used here for referred pain. Furthermore, once the condition causing the pain is diagnosed, prescriptions change to address the cause, rather than the pain, as shown in the table.

Table 1.17. Herbal prescriptions for referred pain

Referred Pain: https://meshb.nlm.nih.gov/record/ui?ui=D053591	
Common prescriptions:	
Sìnìtāng 5g yánhúsuǒ 1g xiāngfù 1g yùjīn 1g Sìnìtāng 5g yánhúsuǒ 1g Sìnìtāng 5g yánhúsuǒ 1g guìzhī 1g Sìnìtāng 5g yánhúsuǒ 1g xiāngfù 1g	
Alternative prescriptions:	
Sìnìtāng 5g yánhúsuǒ 1g dàhuáng 0g Sìnìtāng 5g bànxià 1g dàhuáng 0g Sìnìtāng 5g wúzhūyú 1g dàhuáng 0g Xiǎocháihútāng 5g báizhú 1g fúlíng 1g tiáowèichéngqìtāng 0g Sìnìtāng 5g yánhúsuǒ 2g xiāngfù 2g	
Indicated diseases:	
Unspecified disorder of intestine 569.9 (Disease of intestine, unspecified K639); Diseases of the jaws 526; Diseases of the oral soft tissues, excluding lesions specific for gingiva and tongue 528; Myopathy, unspecified 359.9 (Myopathy, unspecified G729); Myoneural disorders 358; Unspecified disorders of nervous system 349.9 (Disorder of central nervous system, unspecified G969); Heart disease, unspecified 429.9 (Heart disease, unspecified I519); Cardiovascular disease, unspecified 429.2 (Atherosclerotic heart disease of native coronary artery without angina pectoris I2510)	
Unspecified disorder of intestine 569.9/K639 with pain, referred D053591:	
Mázǐrénwán 5g to ♀	Xiāngshāliùjūnzǐtāng 5g cānlíngbáizhúsǎn 5g to ♂
Myopathy, unspecified 359.9/G729 with pain, referred D053591:	
Sháoyàogāncǎotāng 5g shēntòngzhúyūtāng 5g shūjīnghuóxuètāng 5g + acupuncture to ♀	Sháoyàogāncǎotāng 5g shūjīnghuóxuètāng 5g to ♂
Heart disease, unspecified 429.9/I519 with pain, referred D053591:	
Sìnìtāng 5g gānlùyǐn 5g mǔdānpí 1g zhīzǐ 1g huánglián 0g to ♀	Sìnìtāng 5g gānlùyǐn 5g mǔdānpí 1g zhīzǐ 1g huánglián 0g to ♂

1.18. Flank Pain

Pain on the side of the back below the ribs and above the waist is called flank pain. Flank pain is usually an indication of muscle or urinary tract problems, including issues with the kidneys.

Bāzhèngsǎn has traditionally been used for urological infections, so has Wǔlíngsǎn, which is best known for its effect on 'fluid metabolism regulation.' Both herbal formulas promote urination. Most kidney problems also manifest oral lesions (Oyetola et al., 2015). Also, as kidney disease disturbs mineral metabolism, jaw bones can be affected (Kanjevac et al., 2018), as we also see in the table. On the other hand, if the flank pain is caused by muscle strain, Sháoyàogāncǎotāng and Shūjīnghuóxuètāng are prescribed, as shown in the list of alternative prescriptions in Table 1.18.

Table 1.18. Herbal prescriptions for flank pain

Flank Pain: https://meshb.nlm.nih.gov/record/ui?ui=D021501.	
Common prescriptions:	
Bāzhèngsǎn 5g wǔlínsǎn 5g dǐdāngtāng 5g Bāzhèngsǎn 5g dǐdāngtāng 5g tiáowèichéngqìtāng 5g Bāzhèngsǎn 5g wǔlínsǎn 5g táohéchéngqìtāng 5g Bāzhèngsǎn 5g dǐdāngtāng 5g Bāzhèngsǎn 5g wǔlínsǎn 5g	
Alternative prescriptions:	
Bāzhèngsǎn 5g cháihújiālónggǔmǔlìtāng 5g dāngguīlónghuìwán 5g Bāzhèngsǎn 5g lóngdǎnxiègāntāng 5g Bāzhèngsǎn 5g wǔlínsǎn 5g dǐdāngtāng 5g tiáowèichéngqìtāng 5g + acupuncture Sháoyàogāncǎotāng 5g shūjīnghuóxuètāng 5g niúxī 1g yánhúsuǒ 1g + acupuncture	
Indicated diseases:	
Hydronephrosis 591 (Unspecified hydronephrosis N1330); Malignant neoplasm of kidney, except pelvis 189.0 (Malignant neoplasm of unspecified kidney, except renal pelvis C649); Unspecified disorder of intestine 569.9 (Disease of intestine, unspecified K639); Diseases of the jaws 526; Diseases of the oral soft tissues, excluding lesions specific for gingiva and tongue 528; Neuroendocrine tumors 209; Malignant neoplasm of nervous system, part unspecified 192.9 (Malignant neoplasm of central nervous system, unspecified C729)	
Hydronephrosis 591/N1330 with flank pain D021501:	
Wǔlíngsǎn 5g jìshēngshènqìwán 5g to ♀	Wǔlíngsǎn 5g jìshēngshènqìwán 5g to ♂
Malignant neoplasm of kidney, except pelvis 189.0/C649 with flank pain D021501:	
Wǔlíngsǎn 5g jìshēngshènqìwán 5g to ♀	Zhūlíngtāng 5g jìshēngshènqìwán 5g dānshēn 1g dōngguāzǐ 1g báimáogēn 1g zélán 1g to ♂
Unspecified disorder of intestine 569.9/K639 with flank pain D021501:	
Lǐzhōngtāng 5g báisháo 1g guìzhī 1g to ♀	Lǐzhōngtāng 5g báisháo 1g guìzhī 1g to ♂

1.19. Visceral Pain

Visceral pain is pain of the internal organs and tissues in the middle of the body. Because the viscera are diffusely innervated, visceral pain is not perceived locally and the feel is often described as dull, squeezing and sickening.

A pattern of visceral pain is that since the pain is not localized, the pain becomes referred to distal somatic sites. This characteristic may explain why herbalist doctors treat visceral pain with Sìnìtāng, which is also used for referred pain. Pancreatitis is treated by Dàcháihútāng, which has traditionally been used for hepatobiliary conditions. Note that it was suggested that referred orofacial pain could be the chief symptom of visceral diseases of the throat and chest (Myers, 2022).

Table 1.19. Herbal prescriptions for visceral pain

Visceral Pain: https://meshb.nlm.nih.gov/record/ui?ui=D059265.	
Common prescriptions:	
Sìnìtāng 5g wúzhūyútāng 5g Sìnìtāng 5g cháihúguìzhītāng 5g Sìnìtāng 5g guìzhītāng 5g	
Alternative prescriptions:	
Dāngguīsìnìtāng 5g shēngjiāng 1g wúzhūyú 1g Sìnìtāng 5g sháoyàogāncǎotāng 5g chuānliànzǐ 1g yánhúsuǒ 1g xiāngfù 1g Sháoyàogāncǎotāng 5g guìzhīfúlíngwán 5g chuānqī 1g yánhúsuǒ 1g Guìzhītāng 5g fùzǐ 2g Sìnìtāng 5g dāngguīsìnìtāng 4g wúzhūyú 1g gānjiāng 1g	
Indicated diseases:	
Unspecified disorder of intestine 569.9 (Disease of intestine, unspecified K639); Diseases of the jaws 526; Diseases of the oral soft tissues, excluding lesions specific for gingiva and tongue 528; Gastric ulcer 531; Acute pancreatitis 577.0 (Acute pancreatitis without necrosis or infection, unspecified K8590, Acute pancreatitis with uninfected necrosis, unspecified K8591, Acute pancreatitis with infected necrosis, unspecified K8592); Cystitis 595; Unspecified disorder of bladder 596.9 (Bladder disorder, unspecified N329)	
Unspecified disorder of intestine 569.9/K639 with visceral pain D059265:	
Lǐzhōngtāng 5g báisháo 1g guìzhī 1g to ♀	Xiāngshāliùjūnzǐtāng 5g cānlíngbáizhúsǎn 5g to ♂
Diseases of the jaws 526 with Visceral pain D059265:	
Guìzhītāng 5g báisháo 1g dàhuáng 0g to ♀	Gégēnhuángqínhuángliántāng 5g bànxià 1g fúlíng 1g dàhuáng 0g to ♂
Acute pancreatitis 577.0/K8590,K8591,K8592 with visceral pain D059265:	
Dàcháihútāng 5g bànxiàxièxīntāng 5g píngwèisǎn 5g to ♀	Dàcháihútāng 5g píngwèisǎn 5g to ♂
Cystitis 595 with visceral pain D059265:	
Bāzhèngsǎn 5g wǔlínsǎn 5g dǐdāngtāng 5g to ♀	Bāzhèngsǎn 5g wǔlínsǎn 5g dǐdāngtāng 5g to ♂

1.20. Myalgia

Myalgia means muscle pain and can include pain in the muscles, ligaments, tendons and fascia. It can be caused by injuries, overuses and diseases.

We learn in Section 1.1 the use of Huángqíwǔwùtāng for myopathy. Its use here for myalgia is no surprise. Xuèfǔzhúyūtāng 'activates Blood, transforms stasis' and 'moves Qi, stops pain.' Combining Xuèfǔzhúyūtāng and Huángqíwǔwùtāng here is believed to enhance myalgia relieving.

Table 1.20. Herbal prescriptions for myalgia

Myalgia: https://meshb.nlm.nih.gov/record/ui?ui=D063806.
Common prescriptions:
Huángqíwǔwùtāng 5g juānbìtāng 5g dānshēn 1g zhúrú 1g sāngzhī 1g jiānghuáng 1g Xuèfǔzhúyūtāng 5g huángqíwǔwùtāng 5g dānshēn 1g zhúrú 1g sāngzhī 1g jiānghuáng 1g Xuèfǔzhúyūtāng 5g huángqíwǔwùtāng 5g dānshēn 2g zhúrú 2g sāngzhī 2g jiānghuáng 2g Xuèfǔzhúyūtāng 5g huángqíwǔwùtāng 5g dānshēn 1g zhúrú 1g sāngzhī 1g jiānghuáng 1g + acupuncture Huángqíwǔwùtāng 5g juānbìtāng 5g dānshēn 1g zhúrú 1g sāngzhī 1g jiānghuáng 1g + acupuncture

Table 1.20. (Continued)

Myalgia: https://meshb.nlm.nih.gov/record/ui?ui=D063806.	
Alternative prescriptions:	
Huángqíwǔwùtāng 5g chuānxiōng 1g dānshēn 1g zhúrú 1g sāngzhī 1g dāngguī 1g jiānghuáng 1g Huángqíwǔwùtāng 5g juānbìtāng 5g dānshēn 1g zhúrú 1g yánhúsuǒ 1g sāngzhī 1g jiānghuáng 1g Guìzhītāng 5g chuānwū 1g + acupuncture Huángqíwǔwùtāng 5g sháoyàogāncǎotāng 4g dānshēn 2g zhúrú 2g sāngzhī 2g jiānghuáng 2g Huángqíwǔwùtāng 5g chuānxiōng 2g dānshēn 2g zhúrú 2g sāngzhī 2g qínjiāo 2g jiānghuáng 2g	
Indicated diseases:	
Myopathy, unspecified 359.9 (Myopathy, unspecified G729); Myoneural disorders 358; Unspecified disorders of nervous system 349.9 (Disorder of central nervous system, unspecified G969); Other dermatoses 702; Dermatomyositis 710.3 (Juvenile dermatomyositis without myopathy M3303, Other dermatomyositis without myopathy M3313, Dermatopolymyositis, unspecified, organ involvement unspecified M3390, Dermatopolymyositis, unspecified without myopathy M3393); Unspecified disorder of joint, site unspecified 719.90 (Joint disorder, unspecified M259)	
Myopathy, unspecified 359.9/G729 with myalgia D063806:	
Huángqíwǔwùtāng 5g dāngguīsìnìtāng 5g dānshēn 1g zhúrú 1g sāngzhī 1g jiānghuáng 1g to ♀	Huángqíwǔwùtāng 5g juānbìtāng 5g dānshēn 1g zhúrú 1g sāngzhī 1g jiānghuáng 1g to ♂
Other dermatoses 702 with myalgia D063806:	
Xiāofēngsǎn 5g zhēnrénhuómìngyǐnqùchuānshānjiǎ 5g qīngshàngfángfēngtāng 5g jīnyínhuā 1g liánqiáo 1g to ♀	Xiāofēngsǎn 5g dāngguīyǐnzǐ 5g tǔfúlíng 1g báixiānpí 1g dìfūzǐ 1g to ♂

1.21. Neuralgia

Unlike the pain we have met so far where damage occurs to the tissues and is detected by pain receptors which are distributed throughout the body, neuralgia is a result of damage or pathology of the nerve. Causes of neuropathy include traumatic injuries, metabolic problems such as high blood sugar, autoimmune diseases, viral infections, toxic exposures and medication side-effects. Figure 1.1 shows four forms of neuralgia.

Table 1.21. Herbal prescriptions for neuralgia

Neuralgia: https://meshb.nlm.nih.gov/record/ui?ui=D009437.
Common prescriptions:
Èrshùtāng 5g zhènggǔzǐjīndān 5g shūjīnghuóxuètāng 5g yánhúsuǒ 1g Èrshùtāng 5g sháoyàogāncǎotāng 5g shūjīnghuóxuètāng 5g + acupuncture Èrshùtāng 5g shūjīnghuóxuètāng 5g + acupuncture
Alternative prescriptions:
Èrshùtāng 5g dāngguīniāntòngtāng 5g sāngzhī 1g jiānghuáng 1g + acupuncture Èrshùtāng 5g zhènggǔzǐjīndān 5g wūyàoshùnqìsǎn 5g xùduàn 1g Èrshùtāng 5g shūjīnghuóxuètāng 5g yánhúsuǒ 1g jiānghuáng 1g jīxuèténg 1g + acupuncture Èrshùtāng 5g dāngguīniāntòngtāng 5g yánhúsuǒ 1g jiānghuáng 1g + acupuncture Èrshùtāng 5g shūjīnghuóxuètāng 5g mòyào 1g rǔxiāng 1g
Indicated diseases:
Other dermatoses 702; Myoneural disorders 358; Deformity and disproportion of reconstructed breast 612; Unspecified disorders of nervous system 349.9 (Disorder of central nervous system, unspecified G969); Other disorders of breast 611; Benign mammary dysplasias 610; Polyneuropathy in diabetes 357.2 (Diabetes mellitus due to underlying condition with diabetic polyneuropathy E0842, Drug or chemical induced diabetes mellitus with neurological complications with diabetic polyneuropathy E0942, Type 1 diabetes mellitus with diabetic polyneuropathy E1042, Type 2 diabetes mellitus with diabetic polyneuropathy E1142, Other specified diabetes mellitus with diabetic

Neuralgia: https://meshb.nlm.nih.gov/record/ui?ui=D009437.	
polyneuropathy E1342); Diabetes with neurological manifestations 250.6; Diabetes mellitus 250; Unspecified endocrine disorder 259.9 (Endocrine disorder, unspecified E349); Unspecified cerebrovascular disease 437.9 (Cerebrovascular disease, unspecified I679); Other disorders of lipoid metabolism 272.8 (Lipoid dermatoarthritis E7881, Other lipoprotein metabolism disorders E7889, Other specified metabolic disorders E8889); Cardiovascular disease, unspecified 429.2 (Atherosclerotic heart disease of native coronary artery without angina pectoris I2510); Unspecified condition of brain 348.9 (Disorder of brain, unspecified G939); Unspecified disorder of metabolism 277.9 (Metabolic disorder, unspecified E889); Herpes simplex 054; Herpes zoster 053	
Other dermatoses 702 with neuralgia D009437:	
Xiāofēngsǎn 5g bàidúsǎn 5g zhēnrénhuómìngyǐnqùchuānshānjiǎ 4g huángliánjiědútāng 4g to ♀	Xiāofēngsǎn 5g bàidúsǎn 5g zhēnrénhuómìngyǐnqùchuānshānjiǎ 4g huángliánjiědútāng 4g to ♂
Polyneuropathy in diabetes 357.2/E0842,E0942,E1042,E1142,E1342 with neuralgia D009437:	
Huángqíwǔwùtāng 5g dāngguīsìnìtāng 5g dānshēn 1g zhúrú 1g sāngzhī 1g jiānghuáng 1g to ♀	Huángqíwǔwùtāng 5g dāngguīsìnìtāng 5g dānshēn 1g zhúrú 1g sāngzhī 1g jiānghuáng 1g to ♂
Unspecified cerebrovascular disease 437.9/I679 with neuralgia D009437:	
Huángqíwǔwùtāng 5g bǔyánghuánwǔtāng 5g dānshēn 1g sāngzhī 1g jīxuèténg 1g + acupuncture to ♀	Huángqíwǔwùtāng 5g bǔyánghuánwǔtāng 5g dānshēn 1g sāngzhī 1g jīxuèténg 1g + acupuncture to ♂

We see in Section 1.2 that Shūjīnghuóxuètāng opens up meridians, promotes blood circulation and is used for chronic pain. As neuropathy can be permanent, many neuralgias are chronic. Zhènggǔzǐjīndān has primaritly been used to treat injuries caused by blunt trauma, such as those resulting from boxing, falls from heights, or being hit by a vehicle, which can cause nerve damage leading to neuralgia.

1.22. Postherpetic Neuralgia

Postherpetic neuralgia is persisting nerve pain, in the area of the skin where one had shingles, after the shingles resolved. Persistence of the pain is due to damage to the nerves affected by the shingles. Postherpetic neuralgia is the most common long-term complication of shingles infection.

Table 1.22. Herbal prescriptions for postherpetic neuralgia

Postherpetic Neuralgia: https://meshb.nlm.nih.gov/record/ui?ui=D051474.
Common prescriptions:
Èrshùtāng 5g wūyàoshùnqìsǎn 5g shūjīnghuóxuètāng 5g xùduàn 1g Èrshùtāng 5g wūyàoshùnqìsǎn 5g shūjīnghuóxuètāng 5g yánhúsuǒ 1g Èrshùtāng 5g sháoyàogāncǎotāng 5g shūjīnghuóxuètāng 5g + acupuncture
Alternative prescriptions:
Èrshùtāng 5g wūyàoshùnqìsǎn 5g xùduàn 1g Èrshùtāng 5g wūyàoshùnqìsǎn 5g juānbìtāng 5g yánhúsuǒ 1g Èrshùtāng 5g shūjīnghuóxuètāng 5g dāngguīniāntòngtāng 5g Èrshùtāng 5g shūjīnghuóxuètāng 5g gégēntāng 5g Wūyàoshùnqìsǎn 5g yánhúsuǒ 1g guìzhī 1g + acupuncture
Indicated and related diseases:
Myoneural disorders 358; Herpes zoster 053; Disorder of eye, unspecified 379.90 (Unspecified disorder of eye and adnexa H579); Unspecified disorders of nervous system 349.9 (Disorder of central nervous system, unspecified G969); Polyneuropathy in diabetes 357.2 (Diabetes mellitus due to underlying condition with diabetic polyneuropathy E0842, Drug or chemical induced diabetes mellitus with neurological complications with diabetic polyneuropathy E0942,

Table 1.22. (Continued)

Postherpetic Neuralgia: https://meshb.nlm.nih.gov/record/ui?ui=D051474.	
Type 1 diabetes mellitus with diabetic polyneuropathy E1042, Type 2 diabetes mellitus with diabetic polyneuropathy E1142, Other specified diabetes mellitus with diabetic polyneuropathy E1342); Diabetes with neurological manifestations 250.6; Diabetes mellitus 250; Unspecified endocrine disorder 259.9 (Endocrine disorder, unspecified E349); Other dermatoses 702; Rash and other nonspecific skin eruption 782.1 (Rash and other nonspecific skin eruption R21); Herpes simplex 054	
Myoneural disorders 358 with neuralgia, postherpetic D051474:	
Huángqíwǔwùtāng 5g dānshēn 1g zhúrú 1g sāngzhī 1g jiānghuáng 1g + acupuncture to ♀	Èrshùtāng 5g huángqíwǔwùtāng 5g dānshēn 1g zhúrú 1g sāngzhī 1g jiānghuáng 1g + acupuncture to ♂
Polyneuropathy in diabetes 357.2/E0842,E0942,E1042,E1142,E1342 with neuralgia, postherpetic D051474:	
Huángqíwǔwùtāng 5g dāngguīsìnìtāng 5g dānshēn 1g zhúrú 1g sāngzhī 1g jiānghuáng 1g to ♀	Bāwèidìhuángwán 5g báihǔjiārénshēntāng 5g dānshēn 1g tiānhuā 1g shíhú 1g to ♂
Other dermatoses 702 with neuralgia, postherpetic D051474:	
Xiāofēngsǎn 5g bàidúsǎn 5g zhēnrénhuómìngyǐnqùchuānshānjiǎ 4g huángliánjiědútāng 4g to ♀	Xiāofēngsǎn 5g bàidúsǎn 5g zhēnrénhuómìngyǐnqùchuānshānjiǎ 4g huángliánjiědútāng 4g to ♂

In addition to 'drying up Dampness and dissolving Phlegm,' Èrshùtāng also 'dredges meridians.' Ther term shùnqì in Wūyàoshùnqìsǎn reads 'to unchoke Qi.' Combining these formulas is believed to strengthen the prescription. Shingles rashes commonly occur on one side of the body and face including the eye.

1.23. Sciatica

Sciatica is nerve pain caused by irritation, inflammation, compression or damage of the sciatic nerve which originates from the lower back, splits and runs through the back of each of the hips, buttocks, legs and feet. Most commonly, slipped or herniated discs in the lumbar spine press against the sciatic nerve root, causing sciatica pain. Although nerve compression occurs in the lower back, pain radiates and is felt along the path of the sciatic nerve. The radiating pain is a hallmark of sciatica.

We learn in Section 1.14 the use of Sháoyàogāncǎotāng for failed lumbar spine surgery syndrome. Its use for sciatica here and for pains of the pudendal nerve, pelvic girdle and piriformis muscle in later sections suggests that Sháoyàogāncǎotāng also ameliorates pain in the lower body.

Table 1.23. Herbal prescriptions for sciatica

Sciatica: https://meshb.nlm.nih.gov/record/ui?ui=D012585.
Common prescriptions:
Sháoyàogāncǎotāng 5g shūjīnghuóxuètāng 5g dāngguīniāntòngtāng 5g + acupuncture Sháoyàogāncǎotāng 5g shūjīnghuóxuètāng 5g + acupuncture
Alternative prescriptions:
Shūjīnghuóxuètāng 5g sháoyàogāncǎotāng 2g niúxī 1g mòyào 1g rǔxiāng 1g + acupuncture Shūjīnghuóxuètāng 5g sháoyàogāncǎotāng 2g yánhúsuǒ 1g + acupuncture Sháoyàogāncǎotāng 5g shūjīnghuóxuètāng 5g mòyào 1g rǔxiāng 1g Sháoyàogāncǎotāng 5g niúxī 1g Dāngguīniāntòngtāng 5g sháoyàogāncǎotāng 2g mòyào 1g rǔxiāng 1g yánhúsuǒ 1g + acupuncture

Sciatica: https://meshb.nlm.nih.gov/record/ui?ui=D012585.	
Indicated diseases:	
Lesion of sciatic nerve 355.0 (Lesion of sciatic nerve, unspecified lower limb G5700); Malignant neoplasm of spinal cord 192.2 (Malignant neoplasm of spinal cord C720, Malignant neoplasm of cauda equina C721); Mononeuritis multiplex 354.5 (Mononeuritis multiplex G587); Mononeuritis of unspecified site 355.9 (Mononeuropathy, unspecified G589); Unspecified disease of spinal cord 336.9 (Disease of spinal cord, unspecified G959); Myoneural disorders 358; Unspecified disorders of nervous system 349.9 (Disorder of central nervous system, unspecified G969); Neuroendocrine tumors 209; Malignant neoplasm of nervous system, part unspecified 192.9 (Malignant neoplasm of central nervous system, unspecified C729); Unspecified disorder of joint, site unspecified 719.90 (Joint disorder, unspecified M259)	
Lesion of sciatic nerve 355.0/G5700 with sciatica D012585:	
Shūjīnghuóxuètāng 5g dúhuójìshēngtāng 5g + acupuncture to ♀	Shūjīnghuóxuètāng 5g dúhuójìshēngtāng 5g niúxī 1g dùzhòng 1g xùduàn 1g + acupuncture to ♂

1.24. Pudendal Neuralgia

The pudendal nerve, a main nerve in the pelvis, runs from the pubic bone to tailbone and its damage causes discomfort, including pain, tingling or numbness, in the areas from the genitals to buttocks. Males can injure the pudendal nerve in sports like cycling and riding, and females in giving birth.

Table 1.24. Herbal prescriptions for pudendal neuralgia

Pudendal Neuralgia: https://meshb.nlm.nih.gov/record/ui?ui=D060545.	
Common prescriptions:	
Sháoyàogāncǎotāng 5g shūjīnghuóxuètāng 5g dāngguīniāntòngtāng 5g + acupuncture Sháoyàogāncǎotāng 5g shūjīnghuóxuètāng 5g + acupuncture	
Alternative prescriptions:	
Sháoyàogāncǎotāng 5g shūjīnghuóxuètāng 5g Jiāwèixiāoyáosǎn 5g xiāngshāliùjūnzǐtāng 5g gāncǎoxiǎomàidàzǎotāng 2g héhuānpí 1g xiāngfù 1g Jiāwèixiāoyáosǎn 5g xiāngshāliùjūnzǐtāng 3g bànxiàxièxīntāng 2g héhuānpí 1g yánhúsuǒ 1g Zhènggǔzǐjīndān 5g sháoyàogāncǎotāng 3g dāngguīniāntòngtāng 3g sānqī 2g dàdīnghuáng 2g gāncǎo 2g dǎodìwúgōng 2g sūmù 2g xùduàn 2g + acupuncture Shūjīnghuóxuètāng 5g sháoyàogāncǎotāng 4g niúxī 1g dùzhòng 1g xùduàn 1g + acupuncture	
Associated diseases:	
Cardiovascular disease, unspecified 429.2 (Atherosclerotic heart disease of native coronary artery without angina pectoris I2510); Multiple myeloma 203.0; Unspecified hemorrhagic conditions 287.9 (Hemorrhagic condition, unspecified D699); Unspecified diseases of blood and blood-forming organs 289.9 (Disease of blood and blood-forming organs, unspecified D759);	
Unspecified condition of brain 348.9 (Disorder of brain, unspecified G939); Unspecified disorder of metabolism 277.9 (Metabolic disorder, unspecified E889); Alexia 315.01 (Dyslexia and alexia R480); Unspecified disorders of nervous system 349.9 (Disorder of central nervous system, unspecified G969); Heart disease, unspecified 429.9 (Heart disease, unspecified I519)	
Cardiovascular disease, unspecified 429.2/I2510 with pudendal neuralgia D060545:	
Sìnìtāng 5g gānlùyǐn 5g mǔdānpí 1g zhīzǐ 1g huánglián 0g to ♀	Xuèfǔzhúyūtāng 5g zhìgāncǎotāng 5g dānshēn 1g to ♂
Unspecified condition of brain 348.9/G939 with pudendal neuralgia D060545:	
Bǔyánghuánwǔtāng 5g dānshēn 1g tiānmá 1g shíchāngpú 1g yuǎnzhì 1g + acupuncture to ♀	Bǔyánghuánwǔtāng 5g dānshēn 1g tiānmá 1g shíchāngpú 1g yuǎnzhì 1g + acupuncture to ♂

Table 1.24. (Continued)

Pudendal Neuralgia: https://meshb.nlm.nih.gov/record/ui?ui=D060545.	
Unspecified disorder of metabolism 277.9/E889 with pudendal neuralgia D060545:	
Rénshēnbàidúsǎn 5g xiǎocháihútāngqùrénshēn 5g yīnchénhāotāng 2g mùxiāng 1g yùjīn 1g to ♀	Liùwèidìhuángwán 5g bǔzhōngyìqìtāng 5g to ♂
Heart disease, unspecified 429.9/I519 with pudendal neuralgia D060545:	
Sìnìtāng 5g gānlùyǐn 5g mǔdānpí 1g zhīzǐ 1g huánglián 0g to ♀	Xuèfǔzhúyūtāng 5g zhìgāncǎotāng 5g dānshēn 2g chuānqī 1g báijí 1g guìzhī 1g guālóurén 1g xièbái 1g to ♂

Here we see another example of combining Sháoyàogāncǎotāng and Shūjīnghuóxuètāng for the treatment of neuralgia. Dāngguīniāntòngtāng is also seen for its used for such chronic pain as low back pain, flank pain, and sciatica in previous sections. Classical medical texts say that it is used for pain resulting from 'a clash between the pouring Dampness and Heat' to the area of the pain.

1.25. Pelvic Girdle Pain

The pelvic girdle, or hip bone, is made up of a complex of bones to support the linkage of the axial skeleton to the lower limbs. About one in five women develop pelvic girdle pain in the front or back of the pelvis during pregnancy. Pregnancy-related pelvic girdle pain goes away after childbirth. Other causes include osteoarthritis, arthritis and sports injuries. Pelvic girdle pain is a type of musculoskeletal pain, as shown in Figure 1.1.

A modern use of Jiāwèixiāoyáosǎn is for menopause (Wang, 2019). Multiple myeloma, a type of bone marrow cancer, can cause pain in any bone including pelvic bones.

Table 1.25. Herbal prescriptions for pelvic girdle pain

Pelvic Girdle Pain: https://meshb.nlm.nih.gov/record/ui?ui=D059388.	
Common prescriptions:	
Sháoyàogāncǎotāng 5g shūjīnghuóxuètāng 5g dāngguīniāntòngtāng 5g + acupuncture Sháoyàogāncǎotāng 5g shūjīnghuóxuètāng 5g + acupuncture	
Alternative prescriptions:	
Jiāwèixiāoyáosǎn 5g gāncǎoxiǎomàidàzǎotāng 5g sháoyàogāncǎotāng 5g Jiāwèixiāoyáosǎn 5g zhībódìhuángwán 5g suānzǎoréntāng 5g héhuānpí 1g yèjiāoténg 1g fúshén 1g Shūjīnghuóxuètāng 5g sháoyàogāncǎotāng 4g + acupuncture	
Xuèfǔzhúyūtāng 5g sháoyàogāncǎotāng 4g chuānliànzǐ 1g dānshēn 1g mòyào 1g rǔxiāng 1g yánhúsuǒ 1g	
Indicated diseases:	
Multiple myeloma 203.0; Unspecified diseases of blood and blood-forming organs 289.9 (Disease of blood and blood-forming organs, unspecified D759); Unspecified disorder of metabolism 277.9 (Metabolic disorder, unspecified E889); Unspecified disorders of nervous system 349.9 (Disorder of central nervous system, unspecified G969)	
Unspecified disorder of metabolism 277.9/E889 with pelvic girdle pain D059388:	
Rénshēnbàidúsǎn 5g xiǎocháihútāngqùrénshēn 5g yīnchénhāotāng 2g mùxiāng 1g yùjīn 1g to ♀	Dānshēn 5g tiānmágōuténgyǐn 5g sǎnzhǒngkuìjiāntāng 5g bǔyánghuánwǔtāng 5g to ♂

1.26. Colic

Colic is a type of pain that starts and stops abruptly, resulting from spasm of the smooth muscle of a hollow tube organ, e.g., the small, large intestine and ureter, which normally moves in an earthworm-like fashion to propel the content of the tube, i.e., food or urine. Obstruction in the hollow tube organ causes the muscular spasm.

Table 1.26. Herbal prescriptions for colic

Colic: https://meshb.nlm.nih.gov/record/ui?ui=D003085.	
Common prescriptions:	
Bāzhèngsǎn 5g wǔlínsǎn 5g dǐdāngtāng 5g Wǔlínsǎn 5g huàshícǎo 1g huángqín 1g Wǔlínsǎn 5g huàshícǎo 1g	
Alternative prescriptions:	
Bāzhèngsǎn 5g yánhúsuǒ 1g jīnèijīn 1g yùjīn 1g gāncǎo 0g Bāzhèngsǎn 5g yánhúsuǒ 1g jīnèijīn 1g bèimǔ 1g yùjīn 1g gāncǎo 0g Zhūlíngtāng 5g huàshícǎo 1g niúxī 1g jīnqiáncǎo 1g jīnèijīn 1g Zhūlíngtāng 5g huàshícǎo 1g niúxī 1g dōngkuízǐ 1g jīnqiáncǎo 1g jīnèijīn 1g Zhūlíngtāng 5g jīnqiáncǎo 1g jīnèijīn 1g yùjīn 1g	
Indicated diseases:	
Cholecystitis, unspecified 575.10 (Cholecystitis, unspecified K819); Unspecified disorder of gallbladder 575.9 (Disease of gallbladder, unspecified K829); Unspecified disorder of biliary tract 576.9 (Disease of biliary tract, unspecified K839); Diseases of the jaws 526;	
Diseases of the oral soft tissues, excluding lesions specific for gingiva and tongue 528; Unspecified intestinal obstruction 560.9 (Partial intestinal obstruction, unspecified as to cause K56600, Complete intestinal obstruction, unspecified as to cause K56601, Unspecified intestinal obstruction, unspecified as to partial versus complete obstruction K56609); Unspecified disorder of intestine 569.9 (Disease of intestine, unspecified K639); Malignant neoplasm of appendix vermiformis 153.5 (Malignant neoplasm of appendix C181)	
Cholecystitis, unspecified 575.10/K819 with colic D003085:	
Dàcháihútāng 5g chìsháo 1g jīnqiáncǎo 1g yùjīn 1g huǒmárén 0g to ♀	Dàcháihútāng 5g chìsháo 1g jīnqiáncǎo 1g yùjīn 1g huǒmárén 0g to ♂
Unspecified disorder of gallbladder 575.9/K829 with colic D003085:	
Dàcháihútāng 5g chìsháo 1g jīnqiáncǎo 1g yùjīn 1g huǒmárén 0g to ♀	Dàcháihútāng 5g jīnqiáncǎo 1g jīnèijīn 1g yùjīn 1g to ♂
Unspecified disorder of biliary tract 576.9/K839 with colic D003085:	
Dàcháihútāng 5g jīnqiáncǎo 1g jīnèijīn 1g yùjīn 1g to ♀	Dàcháihútāng 5g jīnqiáncǎo 1g jīnèijīn 1g yùjīn 1g to ♂
Unspecified intestinal obstruction 560.9/K56600,K56601,K56609 with colic D003085:	
Mázǐrénwán 5g dàhuáng 1g to ♀	Mázǐrénwán 5g rùnchángwán 5g to ♂
Unspecified disorder of intestine 569.9/K639 with colic D003085:	
Lǐzhōngtāng 5g báisháo 1g guìzhī 1g to ♀	Lǐzhōngtāng 5g báisháo 1g guìzhī 1g to ♂

Bāzhèngsǎn and Wǔlínsǎn are used for flank pain, which most likely results from cystic duct or urinary tract obstruction. Dǐdāngtāng 'removes Blood stasis' and Zhūlíngtāng 'helps urinate and dehydrate.' Zhūlíng, the major herb in Zhūlíngtāng, is today used for chronic glomerulonephritis (Wang, 2019).

1.27. Renal Colic

Stones, i.e., concretions of mineral salts, form in the kidney, dislodge into urine stream and pass through the ureter without symptoms. However, when kidney stones are too large, the ureter can be blocked. Restricted urine flow makes the ureter to spasm, causing renal colic.

Ideally, treatment for renal colic should consider the type of stones, which depends on patient's metabolism and digestion, which are indicated by Guìzhītāng. Furthermore, it was found that renal colic increases the risk of coronary heart diseases and stroke (Peng and Zheng, 2017). This association might explain the use of Sìnìtāng, which is used for a variety of cardiovascular diseases, for renal colic.

Table 1.27. Herbal prescriptions for renal colic

Renal Colic: https://meshb.nlm.nih.gov/record/ui?ui=D056844.	
Common prescriptions:	
Sìnìtāng 5g sháoyàogāncǎotāng 5g Xiǎocháihútāng 5g guìzhītāng 5g gégēn 2g Sìnìtāng 5g sháoyàogāncǎotāng 5g yánhúsuǒ 2g	
Alternative prescriptions:	
Guìzhītāng 5g báisháo 1g dàhuáng 0g Guìzhītāng 5g shēngjiāng 1g báisháo 1g dàhuáng 0g Guìzhītāng 5g gégēn 2g bànxià 1g dàhuáng 0g Sìnìtāng 5g bǔzhōngyìqìtāng 5g Sìnìtāng 5g shēngjiāng 1g guìzhī 1g bànxià 1g	
Indicated and associated diseases:	
Unspecified disorder of intestine 569.9 (Disease of intestine, unspecified K639); Other diseases of appendix 543; Heart disease, unspecified 429.9 (Heart disease, unspecified I519); Unspecified congenital anomaly of heart 746.9 (Congenital malformation of cardiac chambers and connections, unspecified Q209, Congenital malformation of heart, unspecified Q249); Cardiovascular disease, unspecified 429.2 (Atherosclerotic heart disease of native coronary artery without angina pectoris I2510); Malignant neoplasm of kidney, except pelvis 189.0 (Malignant neoplasm of unspecified kidney, except renal pelvis C649); Unspecified disorder of metabolism 277.9 (Metabolic disorder, unspecified E889)	
Unspecified disorder of intestine 569.9/K639 with renal colic D056844:	
Xiāngshāliùjūnzǐtāng 5g cānlíngbáizhúsǎn 5g to ♀	Xiāngshāliùjūnzǐtāng 5g cānlíngbáizhúsǎn 5g to ♂
Heart disease, unspecified 429.9/I519 with renal colic D056844:	
Sìnìtāng 5g gānlùyǐn 5g mǔdānpí 1g zhīzǐ 1g huánglián 0g to ♀	Sìnìtāng 5g gānlùyǐn 5g mǔdānpí 1g zhīzǐ 1g huánglián 0g to ♂
Malignant neoplasm of kidney, except pelvis 189.0/C649 with renal colic D056844:	
Zhūlíngtāng 5g jìshēngshènqìwán 5g dānshēn 1g dōngguāzǐ 1g báimáogēn 1g zélán 1g to ♀	Zhūlíngtāng 5g jìshēngshènqìwán 5g dōngguāzǐ 1g báimáogēn 1g chēqiánzǐ 1g bìxiè 1g to ♂
Unspecified disorder of metabolism 277.9/E889 with renal colic D056844:	
Fángfēngtōngshèngsǎn 5g shānzhā 1g cǎojuémíng 1g chénpí 1g to ♀	Shàngzhōngxiàtōngyòngtòngfēngwán 5g dāngguīniāntòngtāng 5g niúxī 1g huángbò 1g cāngzhú 1g yìyǐrén 1g to ♂

1.28. Piriformis Muscle Syndrome

The piriformis muscle runs from the lower spine through the buttock to the top of the thigh to laterally rotate the femur in the hip joint. Piriformis muscle spasm and swelling can compress the sciatic nerve which comes beneath the piriformis muscle, causing pain and numbness in the buttocks and referred pain along the sciatic nerve. Overuse and trauma can cause muscle spasm.

Table 1.28. Herbal prescriptions for piriformis muscle syndrome

Piriformis Muscle Syndrome: https://meshb.nlm.nih.gov/record/ui?ui=D055958.	
Common prescriptions:	
Sháoyàogāncǎotāng 5g shūjīnghuóxuètāng 5g dāngguīniāntòngtāng 5g + acupuncture Sháoyàogāncǎotāng 5g shūjīnghuóxuètāng 5g + acupuncture	
Alternative prescriptions:	
Shēntòngzhúyūtāng 5g dāngguīniāntòngtāng 5g huángbò 1g cāngzhú 1g + acupuncture Jiāwèixiāoyáosǎn 5g xiāngshāliùjūnzǐtāng 5g bànxiàxièxīntāng 1g héhuānpí 1g yánhúsuǒ 1g Sháoyàogāncǎotāng 5g zhībódìhuángwán 5g shūjīnghuóxuètāng 5g + acupuncture Liùwèidìhuángwán 5g shūjīnghuóxuètāng 5g mùguā 1g niúxī 1g	
Indicated diseases:	
Unspecified disorders of nervous system 349.9 (Disorder of central nervous system, unspecified G969)	
Unspecified disorders of nervous system 349.9/G969 with piriformis muscle syndrome D055958:	
Shūjīnghuóxuètāng 5g píngwèisǎn 2g mùguā 1g sāngzhī 1g jīxuèténg 1g to ♀	Shūjīnghuóxuètāng 5g píngwèisǎn 2g mùguā 1g sāngzhī 1g jīxuèténg 1g to ♂

It is not surprising that many of the herbal prescriptions here are also used for sciatica. Moreover, it happens that Sháoyàogāncǎotāng, Shūjīnghuóxuètāng and Dāngguīniāntòngtāng are the herbal formulas commonly used for neuralgia. Indeed, the modern uses of Sháoyàogāncǎotāng and Shūjīnghuóxuètāng include unspecified neuralgia, neuritis and radiculitis (Wang, 2019).

1.29. Dysmenorrhea

Dysmenorrhea, or menstrual cramps, is pain in the lower abdomen and pelvis due to uterine contractions from menstruation. Over half of women who menstruate experience menstrual cramps before or during the period every month. Other causes of dysmenorrhea include endometriosis, uterine fibroids, and pelvic inflammation.

Table 1.29. Herbal prescriptions for dysmenorrhea

Dysmenorrhea: https://meshb.nlm.nih.gov/record/ui?ui=D004412.
Common prescriptions:
Guìzhīfúlíngwán 5g dāngguīsháoyàosǎn 5g yánhúsuǒ 1g xiāngfù 1g Guìzhīfúlíngwán 5g dāngguīsháoyàosǎn 5g yánhúsuǒ 1g xiāngfù 1g yìmǔcǎo 1g Guìzhīfúlíngwán 5g dāngguīsháoyàosǎn 5g Guìzhīfúlíngwán 5g dāngguīsháoyàosǎn 5g yánhúsuǒ 1g Guìzhīfúlíngwán 5g dāngguīsháoyàosǎn 5g yánhúsuǒ 2g xiāngfù 2g yìmǔcǎo 2g
Alternative prescriptions:
Guìzhīfúlíngwán 5g wēnjīngtāng 5g hónghuā 1g táorén 1g Guìzhīfúlíngwán 5g dāngguīsháoyàosǎn 5g xiāngfù 1g Guìzhīfúlíngwán 5g cháihúshūgāntāng 5g yánhúsuǒ 1g yìmǔcǎo 1g Wēnjīngtāng 5g yánhúsuǒ 0g xiāngfù 0g wūyào 0g Guìzhīfúlíngwán 5g dāngguīsháoyàosǎn 4g wǔlíngzhī 1g xiāngfù 1g púhuáng 1g

Table 1.29. (Continued)

Dysmenorrhea: https://meshb.nlm.nih.gov/record/ui?ui=D004412.
Indicated diseases:
Uterine leiomyoma 218; Unspecified disorder of uterus 621.9 (Noninflammatory disorder of uterus, unspecified N859); Malignant neoplasm of uterus, part unspecified 179 (Malignant neoplasm of uterus, part unspecified C55); Malignant neoplasm of other and unspecified female genital organs 184; Unspecified disorder of female genital organs 629.9 (Unspecified condition associated with female genital organs and menstrual cycle N949); Endometriosis 617; Unspecified endocrine disorder 259.9 (Endocrine disorder, unspecified E349); Absence of menstruation 626.0 (Amenorrhea, unspecified N912)
Uterine leiomyoma 218 with dysmenorrhea D004412:
Jiāwèixiāoyáosǎn 5g guìzhīfúlíngwán 5g sānléng 1g éshù 1g to ♀
Malignant neoplasm of uterus, part unspecified 179/C55 with dysmenorrhea D004412:
Guìzhīfúlíngwán 5g dāngguīsháoyàosǎn 5g dānshēn 1g yánhúsuǒ 1g xiāngfù 1g to ♀
Unspecified endocrine disorder 259.9/E349 with dysmenorrhea D004412:
Jiāwèixiāoyáosǎn 5g dāngguīsháoyàosǎn 5g dānshēn 1g xiāngfù 1g yìmǔcǎo 1g to ♀

Guìzhīfúlíngwán 'removes stasis, dissolves masses,' and has traditionally been used for gynecological conditions. Dāngguīsháoyàosǎn, which 'nourishes Blood,' has traditionally been used to improve women's health during pregnancy. Note that although Guìzhīfúlíngwán and Dāngguīsháoyàosǎn were originally composed for women, they are nowadays used for both women and men for their urological conditions as we will see in Chapter 9.

1.30. Glossalgia

Glossalgia is pain in the tongue. Causes of glossalgia are various, ranging from fungal infections in the oral cavity to psychological conditions.

Gānlùyǐn 'nourishes Yin, moistens dryness,' 'clears Heat, neutralizes pathogens,' and is used for dental caries with toothache in Section 1.9. As it is cooling, i.e., anti-inflammatory, it is widely used for infection and inflammation of the upper digestive tract and skin.

Table 1.30. Herbal prescriptions for glossalgia

Glossalgia: https://meshb.nlm.nih.gov/record/ui?ui=D005926.
Common prescriptions:
Guìzhītāng 5g shēngjiāng 1g guìzhī 1g Guìzhītāng 5g shēngjiāng 1g báisháo 1g dàhuáng 0g Guìzhītāng 5g bànxià 1g dàhuáng 0g Guìzhītāng 5g shēngjiāng 1g guìzhī 1g dàhuáng 0g Guìzhītāng 5g shēngjiāng 1g báisháo 1g
Alternative prescriptions:
Sìnìtāng 5g bànxià 1g dàhuáng 0g Guìzhītāng 5g gégēn 2g bànxià 1g dàhuáng 0g Jiégěngtāng 5g xuánshēn 2g mǔlì 2g bèimǔ 2g huángqín 2g shānzhīzǐ 1g liánqiáo 1g dàhuáng 0g Guìzhītāng 5g jiégěng 1g huángqín 1g dàhuáng 0g
Indicated diseases:
Unspecified condition of the tongue 529.9 (Disease of tongue, unspecified K149); Candidiasis 112; Coccidioidomycosis 114; Histoplasmosis 115; Blastomycotic infection 116; Other mycoses 117; Opportunistic mycoses 118 (Other specified mycoses B488); Dermatophytosis 110; Dermatomycosis, other and unspecified 111; Candidiasis of mouth 112.0 (Candidal stomatitis B370, Candidal cheilitis B3783); Human immunodeficiency virus [HIV] disease 042 (Human immunodeficiency virus [HIV] disease B20); Geographic tongue 529.1 (Geographic tongue K141); Glossitis 529.0 (Glossitis K140)

Glossalgia: https://meshb.nlm.nih.gov/record/ui?ui=D005926.	
Unspecified condition of the tongue 529.9/K149 with glossalgia D005926:	
Gānlùyǐn 5g dǎochìsǎn 5g to ♀	Gānlùyǐn 5g dǎochìsǎn 5g to ♂
Geographic tongue 529.1/K141 with glossalgia D005926:	
Gānlùyǐn 5g qīngwèisǎn 5g dǎochìsǎn 5g to ♀	Gānlùyǐn 5g qīngwèisǎn 5g dǎochìsǎn 5g to ♂

1.31. Chest Pain

Pain in the chest can be caused by lung infection, rib injury, heart disease, pulmonary embolism, gastric reflux, and anxiety.

Table 1.31. Herbal prescriptions for chest pain

Chest Pain: https://meshb.nlm.nih.gov/record/ui?ui=D002637.	
Common prescriptions:	
Fùyuánhuóxuètāng 5g mùxiāng 0g gāncǎo 0g hòupò 0g cāngzhú 0g + acupuncture Fùyuánhuóxuètāng 5g dānshēn 1g yánhúsuǒ 1g yùjīn 1g + acupuncture	
Alternative prescriptions:	
Fùyuánhuóxuètāng 5g sháoyàogāncǎotāng 4g mùxiāng 1g niúxī 1g rǔxiāng 1g yánhúsuǒ 1g + acupuncture Zhènggǔzǐjīndān 5g fùyuánhuóxuètāng 4g yánhúsuǒ 2g mòyào 1g rǔxiāng 1g + acupuncture Xuèfǔzhúyūtāng 5g yánhúsuǒ 1g zhǐqiào 1g yùjīn 1g + acupuncture	
Indicated diseases:	
Heart disease, unspecified 429.9 (Heart disease, unspecified I519); Malignant neoplasm of heart 164.1 (Malignant neoplasm of heart C380); Cardiovascular disease, unspecified 429.2 (Atherosclerotic heart disease of native coronary artery without angina pectoris I2510); Reticulosarcoma 200.0; Malignant neoplasm of thorax 195.1 (Malignant neoplasm of thorax C761); Aneurysm of coronary vessels 414.11 (Coronary artery aneurysm I2541); Aneurysm of unspecified site 442.9 (Aneurysm of unspecified site I729); Unspecified congenital anomaly of heart 746.9 (Congenital malformation of cardiac chambers and connections, unspecified Q209, Congenital malformation of heart, unspecified Q249)	
Heart disease, unspecified 429.9/I519 with chest pain D002637:	
Xuèfǔzhúyūtāng 5g dānshēn 2g chuānqī 1g guìzhī 1g guālóurén 1g xièbái 1g to ♀	Xuèfǔzhúyūtāng 5g bǔzhōngyìqìtāng 5g dānshēn 2g chuānqī 1g guìzhī 1g guālóurén 1g xièbái 1g to ♂
Aneurysm of coronary vessels 414.11/I2541 with chest pain D002637:	
Xuèfǔzhúyūtāng 5g zhìgāncǎotāng 5g dānshēn 1g yùjīn 1g to ♀	Xuèfǔzhúyūtāng 5g zhìgāncǎotāng 5g dānshēn 1g yùjīn 1g to ♂

The modern uses of Fùyuánhuóxuètāng are for unspecified chronic bronchitis, and unspecified chest pain (Wang, 2019).

1.32. Variant Angina Pectoris

Variant angina pectoris is a form of angina pectoris that is caused by a spasm of the coronary arteries which bring blood and oxygen to the heart. Insufficient oxygen to the heart triggers chest pain. A characteristic of variant angina is that it occurs when one is at rest or asleep. Causes of coronary artery spasms include temperature drop, stress, and medications that constrict blood vessels. Variant angina is not common.

Table 1.32. Herbal prescriptions for variant angina pectoris

Variant Angina Pectoris: https://meshb.nlm.nih.gov/record/ui?ui=D000788.	
Common prescriptions:	
Xuèfǔzhúyūtāng 5g chuānqī 1g dānshēn 1g Xuèfǔzhúyūtāng 5g dānshēn 1g guālóurén 1g xièbái 1g Xuèfǔzhúyūtāng 5g dānshēn 1g guālóurén 1g xièbái 1g yùjīn 1g Xuèfǔzhúyūtāng 5g sānqī 1g dānshēn 1g	
Alternative prescriptions:	
Xuèfǔzhúyūtāng 5g guālóurén 1g xièbái 1g Xuèfǔzhúyūtāng 5g dānshēn 1g guālóurén 1g xièbái 1g + acupuncture Fùfāngdānshēnpiàn 5g yánhúsuǒ 1g gāncǎo 0g	
Xuèfǔzhúyūtāng 5g dānshēn 0g Xuèfǔzhúyūtāng 5g sānqī 2g dānshēn 1g + acupuncture	
Indicated and associated diseases:	
Intermediate coronary syndrome 411.1 (Unstable angina I200); Unspecified condition of brain 348.9 (Disorder of brain, unspecified G939); Unspecified cerebrovascular disease 437.9 (Cerebrovascular disease, unspecified I679); Heart disease, unspecified 429.9 (Heart disease, unspecified I519); Cardiovascular disease, unspecified 429.2 (Atherosclerotic heart disease of native coronary artery without angina pectoris I2510); Unspecified disorders of nervous system 349.9 (Disorder of central nervous system, unspecified G969); Diabetes with peripheral circulatory disorders 250.7; Diabetes mellitus 250; Unspecified endocrine disorder 259.9 (Endocrine disorder, unspecified E349); Unspecified disorder of metabolism 277.9 (Metabolic disorder, unspecified E889); Unspecified congenital anomaly of heart 746.9 (Congenital malformation of cardiac chambers and connections, unspecified Q209, Congenital malformation of heart, unspecified Q249)	
Intermediate coronary syndrome 411.1/I200 with angina pectoris, variant D000788:	
Xuèfǔzhúyūtāng 5g dānshēn 1g guālóurén 1g xièbái 1g to ♀	Xuèfǔzhúyūtāng 5g dānshēn 1g guālóurén 1g xièbái 1g to ♂

Dānshēn 'activates Blood and opens meridians.' It is the most commonly prescribed single herbs in clinical practice, in terms of the quantity prescribed in grams. We will witness its predominant uses throughout the chapters in the book, except the body weight and bleeding chapters. Note that narrowing of blood vessels can happen to the carotid arteries at the base of the brain which carry blood to the neck and head, and there was a report of cerebral vasoconstriction and coronary artery vasospasm in a diabetic patient (Laeeq et al., 2019), as we see the association in the table.

1.33. Stable Angina

Coronary arteries can become progressively narrowed by the buildup of fatty substances in the artery walls, a condition called atherosclerosis. Chest pain then starts to occur while one exerts, as the heart does not get enough blood to function properly. Because the pain follows physical activity, it is predictable and called stable angina.

Table 1.33. Herbal prescriptions for stable angina

Stable Angina: https://meshb.nlm.nih.gov/record/ui?ui=D060050.
Common prescriptions:
Xuèfǔzhúyūtāng 5g cháihúshūgāntāng 5g chuānliànzǐ 1g yánhúsuǒ 1g Xuèfǔzhúyūtāng 5g chuānqī 1g dānshēn 1g Xuèfǔzhúyūtāng 5g sānqī 1g dānshēn 1g yánhúsuǒ 1g xiāngfù 1g yùjīn 1g Xuèfǔzhúyūtāng 5g sānqī 1g dānshēn 1g yánhúsuǒ 1g yùjīn 1g Xuèfǔzhúyūtāng 5g sānqī 1g dānshēn 1g

Stable Angina: https://meshb.nlm.nih.gov/record/ui?ui=D060050.	
Alternative prescriptions:	
Xuèfŭzhúyūtāng 5g chuānqī 1g dānshēn 1g yánhúsuŏ 1g yùjīn 1g + acupuncture Xuèfŭzhúyūtāng 5g chuānqī 1g dānshēn 1g mùxiāng 1g yùjīn 1g Xuèfŭzhúyūtāng 5g sānqī 1g dānshēn 1g + acupuncture Xuèfŭzhúyūtāng 5g dānshēn 1g guālóurén 1g xièbái 1g yùjīn 1g + acupuncture	
Indicated and associated diseases:	
Chronic ischemic heart disease, unspecified 414.9 (Chronic ischemic heart disease, unspecified I259); Peripheral angiopathy in diseases classified elsewhere 443.81 (Other disorders of arteries, arterioles and capillaries in diseases classified elsewhere I798); Heart disease, unspecified 429.9 (Heart disease, unspecified I519); Cardiovascular disease, unspecified 429.2 (Atherosclerotic heart disease of native coronary artery without angina pectoris I2510); Unspecified disorder of metabolism 277.9 (Metabolic disorder, unspecified E889); Unspecified cerebrovascular disease 437.9 (Cerebrovascular disease, unspecified I679); Unspecified condition of brain 348.9 (Disorder of brain, unspecified G939); Unspecified disorders of nervous system 349.9 (Disorder of central nervous system, unspecified G969)	
Chronic ischemic heart disease, unspecified 414.9/I259 with angina, stable D060050:	
Xuèfŭzhúyūtāng 5g zhìgāncăotāng 5g dānshēn 1g yùjīn 1g to ♀	Xuèfŭzhúyūtāng 5g zhìgāncăotāng 5g dānshēn 1g yùjīn 1g to ♂
Unspecified cerebrovascular disease 437.9/I679 with angina, stable D060050:	
Bŭyánghuánwŭtāng 5g dānshēn 1g shíchāngpú 1g yuănzhì 1g + acupuncture to ♀	Bŭyánghuánwŭtāng 5g dānshēn 1g shíchāngpú 1g yuănzhì 1g + acupuncture to ♂

Chuānqī, a food, is believed to improve sugar and lipid metabolism. Sānqī 'invigorates Blood, stops pain,' and has traditionally been used for the treatment of pain and paralysis.

1.34. Labor Pain

Labor pain occurs when during childbirth the uterus contracts to push the baby out. Pain is felt in the parts of the lower back, lower abdomen and pelvis.

The formulas for labor pain are also used for pains in the lower body such as sciatica.

Table 1.34. Herbal prescriptions for labor pain

Labor Pain: https://meshb.nlm.nih.gov/record/ui?ui=D048949.
Common prescriptions:
Sháoyàogāncăotāng 5g shūjīnghuóxuètāng 5g dāngguīniāntòngtāng 5g + acupuncture Sháoyàogāncăotāng 5g shūjīnghuóxuètāng 5g + acupuncture
Alternative prescriptions:
Jiāwèixiāoyáosăn 5g xiāngshāliùjūnzĭtāng 5g bànxiàxièxīntāng 2g dānshēn 1g héhuānpí 1g Shūjīnghuóxuètāng 5g dāngguīniāntòngtāng 5g dúhuójìshēngtāng 5g + acupuncture Jiāwèixiāoyáosăn 5g gāncăoxiăomàidàzăotāng 3g héhuānpí 1g yèjiāoténg 1g Shūjīnghuóxuètāng 5g dāngguīniāntòngtāng 5g + acupuncture Zhībódìhuángwán 5g dāngguīniāntòngtāng 5g mòyào 1g rŭxiāng 1g + acupuncture

1.35. Mastodynia

Mastodynia refers to breast pain. Changes in hormones can cause mastodynia, and therefore most premenopausal women experience mastodynia monthly. The pain usually starts shortly before the period and lasts a few days. Breast cancer is a common cause of noncyclic mastodynia in females, while injuries can be a common cause in males.

Table 1.35. Herbal prescriptions for mastodynia

Mastodynia https://meshb.nlm.nih.gov/record/ui?ui=D059373
Common prescriptions:
Sháoyàogāncǎotāng 5g shūjīnghuóxuètāng 5g dāngguīniāntòngtāng 5g + acupuncture Sháoyàogāncǎotāng 5g shūjīnghuóxuètāng 5g + acupuncture
Alternative prescriptions:
Sháoyàogāncǎotāng 5g yánhúsuǒ 1g mòyào 0g rǔxiāng 0g + acupuncture Jiāwèixiāoyáosǎn 5g xiāngshāliùjūnzǐtāng 5g liùwèidìhuángwán 3g dānshēn 1g héhuānpí 1g Sháoyàogāncǎotāng 5g shūjīnghuóxuètāng 5g niúxī 1g yánhúsuǒ 1g + acupuncture Zhènggǔzǐjīndān 5g shūjīnghuóxuètāng 5g dāngguīniāntòngtāng 5g + acupuncture Sháoyàogāncǎotāng 5g shūjīnghuóxuètāng 5g mùguā 1g niúxī 1g + acupuncture

Yánhúsuǒ, Mòyào, Niúxī and Mùguā have long been known for their pain killing. One of Yánhúsuǒ's, Niúxī's and Mùguā's modern uses is for disorder of joint (Wang, 2019). Niúxī's modern uses also include disorders of back (Wang, 2019). Mùguā's modern uses include peripheral enthesopathies and allied syndromes, intervertebral disc disorders, and spondylosis and allied disorders (Wang, 2019). Finally, Mòyào's modern uses consist of rheumatoid arthritis and other inflammatory polyarthropathies, disorders of the nervous system, and osteoarthrosis and allied disorders (Wang, 2019).

1.36. Breakthrough Pain

Pain that flares in people who have been taking pain medicine regularly for the control of chronic pain or disease is called breakthrough pain. The pain is usually more severe and can occur with no patterns, suggesting that the pain medicine that has been taken becomes tolerated. A higher dose of the pain medicine or a different pain medicine are needed for the pain management. Table 1.36 shows some herbal pain medicines for such alternative choices.

Table 1.36. Herbal prescriptions for breakthrough pain

Breakthrough Pain: https://meshb.nlm.nih.gov/record/ui?ui=D059390.
Common prescriptions:
Sháoyàogāncǎotāng 5g shūjīnghuóxuètāng 5g dāngguīniāntòngtāng 5g + acupuncture Sháoyàogāncǎotāng 5g shūjīnghuóxuètāng 5g + acupuncture
Alternative prescriptions:
Zhènggǔzǐjīndān 5g dāngguīniāntòngtāng 5g sānqī 2g mòyào 2g rǔxiāng 2g yánhúsuǒ 2g sūmù 2g xùduàn 2g mòyào 1g rǔxiāng 1g + acupuncture Jiāwèixiāoyáosǎn 5g cháihúshūgāntāng 5g héhuānpí 4g shíchāngpú 1g yuǎnzhì 1g Jiāwèixiāoyáosǎn 5g cháihúshūgāntāng 5g yèjiāoténg 2g dānshēn 1g yuǎnzhì 1g Jiāwèixiāoyáosǎn 5g gāncǎoxiǎomàidàzǎotāng 5g héhuānpí 1g xiāngfù 1g yùjīn 1g + acupuncture Jiāwèixiāoyáosǎn 5g cháihúshūgāntāng 5g shíchāngpú 1g dìlóng 1g yuǎnzhì 1g suānzǎorén 1g
Associated diseases:
Cardiovascular disease, unspecified 429.2 (Atherosclerotic heart disease of native coronary artery without angina pectoris I2510); Multiple myeloma 203.0; Unspecified hemorrhagic conditions 287.9 (Hemorrhagic condition, unspecified D699); Unspecified diseases of blood and blood-forming organs 289.9 (Disease of blood and blood-forming organs, unspecified D759); Unspecified disorder of metabolism 277.9 (Metabolic disorder, unspecified E889); Unspecified condition of brain 348.9 (Disorder of brain, unspecified G939); Unspecified disorders of nervous system 349.9 (Disorder of central nervous system, unspecified G969)

Breakthrough Pain: https://meshb.nlm.nih.gov/record/ui?ui=D059390.	
Cardiovascular disease, unspecified 429.2/I2510 with breakthrough pain D059390:	
Sìnìtāng 5g gānlùyǐn 5g mǔdānpí 1g zhīzǐ 1g huánglián 0g to ♀	Xuèfǔzhúyūtāng 5g zhìgāncǎotāng 5g to ♂
Unspecified disorder of metabolism 277.9/E889 with breakthrough pain D059390:	
Rénshēnbàidúsǎn 5g xiǎocháihútāngqùrénshēn 5g yīnchénhāotāng 2g mùxiāng 1g yùjīn 1g to ♀	Dānshēn 5g tiānmágōuténgyǐn 5g sǎnzhǒngkuìjiāntāng 5g bǔyánghuánwǔtāng 5g to ♂
Unspecified condition of brain 348.9/G939 with breakthrough pain D059390:	
Bǔyánghuánwǔtāng 5g + acupuncture to ♀	Bǔyánghuánwǔtāng 5g shíchāngpú 1g yuǎnzhì 1g + acupuncture to ♂

Jiāwèixiāoyáosǎn has been known for its traditional use for the hormone-variation related psychophysiological conditions of women during their menstruation, pregnancy, delivery, postpartum and menopause. As the formula addresses the conditions of 'Liver depression, Blood depletion' and 'Liver impairment due to anger,' Jiāwèixiāoyáosǎn has found wide applications in modern times when both women and men face high levels of stress in their daily lives.

1.37. Metatarsalgia

Metatarsal bones are bones of the forefoot, connecting toes to the ankle. Pain or inflammation of the metatarsal bone are called metatarsalgia. Metatarsalgia occurs when one spends too much time on the forefoot, which can happen when one wears high-heeled shoes for long hours.

Table 1.37. Herbal prescriptions for metatarsalgia

Metatarsalgia https://meshb.nlm.nih.gov/record/ui?ui=D037061
Common prescriptions:
Sháoyàogāncǎotāng 5g shūjīnghuóxuètāng 5g dāngguīniāntòngtāng 5g + acupuncture Sháoyàogāncǎotāng 5g shūjīnghuóxuètāng 5g + acupuncture
Alternative prescriptions:
Zhènggǔzǐjīndān 5g dāngguīniāntòngtāng 5g mòyào 1g rǔxiāng 1g yánhúsuǒ 1g sūmù 1g xùduàn 1g sānqī 1g + acupuncture Zhènggǔzǐjīndān 5g dāngguīniāntòngtāng 5g sānqī 2g mòyào 2g rǔxiāng 2g yánhúsuǒ 2g sūmù 2g xùduàn 2g + acupuncture Sháoyàogāncǎotāng 5g shūjīnghuóxuètāng 5g gégēntāng 5g + acupuncture Bǔzhōngyìqìtāng 5g Shūjīnghuóxuètāng 5g dāngguīniāntòngtāng 5g dúhuójìshēngtāng 5g
Indicated diseases:
Secondary cardiomyopathy, unspecified 425.9 (Cardiomyopathy due to drug and external agent I427); Unspecified disorders of nervous system 349.9 (Disorder of central nervous system, unspecified G969); Glycogenosis 271.0 (Glycogen storage disease, unspecified E7400, von Gierke disease E7401, McArdle disease E7404, Other glycogen storage disease E7409, Disorders of pyruvate metabolism and gluconeogenesis E744); Congenital stenosis of aortic valve 746.3 (Congenital stenosis of aortic valve Q230); Heart disease, unspecified 429.9 (Heart disease, unspecified I519); Cardiovascular disease, unspecified 429.2 (Atherosclerotic heart disease of native coronary artery without angina pectoris I2510); Unspecified disorder of metabolism 277.9 (Metabolic disorder, unspecified E889); Congestive heart failure, unspecified 428.0 (Right heart failure due to left heart failure I50814, Heart failure, unspecified I509); Unspecified condition of brain 348.9 (Disorder of brain, unspecified G939); Peroxisomal disorders 277.86 (Peroxisomal disorder, unspecified E7150, Zellweger syndrome E71510, Neonatal adrenoleukodystrophy E71511, Adrenomyeloneuropathy E71522, X-linked adrenoleukodystrophy, unspecified type E71529, Other peroxisomal disorders E71548);

Table 1.37. (Continued)

Metatarsalgia: https://meshb.nlm.nih.gov/record/ui?ui=D037061.	
Unspecified diseases of blood and blood-forming organs 289.9 (Disease of blood and blood-forming organs, unspecified D759)	
Secondary cardiomyopathy, unspecified 425.9/I427 with metatarsalgia D037061:	
Xuèfǔzhúyūtāng 5g dānshēn 2g chuānqī 1g báijí 1g rénshēn 1g guìzhī 1g guālóurén 1g xièbái 1g to ♀	Xuèfǔzhúyūtāng 5g dānshēn 2g chuānqī 1g báijí 1g rénshēn 1g guìzhī 1g guālóurén 1g xièbái 1g to ♂
Unspecified condition of brain 348.9/G939 with metatarsalgia D037061:	
Cháihújiālónggǔmǔlìtāng 5g wēndǎntāng 5g zhúrú 1g yèjiāoténg 1g yuǎnzhì 1g to ♀	Bǔyánghuánwǔtāng 5g dānshēn 1g tiānmá 1g shíchāngpú 1g yuǎnzhì 1g + acupuncture to ♂

Zhènggǔzǐjīndān is used for neuralgia in Section 1.21. Neuralgia of the interdigital nerve is a common cause of metatarsalgia. Note that as the foot is farthest away from the heart, conditions of the foot can serve as an early sign of heart deficiencies which fail to push enough blood to the foot. Glycogen is a form of glucose stored in and used by the skeletal muscles. Glycogen storage diseases develop myopathies (Kishnani et al., 2010). Forefoot deformities can result from cerebral palsy which abnormally keeps muscle contraction for a prolonged period of time. Peroxisomal disorders are a group of related metabolic disorders whose clinical features vary considerably and include foot deformation (Lucaccioni et al., 2020).

1.38. Headache

Almost all people experience headache in their lives. The ache varies in terms of location, duration, frequency and intensity. Alcohol overconsumption, caffeine withdrawal, emotional stress, sleep deprivation, viral infection such as colds, and tension of the muscle supporting the head can give rise to headache. Table 1.38 shows herbal headache medicines and illnesses related to headache. Herbal prescriptions for migraine appear in Table 2.8 of Chapter 2.

Table 1.38. Herbal prescriptions for headache

Headache: https://meshb.nlm.nih.gov/record/ui?ui=D006261.
Common prescriptions:
Guìzhītāng 5g yánhúsuǒ 1g + acupuncture Guìzhītāng 5g chuānwū 1g Guìzhītāng 5g chuānwū 1g yánhúsuǒ 1g Guìzhītāng 5g gégēn 1g Guìzhītāng 5g yánhúsuǒ 1g
Alternative prescriptions:
Guìzhītāng 5g chuānwū 1g yánhúsuǒ 1g + acupuncture Guìzhītāng 5g fùzǐ 0g + acupuncture Guìzhītāng 5g gégēn 2g bànxià 1g dàhuáng 0g Guìzhītāng 5g huángqí 1g dāngguī 0g
Indicated diseases:
Cardiovascular disease, unspecified 429.2 (Atherosclerotic heart disease of native coronary artery without angina pectoris I2510); Vascular disorders of skin 709.1 (Vasculitis limited to the skin, unspecified L959); Panuveitis 360.12 (Panuveitis, unspecified eye H44119); Behcet's syndrome 136.1 (Behcet's disease M352); Other dermatoses 702; Disorder of eye, unspecified 379.90 (Unspecified disorder of eye and adnexa H579); Unspecified condition of brain

Headache: https://meshb.nlm.nih.gov/record/ui?ui=D006261.	
348.9 (Disorder of brain, unspecified G939); Unspecified endocrine disorder 259.9 (Endocrine disorder, unspecified E349); Malignant neoplasm of endocrine gland, site unspecified 194.9 (Malignant neoplasm of endocrine gland, unspecified C759); Unspecified disorders of nervous system 349.9 (Disorder of central nervous system, unspecified G969); Neoplasm of unspecified nature of brain 239.6 (Neoplasm of unspecified behavior of brain D496); Unspecified cerebrovascular disease 437.9 (Cerebrovascular disease, unspecified I679); Migraine 346	
Cardiovascular disease, unspecified 429.2/I2510 with headache D006261:	
Sìnìtāng 5g gānlùyǐn 5g mǔdānpí 1g zhīzǐ 1g huánglián 0g to ♀	Sìnìtāng 5g gānlùyǐn 5g mǔdānpí 1g zhīzǐ 1g huánglián 1g to ♂
Unspecified condition of brain 348.9/G939 with headache D006261:	
Huángqíwǔwùtāng 5g chuānxiōng 1g dānshēn 1g zhúrú 1g sāngzhī 1g dāngguī 1g jiānghuáng 1g to ♀	Xiǎoxùmìngtāng 5g bǔyánghuánwǔtāng 5g + acupuncture to ♂
Unspecified cerebrovascular disease 437.9/I679 with headache D006261:	
Bǔyánghuánwǔtāng 5g dānshēn 1g niúxī 1g sāngzhī 1g jīxuèténg 1g + acupuncture to ♀	Bǔyánghuánwǔtāng 5g dānshēn 1g niúxī 1g sāngzhī 1g huángqín 1g jīxuèténg 1g + acupuncture to ♂

We have seen, in previous sections, Guìzhītāng's use for neck pain, acute pain and glossalgia. Here we add headache to its applications. Gégēn has been well known for its use for fever and headache due to colds. When headache is the only manifestation of an ischemic cardiovascular event, it is called cardiac cephalgia. Also noted is that skin pain and headache are linked through the so-called skin-brain axis (Bigal et al., 2008).

1.39. Intermittent Claudication

Intermittent claudication is pain in one's legs when he walks or exercises. The pain goes away when he rests. Intermittent claudication is caused by blockage or narrowing of the arteries, due mainly to atherosclerosis, to the legs.

Table 1.39. Herbal prescriptions for intermittent claudication

Intermittent Claudication: https://meshb.nlm.nih.gov/record/ui?ui=D007383.
Common prescriptions:
Xuèfǔzhúyūtāng 5g sháoyàogāncǎotāng 5g shēntòngzhúyūtāng 5g Xuèfǔzhúyūtāng 5g sháoyàogāncǎotāng 5g shūjīnghuóxuètāng 5g + acupuncture Xuèfǔzhúyūtāng 5g shūjīnghuóxuètāng 5g + acupuncture
Alternative prescriptions:
Xuèfǔzhúyūtāng 5g dānshēn 1g yùjīn 1g + acupuncture Xuèfǔzhúyūtāng 5g chuānqī 1g mòyào 1g rǔxiāng 1g yánhúsuǒ 1g + acupuncture Xuèfǔzhúyūtāng 5g sháoyàogāncǎotāng 5g chuānqī 1g mòyào 1g rǔxiāng 1g + acupuncture Xuèfǔzhúyūtāng 5g chuānqī 0g mòyào 0g rǔxiāng 0g Shūjīnghuóxuètāng 5g chuānqī 0g dānshēn 0g + acupuncture
Indicated diseases:
Peripheral angiopathy in diseases classified elsewhere 443.81 (Other disorders of arteries, arterioles and capillaries in diseases classified elsewhere I798); Unspecified disease of spinal cord 336.9 (Disease of spinal cord, unspecified G959); Cardiovascular disease, unspecified 429.2 (Atherosclerotic heart disease of native coronary artery without angina pectoris I2510); Unspecified disorders of nervous system 349.9 (Disorder of central nervous system, unspecified G969); Myoneural disorders 358; Spinal stenosis, unspecified region 724.00 (Spinal stenosis, site unspecified M4800); Myopathy, unspecified 359.9 (Myopathy, unspecified G729); Compartment syndrome, unspecified 958.90 (Compartment syndrome, unspecified, initial encounter T79A0XA)

Table 1.39. (Continued)

Intermittent Claudication: https://meshb.nlm.nih.gov/record/ui?ui=D007383.	
Peripheral angiopathy in diseases classified elsewhere 443.81/I798 with intermittent claudication D007383:	
Huángqíwǔwùtāng 5g dāngguīsìnìtāng 5g dānshēn 1g zhúrú 1g sāngzhī 1g jiānghuáng 1g to ♀	Dānshēn 5g tiānmágōuténgyǐn 5g sǎnzhǒngkuìjiāntāng 5g bǔyánghuánwǔtāng 5g to ♂

The term zhúyū in both Xuèfǔzhúyūtāng and Shēntòngzhúyūtāng literally means Blood stasis-removing. The prescriptions therefore intend to declot the blocked arteries in patients with intermittent claudication.

1.40. Postoperative Pain

Postoperative pain is acute or chronic pain after surgery. Inflammation and nerve injury can change synaptic plasticity to amplify and maintain pain signalling in a process called pain sensitization. Surgical incision can sensitize the peripheral nerve and spinal cord, causing postoperative pain.

Table 1.40. Herbal prescriptions for postoperative pain

Postoperative Pain: https://meshb.nlm.nih.gov/record/ui?ui=D010149.	
Common prescriptions:	
Shēntòngzhúyūtāng 5g shūjīnghuóxuètāng 5g Xiǎohuóluòdān 5g shēntòngzhúyūtāng 5g shūjīnghuóxuètāng 5g + acupuncture Xiǎohuóluòdān 5g shēntòngzhúyūtāng 5g shūjīnghuóxuètāng 5g Shēntòngzhúyūtāng 5g shūjīnghuóxuètāng 5g + acupuncture	
Alternative prescriptions:	
Shūjīnghuóxuètāng 5g niúxī 1g huángbò 1g cāngzhú 1g yìyǐrén 1g + acupuncture Shēntòngzhúyūtāng 5g shūjīnghuóxuètāng 4g huángqí 1g + acupuncture Shūjīnghuóxuètāng 5g dāngguīniāntòngtāng 5g niúxī 1g mòyào 1g rǔxiāng 1g yánhúsuǒ 1g fùzǐ 1g guìzhī 1g huángqín 1g jīxuèténg 1g + acupuncture Sānbìtāng 5g shūjīnghuóxuètāng 2g Shēntòngzhúyūtāng 5g dāngguīniāntòngtāng 5g niúxī 1g dùzhòng 1g xùduàn 1g + acupuncture	
Indicated diseases:	
Heart disease, unspecified 429.9 (Heart disease, unspecified I519); Unspecified congenital anomaly of heart 746.9 (Congenital malformation of cardiac chambers and connections, unspecified Q209, Congenital malformation of heart, unspecified Q249); Cardiovascular disease, unspecified 429.2 (Atherosclerotic heart disease of native coronary artery without angina pectoris I2510); Unspecified endocrine disorder 259.9 (Endocrine disorder, unspecified E349); Unspecified disorder of male genital organs 608.9 (Disorder of male genital organs, unspecified N509, Pelvic and perineal pain R102); Undescended testis 752.51 (Unilateral high scrotal testis Q5313, Undescended testicle, unspecified Q539); Unspecified disorder of intestine 569.9 (Disease of intestine, unspecified K639); Malignant neoplasm of sigmoid colon 153.3 (Malignant neoplasm of sigmoid colon C187); Diseases of the jaws 526; Malignant neoplasm of colon 153; Myopathy, unspecified 359.9 (Myopathy, unspecified G729); Unspecified disorder of joint, site unspecified 719.90 (Joint disorder, unspecified M259)	
Heart disease, unspecified 429.9/I519 with pain, postoperative D010149:	
Sìnìtāng 5g gānlùyǐn 5g mǔdānpí 1g zhǐzǐ 1g huánglián 0g to ♀	Sìnìtāng 5g gānlùyǐn 5g to ♂
Unspecified endocrine disorder 259.9/E349 with pain, postoperative D010149:	
Jiāwèixiāoyáosǎn 5g zuǒguīwán 5g nǚzhēnzǐ 1g hànliáncǎo 1g to ♀	Huánshǎodān 5g bājǐtiān 1g ròucōngróng 1g yínyánghuò 1g to ♂

Postoperative Pain: https://meshb.nlm.nih.gov/record/ui?ui=D010149.	
Unspecified disorder of intestine 569.9/K639 with pain, postoperative D010149:	
Lǐzhōngtāng 5g báisháo 1g guìzhī 1g to ♀	Gégēnhuángqínhuángliántāng 5g mùxiāng 1g bànxià 1g fúlíng 1g to ♂
Myopathy, unspecified 359.9/G729 with pain, postoperative D010149:	
Huángqíwǔwùtāng 5g báizhú 2g fùzǐ 2g báisháo 2g fúlíng 2g dǎngshēn 1g shēngjiāng 1g gānjiāng 1g dàhuáng 0g to ♀	Huángqíwǔwùtāng 5g báizhú 1g fùzǐ 1g báisháo 1g fúlíng 1g gānjiāng 1g dǎngshēn 1g gāncǎo 1g to ♂

Shēntòngzhúyūtāng literally translates to 'decoction for relieving body pain and removing Blood stasis.' Its modern use is for unspecified neuralgia, neuritis, and radiculitis (Wang, 2019). Xiǎohuóluòdān is used in Section 1.2 for chronic pain.

References

Bigal, M. E., Ashina, S., Burstein, R., Reed, M. L., Buse, D., Serrano, D., Lipton, R. B., & AMPP Group. (2008). Prevalence and characteristics of allodynia in headache sufferers: a population study. *Neurology, 70*(17), 1525–1533. https://doi.org/10.1212/01.wnl.0000310645.31020.b1.

Fernandez, M., Ordoñana, J. R., Hartvigsen, J., Ferreira, M. L., Refshauge, K. M., Sánchez-Romera, J. F., Pinheiro, M. B., Simpson, S. J., Hopper, J. L., & Ferreira, P. H. (2016). Is Chronic Low Back Pain Associated with the Prevalence of Coronary Heart Disease when Genetic Susceptibility Is Considered? A Co-Twin Control Study of Spanish Twins. *PLOS ONE*, *11*(5), e0155194. https://doi.org/10.1371/journal.pone.0155194.

Flammer, J., Konieczka, K., Bruno, R. M., Virdis, A., Flammer, A. J., & Taddei, S. (2013). The eye and the heart. *European Heart Journal*, *34*(17), 1270–1278. https://doi.org/10.1093/eurheartj/eht023.

Jagadeesan, S., & Shenoy, P. (2017). Arthropathy in dermatology: A comprehensive review. *Indian Dermatology Online Journal*, *8*(2), 79–93. https://doi.org/10.4103/idoj.idoj_25_17.

Kanjevac, T., Bijelic, B., Brajkovic, D., Vasovic, M., & Stolic, R. (2018). Impact of Chronic Kidney Disease Mineral and Bone Disorder on Jaw and Alveolar Bone Metabolism: A Narrative Review. *Oral Health and Preventive Dentistry, 16*(1), 79-85. https://doi.org/10.3290/j.ohpd.a39858.

Kishnani, P. S., Austin, S. L., Arn, P., Bali, D. S., Boney, A., Case, L. E., Chung, W. K., Desai, D. M., El-Gharbawy, A., Haller, R., Smit, G. P. A., Smith, A. D., Hobson-Webb, L. D., Wechsler, S. B., Weinstein, D. A., & Watson, M. S. (2010). Glycogen Storage Disease Type III diagnosis and management guidelines. *Genetics in Medicine*, *12*(7), 446–463. https://doi.org/10.1097/gim.0b013e3181e655b6.

Laeeq, R., Berman, J. S., Khalid, U., Lakkis, N. M., & Tabbaa, R. (2019). Reversible Cerebral Vasoconstriction Syndrome Associated with Coronary Artery Vasospasm. *Texas Heart Institute Journal*, *46*(2), 139–142. https://doi.org/10.14503/thij-17-6403.

Lucaccioni, L., Righi, B., Cingolani, G. M., Lugli, L., Della Casa, E., Torcetta, F., Iughetti, L., & Berardi, A. (2020). Overwhelming sepsis in a neonate affected by Zellweger syndrome due to a compound heterozygosis in PEX 6 gene: a case report. *BMC Medical Genetics*, *21*, 229. https://doi.org/10.1186/s12881-020-01175-y.

Myers, D. E. (2022). Review of visceral throat and chest disorders causing nonodontogenic orofacial pain. *The Journal of the American Dental Association*, *153*(8), 769–775. https://doi.org/10.1016/j.adaj.2022.01.007.

Oyetola, E. O., Owotade, F. J., Agbelusi, G. A., Fatusi, O. A., & Sanusi, A. A. (2015). Oral findings in chronic kidney disease: implications for management in developing countries. *BMC Oral Health*, *15*, 24. https://doi.org/10.1186/s12903-015-0004-z.

Peng, J.-P., & Zheng, H. (2017). Kidney stones may increase the risk of coronary heart disease and stroke. *Medicine*, *96*(34), e7898. https://doi.org/10.1097/md.0000000000007898.

Wang, S. C. (2019). *Clinical Herbal Prescriptions: Principles and Practices of Herbal Formulations from Deep Learning Health Insurance Herbal Prescription Big Data*. WSPC. https://doi.org/10.1142/11211.

Wehrhahn, T., Bargetzi, M., Buitrago-Tellez, C., & Cantelmi, G. (2018). Toothache as the initial symptom of plasma cell myeloma. *European Journal of Dentistry*, *12*(03), 443–445. https://doi.org/10.4103/ejd.ejd_412_17.

Chapter 2

Sensation Disorders

As a member of the animal kingdom, we, unlike plants which synthesize their own food, feed on other organisms including plants and other animals. To achieve goals such as feeding and mating, our body's specialized organs gather information about the surrounding environment through sensory receptors in a process called sensation. Human sensory information includes, in the order of distance from our body, vision, hearing, smell, taste and touch, mediated respectively by electromagnetic waves, sound waves, odor chemicals in the air, taste chemicals in the saliva, and pressure and temperature on the body surface. Additionally, sensory receptors within the body allow for detection of changes, pain (which is dealt with in the previous chapter), and sensations in the muscles, joints and internal organs.

Sensory information is sent first to the brainstem and midbrain for preprocessing and finally to higher regions of the brain for interpretation, after which our motor nerves are activated in response to the sensed environmental cues. The human organs and systems responsible for detecting the cues are the eyes, ears, nose, tongue and the somatosensory system. Impairment of their structures or functions can cause sensation disorders. The signs and symptoms produced by the sensation disorders are shown in Figure 2.1.

As sensation is so rudimentary to the survival of human beings, herbalists have found herbs and also composed multi-herb formulas for the relief and removal of sensory signs and symptoms. The sensation benefiting herbal formulas include Língguìshùgāntāng, Huángqíwǔwùtāng, Guìzhītāng, Sìnìtāng, Qǐjúdìhuángwán, Sháoyàogāncǎotāng, Bǔzhōngyìqìtāng, Dāngguīsìnìtāng, Huánshǎodān, Shūjīnghuóxuètāng and Zīshènmíngmùtāng. The herbs supporting the formulas in the prescriptions include Fùzǐ, Dàhuáng, Shārén, Xìxīn, Bànxià, Shēngjiāng, Sāngzhī, Dānshēn, Zhúrú, Jiānghuáng, Xiǎohuíxiāng and Guìzhī.

Some of the above formulas are for specific sense organs. For example, Qǐjúdìhuángwán, Zīshènmíngmùtāng and Xǐgānmíngmùtāng are for the eye. Others are for the health of the brain. For example, Bǔyánghuánwǔtāng is for stroke sequelae. Composition of sensation disorder prescriptions will depend on the affected anatomical site (i.e., eye or brain), not the superficial organ of the sense (eye). Details will be shown in individual tables. Note that acupuncture is an important modality of traditional treatment for some of the sensation signs and symptoms, along with herbs and formulas.

The diseases commonly resulting in or associated with the signs and symptoms of Figure 2.1 are unspecified disorders of nervous system, unspecified disorder of ear, unspecified disorder of eye, unspecified cardiovascular disease, unspecified condition of brain, unspecified endocrine disorder, unspecified retinal disorder, unspecified disorder of cranial nerves, sensorineural hearing loss, unspecified disorder of metabolism, diabetes mellitus, part unspecified malignant neoplasm of nervous system, unspecified cerebrovascular disease, other dermatoses, malignant neoplasm of cranial nerves, neuroendocrine tumors, and disorders of acoustic nerve.

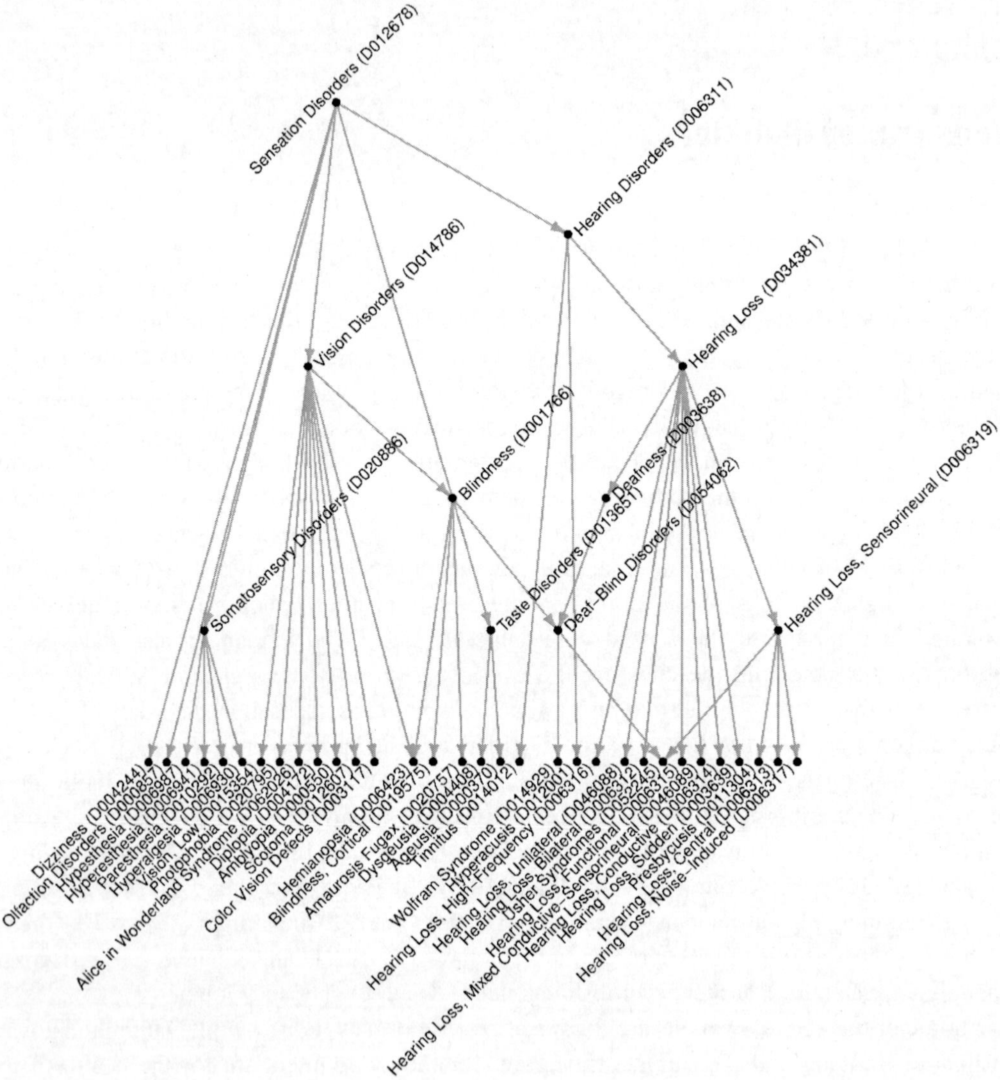

Figure 2.1. Conditions that affect the perception of light, sound, balance, smell, taste and touch, and the presenting signs and symptoms.

2.1. Dizziness

Dizziness is the feeling of lightheadedness, off-balance or faint. Many parts of the body including the eyes, ears, brain, and nerves in the spine and feet work together to keep one balanced. Causes of dizziness can involve any of the organs and systems.

Língguìshùgāntāng has been used, since the Eastern Han dynasty of China (25–220 A.D.), for dizziness and palpitations due to 'dysmetabolic fluids that precipitate in the upper body.' Its modern use is indeed for dizziness and giddiness (Wang, 2019). Cardiovascular conditions that affect circulation can also be a cause of dizziness as the brain needs a steady supply of oxygen-rich nutrients from the blood.

Table 2.1. Herbal prescriptions for dizziness

<table>
<tr><td colspan="2">Dizziness: https://meshb.nlm.nih.gov/record/ui?ui=D004244.</td></tr>
<tr><td colspan="2">Common prescriptions:</td></tr>
<tr><td colspan="2">Língguìshùgāntāng 5g báisháo 1g fùzǐ 1g
Língguìshùgāntāng 5g fùzǐ 1g gānjiāng 1g
Língguìshùgāntāng 5g fùzǐ 1g shārén 1g bànxià 1g dàhuáng 0g
Língguìshùgāntāng 5g bànxià 1g shēngjiāng 1g
Língguìshùgāntāng 5g fùzǐ 1g gānjiāng 1g tiáowèichéngqìtāng 1g</td></tr>
<tr><td colspan="2">Alternative prescriptions:</td></tr>
<tr><td colspan="2">Língguìshùgāntāng 5g xiǎohuíxiāng 1g fùzǐ 1g shārén 1g dàhuáng 0g
Língguìshùgāntāng 5g xiǎohuíxiāng 1g fùzǐ 1g shārén 1g xìxīn 1g dàhuáng 0g
Língguìshùgāntāng 5g shārén 1g huíxiāng 1g fùzǐ 1g dàhuáng 0g
Língguìshùgāntāng 5g fùzǐ 1g shārén 1g xìxīn 1g dàhuáng 0g
Língguìshùgāntāng 5g bànxià 1g shārén 1g dàhuáng 0g</td></tr>
<tr><td colspan="2">Indicated diseases:</td></tr>
<tr><td colspan="2">Unspecified cerebrovascular disease 437.9 (Cerebrovascular disease, unspecified I679); Unspecified condition of brain 348.9 (Disorder of brain, unspecified G939); Cardiovascular disease, unspecified 429.2 (Atherosclerotic heart disease of native coronary artery without angina pectoris I2510); Unspecified disorders of nervous system 349.9 (Disorder of central nervous system, unspecified G969); Unspecified endocrine disorder 259.9 (Endocrine disorder, unspecified E349); Malignant neoplasm of endocrine gland, site unspecified 194.9 (Malignant neoplasm of endocrine gland, unspecified C759); Neoplasm of unspecified nature of brain 239.6 (Neoplasm of unspecified behavior of brain D496); Malignant neoplasm of nervous system, part unspecified 192.9 (Malignant neoplasm of central nervous system, unspecified C729)</td></tr>
<tr><td colspan="2">Unspecified cerebrovascular disease 437.9/I679 with dizziness D004244:</td></tr>
<tr><td>Xiǎoxùmìngtāng 5g bǔyánghuánwǔtāng 5g to ♀</td><td>Bǔyánghuánwǔtāng 5g dānshēn 1g niúxī 1g sāngzhī 1g jīxuèténg 1g + acupuncture to ♂</td></tr>
<tr><td colspan="2">Unspecified condition of brain 348.9/G939 with dizziness D004244:</td></tr>
<tr><td>Xiǎoxùmìngtāng 5g bǔyánghuánwǔtāng 5g to ♀</td><td>Bǔyánghuánwǔtāng 5g dānshēn 1g shíchāngpú 1g yuǎnzhì 1g + acupuncture to ♂</td></tr>
</table>

2.2. Olfaction Disorders

Olfaction disorders include a reduction, loss, or distortion of the sense of smell, which is firstly sensed in a region of the forebrain called the olfactory bulb. Olfactory information is further processed in other regions of the brain including the anterior ventral insula, amygdala and hippocampus. Aging can cause olfactory problems due to neurodegeneration such as dementia.

We see in the previous chapter the use of Sìnìtāng for phantom limb and referred pain, both of which have to do with a compromised central nervous system. Bǔzhōngyìqìtāng has traditionally been used for people who have been weak, resulting in or from a lack of energy and appetite. Combination of the two formulas here is believed to help patients with olfaction disorders. Olfactory dysfunction and cardiovascular diseases were found to be associated (Roh et al., 2021). Note also that since olfactory signals play an importance role in sexual differentiation, sexual development conditions including pseudohermaphroditism, gonadal dysgenesis, and Klinefelter's syndrome are associated with olfaction disorders (Bodo, 2008; Henkin, 1967; Melinte and Sarafoleanu, 2019). Finally, because the neuroanatomies affected by olfactory disorders and schizoaffective disorders are adjacent, there is suggestion of an association between the two (Turetsky et al., 2009), as we also see in the table.

Table 2.2. Herbal prescriptions for olfaction disorders

Olfaction Disorders: https://meshb.nlm.nih.gov/record/ui?ui=D000857.	
Common prescriptions:	
Bǔzhōngyìqìtāng 5g Sìnìtāng 5g bǔzhōngyìqìtāng 5g Sìnìtāng 5g bǔzhōngyìqìtāng 5g chuānxiōng 1g ròuguì 1g yánhúsuǒ 1g zhìgāncǎotāng 1g Sìnìtāng 5g bǔzhōngyìqìtāng 5g chuānxiōng 1g ròuguì 1g zhìgāncǎotāng 1g Sìnìtāng 5g lǐzhōngtāng 5g ròuguì 1g yánhúsuǒ 1g zhìgāncǎotāng 1g	
Alternative prescriptions:	
Sìnìtāng 5g rénshēn 1g wúzhūyú 1g dàhuáng 0g Sìnìtāng 5g shēngjiāng 1g guìzhī 1g xìxīn 1g máhuáng 1g Sìnìtāng 5g dāngguīsìnìtāng 5g shēngjiāng 1g wúzhūyú 1g Máhuángfùzǐxìxīntāng 5g dàzǎo 2g shēngjiāng 2g zhìgāncǎo 2g guìzhī 2g Sìnìtāng 5g lǐzhōngtāng 4g chuānxiōng 1g ròuguì 1g yánhúsuǒ 1g zhìgāncǎotāng 1g	
Indicated and associated diseases:	
Heart disease, unspecified 429.9 (Heart disease, unspecified I519); Unspecified disorders of nervous system 349.9 (Disorder of central nervous system, unspecified G969); Unspecified endocrine disorder 259.9 (Endocrine disorder, unspecified E349); Gonadal dysgenesis 758.6 (Turner's syndrome, unspecified Q969); Cardiovascular disease, unspecified 429.2 (Atherosclerotic heart disease of native coronary artery without angina pectoris I2510); Indeterminate sex and pseudohermaphroditism 752.7 (Pseudohermaphroditism, unspecified Q563, Indeterminate sex, unspecified Q564); Unspecified congenital anomaly of heart 746.9 (Congenital malformation of cardiac chambers and connections, unspecified Q209, Congenital malformation of heart, unspecified Q249); Unspecified condition of brain 348.9 (Disorder of brain, unspecified G939); Malignant neoplasm of endocrine gland, site unspecified 194.9 (Malignant neoplasm of endocrine gland, unspecified C759); Neoplasm of unspecified nature of brain 239.6 (Neoplasm of unspecified behavior of brain D496); Klinefelter's syndrome 758.7 (Klinefelter syndrome, unspecified Q984); Schizoaffective disorder 295.7; Schizophreniform disorder 295.4; Malignant neoplasm of nervous system, part unspecified 192.9 (Malignant neoplasm of central nervous system, unspecified C729)	
Heart disease, unspecified 429.9/I519 with olfaction disorders D000857:	
Sìnìtāng 5g gānlùyǐn 5g mǔdānpí 1g zhīzǐ 1g huánglián 0g to ♀	Sìnìtāng 5g gānlùyǐn 5g shēngmàiyǐn 2g to ♂
Unspecified condition of brain 348.9/G939 with olfaction disorders D000857:	
Xiǎoxùmìngtāng 5g bǔyánghuánwǔtāng 5g to ♀	Bǔyánghuánwǔtāng 5g chuānqī 1g dānshēn 1g shíchāngpú 1g yuǎnzhì 1g + acupuncture to ♂
Unspecified disorders of nervous system 349.9/G969 with olfaction disorders D000857:	
Huángqíwǔwùtāng 5g chuānxiōng 1g dānshēn 1g zhúrú 1g sāngzhī 1g dāngguī 1g jiānghuáng 1g to ♀	Huángqíwǔwùtāng 5g chuānxiōng 1g dānshēn 1g zhúrú 1g sāngzhī 1g dāngguī 1g jiānghuáng 1g to ♂

2.3. Hypesthesia

Hypesthesia or numbness indicate a reduced sensibility to touch. Causes of hypesthesia are nerve damage, which in turn can result from injuries or blockages of the blood vessels that supply blood to the affected tissue and nerve.

The approach of herbal medicine to hypesthesia includes the use of Shūjīnghuóxuètāng to 'open up Qi channels' and at the same time Huángqíwǔwùtāng to 'supply Qi.' A case was reported that Burkitt's lymphoma manifests numb chin as the only symptom (Benites et al., 2020). Cranial nerves affected by tumor can numb the face. Similarly, nerves in the thoracic outlet compressed by trauma can numb the arms and fingers.

Table 2.3. Herbal prescriptions for hypesthesia

Hypesthesia: https://meshb.nlm.nih.gov/record/ui?ui=D006987.	
Common prescriptions:	
Shūjīnghuóxuètāng 5g huángqíwǔwùtāng 5g + acupuncture Xiǎohuóluòdān 5g shūjīnghuóxuètāng 5g + acupuncture	
Alternative prescriptions:	
Sháoyàogāncǎotāng 5g huángqíwǔwùtāng 5g dānshēn 2g zhúrú 2g sāngzhī 2g jiānghuáng 2g Huángqíwǔwùtāng 5g dānshēn 1g zhúrú 1g sāngzhī 1g qínjiāo 1g jiānghuáng 1g Huángqíwǔwùtāng 5g jīxuèténg 1g + acupuncture Huángqíwǔwùtāng 5g sháoyàogāncǎotāng 2g mùguā 1g jīxuèténg 1g + acupuncture Táohóngsìwùtāng 5g huángqí 1g + acupuncture	
Indicated diseases:	
Unspecified disorders of nervous system 349.9 (Disorder of central nervous system, unspecified G969); Burkitt's tumor or lymphoma 200.2; Reticulosarcoma 200.0; Unspecified disorder of cranial nerves 352.9 (Cranial nerve disorder, unspecified G529); Malignant neoplasm of thorax 195.1 (Malignant neoplasm of thorax C761)	
Unspecified disorders of nervous system 349.9/G969 with hypesthesia D006987:	
Huángqíwǔwùtāng 5g chuānxiōng 1g dānshēn 1g zhúrú 1g sāngzhī 1g dāngguī 1g jiānghuáng 1g to ♀	Huángqíwǔwùtāng 5g chuānxiōng 1g dānshēn 1g zhúrú 1g sāngzhī 1g dāngguī 1g jiānghuáng 1g to ♂
Unspecified disorder of cranial nerves 352.9/G529 with hypesthesia D006987:	
Wūyàoshùnqìsǎn 5g huángqíwǔwùtāng 5g dānshēn 1g zhúrú 1g sāngzhī 1g jiānghuáng 1g to ♀	Xiǎoxùmìngtāng 5g wūyàoshùnqìsǎn 5g bǔyánghuánwǔtāng 5g + acupuncture to ♂

2.4. Hyperesthesia

Excessively increased sensitivity to any of the five senses including sound, sight, touch, taste and smell is called hyperesthesia. Hyperesthesia typically develops secondarily to a disease, such as diabetes mellitus and viral infection, that affects the somatosensory nervous system.

Huángqíwǔwùtāng 'benefits Qi, warms up meridians,' 'harmonizes Blood, clears paralysis,' and is used here for hyperesthesia, presumably via the concept of restoring homeostasis.

Table 2.4. Herbal prescriptions for hyperesthesia

Hyperesthesia: https://meshb.nlm.nih.gov/record/ui?ui=D006941.
Common prescriptions:
Huángqíwǔwùtāng 5g dānshēn 1g zhúrú 1g sāngzhī 1g jiānghuáng 1g Huángqíwǔwùtāng 5g dānshēn 1g zhúrú 1g sāngzhī 1g jiānghuáng 1g + acupuncture Huángqíwǔwùtāng 5g dānshēn 1g zhúrú 1g sāngzhī 1g dāngguī 1g jiānghuáng 1g Huángqíwǔwùtāng 5g dānshēn 1g zhúrú 1g sāngzhī 1g jiānghuáng 1g jīxuèténg 1g
Alternative prescriptions:
Huángqíwǔwùtāng 5g dānshēn 1g zhúrú 1g yánhúsuǒ 1g sāngzhī 1g jiānghuáng 1g Huángqíwǔwùtāng 5g dānshēn 1g zhúrú 1g sāngzhī 1g jiānghuáng 1g jīxuèténg 1g + acupuncture Huángqíwǔwùtāng 5g dāngguīsìnìtāng 5g dānshēn 1g zhúrú 1g sāngzhī 1g jiānghuáng 1g Huángqíwǔwùtāng 5g sháoyàogāncǎotāng 2g chuānxiōng 1g dānshēn 1g zhúrú 1g sāngzhī 1g dāngguī 1g jiānghuáng 1g
Indicated diseases:
Unspecified disorders of nervous system 349.9 (Disorder of central nervous system, unspecified G969); Other dermatoses 702

Table 2.4. (Continued)

Hyperesthesia: https://meshb.nlm.nih.gov/record/ui?ui=D006941.	
Unspecified disorders of nervous system 349.9/G969 with hyperesthesia D006941:	
Huángqíwǔwùtāng 5g chuānxiōng 1g dānshēn 1g zhúrú 1g sāngzhī 1g dāngguī 1g jiānghuáng 1g to ♀	Huángqíwǔwùtāng 5g chuānxiōng 1g dānshēn 1g zhúrú 1g sāngzhī 1g dāngguī 1g jiānghuáng 1g to ♂
Other dermatoses 702 with hyperesthesia D006941:	
Yùnǚjiān 5g xuèfǔzhúyūtāng 3g dāngguīsháoyàosǎn 3g báijiāngcán 1g to ♀	Yùnǚjiān 5g xuèfǔzhúyūtāng 3g dāngguīsháoyàosǎn 3g báijiāngcán 1g to ♂

2.5. Paresthesia

Paresthesia refers to abnormal, e.g., pins and needles, sensation of the skin. When one takes a nap on one hand or sits with legs crossed for too long, he or she can temporarily experience hand and leg paresthesia because of the compressed nerves. Chronic paresthesia can be a symptom or consequence of a more serious condition.

Table 2.5. Herbal prescriptions for paresthesia

Paresthesia: https://meshb.nlm.nih.gov/record/ui?ui=D010292.	
Common prescriptions:	
Xiǎohuóluòdān 5g shūjīnghuóxuètāng 5g huángqíwǔwùtāng 5g + acupuncture Xiǎohuóluòdān 5g shūjīnghuóxuètāng 5g huángqíwǔwùtāng 5g Shūjīnghuóxuètāng 5g huángqíwǔwùtāng 5g + acupuncture	
Alternative prescriptions:	
Huángqíwǔwùtāng 5g + acupuncture Dāngguīsìnìtāng 5g Huángqíwǔwùtāng 5g juānbìtāng 5g dānshēn 1g sāngzhī 1g jīxuèténg 1g Shēntòngzhúyūtāng 5g huángqíwǔwùtāng 5g Huángqíwǔwùtāng 5g jīxuèténg 1g sāngzhī 1g jiānghuáng 1g + acupuncture	
Indicated diseases:	
Cardiovascular disease, unspecified 429.2 (Atherosclerotic heart disease of native coronary artery without angina pectoris I2510); Unspecified disorders of nervous system 349.9 (Disorder of central nervous system, unspecified G969); Multiple myeloma 203.0; Unspecified hemorrhagic conditions 287.9 (Hemorrhagic condition, unspecified D699); Unspecified diseases of blood and blood-forming organs 289.9	
(Disease of blood and blood-forming organs, unspecified D759); Other dermatoses 702; Malignant neoplasm of mandible 170.1 (Malignant neoplasm of mandible C411); Deformity and disproportion of reconstructed breast 612; Other disorders of breast 611; Benign mammary dysplasias 610; Unspecified disease of spinal cord 336.9 (Disease of spinal cord, unspecified G959); Malignant neoplasm of spinal cord 192.2 (Malignant neoplasm of spinal cord C720, Malignant neoplasm of cauda equina C721); Unspecified disorder of male genital organs 608.9 (Disorder of male genital organs, unspecified N509, Pelvic and perineal pain R102); Hypoactive sexual desire disorder 302.71 (Hypoactive sexual desire disorder F520)	
Cardiovascular disease, unspecified 429.2/I2510 with paresthesia D010292:	
Yùzhú 5g sìnìtāng 5g mǔdānpí 1g zhīzǐ 1g huánglián 0g to ♀	Sìnìtāng 5g gānlùyǐn 5g mǔdānpí 1g zhīzǐ 1g huánglián 0g to ♂
Other dermatoses 702 with paresthesia D010292:	
Dāngguīsìnìtāng 5g shēngjiāng 1g wúzhūyú 1g to ♀	Xiāofēngsǎn 5g jiědúsìwùtāng 5g zhēnrénhuómìngyǐnqùchuānshānjiǎ 4g huángliánjiědútāng 4g to ♂

Paresthesia: https://meshb.nlm.nih.gov/record/ui?ui=D010292.	
Unspecified disease of spinal cord 336.9/G959 with paresthesia D010292:	
Xiǎohuóluòdān 5g shūjīnghuóxuètāng 5g dāngguīniāntòngtāng 5g dúhuójìshēngtāng 5g to ♀	Guīlùèrxiānjiāo 5g to ♂
Unspecified disorders of nervous system 349.9/G969 with paresthesia D010292:	
Huángqíwǔwùtāng 5g chuānxiōng 1g dānshēn 1g zhúrú 1g sāngzhī 1g dāngguī 1g jiānghuáng 1g to ♀	Huángqíwǔwùtāng 5g chuānxiōng 1g dānshēn 1g zhúrú 1g sāngzhī 1g dāngguī 1g jiānghuáng 1g to ♂

Xiǎohuóluòdān 'dissolves Phlegm, opens meridians' and 'enlivens Blood, stops pain.' Its modern use is for rheumatoid arthritis (Wang, 2019) and it is used here, together with Shūjīnghuóxuètāng and Huángqíwǔwùtāng, for paresthesia. Chest pain due to cardiovascular diseases can occur along with left arm tingling. Malignant plasma cells of myeloma produce proteins that are toxic to nerves, causing paresthesia. Dental procedures can cause dental paresthesia, so can breast surgery cause tingling in the armpit. Cauda equina syndrome can manifest pelvic and genital paresthesia, making one to lose interest in sex.

2.6. Hyperalgesia

Hyperalgesia overreacts to normally painful stimuli such that the pain felt becomes more severe than usual. Causes that either lower the pain threshold or enhance pain intensity in hyperalgesia vary and include complications from medication, peripheral neuropathy in diabetes, chronic pain syndrome such as postherpetic neuralgia, autoimmune inflammatory disorders such as rheumatoid arthritis, and so on.

Table 2.6. Herbal prescriptions for hyperalgesia

Hyperalgesia: https://meshb.nlm.nih.gov/record/ui?ui=D006930.	
Common prescriptions:	
Huángqíwǔwùtāng 5g dānshēn 1g zhúrú 1g sāngzhī 1g jiānghuáng 1g Huángqíwǔwùtāng 5g dānshēn 1g zhúrú 1g sāngzhī 1g jiānghuáng 1g + acupuncture Huángqíwǔwùtāng 5g dānshēn 1g zhúrú 1g sāngzhī 1g jiānghuáng 1g jīxuèténg 1g Huángqíwǔwùtāng 5g dānshēn 1g zhúrú 1g sāngzhī 1g dāngguī 1g jiānghuáng 1g	
Alternative prescriptions:	
Guìzhītāng 5g yánhúsuǒ 1g dàhuáng 0g Guìzhītāng 5g chuānwū 1g Guìzhītāng 5g shēngjiāng 0g guìzhī 0g Huángqíwǔwùtāng 5g + acupuncture	
Indicated diseases:	
Lesion of sciatic nerve 355.0 (Lesion of sciatic nerve, unspecified lower limb G5700); Mononeuritis multiplex 354.5 (Mononeuritis multiplex G587); Mononeuritis of unspecified site 355.9 (Mononeuropathy, unspecified G589); Myoneural disorders 358; Unspecified disorders of nervous system 349.9 (Disorder of central nervous system, unspecified G969); Unspecified disorder of joint, site unspecified 719.90 (Joint disorder, unspecified M259); Gouty arthropathy 274.0; Unspecified disorder of metabolism 277.9 (Metabolic disorder, unspecified E889); Diabetes mellitus 250; Unspecified endocrine disorder 259.9 (Endocrine disorder, unspecified E349)	
Lesion of sciatic nerve 355.0/G5700 with hyperalgesia D006930:	
Dúhuójìshēngtāng 5g dùzhòng 1g xùduàn 1g + acupuncture to ♀	Dúhuójìshēngtāng 5g dùzhòng 1g xùduàn 1g + acupuncture to ♂

Table 2.6. (Continued)

Hyperalgesia: https://meshb.nlm.nih.gov/record/ui?ui=D006930.	
Unspecified disorders of nervous system 349.9/G969 with hyperalgesia D006930:	
Huángqíwǔwùtāng 5g chuānxiōng 1g dānshēn 1g zhúrú 1g sāngzhī 1g dāngguī 1g jiānghuáng 1g to ♀	Huángqíwǔwùtāng 5g chuānxiōng 1g dānshēn 1g zhúrú 1g sāngzhī 1g dāngguī 1g jiānghuáng 1g to ♂

We see in Section 2.4 the use of Huángqíwǔwùtāng for hyperesthesia which encompasses hyperalgesia. The use of Huángqíwǔwùtāng for hyperalgesia is comprehensible. In addition, as Guìzhītāng is antipyretic, it is presumably used here for inflammatory hyperalgesia.

2.7. Low Vision

Low vision means partial loss of vision that cannot be corrected by conventional treatments such as eyeglasses, contact lenses, medicine or surgery. Common causes of low vision are diabetes, glaucoma and aging.

Table 2.7. Herbal prescriptions for low vision

Low Vision: https://meshb.nlm.nih.gov/record/ui?ui=D015354.
Common prescriptions:
Qǐjúdìhuángwán 5g zīshènmíngmùtāng 5g Qǐjúdìhuángwán 5g Qǐjúdìhuángwán 5g xǐgānmíngmùtāng 5g Qǐjúdìhuángwán 5g xǐgānmíngmùtāng 5g zīshènmíngmùtāng 5g
Alternative prescriptions:
Qǐjúdìhuángwán 5g xǐgānmíngmùtāng 5g qiānlǐguāng 1g Qǐjúdìhuángwán 5g bǔzhōngyìqìtāng 5g Xǐgānmíngmùtāng 5g zīshènmíngmùtāng 5g qiānlǐguāng 1g mùzéicǎo 1g xiàkūcǎo 1g
Indicated diseases:
Macular degeneration (senile), unspecified 362.50 (Unspecified macular degeneration H3530); Unspecified retinal disorder 362.9 (Unspecified retinal disorder H359); Disorder of eye, unspecified 379.90 (Unspecified disorder of eye and adnexa H579); Unspecified disorders of nervous system 349.9 (Disorder of central nervous system, unspecified G969); Primary open angle glaucoma 365.11 (Primary open-angle glaucoma, right eye, stage unspecified H401110, Primary open-angle glaucoma, right eye, mild stage H401111, Primary open-angle glaucoma, right eye, moderate stage H401112, Primary open-angle glaucoma, right eye, severe stage H401113, Primary open-angle glaucoma, right eye, indeterminate stage H401114, Primary open-angle glaucoma, left eye, stage unspecified H401120, Primary open-angle glaucoma, left eye, mild stage H401121, Primary open-angle glaucoma, left eye, moderate stage H401122, Primary open-angle glaucoma, left eye, severe stage H401123, Primary open-angle glaucoma, left eye, indeterminate stage H401124, Primary open-angle glaucoma, bilateral, stage unspecified H401130, Primary open-angle glaucoma, bilateral, mild stage H401131, Primary open-angle glaucoma, bilateral, moderate stage H401132, Primary open-angle glaucoma, bilateral, severe stage H401133, Primary open-angle glaucoma, bilateral, indeterminate stage H401134, Primary open-angle glaucoma, unspecified eye, stage unspecified H401190, Primary open-angle glaucoma, unspecified eye, mild stage H401191, Primary open-angle glaucoma, unspecified eye, moderate stage H401192, Primary open-angle glaucoma, unspecified eye, severe stage H401193, Primary open-angle glaucoma, unspecified eye, indeterminate stage H401194); Open-angle glaucoma 365.1; Glaucoma 365; Ocular hypertension 365.04 (Ocular hypertension, unspecified eye H40059); Cardiovascular disease, unspecified 429.2 (Atherosclerotic heart disease of native coronary artery without angina pectoris I2510); Diabetes with peripheral circulatory disorders 250.7; Diabetic retinopathy 362.0; Diabetes mellitus 250; Unspecified endocrine disorder 259.9 (Endocrine disorder, unspecified E349); Unspecified disorder of metabolism 277.9 (Metabolic disorder, unspecified E889) Macular degeneration (senile), unspecified 362.50/H3530 with Vision, low D015354:

Low Vision: https://meshb.nlm.nih.gov/record/ui?ui=D015354.	
Qǐjúdìhuángwán 5g zīshènmíngmùtāng 5g to ♀	Qǐjúdìhuángwán 5g zīshènmíngmùtāng 5g to ♂
Primary open angle glaucoma 365.11/H401110,H401111,H401112,H401113,H401114, H401120,H401121,H401122,H401123,H401124,H401130,H401131,H401132,H401133, H401134,H401190,H401191,H401192,H401193,H401194 with Vision, low D015354:	
Qǐjúdìhuángwán 5g xǐgānmíngmùtāng 5g zīshènmíngmùtāng 5g to ♀	Qǐjúdìhuángwán 5g xǐgānmíngmùtāng 5g zīshènmíngmùtāng 5g to ♂
Cardiovascular disease, unspecified 429.2/I2510 with vision, low D015354:	
Yùzhú 5g sìnìtāng 5g mǔdānpí 1g zhīzǐ 1g huánglián 1g to ♀	Yùzhú 5g sìnìtāng 5g zhìgāncǎotāng 5g to ♂

Qǐjúdìhuángwán has traditionally been used for people with blurred vision and dry eyes, improving and maintaining eye health.

2.8. Photophobia

Photophobia is increased sensitivity, and therefore aversion, to light. Migraine headache and dry eyes can cause photophobia.

Table 2.8. Herbal prescriptions for photophobia

Photophobia: https://meshb.nlm.nih.gov/record/ui?ui=D020795.	
Common prescriptions:	
Xǐgānmíngmùtāng 5g zīshènmíngmùtāng 5g Qǐjúdìhuángwán 5g Qǐjúdìhuángwán 5g zīshènmíngmùtāng 5g Xǐgānmíngmùtāng 5g Qǐjúdìhuángwán 5g xǐgānmíngmùtāng 5g	
Alternative prescriptions:	
Liùwèidìhuángwán 5g Rénshēnbàidúsǎn 5g dānshēn 0g niúxī 0g Xǐgānmíngmùtāng 5g zīshènmíngmùtāng 4g mùzéicǎo 1g cǎojuémíng 1g	
Indicated diseases:	
Migraine without aura 346.1; Migraine with aura 346.0; Migraine 346; Disorder of eye, unspecified 379.90 (Unspecified disorder of eye and adnexa H579); Unspecified condition of brain 348.9 (Disorder of brain, unspecified G939); Unspecified disorders of nervous system 349.9 (Disorder of central nervous system, unspecified G969); Unspecified corneal disorder 371.9 (Unspecified disorder of cornea H189); Diabetic retinopathy 362.0; Diabetes with peripheral circulatory disorders 250.7; Unspecified retinal disorder 362.9 (Unspecified retinal disorder H359); Diabetes mellitus 250; Unspecified endocrine disorder 259.9 (Endocrine disorder, unspecified E349)	
Migraine without aura 346.1 with photophobia D020795:	
Chuānxiōngchádiàosǎn 5g bànxiàbáizhútiānmátāng 5g to ♀	Chuānxiōngchádiàosǎn 5g qiānghuóshèngshītāng 5g to ♂
Disorder of eye, unspecified 379.90/H579 with photophobia D020795:	
Qǐjúdìhuángwán 5g xǐgānmíngmùtāng 5g zīshènmíngmùtāng 5g to ♀	Qǐjúdìhuángwán 5g xǐgānmíngmùtāng 5g zīshènmíngmùtāng 5g to ♂
Unspecified corneal disorder 371.9/H189 with photophobia D020795:	
Qǐjúdìhuángwán 5g zīshènmíngmùtāng 5g to ♀	Qǐjúdìhuángwán 5g xǐgānmíngmùtāng 5g zīshènmíngmùtāng 5g to ♂

Xǐgānmíngmùtāng, the other eye formulas in traditional Chinese medicine, is primarily used for acute conditions such as swelling and inflammation of the eye due to infection.

2.9. Alice in Wonderland Syndrome

People with Alice in Wonderland syndrome experience episodes of distorted visual perception where objects or parts of their own bodies appear smaller or larger and closer or farther than they actually are. The cause of this neuropathic condition is poorly known but it was reported to be associated with migraine, epilepsy, psychoactive substance use, brain tumor, and Epstein-Barr viral infection.

Table 2.9. Herbal prescriptions for Alice in Wonderland syndrome

Alice in Wonderland Syndrome: https://meshb.nlm.nih.gov/record/ui?ui=D062026.	
Common prescriptions:	
Sháoyàogāncǎotāng 5g shūjīnghuóxuètāng 5g dāngguīniāntòngtāng 5g + acupuncture Sháoyàogāncǎotāng 5g shūjīnghuóxuètāng 5g + acupuncture	
Alternative prescriptions:	
Jiāwèixiāoyáosǎn 5g xiāngshāliùjūnzǐtāng 5g gāncǎoxiǎomàidàzǎotāng 2g héhuānpí 1g yánhúsuǒ 1g Jiāwèixiāoyáosǎn 5g xiāngshāliùjūnzǐtāng 5g bànxiàxièxīntāng 2g héhuānpí 1g yánhúsuǒ 1g Sháoyàogāncǎotāng 5g shūjīnghuóxuètāng 5g dāngguīniāntòngtāng 5g Shūjīnghuóxuètāng 5g sháoyàogāncǎotāng 4g mùguā 1g niúxī 1g + acupuncture Shūjīnghuóxuètāng 5g dāngguīniāntòngtāng 5g mòyào 1g rǔxiāng 1g	
Indicated diseases:	
Unspecified condition of brain 348.9 (Disorder of brain, unspecified G939); Unspecified disorders of nervous system 349.9 (Disorder of central nervous system, unspecified G969)	
Unspecified condition of brain 348.9/G939 with Alice in Wonderland syndrome D062026:	
Bǔyánghuánwǔtāng 5g + acupuncture to ♀	Bǔyánghuánwǔtāng 5g shíchāngpú 1g yuǎnzhì 1g + acupuncture to ♂

The combination of Sháoyàogāncǎotāng, Shūjīnghuóxuètāng and Dāngguīniāntòngtāng is used in the previous chapter for neuralgia. That the same combination is used here for Alice in Wonderland syndrome may be related to the finding that visual distortion of body size modulates pain perception (Mancini et al., 2011).

2.10. Diplopia

People with diplopia see two images of a single object. Diplopia can be caused by injuries, inflammation, or autoimmune diseases that damage the tissues surrounding the eye.

Table 2.10. Herbal prescriptions for diplopia

Diplopia: https://meshb.nlm.nih.gov/record/ui?ui=D004172.
Common prescriptions:
Bǎnlángēn 5g huángqín 5g báihǔtāng 5g sháoyàogāncǎotāng 5g yínqiàosǎn 5g xièbáisǎn 5g púgōngyīng 3g mǔdānpí 2g jiāngcán 2g zhīzǐchǐtāng 2g Bǎnlángēn 5g huángqín 5g báihǔtāng 5g sháoyàogāncǎotāng 5g yínqiàosǎn 5g xièbáisǎn 5g púgōngyīng 3g mǔdānpí 2g jiāngcán 2g zhīzǐ 2g Bǎnlángēn 5g huángqín 5g púgōngyīng 5g báihǔtāng 5g sháoyàogāncǎotāng 5g yínqiàosǎn 5g xièbáisǎn 5g mǔdānpí 2g jiāngcán 2g zhīzǐchǐtāng 2g Bǎnlángēn 5g huángqín 5g báihǔtāng 5g sháoyàogāncǎotāng 5g yínqiàosǎn 5g xièbáisǎn 5g púgōngyīng 3g mǔdānpí 2g zhīzǐ 2g jiāngcán 2g Bǎnlángēn 5g huángqín 5g púgōngyīng 5g báihǔtāng 5g sháoyàogāncǎotāng 5g yínqiàosǎn 5g xièbáisǎn 5g mǔdānpí 2g jiāngcán 2g zhīzǐ 2g

Diplopia: https://meshb.nlm.nih.gov/record/ui?ui=D004172.	
Alternative prescriptions:	
Huángqín 5g báihǔtāng 5g sháoyàogāncǎotāng 5g yínqiàosǎn 5g xièbáisǎn 5g púgōngyīng 3g mǔdānpí 2g jiāngcán 2g zhīzǐchǐtāng 2g Bǎnlángēn 5g huángqín 5g púgōngyīng 5g báihǔtāng 5g sháoyàogāncǎotāng 5g yínqiàosǎn 5g xièbáisǎn 5g mǔdānpí 2g jiāngcán 2g zhīzǐchǐtāng 2g qīngzàojiùfèitāng 2g Yínqiàosǎn 5g bǎnlángēn 1g shígāo 1g shègān 1g sāngbáipí 1g chénpí 1g Bǎnlángēn 5g huángqín 5g púgōngyīng 5g báihǔtāng 5g sháoyàogāncǎotāng 5g yínqiàosǎn 5g xièbáisǎn 5g mǔdānpí 2g jiāngcán 2g	
Indicated diseases:	
Exophthalmos, unspecified 376.30 (Unspecified exophthalmos H0520); Goiter, unspecified 240.9 (Iodine-deficiency related (endemic) goiter, unspecified E012, Nontoxic goiter, unspecified E049); Unspecified disorder of orbit 376.9 (Unspecified disorder of orbit H059); Disorder of eye, unspecified 379.90 (Unspecified disorder of eye and adnexa H579); Unspecified disorder of thyroid 246.9 (Disorder of thyroid, unspecified E079); Unspecified endocrine disorder 259.9 (Endocrine disorder, unspecified E349); Unspecified disorders of nervous system 349.9 (Disorder of central nervous system, unspecified G969); Unspecified disorder of cranial nerves 352.9 (Cranial nerve disorder, unspecified G529); Multiple myeloma 203.0; Unspecified hemorrhagic conditions 287.9 (Hemorrhagic condition, unspecified D699); Unspecified diseases of blood and blood-forming organs 289.9 (Disease of blood and blood-forming organs, unspecified D759); Malignant neoplasm of orbit 190.1 (Malignant neoplasm of unspecified orbit C6960); Malignant neoplasm of other specified sites of eye 190.8 (Malignant neoplasm of overlapping sites of unspecified eye and adnexa C6980); Reticulosarcoma 200.0	
Exophthalmos, unspecified 376.30/H0520 with diplopia D004172:	
Qǐjúdìhuángwán 5g xǐgānmíngmùtāng 5g zīshènmíngmùtāng 5g to ♀	Xǐgānmíngmùtāng 5g zīshènmíngmùtāng 5g to ♂
Unspecified disorder of orbit 376.9/H059 with diplopia D004172:	
Qǐjúdìhuángwán 5g xǐgānmíngmùtāng 5g to ♀	Qǐjúdìhuángwán 5g xǐgānmíngmùtāng 5g zīshènmíngmùtāng 5g to ♂

Any of Bǎnlángēn, Huángqín, Báihǔtāng, Yínqiàosǎn, Xièbáisǎn, and Púgōngyīng 'clears Heat and neutralizes pathogens.' Combining them in the prescriptions is thought to treat diplopia resulting mainly from inflammation. Notice that diplopia was reported to be the initial symptom of multiple myeloma (Yazdanpanah et al., 2020) and reticulosarcoma (Claeys et al., 2002).

2.11. Amblyopia

Amblyopia is a childhood condition where one of the eyes is weaker than the other. Children with amblyopia will favor the use of the better eye, making the weak one to become worse. Causes of amblyopia involve problems with coordination between the affected eye and the brain during development.

Table 2.11. Herbal prescriptions for amblyopia

Amblyopia: https://meshb.nlm.nih.gov/record/ui?ui=D000550.
Common prescriptions:
Qǐjúdìhuángwán 5g zīshènmíngmùtāng 5g
Alternative prescriptions:
Qǐjúdìhuángwán 5g yìqìcōngmíngtāng 5g zīshènmíngmùtāng 5g mùzéicǎo 1g cǎojuémíng 1g Bāwèidìhuángwán 5g gǒuqǐzǐ 1g tùsīzǐ 1g Huánshǎodān 5g gǒuqǐzǐ 0g júhuā 0g Bāwèidìhuángwán 5g gǒuqǐzǐ 1g júhuā 1g Qǐjúdìhuángwán 5g shūjīnghuóxuètāng 5g dúhuójìshēngtāng 5g dùzhòng 1g sāngjìshēng 1g xùduàn 1g

Table 2.11. (Continued)

Amblyopia: https://meshb.nlm.nih.gov/record/ui?ui=D000550.	
Indicated diseases:	
Monocular esotropia 378.01 (Monocular esotropia, right eye H50011, Monocular esotropia, left eye H50012); Esotropia 378.0; Strabismic amblyopia 368.01 (Strabismic amblyopia, unspecified eye H53039); Amblyopia, unspecified 368.00 (Unspecified amblyopia, unspecified eye H53009); Hypertropia 378.31 (Vertical strabismus, right eye H5021, Vertical strabismus, left eye H5022); Mechanical strabismus 378.6; Brown's (tendon) sheath syndrome 378.61 (Brown's sheath syndrome, right eye H50611, Brown's sheath syndrome, left eye H50612); Internuclear ophthalmoplegia 378.86 (Internuclear ophthalmoplegia, unspecified eye H5120); Unspecified disorder of eye movements 378.9 (Unspecified disorder of binocular movement H519); Unspecified disorder of cranial nerves 352.9 (Cranial nerve disorder, unspecified G529); Disorder of eye, unspecified 379.90 (Unspecified disorder of eye and adnexa H579); Unspecified condition of brain 348.9 (Disorder of brain, unspecified G939); Unspecified disorders of nervous system 349.9 (Disorder of central nervous system, unspecified G969); Anisometropia 367.31 (Anisometropia H5231)	
Monocular esotropia 378.01/H50011,H50012 with amblyopia D000550:	
Qǐjúdìhuángwán 5g zīshènmíngmùtāng 5g to ♀	Qǐjúdìhuángwán 5g zīshènmíngmùtāng 5g to ♂
Amblyopia, unspecified 368.00/H53009 with amblyopia D000550:	
Bànxiàbáizhútiānmátāng 5g wǔlíngsǎn 1g huòxiāng 0g to ♀	Qǐjúdìhuángwán 5g zīshènmíngmùtāng 5g to ♂
Anisometropia 367.31/H5231 with amblyopia D000550:	
Qǐjúdìhuángwán 5g zīshènmíngmùtāng 5g to ♀	Qǐjúdìhuángwán 5g zīshènmíngmùtāng 5g to ♂

Zīshènmíngmùtāng, another traditional eye formula, 'nourishes the Kidney,' whose functions, in traditional medicine, concern mainly with development. We therefore see its use, rather than Xǐgānmíngmùtāng's, here for amblyopia, which begins in infancy or early childhood.

2.12. Scotoma

Scotoma is a dark or blurry spot in one's field of vision. Causes of scotoma are vast, including aging, stroke, brain tumor, multiple sclerosis, or diabetic retinopathy that damage the visual system.

Table 2.12. Herbal prescriptions for scotoma

Scotoma: https://meshb.nlm.nih.gov/record/ui?ui=D012607.
Common prescriptions:
Dāngguīsìnìtāng 5g shēngjiāng 1g wúzhūyú 1g Dāngguīsìnìtāng 5g shēngjiāng 1g wúzhūyú 1g fùzǐ 1g Guìzhītāng 5g gégēn 1g
Alternative prescriptions:
Guìzhītāng 5g shēngjiāng 0g guìzhī 0g dàhuáng 0g Guìzhītāng 5g gégēn 2g bànxià 1g dàhuáng 0g Dāngguīsìnìtāng 5g shēngjiāng 0g wúzhūyú 0g Huángqíwǔwùtāng 5g chuānxiōng 1g dānshēn 1g zhúrú 1g sāngzhī 1g dāngguī 1g jiānghuáng 1g jīxuèténg 1g + acupuncture Sìnìtāng 5g gǒuqǐzǐ 1g júhuā 1g

Scotoma: https://meshb.nlm.nih.gov/record/ui?ui=D012607.	
Indicated diseases:	
Optic neuritis 377.3; Foster-Kennedy syndrome 377.04 (Foster-Kennedy syndrome, unspecified eye H47149); Unspecified disorder of cranial nerves 352.9 (Cranial nerve disorder, unspecified G529); Disorder of eye, unspecified 379.90 (Unspecified disorder of eye and adnexa H579); Unspecified disorders of nervous system 349.9 (Disorder of central nervous system, unspecified G969); Macular degeneration (senile), unspecified 362.50 (Unspecified macular degeneration H3530); Unspecified retinal disorder 362.9 (Unspecified retinal disorder H359); Cardiovascular disease, unspecified 429.2 (Atherosclerotic heart disease of native coronary artery without angina pectoris I2510); Diabetes with peripheral circulatory disorders 250.7; Diabetic retinopathy 362.0; Diabetes mellitus 250; Unspecified endocrine disorder 259.9 (Endocrine disorder, unspecified E349); Malignant neoplasm of endocrine gland, site unspecified 194.9 (Malignant neoplasm of endocrine gland, unspecified C759); Unspecified condition of brain 348.9 (Disorder of brain, unspecified G939); Neoplasm of unspecified nature of brain 239.6 (Neoplasm of unspecified behavior of brain D496)	
Optic neuritis 377.3 with scotoma D012607:	
Qǐjúdìhuángwán 5g to ♀	Qǐjúdìhuángwán 5g zīshènmíngmùtāng 5g gǒuqǐzǐ 1g júhuā 1g to ♂
Macular degeneration (senile), unspecified 362.50/H3530 with scotoma D012607:	
Qǐjúdìhuángwán 5g zīshènmíngmùtāng 5g to ♀	Qǐjúdìhuángwán 5g zīshènmíngmùtāng 5g to ♂
Cardiovascular disease, unspecified 429.2/I2510 with scotoma D012607:	
Yùzhú 5g sìnìtāng 5g mǔdānpí 1g zhīzǐ 1g huánglián 0g to ♀	Sìnìtāng 5g gānlùyǐn 5g lóngdǎnxiègāntāng 5g to ♂
Disorder of eye, unspecified 379.90/H579 with scotoma D012607:	
Qǐjúdìhuángwán 5g xǐgānmíngmùtāng 5g zīshènmíngmùtāng 5g to ♀	Qǐjúdìhuángwán 5g xǐgānmíngmùtāng 5g zīshènmíngmùtāng 5g to ♂

Dāngguīsìnìtāng ‘nourishes Blood, links meridians,’ ‘warms up meridians, dispels chills,’ and is used here for scotoma, presumably based on its benefits to aged people with chronic conditions.

2.13. Color Vision Defects

People affected by color vision defects, i.e., color blindness, do not see difference between certain shades of color (usually red and green). Most color vision defect cases are hereditary. However, color vision defects can be acquired through such chronic diseases as Alzheimer’s disease, diabetes mellitus, glaucoma, alcohol intake, liver cirrhosis, multiple sclerosis, and Parkinson’s disease.

Table 2.13. Herbal prescriptions for color vision defects

Color Vision Defects: https://meshb.nlm.nih.gov/record/ui?ui=D003117.
Common prescriptions:
Huánshǎodān 5g yínyánghuò 1g tùsīzǐ 1g Huánshǎodān 5g yínyánghuò 1g Huánshǎodān 5g jīnsuǒgùjīngwán 4g yínyánghuò 1g shéchuángzǐ 1g Huánshǎodān 5g jīnsuǒgùjīngwán 4g yínyánghuò 1g
Alternative prescriptions:
Bāwèidìhuángwán 5g huánshǎodān 5g yínyánghuò 2g Liùwèidìhuángwán 5g huánshǎodān 5g bājǐtiān 1g yínyánghuò 1g tùsīzǐ 1g Huánshǎodān 5g yòuguīwán 4g yínyánghuò 1g shéchuángzǐ 1g Huánshǎodān 5g yínyánghuò 1g shéchuángzǐ 1g ròucōngróng 1g tùsīzǐ 1g Huánshǎodān 5g jīnsuǒgùjīngwán 2g

Table 2.13. (Continued)

Color Vision Defects: https://meshb.nlm.nih.gov/record/ui?ui=D003117.	
Indicated diseases:	
Cardiovascular disease, unspecified 429.2 (Atherosclerotic heart disease of native coronary artery without angina pectoris I2510); Achromatopsia 368.54 (Achromatopsia H5351); Diabetes with peripheral circulatory disorders 250.7; Acquired color vision deficiencies 368.55 (Acquired color vision deficiency H5352); Tritan defect 368.53 (Tritanomaly H5355); Protan defect 368.51 (Protanomaly H5354); Deutan defect 368.52 (Deuteranomaly H5353); Color vision deficiencies 368.5; Diabetic retinopathy 362.0; Unspecified retinal disorder 362.9	
(Unspecified retinal disorder H359); Disorder of eye, unspecified 379.90 (Unspecified disorder of eye and adnexa H579); Unspecified disorders of nervous system 349.9 (Disorder of central nervous system, unspecified G969); Diabetes mellitus 250; Unspecified endocrine disorder 259.9 (Endocrine disorder, unspecified E349); Unspecified disorder of metabolism 277.9 (Metabolic disorder, unspecified E889)	
Cardiovascular disease, unspecified 429.2/I2510 with color vision defects D003117:	
Yùzhú 5g sìnìtāng 5g mǔdānpí 1g zhīzǐ 1g huánglián 1g to ♀	Yùzhú 5g sìnìtāng 5g shēngmàiyǐn 2g to ♂
Tritan defect 368.53/H5355 with color vision defects D003117:	
Qǐjúdìhuángwán 5g zīshènmíngmùtāng 5g to ♀	Qǐjúdìhuángwán 5g zīshènmíngmùtāng 5g to ♂
Deutan defect 368.52/H5353 with color vision defects D003117:	
Jiāwèixiāoyáosǎn 5g qǐjúdìhuángwán 5g nǔzhēnzǐ 1g héhuānpí 1g hànliáncǎo 1g yèjiāoténg 1g to ♀	Qǐjúdìhuángwán 5g zīshènmíngmùtāng 5g to ♂

A word-for-word translation of Huánshǎodān gives 'restoring youth pill.' It is therefore thought to treat color vision defects caused by age debilitating chronic conditions.

2.14. Hemianopsia

Hemianopsia is loss of one half of the visual field in one or both eyes. Because the left brain receives, via optic nerve, visual information from the right side of both eyes and vice versa, the half refers to left or right, depending on which side of the brain is damaged. However, in case the brain damage occurs in the intersection of the optic nerves, superior or inferior hemianopsia can occur.

Table 2.14. Herbal prescriptions for hemianopsia

Hemianopsia: https://meshb.nlm.nih.gov/record/ui?ui=D006423.
Common prescriptions:
Huángqíwǔwùtāng 5g dānshēn 1g zhúrú 1g sāngzhī 1g jiānghuáng 1g Huángqíwǔwùtāng 5g dānshēn 1g zhúrú 1g sāngzhī 1g jiānghuáng 1g + acupuncture Huángqíwǔwùtāng 5g dānshēn 1g zhúrú 1g sāngzhī 1g dāngguī 1g jiānghuáng 1g Huángqíwǔwùtāng 5g dānshēn 1g zhúrú 1g sāngzhī 1g jiānghuáng 1g jīxuèténg 1g Huángqíwǔwùtāng 5g dānshēn 1g zhúrú 1g sāngzhī 1g qínjiāo 1g jiānghuáng 1g
Alternative prescriptions:
Huángqíwǔwùtāng 5g dānshēn 1g zhúrú 1g sāngzhī 1g Huángqíwǔwùtāng 5g dānshēn 1g zhúrú 1g sāngzhī 1g dāngguī 1g jiānghuáng 1g chuānxiōng 1g
Huángqíwǔwùtāng 5g chuānxiōng 2g dānshēn 2g zhúrú 2g sāngzhī 2g qínjiāo 2g dāngguī 2g jiānghuáng 2g gōuténg 2g Dāngguīsìnìtāng 5g shēngjiāng 1g wúzhūyú 1g fùzǐ 1g Huángqíwǔwùtāng 5g dāngguīsìnìtāng 4g dānshēn 1g sāngzhī 1g jīxuèténg 1g + acupuncture

<table>
<tr><td colspan="2">Hemianopsia: https://meshb.nlm.nih.gov/record/ui?ui=D006423.</td></tr>
<tr><td colspan="2">Indicated diseases:</td></tr>
<tr><td colspan="2">Unspecified cerebrovascular disease 437.9 (Cerebrovascular disease, unspecified I679); Disorder of eye, unspecified 379.90 (Unspecified disorder of eye and adnexa H579); Cardiovascular disease, unspecified 429.2 (Atherosclerotic heart disease of native coronary artery without angina pectoris I2510); Unspecified condition of brain 348.9 (Disorder of brain, unspecified G939); Unspecified disorders of nervous system 349.9 (Disorder of central nervous system, unspecified G969); Unspecified endocrine disorder 259.9 (Endocrine disorder, unspecified E349); Malignant neoplasm of endocrine gland, site unspecified 194.9 (Malignant neoplasm of endocrine gland, unspecified C759); Neoplasm of unspecified nature of brain 239.6 (Neoplasm of unspecified behavior of brain D496); Migraine 346</td></tr>
<tr><td colspan="2">Unspecified cerebrovascular disease 437.9/I679 with hemianopsia D006423:</td></tr>
<tr><td>Bǔyánghuánwǔtāng 5g dānshēn 1g shíchāngpú 1g yuǎnzhì 1g + acupuncture to ♀</td><td>Bǔyánghuánwǔtāng 5g dānshēn 1g shíchāngpú 1g yuǎnzhì 1g + acupuncture to ♂</td></tr>
<tr><td colspan="2">Unspecified condition of brain 348.9/G939 with hemianopsia D006423:</td></tr>
<tr><td>Bǔyánghuánwǔtāng 5g dānshēn 1g tiānmá 1g shíchāngpú 1g yuǎnzhì 1g to ♀</td><td>Bǔyánghuánwǔtāng 5g dānshēn 1g tiānmá 1g shíchāngpú 1g yuǎnzhì 1g + acupuncture to ♂</td></tr>
<tr><td colspan="2">Disorder of eye, unspecified 379.90/H579 with hemianopsia D006423:</td></tr>
<tr><td>Qǐjúdìhuángwán 5g zīshènmíngmùtāng 5g to ♀</td><td>Qǐjúdìhuángwán 5g xǐgānmíngmùtāng 5g zīshènmíngmùtāng 5g to ♂</td></tr>
</table>

Bǔyánghuánwǔtāng 'nourishes Qi, invigorates blood, and interlinks meridians.' Its primary use today is for stroke sequelae.

2.15. Cortical Blindness

Cortical blindness describes a loss of vision due to damage to the visual part of the brain called the occipital cortex. Acquired cortical blindness is most often caused by blockage of blood flow to and thus damage of the occipital lobe. Transient cortical blindness can be caused by brain surgery.

Table 2.15. Herbal prescriptions for cortical blindness

Cortical Blindness: https://meshb.nlm.nih.gov/record/ui?ui=D019575.
Common prescriptions:
Guìzhītāng 5g shēngjiāng 1g báisháo 1g dàhuáng 0g Guìzhītāng 5g shēngjiāng 1g guìzhī 1g Guìzhītāng 5g shēngjiāng 1g báisháo 1g Guìzhītāng 5g shēngjiāng 1g báisháo 1g guìzhī 1g
Alternative prescriptions:
Guìzhītāng 5g fùzǐ 0g Guìzhītāng 5g báisháo 1g shēngjiāng 0g dàhuáng 0g Máhuángfùzǐxìxīntāng 5g fùzǐ 3g guìzhī 3g dàzǎo 2g shēngjiāng 2g zhìgāncǎo 2g
Indicated diseases:
Unspecified cerebrovascular disease 437.9 (Cerebrovascular disease, unspecified I679); Cortical blindness 377.75 (Cortical blindness, unspecified side of brain H47619); Cardiovascular disease, unspecified 429.2 (Atherosclerotic heart disease of native coronary artery without angina pectoris I2510); Disorder of eye, unspecified 379.90 (Unspecified disorder of eye and adnexa H579); Unspecified condition of brain 348.9 (Disorder of brain, unspecified G939); Unspecified disorders of nervous system 349.9 (Disorder of central nervous system, unspecified G969); Hypertensive encephalopathy 437.2 (Hypertensive encephalopathy I674); Unspecified disorder of metabolism 277.9 (Metabolic disorder, unspecified E889); Myopathy, unspecified 359.9 (Myopathy, unspecified G729); Myoneural disorders 358; Aneurysm of unspecified site 442.9 (Aneurysm of unspecified site I729)

Table 2.15. (Continued)

Cortical Blindness: https://meshb.nlm.nih.gov/record/ui?ui=D019575.	
Unspecified cerebrovascular disease 437.9/I679 with blindness, cortical D019575:	
Bǔyánghuánwǔtāng 5g chuānqī 1g dānshēn 1g shíchāngpú 1g yuǎnzhì 1g + acupuncture to ♀	Bǔyánghuánwǔtāng 5g dānshēn 1g shíchāngpú 1g yuǎnzhì 1g + acupuncture to ♂
Hypertensive encephalopathy 437.2/I674 with blindness, cortical D019575:	
Xiǎoxùmìngtāng 5g + acupuncture to ♀	Xiǎoxùmìngtāng 5g + acupuncture to ♂
Aneurysm of unspecified site 442.9/I729 with blindness, cortical D019575:	
Guìzhītāng 5g gégēn 2g bànxià 1g dàhuáng 0g to ♀	Xiǎoxùmìngtāng 5g bǔyánghuánwǔtāng 5g + acupuncture to ♂

Guìzhītāng is used in the previous chapter for such acute and intractable pain as headache, glossalgia and neck pain. Its use here looks to consider cortical blindness as a complication resulting from a brain damage or operation. Indeed, transient cortical blindness was reported to be associated with cerebral aneurysm procedures (Niimi et al., 2008; Tong et al., 2018).

2.16. Amaurosis Fugax

Amaurosis fugax is transient loss of vision due to lack of blood flow to the retina of the affected eye. Occlusion of the retinal artery or carotid artery that deliver blood to the side of blinding can cause amaurosis fugax. People with vascular diseases such as atherosclerosis which narrow blood vessels are at high risk of experiencing temporary vision loss.

Table 2.16. Herbal prescriptions for amaurosis fugax

Amaurosis Fugax: https://meshb.nlm.nih.gov/record/ui?ui=D020757.
Common prescriptions:
Wúzhūyútāng 5g máhuángfùzǐxìxīntāng 5g fùzǐ 2g guìzhī 2g gānjiāng 2g Máhuángfùzǐxìxīntāng 5g shēngjiāng 2g guìzhī 2g zhìgāncǎo 1g Máhuángfùzǐxìxīntāng 5g shēngjiāng 2g guìzhī 2g gāncǎo 1g
Alternative prescriptions:
Dāngguīsìnìtāng 5g shēngjiāng 1g wúzhūyú 1g Máhuángfùzǐxìxīntāng 5g fùzǐ 3g guìzhī 3g báizhú 2g wúzhūyú 2g gānjiāng 2g zhìgāncǎotāng 2g Guìzhītāng 5g báizhú 2g fùzǐ 2g báisháo 2g fúlíng 2g dǎngshēn 1g shēngjiāng 1g gānjiāng 1g dàhuáng 0g Máhuángfùzǐxìxīntāng 5g shēngjiāng 1g zhìgāncǎo 1g guìzhī 1g Dāngguīsìnìtāng 5g wúzhūyú 1g fùzǐ 1g gānjiāng 1g
Indicated diseases:
Unspecified cerebrovascular disease 437.9 (Cerebrovascular disease, unspecified I679); Disorder of eye, unspecified 379.90 (Unspecified disorder of eye and adnexa H579); Cardiovascular disease, unspecified 429.2 (Atherosclerotic heart disease of native coronary artery without angina pectoris I2510); Unspecified condition of brain 348.9 (Disorder of brain, unspecified G939); Unspecified disorders of nervous system 349.9 (Disorder of central nervous system, unspecified G969); Heart disease, unspecified 429.9 (Heart disease, unspecified I519); Unspecified congenital anomaly of heart 746.9 (Congenital malformation of cardiac chambers and connections, unspecified Q209, Congenital malformation of heart, unspecified Q249); Peripheral angiopathy in diseases classified elsewhere 443.81 (Other disorders of arteries, arterioles and capillaries in diseases classified elsewhere I798); Retinal arterial branch occlusion 362.32 (Retinal artery branch occlusion, unspecified eye H34239); Central retinal artery occlusion 362.31 (Central retinal artery occlusion, bilateral H3413); Unspecified retinal disorder 362.9 (Unspecified retinal disorder H359)

Amaurosis Fugax: https://meshb.nlm.nih.gov/record/ui?ui=D020757.	
Unspecified cerebrovascular disease 437.9/I679 with amaurosis fugax D020757:	
Bǔyánghuánwǔtāng 5g dānshēn 1g tiānmá 1g shíchāngpú 1g yuǎnzhì 1g to ♀	Bǔyánghuánwǔtāng 5g dānshēn 1g shíchāngpú 1g yuǎnzhì 1g + acupuncture to ♂
Heart disease, unspecified 429.9/I519 with amaurosis fugax D020757:	
Sìnìtāng 5g gānlùyǐn 5g mǔdānpí 1g zhīzǐ 1g huánglián 0g to ♀	Sìnìtāng 5g gānlùyǐn 5g mǔdānpí 1g zhīzǐ 1g huánglián 0g to ♂
Peripheral angiopathy in diseases classified elsewhere 443.81/I798 with amaurosis fugax D020757:	
Huángqíwǔwùtāng 5g dāngguīsìnìtāng 5g dānshēn 1g zhúrú 1g sāngzhī 1g jiānghuáng 1g to ♀	Huángqíwǔwùtāng 5g dāngguīsìnìtāng 5g dānshēn 1g zhúrú 1g sāngzhī 1g jiānghuáng 1g to ♂

Both Wúzhūyútāng and Máhuángfùzǐxìxīntāng warm up the body and have traditionally been used for people who have a weak pulse and feel sleepy all the time. It is thought that herbalists use Wúzhūyútāng and Máhuángfùzǐxìxīntāng to attend to the circulatory cause of amaurosis fugax.

2.17. Night Blindness

Night blindness is reduced or loss of vision in low light conditions. Causes of night blindness include vitamin A deficiency, nearsightedness, cataracts, glaucoma, retinitis pigmentosa, and inheritance.

Table 2.17. Herbal prescriptions for night blindness

Night Blindness: https://meshb.nlm.nih.gov/record/ui?ui=D009755.	
Common prescriptions:	
Qǐjúdìhuángwán 5g zīshènmíngmùtāng 5g Qǐjúdìhuángwán 5g xǐgānmíngmùtāng 5g zīshènmíngmùtāng 5g Qǐjúdìhuángwán 5g xǐgānmíngmùtāng 5g zīshènmíngmùtāng 5g mùzéicǎo 1g cǎojuémíng 1g mìmēnghuā 1g Qǐjúdìhuángwán 5g zīshènmíngmùtāng 5g mùzéicǎo 1g juémíngzǐ 1g mìmēnghuā 1g	
Alternative prescriptions:	
Zīshènmíngmùtāng 5g gǒuqǐzǐ 1g mìmēnghuā 1g júhuā 1g Xǐgānmíngmùtāng 5g zīshènmíngmùtāng 5g mùzéicǎo 1g mìmēnghuā 1g gǔjīngcǎo 1g Qǐjúdìhuángwán 5g zīshènmíngmùtāng 3g cǎojuémíng 1g huángjīng 1g gǔjīngcǎo 1g Xǐgānmíngmùtāng 5g zīshènmíngmùtāng 5g mùzéicǎo 1g mìmēnghuā 1g chántuì 1g Qǐjúdìhuángwán 5g sìwùtāng 4g juémíngzǐ 1g mìmēnghuā 1g gǔjīngcǎo 1g	
Indicated diseases:	
Night blindness 368.6; Unspecified retinal disorder 362.9 (Unspecified retinal disorder H359); Disorder of eye, unspecified 379.90 (Unspecified disorder of eye and adnexa H579); Unspecified disorder of liver 573.9 (Liver disease, unspecified K769); Diseases of the jaws 526; Macular degeneration (senile), unspecified 362.50 (Unspecified macular degeneration H3530);	
Other dermatoses 702; Neuroendocrine tumors 209; Malignant neoplasm of nervous system, part unspecified 192.9 (Malignant neoplasm of central nervous system, unspecified C729); Myopia 367.1 (Myopia, bilateral H5213)	
Night blindness 368.6 with night blindness D009755:	
Qǐjúdìhuángwán 5g zīshènmíngmùtāng 5g to ♀	Qǐjúdìhuángwán 5g zīshènmíngmùtāng 5g to ♂
Unspecified disorder of liver 573.9/K769 with night blindness D009755:	
Jiāwèixiāoyáosǎn 5g qǐjúdìhuángwán 5g cháihúshūgāntāng 5g to ♀	Xiǎocháihútāng 5g qǐjúdìhuángwán 5g dānshēn 1g wǔwèizǐ 1g hǔzhàng 1g to ♂
Other dermatoses 702 with night blindness D009755:	
Jiāwèixiāoyáosǎn 5g qǐjúdìhuángwán 5g nǚzhēnzǐ 1g hànliáncǎo 1g to ♀	Xiāofēngsǎn 5g jiědúsìwùtāng 5g zhēnrénhuómìngyǐn 4g huángliánjiědútāng 4g to ♂

Mùzéicǎo is today used for disorders of lacrimal system (Wang, 2019) and is here added to the prescriptions to support the eye formulas for night blindness.

2.18. Dysgeusia

People with dysgeusia have an altered sense of taste so that food tastes strange. The neural taste pathway begins with the taste receptors in the tongue and throat, through three cranial nerves, to the brain stem, temporal lobes and thalamus. Damage to any part of the pathway can change taste. Common causes of dysgeusia are anti-cancer therapy side-effects, vitamin and mineral deficiencies, and viral infections.

Table 2.18. Herbal prescriptions for dysgeusia

Dysgeusia: https://meshb.nlm.nih.gov/record/ui?ui=D004408.	
Common prescriptions:	
Sìnìtāng 5g bànxià 1g dàhuáng 0g Sìnìtāng 5g guìzhī 1g máhuáng 1g xìxīn 1g Sìnìtāng 5g guìzhī 1g máhuáng 1g xìxīn 0g Sìnìtāng 5g guìzhī 2g máhuáng 2g xìxīn 1g	
Alternative prescriptions:	
Guìzhītāng 5g shēngjiāng 1g báisháo 1g dàhuáng 0g Sìnìtāng 5g bànxià 1g fúlíng 1g dàhuáng 0g Sìnìtāng 5g guìzhī 1g máhuáng 1g xìxīn 0g dàhuáng 0g	
Indicated diseases:	
Other dermatoses 702; Unspecified disorders of nervous system 349.9 (Disorder of central nervous system, unspecified G969); Deformity and disproportion of reconstructed breast 612; Other disorders of breast 611; Benign mammary dysplasias 610; Diabetes mellitus 250; Unspecified endocrine disorder 259.9 (Endocrine disorder, unspecified E349); Unspecified disorder of metabolism 277.9 (Metabolic disorder, unspecified E889); Viral pneumonia 480; Malignant neoplasm of thorax 195.1 (Malignant neoplasm of thorax C761)	
Other dermatoses 702 with dysgeusia D004408:	
Dāngguīsinìtāng 5g wúzhūyú 1g fùzǐ 1g gānjiāng 1g to ♀	Huángliánjiědútāng 5g to ♂
Unspecified disorders of nervous system 349.9/G969 with dysgeusia D004408:	
Huángqíwǔwùtāng 5g chuānxiōng 1g dānshēn 1g zhúrú 1g sāngzhī 1g dāngguī 1g jiānghuáng 1g to ♀	Huángqíwǔwùtāng 5g chuānxiōng 1g dānshēn 1g zhúrú 1g sāngzhī 1g dāngguī 1g jiānghuáng 1g to ♂
Viral pneumonia 480 with dysgeusia D004408:	
Guìzhītāng 5g xìngrén 1g hòupò 1g to ♀	Guìzhītāng 5g xìngrén 1g hòupò 1g to ♂

Sìnìtāng is used in Section 2.2 for olfaction disorders.

Note that information about taste and smell combines in a region of the brain called the orbitofrontal cortex to produce a flavor. If either smell or taste is altered, the food will no longer taste right. Therefore, the use of Sìnìtāng here for dysgeusia comes as no surprise. Low appetite due to bad taste can contribute to nutritional deficiencies which in turn manifest cutaneous signs.

2.19. Ageusia

Ageusia is loss of the taste function of the tongue. Ageusia, rarer than dysgeusia, is mainly caused by viral infections such as COVID-19.

Table 2.19. Herbal prescriptions for ageusia

<table>
<tr><td colspan="2">Ageusia https://meshb.nlm.nih.gov/record/ui?ui=D000370</td></tr>
<tr><td colspan="2">Common prescriptions:</td></tr>
<tr><td colspan="2">Guìzhītāng 5g shēngjiāng 1g báisháo 1g dàhuáng 0g
Guìzhītāng 5g shēngjiāng 1g guìzhī 1g
Máhuángfùzǐxìxīntāng 5g shēngjiāng 2g guìzhī 2g zhìgāncǎo 1g
Guìzhītāng 5g shēngjiāng 1g báisháo 1g</td></tr>
<tr><td colspan="2">Alternative prescriptions:</td></tr>
<tr><td colspan="2">Guìzhītāng 5g gégēn 2g bànxià 1g dàhuáng 0g
Dāngguīsìnìtāng 5g shēngjiāng 1g wúzhūyú 1g
Guìzhītāng 5g bànxià 1g jiégěng 1g dàhuáng 0g
Guìzhītāng 5g shēngjiāng 1g báisháo 1g guìzhī 1g
Guìzhītāng 5g fùzǐ 0g</td></tr>
<tr><td colspan="2">Indicated diseases:</td></tr>
<tr><td colspan="2">Viral pneumonia 480; Unspecified disorders of nervous system 349.9 (Disorder of central nervous system, unspecified G969); Other dermatoses 702; Deformity and disproportion of reconstructed breast 612; Other disorders of breast 611; Benign mammary dysplasias 610</td></tr>
<tr><td colspan="2">Viral pneumonia 480 with ageusia D000370:</td></tr>
<tr><td>Guìzhītāng 5g xìngrén 1g hòupò 1g to ♀</td><td>Guìzhītāng 5g xìngrén 1g hòupò 1g to ♂</td></tr>
<tr><td colspan="2">Other dermatoses 702 with ageusia D000370:</td></tr>
<tr><td>Dāngguīsìnìtāng 5g shēngjiāng 1g wúzhūyú 1g to ♀</td><td>Xiāofēngsǎn 5g jiědúsìwùtāng 5g zhēnrénhuómìngyǐn 4g huángliánjiědútāng 4g
to ♂</td></tr>
</table>

Guìzhītāng is used for not only headache and glossalgia but also upper respiratory tract infections as we will see in Chapter 3. It can be understood that it is used here mainly for infection related ageusia. Note that skin lesions are associated with ageusia in confirmed COVID-19 cases (Birlutiu et al., 2021).

2.20. Tinnitus

Tinnitus is hearing of ringing in the ear while there is actually not such a sound in the outside world. Exposure to loud noise, injuries, or neurodegeneration of the auditory function of the brain can cause tinnitus.

We learn the use of Língguìshùgāntāng for dizziness in Section 2.1. As the ears not only facilitate hearing but also help maintain balance, Língguìshùgāntāng's use here for tinnitus is unsurprising. Tinnitus was found to be associated with somatization disorders (Hiller et al., 1997).

Table 2.20. Herbal prescriptions for tinnitus

<table>
<tr><td colspan="2">Tinnitus: https://meshb.nlm.nih.gov/record/ui?ui=D014012.</td></tr>
<tr><td colspan="2">Common prescriptions:</td></tr>
<tr><td colspan="2">Língguìshùgāntāng 5g fùzǐ 1g shārén 1g xìxīn 1g dàhuáng 0g
Língguìshùgāntāng 5g bànxià 1g fùzǐ 1g shārén 1g dàhuáng 0g
Língguìshùgāntāng 5g bànxià 1g fùzǐ 1g shārén 1g xìxīn 1g dàhuáng 0g
Língguìshùgāntāng 5g fùzǐ 1g shārén 1g dàhuáng 0g</td></tr>
<tr><td colspan="2">Alternative prescriptions:</td></tr>
<tr><td colspan="2">Língguìshùgāntāng 5g fùzǐ 1g shārén 1g bànxià 1g dàhuáng 0g
Língguìshùgāntāng 5g shārén 1g huíxiāng 1g fùzǐ 1g dàhuáng 0g
Língguìshùgāntāng 5g bànxià 1g shēngjiāng 1g zéxiè 1g dàhuáng 0g
Língguìshùgāntāng 5g shārén 1g huíxiāng 1g fùzǐ 1g dàhuáng 0g + acupuncture</td></tr>
<tr><td colspan="2">Indicated diseases:</td></tr>
<tr><td colspan="2">Unspecified cerebrovascular disease 437.9 (Cerebrovascular disease, unspecified I679); Unspecified disorder of ear 388.9 (Unspecified disorder of ear, bilateral H9393); Cardiovascular disease, unspecified 429.2 (Atherosclerotic heart disease of native coronary artery without angina pectoris I2510); Unspecified condition of brain 348.9 (Disorder of brain, unspecified G939); Unspecified disorders of nervous system 349.9 (Disorder of central nervous system, unspecified G969); Disorders of acoustic nerve 388.5 (Disorders of unspecified acoustic nerve H933X9); Malignant neoplasm of cranial nerves 192.0 (Malignant neoplasm of unspecified cranial nerve C7250); Unspecified disorder of cranial nerves 352.9 (Cranial nerve disorder, unspecified G529); Neuroendocrine tumors 209; Malignant neoplasm of nervous system, part unspecified 192.9 (Malignant neoplasm of central nervous system, unspecified C729); Aneurysm of unspecified site 442.9 (Aneurysm of unspecified site I729); Somatization disorder 300.81 (Somatization disorder F450)</td></tr>
<tr><td colspan="2">Unspecified cerebrovascular disease 437.9/I679 with tinnitus D014012:</td></tr>
<tr><td>Bǔyánghuánwǔtāng 5g chuānqī 2g dānshēn 1g shíchāngpú 1g yuǎnzhì 1g + acupuncture to ♀</td><td>Bǔyánghuánwǔtāng 5g chuānqī 2g dānshēn 1g shíchāngpú 1g yuǎnzhì 1g + acupuncture to ♂</td></tr>
<tr><td colspan="2">Disorders of acoustic nerve 388.5/H933X9 with tinnitus D014012:</td></tr>
<tr><td>Xiǎocháihútāng 5g língguìshùgāntāng 5g shíchāngpú 1g yuǎnzhì 1g to ♀</td><td>Xiǎocháihútāng 5g língguìshùgāntāng 5g shíchāngpú 1g yuǎnzhì 1g to ♂</td></tr>
<tr><td colspan="2">Aneurysm of unspecified site 442.9/I729 with tinnitus D014012:</td></tr>
<tr><td>Língguìshùgāntāng 5g bànxià 1g shārén 1g dàhuáng 0g to ♀</td><td>Xiǎocháihútāng 5g língguìshùgāntāng 5g niúxī 1g chēqiánzǐ 1g to ♂</td></tr>
<tr><td colspan="2">Unspecified disorder of ear 388.9/H9393 with tinnitus D014012:</td></tr>
<tr><td>Xiǎocháihútāng 5g yìqìcōngmíngtāng 5g shíchāngpú 1g yuǎnzhì 1g to ♀</td><td>Xiǎocháihútāng 5g yìqìcōngmíngtāng 5g shíchāngpú 1g yuǎnzhì 1g to ♂</td></tr>
</table>

2.21. Wolfram Syndrome

The primary symptoms of Wolfram syndrome are childhood-onset diabetes, optic atrophy, excessive thirst and urination, and deafness. It is a rare genetic disorder caused by a mutated gene on chromosome 4 of the human genome.

Traditionally, Bāwèidìhuángwán 'benefits the Kidney Yang' and Bǔzhōngyìqìtāng 'tonifies the Spleen and Stomach.' The modern use of Bāwèidìhuángwán is for diabetes mellitus and that of Bǔzhōngyìqìtāng is for anemia (Wang, 2019). Combining them here is believed to alleviate the digestive and metabolic problems in patients with Wolfram syndrome.

Table 2.21. Herbal prescriptions for Wolfram syndrome

Wolfram Syndrome: https://meshb.nlm.nih.gov/record/ui?ui=D014929.	
Common prescriptions:	
Bāwèidìhuángwán 5g bǔzhōngyìqìtāng 5g Bǔzhōngyìqìtāng 5g Bǔzhōngyìqìtāng 5g huánshǎodān 5g	
Alternative prescriptions:	
Dāngguīsìnìtāng 5g shēngjiāng 1g wúzhūyú 1g Bǔzhōngyìqìtāng 5g yínyánghuò 1g tùsīzǐ 1g Bǔzhōngyìqìtāng 5g bāwèidìhuángwán 4g Liùwèidìhuángwán 5g huánshǎodān 5g	
Indicated diseases:	
Optic atrophy 377.1; Diabetes insipidus 253.5 (Diabetes insipidus E232); Foster-Kennedy syndrome 377.04 (Foster-Kennedy syndrome, unspecified eye H47149); Unspecified disorder of cranial nerves 352.9 (Cranial nerve disorder, unspecified G529); Unspecified disorder of ear 388.9 (Unspecified disorder of ear, bilateral H9393); Disorder of eye, unspecified 379.90 (Unspecified disorder of eye and adnexa H579); Unspecified disorders of nervous system 349.9 (Disorder of central nervous system, unspecified G969); Diabetes mellitus 250; Unspecified endocrine disorder 259.9 (Endocrine disorder, unspecified E349); Unspecified disorder of metabolism 277.9 (Metabolic disorder, unspecified E889); Heart disease, unspecified 429.9 (Heart disease, unspecified I519); Cardiovascular disease, unspecified 429.2 (Atherosclerotic heart disease of native coronary artery without angina pectoris I2510); Schizophrenic disorders 295	
Optic atrophy 377.1 with Wolfram syndrome D014929:	
Qǐjúdìhuángwán 5g yìqìcōngmíngtāng 5g to ♀	Qǐjúdìhuángwán 5g zīshènmíngmùtāng 5g mùzéicǎo 1g cǎojuémíng 1g to ♂
Heart disease, unspecified 429.9/I519 with Wolfram syndrome D014929:	
Xuèfǔzhúyūtāng 5g wēndǎntāng 5g dānshēn 2g chuānqī 1g báijí 1g guìzhī 1g guālóurén 1g xièbái 1g to ♀	Xuèfǔzhúyūtāng 5g wēndǎntāng 5g dānshēn 2g chuānqī 1g báijí 1g guìzhī 1g guālóurén 1g xièbái 1g to ♂

2.22. Hyperacusis

Hyperacusis is low tolerance for loudness in one or both ears. Causes of hyperacusis include damage to the hair cells in the cochlea in the inner ear which receive and amplify sounds for the auditory processing in the brain.

Hyperacusis and tinnitus are related (Koops and van Dijk, 2021). Língguìshùgāntāng is used for hyperacusis, as it is used for tinnitus.

Table 2.22. Herbal prescriptions for hyperacusis

Hyperacusis: https://meshb.nlm.nih.gov/record/ui?ui=D012001.
Common prescriptions:
Língguìshùgāntāng 5g fùzǐ 1g shārén 1g xìxīn 1g dàhuáng 0g Língguìshùgāntāng 5g fùzǐ 1g shārén 1g bànxià 1g dàhuáng 0g Língguìshùgāntāng 5g fùzǐ 1g gānjiāng 1g xìxīn 1g Língguìshùgāntāng 5g fùzǐ 1g gānjiāng 1g Língguìshùgāntāng 5g fùzǐ 1g shārén 1g xìxīn 1g
Alternative prescriptions:
Língguìshùgāntāng 5g bànxià 1g fùzǐ 1g shārén 1g xìxīn 1g dàhuáng 0g Língguìshùgāntāng 5g bànxià 2g fùzǐ 1g shārén 1g xìxīn 1g dàhuáng 0g Língguìshùgāntāng 5g bànxià 1g fùzǐ 1g xìxīn 1g dàhuáng 0g Língguìshùgāntāng 5g shārén 1g huíxiāng 1g fùzǐ 1g xìxīn 1g dàhuáng 0g + acupuncture Bǔzhōngyìqìtāng 5g fùzǐ 1g

Table 2.22. (Continued)

Hyperacusis: https://meshb.nlm.nih.gov/record/ui?ui=D012001.	
Indicated diseases:	
Unspecified disorder of ear 388.9 (Unspecified disorder of ear, bilateral H9393); Autistic disorder 299.0; Unspecified disorders of nervous system 349.9 (Disorder of central nervous system, unspecified G969); Unspecified condition of brain 348.9 (Disorder of brain, unspecified G939); Schizophrenic disorders 295	
Unspecified disorder of ear 388.9/H9393 with hyperacusis D012001:	
Xiǎocháihútāng 5g língguìshùgāntāng 5g shíchāngpú 1g yuǎnzhì 1g to ♀	Xiǎocháihútāng 5g yìqìcōngmíngtāng 5g shíchāngpú 1g yuǎnzhì 1g to ♂

2.23. High-Frequency Hearing Loss

People with high-frequency hearing loss have difficulty hearing high-pitched sounds, such as squeak, whistle and siren, which are received and transduced to electric impulses by the hair cells in the inner ear. Common causes of high-frequency hearing loss are aging, noise exposure, and diseases including infections.

Table 2.23. Herbal prescriptions for high-frequency hearing loss

High-Frequency Hearing Loss: https://meshb.nlm.nih.gov/record/ui?ui=D006316.	
Common prescriptions:	
Língguìshùgāntāng 5g xiǎohuíxiāng 1g fùzǐ 1g shārén 1g dàhuáng 0g Língguìshùgāntāng 5g xiǎohuíxiāng 1g fùzǐ 1g shārén 1g xìxīn 1g dàhuáng 0g Língguìshùgāntāng 5g fùzǐ 1g shārén 1g xìxīn 1g dàhuáng 0g Língguìshùgāntāng 5g xiǎohuíxiāng 1g fùzǐ 1g shārén 1g	
Alternative prescriptions:	
Língguìshùgāntāng 5g bànxià 1g fùzǐ 1g shārén 1g xìxīn 1g dàhuáng 0g Língguìshùgāntāng 5g bànxià 1g shārén 1g dàhuáng 0g Língguìshùgāntāng 5g xiǎohuíxiāng 1g shārén 1g fùzǐ 0g	
Indicated diseases:	
Disorders of acoustic nerve 388.5 (Disorders of unspecified acoustic nerve H933X9); Malignant neoplasm of cranial nerves 192.0 (Malignant neoplasm of unspecified cranial nerve C7250); Unspecified disorder of cranial nerves 352.9 (Cranial nerve disorder, unspecified G529); Unspecified disorder of ear 388.9 (Unspecified disorder of ear, bilateral H9393); Unspecified disorders of nervous system 349.9 (Disorder of central nervous system, unspecified G969); Neuroendocrine tumors 209; Malignant neoplasm of nervous system, part unspecified 192.9 (Malignant neoplasm of central nervous system, unspecified C729); Ménière's disease 386.0; Human immunodeficiency virus [HIV] disease 042 (Human immunodeficiency virus [HIV] disease B20)	
Disorders of acoustic nerve 388.5/H933X9 with hearing loss, high-frequency D006316:	
Xiǎocháihútāng 5g língguìshùgāntāng 5g shíchāngpú 1g yuǎnzhì 1g to ♀	Xiǎocháihútāng 5g língguìshùgāntāng 5g shíchāngpú 1g yuǎnzhì 1g to ♂
Unspecified disorder of ear 388.9/H9393 with hearing loss, high-frequency D006316:	
Xiǎocháihútāng 5g língguìshùgāntāng 5g shíchāngpú 1g yuǎnzhì 1g to ♀	Xiǎocháihútāng 5g yìqìcōngmíngtāng 5g shíchāngpú 1g yuǎnzhì 1g to ♂
Ménière's disease 386.0 with hearing loss, high-frequency D006316:	
Língguìshùgāntāng 5g cháihújiālónggǔmǔlìtāng 5g dāngguīsháoyàosǎn 5g to ♀	Língguìshùgāntāng 5g chuānxiōng 1g shénqū 1g shānzhā 1g chénpí 1g to ♂

Xiǎohuíxiāng is a food flavoring and used today for neurotic disorders (Wang, 2019). Its inclusion is believed to enhance the digestive and emotional benefits of the prescription.

2.24. Unilateral Hearing Loss

A reduced or complete loss of hearing in one ear, while the other is normal, is called unilateral hearing loss. Causes of unilateral hearing loss include injury to the ear, medication side-effect, and tumor.

Xiǎocháihútāng is used for earache in Section 1.8 of Chapter 1. Its use here may target the traumatic cause of unilateral hearing loss. As functions of the cochlea depend on adequate blood supply, hearing loss and cardiovascular diseases are associated (Tan et al., 2018).

Table 2.24. Herbal prescriptions for unilateral hearing loss

Unilateral Hearing Loss: https://meshb.nlm.nih.gov/record/ui?ui=D046088.	
Common prescriptions:	
Língguìshùgāntāng 5g fùzǐ 1g shārén 1g xìxīn 1g dàhuáng 0g Língguìshùgāntāng 5g fùzǐ 1g shārén 1g dàhuáng 0g Xiǎocháihútāng 5g língguìshùgāntāng 5g niúxī 1g chēqiánzǐ 1g Xiǎocháihútāng 5g língguìshùgāntāng 5g niúxī 1g chēqiánzǐ 1g yuǎnzhì 1g Língguìshùgāntāng 5g bànxià 1g shēngjiāng 1g	
Alternative prescriptions:	
Língguìshùgāntāng 5g xiǎohuíxiāng 2g shārén 2g fùzǐ 1g dàhuáng 0g Língguìshùgāntāng 5g shārén 1g bànxià 1g fùzǐ 1g dàhuáng 0g Língguìshùgāntāng 5g bànxià 1g shēngjiāng 1g dàhuáng 0g	
Indicated diseases:	
Disorders of acoustic nerve 388.5 (Disorders of unspecified acoustic nerve H933X9); Malignant neoplasm of cranial nerves 192.0 (Malignant neoplasm of unspecified cranial nerve C7250); Unspecified disorder of cranial nerves 352.9 (Cranial nerve disorder, unspecified G529); Unspecified disorder of ear 388.9 (Unspecified disorder of ear, bilateral H9393); Unspecified disorders of nervous system 349.9 (Disorder of central nervous system, unspecified G969); Neuroendocrine tumors 209; Malignant neoplasm of nervous system, part unspecified 192.9 (Malignant neoplasm of central nervous system, unspecified C729); Ménière's disease 386.0; Cardiovascular disease, unspecified 429.2 (Atherosclerotic heart disease of native coronary artery without angina pectoris I2510)	
Disorders of acoustic nerve 388.5/H933X9 with hearing loss, unilateral D046088:	
Xiǎocháihútāng 5g língguìshùgāntāng 5g shíchāngpú 1g yuǎnzhì 1g to ♀	Xiǎocháihútāng 5g língguìshùgāntāng 5g shíchāngpú 1g yuǎnzhì 1g to ♂
Ménière's disease 386.0 with hearing loss, unilateral D046088:	
Língguìshùgāntāng 5g cháihújiālónggǔmǔlìtāng 5g dāngguīsháoyàosǎn 5g to ♀	Língguìshùgāntāng 5g cháihújiālónggǔmǔlìtāng 5g dāngguīsháoyàosǎn 5g to ♂
Unspecified disorder of ear 388.9/H9393 with hearing loss, unilateral D046088:	
Xiǎocháihútāng 5g língguìshùgāntāng 5g shíchāngpú 1g yuǎnzhì 1g to ♀	Xiǎocháihútāng 5g yìqìcōngmíngtāng 5g shíchāngpú 1g yuǎnzhì 1g to ♂
Cardiovascular disease, unspecified 429.2/I2510 with hearing loss, unilateral D046088:	
Yùzhú 5g sìnìtāng 5g zhìgāncǎotāng 5g to ♀	Sìnìtāng 5g gānlùyǐn 5g lóngdǎnxiègāntāng 5g to ♂

2.25. Bilateral Hearing Loss

Bilateral hearing loss affects both ears. Infection and inflammation of the protective membranes covering the brain can spread to damage the hair cells in the inner ear, causing bilateral hearing loss.

Table 2.25. Herbal prescriptions for bilateral hearing loss

Bilateral Hearing Loss: https://meshb.nlm.nih.gov/record/ui?ui=D006312.	
Common prescriptions:	
Língguìshùgāntāng 5g xiǎohuíxiāng 1g fùzǐ 1g shārén 1g dàhuáng 0g Língguìshùgāntāng 5g xiǎohuíxiāng 1g fùzǐ 1g shārén 1g xìxīn 1g dàhuáng 0g Língguìshùgāntāng 5g xiǎohuíxiāng 1g fùzǐ 1g shārén 1g	
Alternative prescriptions:	
Língguìshùgāntāng 5g shārén 1g huíxiāng 1g fùzǐ 1g dàhuáng 0g Língguìshùgāntāng 5g shārén 1g fùzǐ 1g xìxīn 1g dàhuáng 0g	
Indicated diseases:	
Disorders of acoustic nerve 388.5 (Disorders of unspecified acoustic nerve H933X9); Malignant neoplasm of cranial nerves 192.0 (Malignant neoplasm of unspecified cranial nerve C7250); Unspecified disorder of cranial nerves 352.9 (Cranial nerve disorder, unspecified G529); Unspecified disorder of ear 388.9 (Unspecified disorder of ear, bilateral H9393); Unspecified disorders of nervous system 349.9 (Disorder of central nervous system, unspecified G969); Neuroendocrine tumors 209; Malignant neoplasm of nervous system, part unspecified 192.9 (Malignant neoplasm of central nervous system, unspecified C729); Meningitis, unspecified 322.9 (Meningitis, unspecified G039); Cryptococcosis 117.5 (Pulmonary cryptococcosis B450, Disseminated cryptococcosis B457, Cryptococcosis, unspecified B459); Candidiasis 112; Coccidioidomycosis 114; Histoplasmosis 115; Blastomycotic infection 116; Other mycoses 117; Opportunistic mycoses 118 (Other specified mycoses B488); Dermatophytosis 110; Human immunodeficiency virus [HIV] disease 042 (Human immunodeficiency virus [HIV] disease B20); Dermatomycosis, other and unspecified 111; Cardiovascular disease, unspecified 429.2 (Atherosclerotic heart disease of native coronary artery without angina pectoris I2510); Multiple myeloma 203.0; Unspecified hemorrhagic conditions 287.9 (Hemorrhagic condition, unspecified D699); Unspecified diseases of blood and blood-forming organs 289.9 (Disease of blood and blood-forming organs, unspecified D759); Ménière's disease 386.0	
Disorders of acoustic nerve 388.5/H933X9 with hearing loss, bilateral D006312:	
Xiǎocháihútāng 5g língguìshùgāntāng 5g shíchāngpú 1g yuǎnzhì 1g to ♀	Yìqìcōngmíngtāng 5g zīshèntōngěrtāng 5g shíchāngpú 1g yuǎnzhì 1g to ♂
Meningitis, unspecified 322.9/G039 with hearing loss, bilateral D006312:	
Bànxiàbáizhútiānmátāng 5g bǔzhōngyìqìtāng 5g guīpítāng 5g to ♀	Bànxiàbáizhútiānmátāng 5g bǔyánghuánwǔtāng 5g dānshēn 1g shíchāngpú 1g yuǎnzhì 1g to ♂
Cardiovascular disease, unspecified 429.2/I2510 with hearing loss, bilateral D006312:	
Yùzhú 5g sìnìtāng 5g zhìgāncǎotāng 5g to ♀	Yùzhú 5g sìnìtāng 5g zhìgāncǎotāng 5g to ♂
Ménière's disease 386.0 with hearing loss, bilateral D006312:	
Língguìshùgāntāng 5g cháihújiālónggǔmǔlìtāng 5g dāngguīsháoyàosǎn 5g to ♀	Língguìshùgāntāng 5g cháihújiālónggǔmǔlìtāng 5g dāngguīsháoyàosǎn 5g to ♂

Fungal infections of the outer ear canal can cause unilateral or bilateral hearing loss. A case of unilateral followed by bilateral hearing loss was reported in a multiple myeloma patient (Keay, 1988).

2.26. Usher Syndromes

Usher syndromes are a rare genetic disorder caused by mutations in genes that are involved in the development of the hair cells in the cochlea and photoreceptors in the retina, resulting in hearing loss and vision impairment in the newborn.

Each of the three formulas Wǔlíngsǎn, Língguìshùgāntāng and Zhēnwǔtāng contains Fúlíng and Báizhú as their major constituent herbs, each of which improves fluid metabolism. Combination or interchange of the formulas here are believed to reinforce the medicinal effects. Note that Bànxià is used for functional hearing loss below and motion sickness of Section 17.26.

Table 2.26. Herbal prescriptions for Usher syndromes

Usher Syndromes: https://meshb.nlm.nih.gov/record/ui?ui=D052245.	
Common prescriptions:	
Língguìshùgāntāng 5g bànxià 1g fùzǐ 1g shārén 1g dàhuáng 0g Língguìshùgāntāng 5g bànxià 1g fùzǐ 1g shārén 1g xìxīn 1g dàhuáng 0g Língguìshùgāntāng 5g bànxià 1g fùzǐ 1g shārén 1g Língguìshùgāntāng 5g bànxià 1g shēngjiāng 1g zéxiè 1g	
Alternative prescriptions:	
Língguìshùgāntāng 5g shārén 1g fùzǐ 1g xìxīn 1g dàhuáng 0g Wǔlíngsǎn 5g língguìshùgāntāng 5g niúxī 1g chēqiánzǐ 1g Zhēnwǔtāng 5g wúzhūyútāng 2g fùzǐ 1g Língguìshùgāntāng 5g bànxià 1g shēngjiāng 1g fùzǐ 1g shārén 1g xìxīn 1g	
Indicated and associated diseases:	
Sensorineural hearing loss 389.1; Unspecified retinal disorder 362.9 (Unspecified retinal disorder H359); Unspecified disorder of ear 388.9 (Unspecified disorder of ear, bilateral H9393); Disorder of eye, unspecified 379.90 (Unspecified disorder of eye and adnexa H579); Unspecified disorders of nervous system 349.9 (Disorder of central nervous system, unspecified G969); Macular degeneration (senile), unspecified 362.50 (Unspecified macular degeneration H3530)	
Sensorineural hearing loss 389.1 with Usher syndromes D052245:	
Yìqìcōngmíngtāng 5g shíchāngpú 1g yuǎnzhì 1g to ♀	Yìqìcōngmíngtāng 5g shíchāngpú 1g yuǎnzhì 1g to ♂
Macular degeneration (senile), unspecified 362.50/H3530 with Usher syndromes D052245:	
Qǐjúdìhuángwán 5g zīshènmíngmùtāng 5g to ♀	Qǐjúdìhuángwán 5g zīshènmíngmùtāng 5g xuèfǔzhúyūtāng 2g to ♂
Unspecified retinal disorder 362.9/H359 with Usher syndromes D052245:	
Qǐjúdìhuángwán 5g zīshènmíngmùtāng 5g xuèfǔzhúyūtāng 2g to ♀	Qǐjúdìhuángwán 5g zīshènmíngmùtāng 3g xuèfǔzhúyūtāng 2g to ♂

2.27. Functional Hearing Loss

Functional hearing loss is loss of hearing with no known organic basis. As physical lesions of the auditory pathway are not detected, causes of functional hearing loss are believed to be psychological or emotional.

Table 2.27. Herbal prescriptions for functional hearing loss

Functional Hearing Loss: https://meshb.nlm.nih.gov/record/ui?ui=D006315.
Common prescriptions:
Sìnìtāng 5g rénshēn 1g wúzhūyú 1g Sìnìtāng 5g rénshēn 1g Sìnìtāng 5g rénshēn 1g bànxià 1g dàhuáng 0g Sìnìtāng 5g rénshēn 1g bànxià 1g Sìnìtāng 5g rénshēn 1g bànxià 1g gānjiāng 1g
Alternative prescriptions:
Guìzhītāng 5g gégēn 2g bànxià 1g dàhuáng 0g Bǔzhōngyìqìtāng 5g shēngmàiyǐn 2g Bǔzhōngyìqìtāng 5g Sìnìtāng 5g rénshēn 1g yánhúsuǒ 1g
Indicated diseases:
Unspecified disorder of ear 388.9 (Unspecified disorder of ear, bilateral H9393); Autistic disorder 299.0; Unspecified disorders of nervous system 349.9 (Disorder of central nervous system, unspecified G969); Disorders of acoustic nerve 388.5 (Disorders of unspecified acoustic nerve H933X9); Malignant neoplasm of cranial nerves 192.0 (Malignant neoplasm of unspecified cranial nerve C7250); Unspecified disorder of cranial nerves 352.9 (Cranial nerve disorder,

Table 2.27. (Continued)

Functional Hearing Loss: https://meshb.nlm.nih.gov/record/ui?ui=D006315.	
unspecified G529); Neuroendocrine tumors 209; Malignant neoplasm of nervous system, part unspecified 192.9 (Malignant neoplasm of central nervous system, unspecified C729); Unspecified condition of brain 348.9 (Disorder of brain, unspecified G939)	
Unspecified disorder of ear 388.9/H9393 with hearing loss, functional D006315:	
Xiǎocháihútāng 5g língguìshùgāntāng 5g shíchāngpú 1g yuǎnzhì 1g to ♀	Xiǎocháihútāng 5g língguìshùgāntāng 5g shíchāngpú 1g yuǎnzhì 1g to ♂
Disorders of acoustic nerve 388.5/H933X9 with hearing loss, functional D006315:	
Xiǎocháihútāng 5g língguìshùgāntāng 5g shíchāngpú 1g yuǎnzhì 1g to ♀	Yìqìcōngmíngtāng 5g zīshèntōngěrtāng 5g shíchāngpú 1g yuǎnzhì 1g to ♂

Sìnìtāng is used for smell and taste problems in Sections 2.2 and 2.18 respectively. The higher regions of the brain integrate smell and taste to produce the sensation of flavor. It can be thought that functional hearing loss involves not only the hearing per se, but also higher-level processing in the brain. Sìnìtāng therefore comes to the help.

2.28. Conductive Hearing Loss

Conductive hearing loss is hearing loss due to problems with the outer or middle ear that impede the propagation of incoming sound waves. Injuries or illnesses that change the structure of the outer or middle ear can cause conductive hearing loss.

Table 2.28. Herbal prescriptions for conductive hearing loss

Conductive Hearing Loss: https://meshb.nlm.nih.gov/record/ui?ui=D006314.
Common prescriptions:
Xiǎocháihútāng 5g língguìshùgāntāng 5g niúxī 1g chēqiánzǐ 1g Xiǎocháihútāng 5g língguìshùgāntāng 5g shíchāngpú 1g yuǎnzhì 1g Xiǎocháihútāng 5g língguìshùgāntāng 5g niúxī 1g shíchāngpú 1g chēqiánzǐ 1g yuǎnzhì 1g Xiǎocháihútāng 5g língguìshùgāntāng 5g niúxī 1g chēqiánzǐ 1g yuǎnzhì 1g Xiǎocháihútāng 5g língguìshùgāntāng 5g niúxī 2g chēqiánzǐ 2g yuǎnzhì 2g
Alternative prescriptions:
Xiǎocháihútāng 5g língguìshùgāntāng 4g shíchāngpú 1g yuǎnzhì 1g gōuténg 1g Xiǎocháihútāng 5g yìqìcōngmíngtāng 5g shíchāngpú 1g yuǎnzhì 1g Língguìshùgāntāng 5g yìqìcōngmíngtāng 5g niúxī 2g chēqiánzǐ 2g yuǎnzhì 2g Xiǎocháihútāng 5g língguìshùgāntāng 5g chuānxiōng 1g niúxī 1g báizhǐ 1g shíchāngpú 1g chēqiánzǐ 1g jīngjiè 1g yuǎnzhì 1g Qǐjúdìhuángwán 5g língguìshùgāntāng 4g shíchāngpú 1g yuǎnzhì 1g
Indicated diseases:
Other dermatoses 702; Cholesteatoma of middle ear 385.32 (Cholesteatoma of tympanum, bilateral H7113, Polyp of middle ear, unspecified ear H7440); Cholesteatoma, unspecified 385.30 (Unspecified cholesteatoma, bilateral H7193); Unspecified disorder of ear 388.9 (Unspecified disorder of ear, bilateral H9393); Unspecified disorders of nervous system 349.9 (Disorder of central nervous system, unspecified G969); Osteogenesis imperfecta 756.51 (Osteogenesis imperfecta Q780); Multiple epiphyseal dysplasia 756.56 (Progressive diaphyseal dysplasia Q783); Chondrodystrophy 756.4 (Thanatophoric short stature Q771, Achondroplasia Q774, Other osteochondrodysplasia with defects of growth of tubular bones and spine Q778, Enchondromatosis Q784); Unspecified otitis media 382.9 (Otitis media, unspecified, unspecified ear H6690)

Conductive Hearing Loss: https://meshb.nlm.nih.gov/record/ui?ui=D006314.	
Other dermatoses 702 with hearing loss, conductive D006314:	
Xiāofēngsǎn 5g jiědúsìwùtāng 5g zhēnrénhuómìngyǐnqùchuānshānjiǎ 4g huángliánjiědútāng 4g to ♀	Xiāofēngsǎn 5g bàidúsǎn 5g zhēnrénhuómìngyǐnqùchuānshānjiǎ 4g huángliánjiědútāng 4g to ♂
Unspecified disorder of ear 388.9/H9393 with hearing loss, conductive D006314:	
Xiǎocháihútāng 5g yìqìcōngmíngtāng 5g shíchāngpú 1g yuǎnzhì 1g to ♀	Yìqìcōngmíngtāng 5g zīshèntōngěrtāng 5g shíchāngpú 1g yuǎnzhì 1g to ♂

Xiǎocháihútāng is used in Section 1.8 for earache. Its use here for conductive hearing loss is conceivable. Yìqìcōngmíngtāng, where the Chinese character cōng means acuity in hearing and the character míng refers to clarity in vision, is a traditional formula for both hearing and vision as it 'supplements Qi and lifts Yang.' Note that multiple epiphyseal dysplasia, osteogenesis imperfecta, and chondrodystrophy were found to be associated with hearing loss (Beighton et al., 1978; Pillion et al., 2011; Yarington and Sprinkle, 1967), as are also revealed in the table.

2.29. Mixed Conductive-Sensorineural Hearing Loss

Hearing loss with both conductive and sensorineural origins is called mixed conductive-sensorineural hearing loss. Sensorineural hearing loss involves problems with the inner ear and nerve pathway which convert and transmit auditory information to the auditory cortex. A foreign object obstructing the ear canal along with an inflammation of the inner ear can cause mixed conductive-sensorineural hearing loss.

Table 2.29. Herbal prescriptions for mixed conductive-sensorineural hearing loss

Mixed Conductive-Sensorineural Hearing Loss: https://meshb.nlm.nih.gov/record/ui?ui=D046089.	
Common prescriptions:	
Língguìshùgāntāng 5g fùzǐ 1g shārén 1g xìxīn 1g dàhuáng 0g Língguìshùgāntāng 5g bànxià 1g fùzǐ 1g shārén 1g dàhuáng 0g Língguìshùgāntāng 5g fùzǐ 1g shārén 1g dàhuáng 0g Língguìshùgāntāng 5g bànxià 1g fùzǐ 1g shārén 1g xìxīn 1g dàhuáng 0g	
Alternative prescriptions:	
Língguìshùgāntāng 5g shārén 1g huíxiāng 1g fùzǐ 1g dàhuáng 0g Língguìshùgāntāng 5g fùzǐ 1g gānjiāng 1g xìxīn 1g Língguìshùgāntāng 5g bànxià 1g fùzǐ 1g shārén 1g dàhuáng 0g + acupuncture Língguìshùgāntāng 5g fùzǐ 1g xìxīn 1g tiáowèichéngqìtāng 1g	
Indicated diseases:	
Disorders of acoustic nerve 388.5 (Disorders of unspecified acoustic nerve H933X9); Malignant neoplasm of cranial nerves 192.0 (Malignant neoplasm of unspecified cranial nerve C7250); Unspecified disorder of cranial nerves 352.9 (Cranial nerve disorder, unspecified G529); Unspecified disorder of ear 388.9 (Unspecified disorder of ear, bilateral H9393); Unspecified disorders of nervous system 349.9 (Disorder of central nervous system, unspecified G969); Neuroendocrine tumors 209; Malignant neoplasm of nervous system, part unspecified 192.9 (Malignant neoplasm of central nervous system, unspecified C729); Other dermatoses 702; Cholesteatoma of middle ear 385.32 (Cholesteatoma of tympanum, bilateral H7113, Polyp of middle ear, unspecified ear H7440); Cholesteatoma, unspecified 385.30 (Unspecified cholesteatoma, bilateral H7193); Ménière's disease 386.0	
Disorders of acoustic nerve 388.5/H933X9 with hearing loss, mixed conductive-sensorineural D046089:	
Xiǎocháihútāng 5g língguìshùgāntāng 5g shíchāngpú 1g yuǎnzhì 1g to ♀	Xiǎocháihútāng 5g língguìshùgāntāng 5g shíchāngpú 1g yuǎnzhì 1g to ♂

Table 2.29. (Continued)

Mixed Conductive-Sensorineural Hearing Loss: https://meshb.nlm.nih.gov/record/ui?ui=D046089.	
Other dermatoses 702 with hearing loss, mixed conductive-sensorineural D046089:	
Dāngguīsìnìtāng 5g shēngjiāng 1g wúzhūyú 1g to ♀	Yùnǚjiān 5g xuèfǔzhúyūtāng 3g dāngguīsháoyàosǎn 3g báijiāngcán 1g to ♂
Ménière's disease 386.0 with hearing loss, mixed conductive-sensorineural D046089:	
Língguìshùgāntāng 5g cháihújiālónggǔmǔlìtāng 5g dāngguīsháoyàosǎn 5g to ♀	Língguìshùgāntāng 5g chuānxiōng 1g shénqū 1g shānzhā 1g chénpí 1g to ♂
Unspecified disorder of ear 388.9/H9393 with hearing loss, mixed conductive-sensorineural D046089:	
Xiǎocháihútāng 5g língguìshùgāntāng 5g shíchāngpú 1g yuǎnzhì 1g to ♀	Xiǎocháihútāng 5g yìqìcōngmíngtāng 5g shíchāngpú 1g yuǎnzhì 1g to ♂

Shíchāngpú 'drains off Dampness.' Its addition to the prescription is believed to help clear ear discharge, building up of which can cause ear infections. Truly, Shíchāngpú's modern uses include tinnitus and Ménière's disease (Wang, 2020).

2.30. Sudden Hearing Loss

Sudden hearing loss occurs rapidly, affecting typically one ear. Sudden hearing loss usually reflects an underlying medical condition such as viral infection, brain tumor, head trauma and vascular disease.

Table 2.30. Herbal prescriptions for sudden hearing loss

Sudden Hearing Loss: https://meshb.nlm.nih.gov/record/ui?ui=D003639.	
Common prescriptions:	
Língguìshùgāntāng 5g xiǎohuíxiāng 1g fùzǐ 1g shārén 1g dàhuáng 0g Língguìshùgāntāng 5g xiǎohuíxiāng 1g fùzǐ 1g shārén 1g xìxīn 1g dàhuáng 0g Língguìshùgāntāng 5g fùzǐ 1g shārén 1g xìxīn 1g dàhuáng 0g Língguìshùgāntāng 5g xiǎohuíxiāng 1g fùzǐ 1g shārén 1g	
Alternative prescriptions:	
Língguìshùgāntāng 5g shārén 1g fùzǐ 1g xìxīn 1g dàhuáng 0g Língguìshùgāntāng 5g shārén 2g xiǎohuíxiāng 1g fùzǐ 1g dàhuáng 0g	
Indicated diseases:	
Disorders of acoustic nerve 388.5 (Disorders of unspecified acoustic nerve H933X9); Malignant neoplasm of cranial nerves 192.0 (Malignant neoplasm of unspecified cranial nerve C7250); Unspecified disorder of cranial nerves 352.9 (Cranial nerve disorder, unspecified G529); Unspecified disorder of ear 388.9 (Unspecified disorder of ear, bilateral H9393); Unspecified disorders of nervous system 349.9 (Disorder of central nervous system, unspecified G969); Neuroendocrine tumors 209; Malignant neoplasm of nervous system, part unspecified 192.9 (Malignant neoplasm of central nervous system, unspecified C729); Ménière's disease 386.0; Unspecified cerebrovascular disease 437.9 (Cerebrovascular disease, unspecified I679); Cardiovascular disease, unspecified 429.2 (Atherosclerotic heart disease of native coronary artery without angina pectoris I2510); Unspecified condition of brain 348.9 (Disorder of brain, unspecified G939)	
Disorders of acoustic nerve 388.5/H933X9 with hearing loss, sudden D003639:	
Xiǎocháihútāng 5g língguìshùgāntāng 5g shíchāngpú 1g yuǎnzhì 1g to ♀	Xiǎocháihútāng 5g língguìshùgāntāng 5g shíchāngpú 1g yuǎnzhì 1g to ♂
Ménière's disease 386.0 with hearing loss, sudden D003639:	
Língguìshùgāntāng 5g cháihújiālónggǔmǔlìtāng 5g dāngguīsháoyàosǎn 5g to ♀	Língguìshùgāntāng 5g cháihújiālónggǔmǔlìtāng 5g dāngguīsháoyàosǎn 5g to ♂
Unspecified cerebrovascular disease 437.9/I679 with hearing loss, sudden D003639:	
Bǔyánghuánwǔtāng 5g dānshēn 1g shíchāngpú 1g yuǎnzhì 1g + acupuncture to ♀	Bǔyánghuánwǔtāng 5g chuānqī 2g dānshēn 1g shíchāngpú 1g yuǎnzhì 1g + acupuncture to ♂

Symptoms of Ménière's disease include vertigo, tinnitus and sudden hearing loss. Vertigo can in turn bring up nausea and vomiting. The causes of Ménière's disease are unclear but its symptoms are related to fluid buildup in the inner ear. Cháihújiālónggǔmǔlìtāng 'quells panic and calms spirits.' Furthermore, Dāngguīsháoyàosǎn 'nourishes Blood and drains Dampness' to enhance the fluid homeostatic effect of Língguìshùgāntāng in the prescription for Ménière's disease with sudden hearing loss.

2.31. Presbycusis

Presbycusis is progressive sensorineural hearing loss in both ears when one gets older. Causes of presbycusis are a combination of harmful environmental accumulations, such as loud noise exposure over time, and age-related degenerative pathologies.

Sìnìtāng is already used for functional hearing loss. As it 'lifts a dying Yang,' its use here, together with Língguìshùgāntāng, is supposed to relieve aging related hearing loss.

Table 2.31. Herbal prescriptions for presbycusis

Presbycusis: https://meshb.nlm.nih.gov/record/ui?ui=D011304.	
Common prescriptions:	
Sìnìtāng 5g língguìshùgāntāng 5g Sìnìtāng 5g wúzhūyútāng 5g língguìshùgāntāng 5g	
Alternative prescriptions:	
Língguìshùgāntāng 5g bànxià 1g fùzǐ 1g shārén 1g xìxīn 1g dàhuáng 0g Língguìshùgāntāng 5g fùzǐ 1g gānjiāng 1g tiáowèichéngqìtāng 1g dàhuáng 0g Zhēnwǔtāng 5g fùzǐ 1g gānjiāng 1g dǐdāngtāng 0g Língguìshùgāntāng 5g fùzǐ 1g xìxīn 1g xiǎochéngqìtāng 1g dàhuáng 0g Bǔzhōngyìqìtāng 5g shēngmàiyǐn 3g	
Indicated diseases:	
Hypertensive heart and chronic kidney disease 404; Sensorineural hearing loss 389.1; Secondary hypertension 405; Essential hypertension 401; Hypertensive chronic kidney disease 403; Hypertensive heart disease 402; Cardiovascular disease, unspecified 429.2 (Atherosclerotic heart disease of native coronary artery without angina pectoris I2510); Unspecified disorder of ear 388.9 (Unspecified disorder of ear, bilateral H9393); Unspecified disorders of nervous system 349.9 (Disorder of central nervous system, unspecified G969); Diabetes mellitus 250; Unspecified endocrine disorder 259.9 (Endocrine disorder, unspecified E349); Unspecified disorder of metabolism 277.9 (Metabolic disorder, unspecified E889)	
Hypertensive heart and chronic kidney disease 404 with presbycusis D011304:	
Tiānmágōuténgyǐn 5g bànxiàbáizhútiānmátāng 5g língguìshùgāntāng 5g to ♀	Tiānmágōuténgyǐn 5g xuèfǔzhúyūtāng 5g zhībódìhuángwán 5g to ♂
Cardiovascular disease, unspecified 429.2/I2510 with presbycusis D011304:	
Yùzhú 5g sìnìtāng 5g zhìgāncǎotāng 2g to ♀	Sìnìtāng 5g gānlùyǐn 5g zhìgāncǎotāng 5g to ♂
Sensorineural hearing loss 389.1 with presbycusis D011304:	
Xiǎocháihútāng 5g língguìshùgāntāng 5g shíchāngpú 1g yuǎnzhì 1g to ♀	Xiǎocháihútāng 5g yìqìcōngmíngtāng 5g shíchāngpú 1g yuǎnzhì 1g to ♂

2.32. Central Hearing Loss

Central hearing loss is hearing loss due to problems with the central auditory pathway in the brain, not in the ear. Illnesses, such as stroke, tumor and infection, affecting the auditory cortex can cause central hearing loss.

Guìzhītāng is used for cortical blindness in Section 2.15. It is not surprising it is used here for central hearing loss, as both conditions involve problems with regions deep inside the brain.

Table 2.32. Herbal prescriptions for central hearing loss

Central Hearing Loss: https://meshb.nlm.nih.gov/record/ui?ui=D006313.	
Common prescriptions:	
Guìzhītāng 5g báizhú 1g fùzǐ 1g fúlíng 1g Guìzhītāng 5g gégēn 1g + acupuncture Guìzhītāng 5g báizhú 1g fùzǐ 1g Guìzhītāng 5g gégēn 1g Guìzhītāng 5g báizhú 1g fúlíng 1g	
Alternative prescriptions:	
Guìzhītāng 5g shēngjiāng 1g guìzhī 1g dàhuáng 0g Guìzhītāng 5g gégēn 3g bànxià 1g dàhuáng 0g Guìzhītāng 5g shēngjiāng 1g báisháo 1g guìzhī 1g Guìzhītāng 5g shēngjiāng 1g báisháo 1g dàhuáng 0g	
Indicated or associated diseases:	
Disorders of acoustic nerve 388.5 (Disorders of unspecified acoustic nerve H933X9); Neurofibromatosis, type 2 [acoustic neurofibromatosis] 237.72 (Neurofibromatosis, type 2 Q8502); Sensorineural hearing loss 389.1; Unspecified disorder of cranial nerves 352.9 (Cranial nerve disorder, unspecified G529); Unspecified disorder of ear 388.9 (Unspecified disorder of ear, bilateral H9393); Unspecified condition of brain 348.9 (Disorder of brain, unspecified G939); Unspecified disorders of nervous system 349.9 (Disorder of central nervous system, unspecified G969); Neurofibromatosis 237.7; Malignant neoplasm of cranial nerves 192.0 (Malignant neoplasm of unspecified cranial nerve C7250); Neuroendocrine tumors 209; Malignant neoplasm of nervous system, part unspecified 192.9 (Malignant neoplasm of central nervous system, unspecified C729); Neoplasm of unspecified nature of brain 239.6 (Neoplasm of unspecified behavior of brain D496)	
Disorders of acoustic nerve 388.5/H933X9 with hearing loss, central D006313:	
Xiǎocháihútāng 5g língguìshùgāntāng 5g shíchāngpú 1g yuǎnzhì 1g to ♀	Yìqìcōngmíngtāng 5g zīshèntōngěrtāng 5g shíchāngpú 1g yuǎnzhì 1g to ♂

2.33. Noise-Induced Hearing Loss

Noise-induced hearing loss is hearing loss due to damage to the hair cells in the inner ear by loud sounds. Examples of loud sounds are repeated loud music from earbuds and impulse noise such as gunshots during military service.

Noise-induced hearing loss can contribute to age-related hearing loss. Noise-induced hearing loss is prescribed Sìnìtāng as presbycusis is prescribed Sìnìtāng.

Table 2.33. Herbal prescriptions for noise-induced hearing loss

Noise-Induced Hearing Loss: https://meshb.nlm.nih.gov/record/ui?ui=D006317.
Common prescriptions:
Sìnìtāng 5g língguìshùgāntāng 5g Sìnìtāng 5g wúzhūyútāng 5g máhuángfùzǐxìxīntāng 5g Sìnìtāng 5g wúzhūyútāng 5g língguìshùgāntāng 5g
Alternative prescriptions:
Língguìshùgāntāng 5g shārén 2g fùzǐ 1g xìxīn 1g dàhuáng 0g Bǔzhōngyìqìtāng 5g chuānxiōng 0g mànjīngzǐ 0g Língguìshùgāntāng 5g bànxià 1g shíchāngpú 1g fùzǐ 1g shārén 1g xìxīn 1g dàhuáng 0g Língguìshùgāntāng 5g bànxià 1g shēngjiāng 1g fùzǐ 1g shārén 1g dàhuáng 0g Língguìshùgāntāng 5g fùzǐ 1g ròuguì 0g

Noise-Induced Hearing Loss: https://meshb.nlm.nih.gov/record/ui?ui=D006317.	
Indicated diseases:	
Hypertensive heart and chronic kidney disease 404; Sensorineural hearing loss 389.1; Secondary hypertension 405; Essential hypertension 401; Hypertensive chronic kidney disease 403; Hypertensive heart disease 402; Cardiovascular disease, unspecified 429.2 (Atherosclerotic heart disease of native coronary artery without angina pectoris I2510); Unspecified disorder of ear 388.9 (Unspecified disorder of ear, bilateral H9393); Unspecified disorders of nervous system 349.9 (Disorder of central nervous system, unspecified G969); Diabetes mellitus 250; Unspecified endocrine disorder 259.9 (Endocrine disorder, unspecified E349); Unspecified disorder of metabolism 277.9 (Metabolic disorder, unspecified E889)	
Hypertensive heart and chronic kidney disease 404 with hearing loss, noise-induced D006317:	
Bànxiàbáizhútiānmátāng 5g bǔyánghuánwǔtāng 5g dānshēn 1g to ♀	Tiānmágōuténgyǐn 5g xuèfǔzhúyūtāng 5g dānshēn 1g to ♂
Cardiovascular disease, unspecified 429.2/I2510 with hearing loss, noise-induced D006317:	
Yùzhú 5g sìnìtāng 5g zhìgāncǎotāng 2g to ♀	Sìnìtāng 5g gānlùyǐn 5g mǔdānpí 1g zhīzǐ 1g huánglián 0g to ♂
Sensorineural hearing loss 389.1 with hearing loss, noise-induced D006317:	
Xiǎocháihútāng 5g língguìshùgāntāng 5g shíchāngpú 1g yuǎnzhì 1g to ♀	Yìqìcōngmíngtāng 5g yìqìcōngmíngtāng 4g shíchāngpú 1g yuǎnzhì 1g to ♂

References

Beighton, P., Goldberg, L., & Hof, J. O. (2008). Dominant inheritance of multiple epiphyseal dysplasia, myopia and deafness. *Clinical Genetics*, *14*(3), 173–177. https://doi.org/10.1111/j.1399-0004.1978.tb02125.x.

Benites, B. M., Miranda-Silva, W., Rocha, A. C., Passos, U. L., Fonseca, F. P., da Silva, C. A. R., & Fregnani, E. R. (2021). Late recurrence of Burkitt s lymphoma in the jaw: numb chin syndrome as the only symptom. *Autopsy Case Reports*, *11*, e2020218. https://doi.org/10.4322/acr.2020.218.

Birlutiu, V., Feiereisz, A. I., Oprinca, G., Dobritoiu, S., Rotaru, M., Birlutiu, R. M., & Iancu, G. M. (2021). Cutaneous manifestations associated with anosmia, ageusia and enteritis in SARS-CoV-2 infection – A possible pattern? Observational study and review of the literature. *International Journal of Infectious Diseases*, *107*, 72–77. https://doi.org/10.1016/j.ijid.2021.04.058.

Bodo, C. (2008). A role for the androgen receptor in the sexual differentiation of the olfactory system in mice. *Brain Research Reviews*, *57*(2), 321–331. https://doi.org/10.1016/j.brainresrev.2007.08.008.

Claeys, A., Trullemans, F., Maes, J., Hennekes, R., & Salu, P. (2002). Diplopia as an initial manifestation of disseminated non-Hodgkin's lymphoma. *Bulletin De La Société Belge D'ophtalmologie*, *286*, 35–38. PMID: 12564315.

Henkin, R. I. (1967). Abnormalities of Taste and Olfaction in Patients with Chromatin Negative Gonadal Dysgenesis. *The Journal of Clinical Endocrinology & Metabolism*, *27*(10), 1436–1440. https://doi.org/10.1210/jcem-27-10-1436.

Hiller, W., Janca, A., & Burke, K. C. (1997). Association between tinnitus and somatoform disorders. *Journal of Psychosomatic Research*, *43*(6), 613–624. https://doi.org/10.1016/s0022-3999(97)00188-8.

Keay, D. (1988). Total bilateral hearing loss as a complication of myeloma. *The Journal of Laryngology & Otology*, *102*(4), 357–358. https://doi.org/10.1017/s0022215100104955.

Koops, E. A., & van Dijk, P. (2021). Hyperacusis in tinnitus patients relates to enlarged subcortical and cortical responses to sound except at the tinnitus frequency. *Hearing Research*, *401*, 108158. https://doi.org/10.1016/j.heares.2020.108158.

Mancini, F., Longo, M. R., Kammers, M. P. M., & Haggard, P. (2011). Visual Distortion of Body Size Modulates Pain Perception. *Psychological Science*, *22*(3), 325–330. https://doi.org/10.1177/0956797611398496.

Melinte, V., & Sarafoleanu, C. (2019). Congenital anosmia: a case report. *Romanian Journal of Rhinology*, *9*(35), 161–164. https://doi.org/10.2478/rjr-2019-0020.

Niimi, Y., Kupersmith, M. J., Ahmad, S., Song, J., & Berenstein, A. (2007). Cortical Blindness, Transient and Otherwise, Associated with Detachable Coil Embolization of Intracranial Aneurysms. *American Journal of Neuroradiology*, *29*(3), 603–607. https://doi.org/10.3174/ajnr.a0858.

Pillion, J. P., Vernick, D., & Shapiro, J. (2011). Hearing Loss in Osteogenesis Imperfecta: Characteristics and Treatment Considerations. *Genetics Research International*, *2011*, 1–6. https://doi.org/10.4061/2011/983942.

Roh, D., Lee, D.-H., Kim, S. W., Kim, S. W., Kim, B.-G., Kim, D. H., & Shin, J.-H. (2021). The association between olfactory dysfunction and cardiovascular disease and its risk factors in middle-aged and older adults. *Scientific Reports*, *11*(1), 1248. https://doi.org/10.1038/s41598-020-80943-5.

Tan, H. E., Lan, N. S. R., Knuiman, M. W., Divitini, M. L., Swanepoel, D. W., Hunter, M., Brennan-Jones, C. G., Hung, J., Eikelboom, R. H., & Santa Maria, P. L. (2018). Associations between cardiovascular disease and its risk factors with hearing loss-A cross-sectional analysis. *Clinical Otolaryngology: Official Journal of ENT-UK; Official Journal of Netherlands Society for Oto-Rhino-Laryngology & Cervico-Facial Surgery*, *43*(1), 172–181. https://doi.org/10.1111/coa.12936.

Tong, X., Hu, P., Hong, T., Li, M., Zhang, P., Li, G., & Zhang, H. (2018). Transient Cortical Blindness Associated with Endovascular Procedures for Intracranial Aneurysms. *World Neurosurgery*, *119*, 123–131. https://doi.org/10.1016/j.wneu.2018.07.234.

Turetsky, B. I., Hahn, C.-G., Borgmann-Winter, K., & Moberg, P. J. (2009). Scents and Nonsense: Olfactory Dysfunction in Schizophrenia. *Schizophrenia Bulletin*, *35*(6), 1117–1131. https://doi.org/10.1093/schbul/sbp111.

Wang, S. C. (2019). *Clinical Herbal Prescriptions: Principles and Practices of Herbal Formulations from Deep Learning Health Insurance Herbal Prescription Big Data*. WSPC. https://doi.org/10.1142/11211.

Wang, S. C. (2020). *Veterinary Herbal Pharmacopoeia*. Nova Science Publishers. https://doi.org/10.52305/GHTR1903.

Yarington, C. T., & Sprinkle, P. (1967). Hearing problems in certain forms of osteodystrophy: the chondrodystrophies. *Eye, Ear, Nose & Throat Monthly*, *46*(9), 1136–1138. PMID: 4965414.

Yazdanpanah, O., Kaur, J., Shafi, I., & Sarakbi, H. A. (2020). Diplopia as the initial symptom of multiple myeloma in a patient with sarcoidosis. *BMJ Case Reports*, *13*(8), e235725. https://doi.org/10.1136/bcr-2020-235725.

Chapter 3

Signs and Symptoms, Respiratory

Our respiratory system takes in oxygen and throws out carbon dioxide. Oxygen is needed by the mitochondria within the cell to metabolize nutrients such as glucose into chemical energy, and carbon dioxide is produced as a waste product during this process. The lungs, where gas exchange takes place, are the major organ of the respiratory system. As cells cannot work without energy, a stable and adequate supply of oxygen is of vital importance. The involuntary and automatic control of ventilatory rhythm is set up by the network of neurons in the so-called respiratory center in the regions of the medulla and pons in the brainstem.

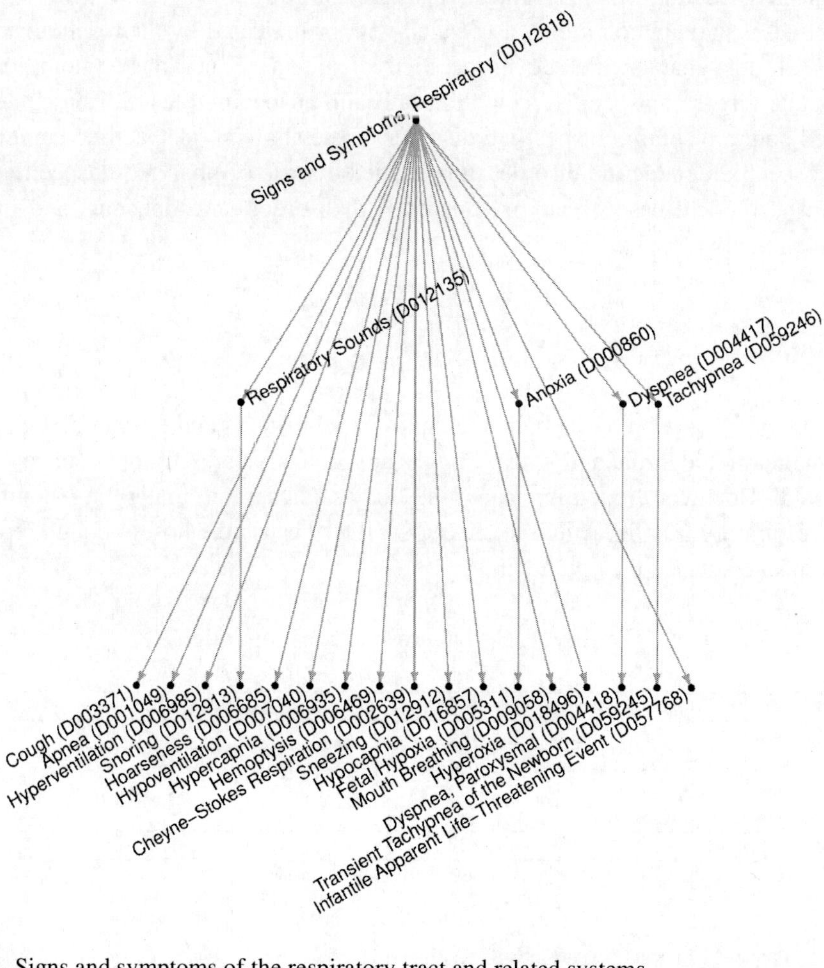

Figure 3.1. Signs and symptoms of the respiratory tract and related systems.

Monitoring of the rhythm is facilitated by signals from the central chemoreceptors in the brainstem and peripheral chemoreceptors in the neck and chest, the former of which are sensitive to changes in the pH and carbon dioxide partial pressure in the brain and the latter of which to changes in the partial pressures of oxygen and carbon dioxide in arterial blood. The respiratory center then responds with activating or inhibiting signals to the respiratory muscles including muscles in the respiratory tract, rib cage and diaphragm. Breathing is also subject to voluntary control, as we can control our breath during activities such as speaking, singing, diving and meditation. Additionally, the interaction of the upper respiratory and digestive tracts further complicates ventilation dynamics. Finally, as oxygen is outside of the body in the air and cells are distributed within the body, circulation of blood is also involved in the functioning of respiration.

The herbal formulas that appear frequently in the herbal prescriptions for the respiratory signs and symptoms in Figure 3.1 include Sìnìtāng, Guìzhītāng, Jiégěngtāng, Sháoyào-gāncǎotāng, Gānlùyǐn, Xiǎoqīnglóngtāng, Gāncǎoxiǎomàidàzǎotāng, Xīnyísǎn, and Sāngjúyǐn. Etiologies of the respiratory signs and symptoms and their comorbidities play a major role in determining the compositions of the herbal prescriptions. The single herbs that play supporting roles in the prescriptions include Dàhuáng, Shēngjiāng, Bànxià, Rénshēn, Guìzhī, Báisháo, Bèimǔ, Zhīzǐ, Liánqiáo, Xuánshēn and Mǔlì.

The diseases that are commonly associated with or indicated by the respiratory signs and symptoms of this chapter include unspecified disorders of nervous system, unspecified cardiovascular disease, unspecified condition of brain, unspecified heart disease, neoplasm of unspecified nature of brain, unspecified disorder of metabolism, unspecified cerebrovascular disease, unspecified endocrine disorder, unspecified disease of pharynx, unspecified disorder of eye, unspecified disease of larynx, unspecified disorder of esophagus, and unspecified congenital anomaly of heart.

3.1. Cough

Coughing is a reflex action of the body that helps expel irritants and foreign particles from the airways, including the throat and lungs. Coughs are protective and disappear once the irritants are removed. However, repetitive coughing may indicate an underlying condition. For example, respiratory tract infections such as COVID-19 cause the host to cough repeatedly as coughs help spreading of the coronaviruses.

Table 3.1. Herbal prescriptions for cough

Cough: https://meshb.nlm.nih.gov/record/ui?ui=D003371.
Common prescriptions:
Sāngjúyǐn 5g máxìnggānshítāng 5g yínqiàosǎn 5g Sāngjúyǐn 5g yínqiàosǎn 5g Sāngjúyǐn 5g máxìnggānshítāng 5g
Alternative prescriptions:
Sāngjúyǐn 5g bèimǔ 1g pípáyè 1g qīngpí 1g qiánhú 1g zhīzǐ 1g huángqín 1g Sāngjúyǐn 5g xīnyíqīngfèitāng 2g pípáyè 1g qīngpí 1g qiánhú 1g zhīzǐ 1g huángqín 1g Sāngjúyǐn 5g máxìnggānshítāng 5g bànxià 1g xīnyí 1g zhīmǔ 1g zhīzǐ 1g huángqín 1g cāngěrzǐ 1g Sāngjúyǐn 5g yínqiàosǎn 4g bèimǔ 1g guālóurén 1g Sāngjúyǐn 5g máxìnggānshítāng 5g jiégěng 1g huángqín 1g dàhuáng 0g
Indicated and associated diseases:
Unspecified disorder of esophagus 530.9 (Disease of esophagus, unspecified K229); Diseases of the jaws 526; Diseases of the oral soft tissues, excluding lesions specific for gingiva and tongue 528; Heart disease, unspecified 429.9 (Heart disease, unspecified I519); Bronchiectasis 494; Situs inversus 759.3 (Situs inversus Q893); Cardiovascular disease,

Cough: https://meshb.nlm.nih.gov/record/ui?ui=D003371.	
unspecified 429.2 (Atherosclerotic heart disease of native coronary artery without angina pectoris I2510); Unspecified congenital anomaly of heart 746.9 (Congenital malformation of cardiac chambers and connections, unspecified Q209, Congenital malformation of heart, unspecified Q249); Unspecified disease of pharynx 478.20 (Other diseases of pharynx J392); Unspecified disease of larynx 478.70 (Other diseases of larynx J387); Esophageal reflux 530.81 (Gastro-esophageal reflux disease without esophagitis K219); Dyskinesia of esophagus 530.5 (Dyskinesia of esophagus K224); Vascular disorders of skin 709.1 (Vasculitis limited to the skin, unspecified L959); Other dermatoses 702	
Unspecified disorder of esophagus 530.9/K229 with cough D003371:	
Jiāwèixiāoyáosǎn 5g xiāngshāliùjūnzǐtāng 5g bànxiàxièxīntāng 3g zhǐqiào 2g hǎipiāoxiāo 2g to ♀	Jiāwèixiāoyáosǎn 5g xuánfùdàizhěshítāng 5g xuánfùdàizhěshítāng 5g dúhuójìshēngtāng 5g hǎipiāoxiāo 2g chuānliànzǐ 1g dānshēn 1g xiāngfù 0g to ♂
Heart disease, unspecified 429.9/I519 with cough D003371:	
Sìnìtāng 5g gānlùyǐn 5g mǔdānpí 1g zhīzǐ 1g huánglián 0g to ♀	Sìnìtāng 5g gānlùyǐn 5g mǔdānpí 1g zhīzǐ 1g huánglián 0g to ♂
Unspecified disease of pharynx 478.20/J392 with cough D003371:	
Bànxiàhòupòtāng 5g màiméndōngtāng 5g jiégěng 1g to ♀	Bànxiàhòupòtāng 5g màiméndōngtāng 5g jiégěng 1g to ♂
Unspecified disease of larynx 478.70/J387 with cough D003371:	
Guìzhītāng 5g xìngrén 1g hòupò 1g to ♀	Guìzhītāng 5g xìngrén 1g hòupò 1g to ♂
Cardiovascular disease, unspecified 429.2/I2510 with cough D003371:	
Sìnìtāng 5g gānlùyǐn 5g mǔdānpí 1g zhīzǐ 1g huánglián 0g to ♀	Sìnìtāng 5g gānlùyǐn 5g mǔdānpí 1g zhīzǐ 1g huánglián 1g to ♂

Sāngjúyǐn has traditionally been used for the common cold and influenza. It is immunosuppressing as it is used nowadays for chronic bronchitis and sinusitis (Wang, 2019). Situs inversus, where the internal organs develop in a mirror-image formation compared with normal human anatomy, does not usually cause health problems. However, if it occurs with ciliary dyskinesia, where the hair-like organelles on the surface of respiratory tract cells which transport mucus do not move properly, in a condition called Kartagener's syndrome, then chronic cough is one of its symptoms.

Respiration interacts with heart functions, a well-known example being the association between sleep apnea and heart failure. Furthermore, cough can be triggered by heart arrhythmia through the hypothesized interaction between reflex and hemodynamics (Grabczak et al., 2020). As the skin also serves as a defense system of our body against environmental factors, skin conditions and cough are associated through shared neuropathic pathways (Misery et al., 2021), as we also see in the table.

3.2. Obstructive Sleep Apnea

Apnea is temporary disruption of breathing. If apnea occurs at night when one sleeps, it is called sleep apnea. Since no air flows in the airways during apnea, people with sleep apnea wake up periodically in the night to take a deep breath in order to get enough oxygen. Sleep quality deteriorates as a result. Causes of obstructive sleep apnea include structural or functional changes in the head and neck such as enlarged tonsils and relaxed throat, obesity, and aging.

Table 3.2. Herbal prescriptions for obstructive sleep apnea

Obstructive Sleep Apnea: https://meshb.nlm.nih.gov/record/ui?ui=D020181.	
Common prescriptions:	
Sìnìtāng 5g bànxià 1g dàhuáng 0g Sìnìtāng 5g shēngjiāng 1g guìzhī 1g Sìnìtāng 5g rénshēn 1g bànxià 1g dàhuáng 0g Sìnìtāng 5g rénshēn 1g Sìnìtāng 5g shēngjiāng 1g guìzhī 1g xìxīn 1g	
Alternative prescriptions:	
Sìnìtāng 5g rénshēn 2g dàhuáng 0g Sìnìtāng 5g rénshēn 1g wúzhūyú 1g dàhuáng 0g Sìnìtāng 5g bànxià 1g guìzhī 1g xìxīn 1g dàhuáng 0g Sìnìtāng 5g rénshēn 2g bànxià 1g dàhuáng 0g	
Indicated diseases:	
Cardiovascular disease, unspecified 429.2 (Atherosclerotic heart disease of native coronary artery without angina pectoris I2510); Diabetic retinopathy 362.0; Diabetes with peripheral circulatory disorders 250.7; Unspecified sleep apnea 780.57 (Sleep apnea, unspecified G4730); Obstructive sleep apnea (adult)(pediatric) 327.23 (Obstructive sleep apnea (adult) (pediatric) G4733); Unspecified retinal disorder 362.9 (Unspecified retinal disorder H359); Disorder of eye, unspecified 379.90 (Unspecified disorder of eye and adnexa H579); Unspecified disorders of nervous system 349.9 (Disorder of central nervous system, unspecified G969); Diabetes mellitus 250; Unspecified endocrine disorder 259.9 (Endocrine disorder, unspecified E349); Unspecified disorder of metabolism 277.9 (Metabolic disorder, unspecified E889); Dysmetabolic syndrome X 277.7 (Metabolic syndrome E8881); Heart disease, unspecified 429.9 (Heart disease, unspecified I519); Unspecified congenital anomaly of heart 746.9 (Congenital malformation of cardiac chambers and connections, unspecified Q209, Congenital malformation of heart, unspecified Q249); Atrial fibrillation 427.31 (Unspecified atrial fibrillation I4891)	
Cardiovascular disease, unspecified 429.2/I2510 with sleep apnea, obstructive D020181:	
Sìnìtāng 5g gānlùyǐn 5g mǔdānpí 1g zhīzǐ 1g huánglián 0g to ♀	Sìnìtāng 5g gānlùyǐn 5g mǔdānpí 1g zhīzǐ 1g huánglián 0g to ♂
Heart disease, unspecified 429.9/I519 with sleep apnea, obstructive D020181:	
Sìnìtāng 5g gānlùyǐn 5g mǔdānpí 1g zhīzǐ 1g huánglián 0g to ♀	Sìnìtāng 5g gānlùyǐn 5g mǔdānpí 1g zhīzǐ 1g huánglián 0g to ♂
Atrial fibrillation 427.31/I4891 with sleep apnea, obstructive D020181:	
Zhìgāncǎotāng 5g zhēnwǔtāng 5g to ♀	Zhìgāncǎotāng 5g zhēnwǔtāng 5g to ♂

Sìnìtāng is used for the signs and symptoms associated with aging and chronic diseases in the previous chapters. It is presumably used here for aging-related obstructive sleep apnea. Low oxygen levels in the blood and tissues resulting from obstructive sleep apnea can stress the heart, aggravating heart diseases. Intermittent hypoxemia and sleep fragmentation in obstructive sleep apnea can worsen glucose dysmetabolism in diabetics. Diabetic neuropathy can affect respiratory reflexes. Diabetes and its complications are therefore frequently comorbid with obstructive sleep apnea, as we see in Table 3.2.

3.3. Hyperventilation

Hyperventilation is fast and deep breathing. With hyperventilation, one exhales more than inhales, dropping the carbon dioxide concentration in the blood. Complications of hyperventilation include dizziness, headache, numbness in hands and feet, spasm of hand and foot muscles. Causes of hyperventilation are usually emotional, including anxiety and panic.

Table 3.3. Herbal prescriptions for hyperventilation

<table>
<tr><td colspan="2">Hyperventilation: https://meshb.nlm.nih.gov/record/ui?ui=D006985.</td></tr>
<tr><td colspan="2">Common prescriptions:</td></tr>
<tr><td colspan="2">Gāncǎoxiǎomàidàzǎotāng 5g cháihújiālónggǔmǔlìtāng 5g zhúrú 1g yèjiāoténg 1g yuǎnzhì 1g
Gāncǎoxiǎomàidàzǎotāng 5g cháihújiālónggǔmǔlìtāng 5g zhúrú 1g yùlǐrén 1g cǎojuémíng 1g yuǎnzhì 1g
Gāncǎoxiǎomàidàzǎotāng 5g cháihújiālónggǔmǔlìtāng 5g zhúrú 1g yèjiāoténg 1g bózǐrén 1g yuǎnzhì 1g
Gāncǎoxiǎomàidàzǎotāng 5g cháihújiālónggǔmǔlìtāng 5g zhúrú 1g yèjiāoténg 1g yuǎnzhì 1g gōuténg 1g</td></tr>
<tr><td colspan="2">Alternative prescriptions:</td></tr>
<tr><td colspan="2">Guīpítāng 5g
Jiāwèixiāoyáosǎn 5g gāncǎoxiǎomàidàzǎotāng 5g
Tiānwángbǔxīndān 5g jiāwèixiāoyáosǎn 5g héhuānpí 1g yèjiāoténg 1g yuǎnzhì 1g
Gāncǎoxiǎomàidàzǎotāng 5g cháihújiālónggǔmǔlìtāng 5g bózǐrén 1g fúshén 1g suānzǎorén 1g yùjīn 1g
Gāncǎoxiǎomàidàzǎotāng 5g suānzǎoréntāng 5g héhuānpí 1g yèjiāoténg 1g</td></tr>
<tr><td colspan="2">Indicated and associated diseases:</td></tr>
<tr><td colspan="2">Unspecified cerebrovascular disease 437.9 (Cerebrovascular disease, unspecified I679); Unspecified condition of brain 348.9 (Disorder of brain, unspecified G939); Cardiovascular disease, unspecified 429.2 (Atherosclerotic heart disease of native coronary artery without angina pectoris I2510); Unspecified disorders of nervous system 349.9 (Disorder of central nervous system, unspecified G969); Neoplasm of unspecified nature of brain 239.6 (Neoplasm of unspecified behavior of brain D496); Malignant neoplasm of nervous system, part unspecified 192.9 (Malignant neoplasm of central nervous system, unspecified C729); Heart disease, unspecified 429.9 (Heart disease, unspecified I519); Unspecified disorder of metabolism 277.9 (Metabolic disorder, unspecified E889); Epilepsy, unspecified 345.9</td></tr>
<tr><td colspan="2">Unspecified cerebrovascular disease 437.9/I679 with hyperventilation D006985.</td></tr>
<tr><td>Bǔyánghuánwǔtāng 5g dānshēn 1g shíchāngpú 1g yuǎnzhì 1g + acupuncture to ♀</td><td>Bǔyánghuánwǔtāng 5g dānshēn 1g shíchāngpú 1g yuǎnzhì 1g + acupuncture to ♂</td></tr>
<tr><td colspan="2">Unspecified condition of brain 348.9/G939 with hyperventilation D006985:</td></tr>
<tr><td>Bǔzhōngyìqìtāng 5g bǔyánghuánwǔtāng 5g to ♀</td><td>Bǔyánghuánwǔtāng 5g dānshēn 1g shíchāngpú 1g yuǎnzhì 1g + acupuncture to ♂</td></tr>
<tr><td colspan="2">Heart disease, unspecified 429.9/I519 with hyperventilation D006985:</td></tr>
<tr><td>Sìnìtāng 5g gānlùyǐn 5g mǔdānpí 1g zhīzǐ 1g huánglián 0g to ♀</td><td>Xuèfǔzhúyūtāng 5g jìshēngshènqìwán 5g dānshēn 2g chuānqī 1g guìzhī 1g guālóurén 1g xièbái 1g to ♂</td></tr>
<tr><td colspan="2">Epilepsy, unspecified 345.9 with hyperventilation D006985:</td></tr>
<tr><td>Tiānwángbǔxīndān 5g jiāwèixiāoyáosǎn 5g tiānmá 1g mǔlì 1g yèjiāoténg 1g gōuténg 1g to ♀</td><td>Tiānwángbǔxīndān 5g tiānmágōuténgyǐn 5g jiāwèixiaoyáosǎn 5g to ♂</td></tr>
</table>

In classical Chinese medical texts, Gāncǎoxiǎomàidàzǎotāng 'nourishes the Heart and calms one's spirits.' Similarly, Cháihújiālónggǔmǔlìtāng 'quells panic and calms one's spirits.' As both are sedative, they are combined here for the panic induced hyperventilation. Heart diseases are associated with hyperventilation through the cardiorespiratory coupling mentioned in previous sections.

Although hyperventilation is known to lower intracranial pressure via hypocapnia, which reduces cerebral blood volume through arterial vasoconstriction, in traumatic brain injury, its effect is not sustained and may cause secondary brain injury such as cerebral ischemia and cerebral hypoxia. Therapeutic use of hyperventilation should therefore carefully weigh its potential benefits and risks (Godoy et al., 2017). Note also that voluntary hyperventilation can trigger seizures in people with absence epilepsy although the mechanism is not known (Salvati and Beenhakker, 2019).

3.4. Snoring

Snoring is hoarse or harsh sound making while one is asleep. It occurs when the parts in the airways, such as the uvula and mouth, relax and then vibrate in breathing. Alcohol consumption may cause snoring as the muscles in the airways are relaxed by alcohol.

Guìzhītāng is used for upper respiratory tract allergy and infection (Wang, 2019) and is thought to be used here for the snoring caused by inflamed and congested airways. Snoring and cerebral infarction were found to be significantly associated (Partinen and Palomaki, 1985). The association could be due to the fact that snoring often co-occurs with obstructive sleep apnea which reduces the amount of oxygen reaching the brain. Tonsillar lymphoma would manifest snoring (Tsou et al., 2004). Qīngyānlìgétāng is today used for pharyngitis, sinusitis and throat pain, and Yínqiàosǎn for sinusitis, rhinitis and throat pain (Wang, 2019).

Table 3.4. Herbal prescriptions for snoring

Snoring: https://meshb.nlm.nih.gov/record/ui?ui=D012913.	
Common prescriptions:	
Guìzhītāng 5g báisháo 1g dàhuáng 0g Guìzhītāng 5g shēngjiāng 1g báisháo 1g dàhuáng 0g Guìzhītāng 5g shēngjiāng 1g guìzhī 1g Guìzhītāng 5g shēngjiāng 1g báisháo 1g guìzhī 1g Guìzhītāng 5g shēngjiāng 1g báisháo 1g	
Alternative prescriptions:	
Guìzhītāng 5g bànxià 1g dàhuáng 0g Guìzhītāng 5g gégēn 1g dàhuáng 0g Guìzhītāng 5g bànxià 1g dàhuáng 0g + acupuncture	
Indicated diseases:	
Unspecified cerebrovascular disease 437.9 (Cerebrovascular disease, unspecified I679); Unspecified condition of brain 348.9 (Disorder of brain, unspecified G939); Cardiovascular disease, unspecified 429.2 (Atherosclerotic heart disease of native coronary artery without angina pectoris I2510); Unspecified disorders of nervous system 349.9 (Disorder of central nervous system, unspecified G969); Unspecified disease of pharynx 478.20 (Other diseases of pharynx J392); Malignant neoplasm of anterior wall of nasopharynx 147.3 (Malignant neoplasm of anterior wall of nasopharynx C113); Reticulosarcoma 200.0; Unspecified disorder of esophagus 530.9 (Disease of esophagus, unspecified K229); Diseases of the jaws 526	
Unspecified cerebrovascular disease 437.9/I679 with snoring D012913:	
Bǔyánghuánwǔtāng 5g chuānqī 1g dānshēn 1g shíchāngpú 1g yuǎnzhì 1g + acupuncture to ♀	Bǔyánghuánwǔtāng 5g chuānqī 1g dānshēn 1g shíchāngpú 1g yuǎnzhì 1g + acupuncture to ♂
Unspecified disease of pharynx 478.20/J392 with snoring D012913:	
Qīngyānligétāng 5g yínqiàosǎn 5g to ♀	Qīngyānligétāng 5g yínqiàosǎn 5g to ♂

3.5. Hoarseness

Hoarseness, or dysphonia, is changes in the vocal voice so that the sound becomes scratchy or raspy. It can be caused by overuse or misuse of the voice. Other causes include laryngitis, acid reflux, vocal nodules, polyps, cysts and tumor.

Jiégěngtāng has long been used for complications of lung abscesses as it 'expels Phlegm and drains abscesses.' Its modern uses are for allergic rhinitis and chronic bronchitis, so are Jiégěng's (Wang, 2019). Thyroid conditions could affect voice quality.

Table 3.5. Herbal prescriptions for hoarseness

Hoarseness: https://meshb.nlm.nih.gov/record/ui?ui=D006685.	
Common prescriptions:	
Jiégěngtāng 5g xuánshēn 2g mǔlì 2g bèimǔ 2g liánqiáo 2g zhīzǐ 1g dàhuáng 0g Jiégěngtāng 5g xuánshēn 2g mǔlì 2g bèimǔ 2g dàzǎo 2g shēngjiāng 2g zhīzǐ 1g liánqiáo 1g dàhuáng 0g Jiégěngtāng 5g xuánshēn 2g mǔlì 2g bèimǔ 2g liánqiáo 2g zhīzǐ 1g Jiégěngtāng 5g xuánshēn 2g mǔlì 2g bèimǔ 2g liánqiáo 2g dàzǎo 1g shēngjiāng 1g zhīzǐ 1g Jiégěngtāng 5g xuánshēn 2g mǔlì 2g bèimǔ 2g dàzǎo 2g shēngjiāng 2g zhīzǐ 1g liánqiáo 1g	
Alternative prescriptions:	
Qīngyānligétāng 5g shāndòugēn 1g shègān 1g Qīngyānligétāng 5g èrchéntāng 3g gégēn 2g dàzǎo 1g liánqiáo 1g Jiégěngtāng 5g dàzǎo 1g shēngjiāng 1g zhīzǐ 1g liánqiáo 1g dàhuáng 0g Guìzhītāng 5g bànxià 1g dàhuáng 0g	
Indicated diseases:	
Unspecified disease of larynx 478.70 (Other diseases of larynx J387); Unspecified disorders of nervous system 349.9 (Disorder of central nervous system, unspecified G969); Unspecified disorder of thyroid 246.9 (Disorder of thyroid, unspecified E079); Malignant neoplasm of endocrine gland, site unspecified 194.9 (Malignant neoplasm of endocrine gland, unspecified C759); Unspecified endocrine disorder 259.9 (Endocrine disorder, unspecified E349); Esophageal reflux 530.81 (Gastro-esophageal reflux disease without esophagitis K219); Malignant neoplasm of larynx 161	
Unspecified disease of larynx 478.70/J387 with hoarseness D006685:	
Yínqiàosǎn 5g jiégěng 3g cāngěrsǎn 3g gānlùyǐn 1g qīngzàojiùfèitāng 1g shíhúsuī 1g yúxīngcǎo 1g to ♀	Yínqiàosǎn 5g jiégěng 2g cāngěrsǎn 2g gānlùyǐn 1g qīngzàojiùfèitāng 1g shíhúsuī 1g yúxīngcǎo 1g to ♂

3.6. Hypoventilation

Hypoventilation is insufficient ventilation to meet the need of respiratory gas exchange required for the cells in our body to function properly. Problems with the central nervous system and muscles of respiration can cause hypoventilation.

Congestion of respiratory airways can cause snoring and hypoventilation. We see here Guìzhītāng's use for hypoventilation, as we see its use for snoring. If myasthenia gravis affects the respiratory system, respiratory muscles are weakened, leading to respiratory dysfunctions including hypoventilation. Obesity hypoventilation can worsen heart diseases because of cardiopulmonary complications (Egea-Santaolalla and Javaheri, 2016).

Table 3.6. Herbal prescriptions for hypoventilation

Hypoventilation: https://meshb.nlm.nih.gov/record/ui?ui=D007040.
Common prescriptions:
Guìzhītāng 5g shēngjiāng 1g báisháo 1g dàhuáng 0g Guìzhītāng 5g báisháo 1g dàhuáng 0g Guìzhītāng 5g shēngjiāng 1g guìzhī 1g Guìzhītāng 5g shēngjiāng 1g guìzhī 1g dàhuáng 0g Guìzhītāng 5g shēngjiāng 1g báisháo 1g
Alternative prescriptions:
Guìzhītāng 5g xìngrén 1g hòupò 1g dàhuáng 0g Guìzhītāng 5g báizhú 2g fùzǐ 2g báisháo 2g fúlíng 2g dǎngshēn 1g shēngjiāng 1g gānjiāng 1g dàhuáng 0g Guìzhītāng 5g gégēn 1g dàhuáng 0g Guìzhītāng 5g báisháo 2g dàhuáng 0g

Table 3.6. (Continued)

Hypoventilation: https://meshb.nlm.nih.gov/record/ui?ui=D007040.	
Indicated diseases:	
Unspecified condition of brain 348.9 (Disorder of brain, unspecified G939); Neoplasm of unspecified nature of brain 239.6 (Neoplasm of unspecified behavior of brain D496); Unspecified disorders of nervous system 349.9 (Disorder of central nervous system, unspecified G969); Malignant neoplasm of nervous system, part unspecified 192.9 (Malignant neoplasm of central nervous system, unspecified C729); Myasthenia gravis without (acute) exacerbation 358.00 (Myasthenia gravis without (acute) exacerbation G7000); Myoneural disorders 358; Heart disease, unspecified 429.9 (Heart disease, unspecified I519); Cardiovascular disease, unspecified 429.2 (Atherosclerotic heart disease of native coronary artery without angina pectoris I2510)	
Unspecified condition of brain 348.9/G939 with hypoventilation D007040:	
Bǔyánghuánwǔtāng 5g + acupuncture to ♀	Bǔyánghuánwǔtāng 5g chuānqī 1g dānshēn 1g shíchāngpú 1g yuǎnzhì 1g + acupuncture to ♂
Myasthenia gravis without (acute) exacerbation 358.00/G7000 with hypoventilation D007040:	
Bǔzhōngyìqìtāng 5g to ♀	Bǔzhōngyìqìtāng 5g jìshēngshènqìwán 5g dùzhòng 1g xùduàn 1g to ♂
Heart disease, unspecified 429.9/I519 with hypoventilation D007040:	
Sìnìtāng 5g gānlùyǐn 5g mǔdānpí 1g zhīzǐ 1g huánglián 0g to ♀	Sìnìtāng 5g gānlùyǐn 5g mǔdānpí 1g zhīzǐ 1g huánglián 0g to ♂

3.7. Hypercapnia

Hypercapnia refers to elevated levels of carbon dioxide in the blood. Hypercapnia is usually caused by lung impairments where the lungs fail to clear carbon dioxide efficiently.

Table 3.7. Herbal prescriptions for hypercapnia

Hypercapnia: https://meshb.nlm.nih.gov/record/ui?ui=D006935.	
Common prescriptions:	
Sìnìtāng 5g bànxià 1g dàhuáng 0g Sìnìtāng 5g bànxià 1g fúlíng 1g dàhuáng 0g Sìnìtāng 5g bànxià 1g yánhúsuǒ 1g dàhuáng 0g Sìnìtāng 5g lǐzhōngtāng 5g bànxià 1g shārén 1g fúlíng 1g	
Alternative prescriptions:	
Zhēnwǔtāng 5g wúzhūyútāng 3g fùzǐ 1g Guìzhītāng 5g gégēn 4g bànxià 2g dàhuáng 0g Sìnìtāng 5g dāngguīsìnìtāng 5g wúzhūyú 1g gānjiāng 1g Sìnìtāng 5g máhuángfùzǐxìxīntāng 5g shēngjiāng 2g guìzhī 2g zhìgāncǎo 1g	
Indicated and associated diseases:	
Unspecified cerebrovascular disease 437.9 (Cerebrovascular disease, unspecified I679); Unspecified condition of brain 348.9 (Disorder of brain, unspecified G939); Cardiovascular disease, unspecified 429.2 (Atherosclerotic heart disease of native coronary artery without angina pectoris I2510); Unspecified disorders of nervous system 349.9 (Disorder of central nervous system, unspecified G969); Heart disease, unspecified 429.9 (Heart disease, unspecified I519); Unspecified congenital anomaly of heart 746.9 (Congenital malformation of cardiac chambers and connections, unspecified Q209, Congenital malformation of heart, unspecified Q249); Unspecified disorder of metabolism 277.9 (Metabolic disorder, unspecified E889); Neoplasm of unspecified nature of brain 239.6 (Neoplasm of unspecified behavior of brain D496)	
Unspecified cerebrovascular disease 437.9/I679 with hypercapnia D006935:	
Bǔyánghuánwǔtāng 5g chuānqī 1g dānshēn 1g shíchāngpú 1g yuǎnzhì 1g + acupuncture to ♀	Bǔyánghuánwǔtāng 5g chuānqī 2g dānshēn 1g shíchāngpú 1g yuǎnzhì 1g + acupuncture to ♂

Hypercapnia: https://meshb.nlm.nih.gov/record/ui?ui=D006935.	
Heart disease, unspecified 429.9/I519 with hypercapnia D006935:	
Sìnìtāng 5g gānlùyǐn 5g mǔdānpí 1g zhīzǐ 1g huánglián 0g to ♀	Sìnìtāng 5g gānlùyǐn 5g mǔdānpí 1g zhīzǐ 1g huánglián 0g to ♂
Unspecified condition of brain 348.9/G939 with hypercapnia D006935:	
Bǔyánghuánwǔtāng 5g chuānqī 1g dānshēn 1g shíchāngpú 1g yuǎnzhì 1g + acupuncture to ♀	Bǔyánghuánwǔtāng 5g chuānqī 1g dānshēn 1g shíchāngpú 1g yuǎnzhì 1g + acupuncture to ♂

Sleep apnea can cause not only nighttime but also daytime hypercapnia (Kawata et al., 2007). Sìnìtāng is used here for hypercapnia as it is used for apnea in Section 3.2. Also noted is that as hypoventilation can lead to hypercapnia, Guìzhītāng is prescribed for hypoventilation-related hypercapnia as we see in the list of alternative prescriptions in the table. Hypercapnia and emergency room length of stay in patients with acute heart failure are associated (Fabre et al., 2021). Hypercapnic acidosis increases the mortality of cerebral injury (Tiruvoipati et al., 2018).

3.8. Hemoptysis

Hemoptysis is coughing up of blood or bloody mucus from the lower respiratory tract including larynx, trachea, bronchi and lungs. Common causes of hemoptysis are bronchitis, lung cancer and lung infections such as tuberculosis and pneumonia. Massive hemoptysis can be caused by fungal infection of the pulmonary system.

Table 3.8. Herbal prescriptions for hemoptysis

Hemoptysis: https://meshb.nlm.nih.gov/record/ui?ui=D006469.	
Common prescriptions:	
Xiǎoqīnglóngtāng 5g xīnyísǎn 5g xiāngshāliùjūnzǐtāng 2g Xiǎoqīnglóngtāng 5g xīnyísǎn 5g xiāngshāliùjūnzǐtāng 5g Xiǎoqīnglóngtāng 5g xīnyísǎn 5g bǔzhōngyìqìtāng 5g	
Alternative prescriptions:	
Xiǎoqīnglóngtāng 5g xīnyísǎn 5g xiāngshāliùjūnzǐtāng 2g yínqiàosǎn 2g Xiǎoqīnglóngtāng 5g xīnyísǎn 3g xiāngshāliùjūnzǐtāng 1g xiāofēngsǎn 1g zhēnrénhuómìngyǐnqùchuānshānjiǎ 1g Xiǎoqīnglóngtāng 5g xīnyísǎn 2g xiāngshāliùjūnzǐtāng 2g bǔzhōngyìqìtāng 2g Xiǎoqīnglóngtāng 5g xīnyísǎn 5g xiāngshāliùjūnzǐtāng 5g gégēntāng 5g	
Indicated diseases:	
Other dermatoses 702; Aspergillosis 117.3 (Aspergillosis, unspecified B449); Dermatomycosis, unspecified 111.9 (Superficial mycosis, unspecified B369); Candidiasis 112; Coccidioidomycosis 114; Histoplasmosis 115; Blastomycotic infection 116; Other mycoses 117; Opportunistic mycoses 118 (Other specified mycoses B488); Dermatophytosis 110; Dermatomycosis, other and unspecified 111; Cardiovascular disease, unspecified 429.2 (Atherosclerotic heart disease of native coronary artery without angina pectoris I2510); Malignant neoplasm of thorax 195.1 (Malignant neoplasm of thorax C761); Pulmonary tuberculosis 011	
Other dermatoses 702 with hemoptysis D006469:	
Jiědúsìwùtāng 5g xiāofēngsǎn 4g zhēnrénhuómìngyǐnqùchuānshānjiǎ 4g huángliánjiědútāng 4g to ♀	Jiědúsìwùtāng 5g xiāofēngsǎn 4g zhēnrénhuómìngyǐn 4g huángliánjiědútāng 4g to ♂
Cardiovascular disease, unspecified 429.2/I2510 with hemoptysis D006469:	
Yùzhú 5g sìnìtāng 5g mǔdānpí 1g zhīzǐ 1g huánglián 1g to ♀	Sìnìtāng 5g gānlùyǐn 5g mǔdānpí 1g zhīzǐ 1g huánglián 0g to ♂
Malignant neoplasm of thorax 195.1/C761 with hemoptysis D006469:	
Xiǎoqīnglóngtāng 5g xiāngshāliùjūnzǐtāng 5g bǔzhōngyìqìtāng 5g to ♀	Xiǎoqīnglóngtāng 5g xiāngshāliùjūnzǐtāng 5g bǔzhōngyìqìtāng 5g to ♂

Xiǎoqīnglóngtāng ‘stops coughs, subdues gasps’ and is used here for hemoptysis. Since both the skin and respiratory tract expose to the air, dermatoses and respiratory disorders can be considered as different demonstrations of a common immune response mediated by neutrophils (Salem et al., 2019). Mitral stenosis reduces blood flow into the heart to congest and then rupture the pulmonary vessels, leading to hemoptysis.

3.9. Cheyne-Stokes Respiration

Cheyne-Stokes respiration is an abnormal pattern of respiration where apnea or shallow breath alternate with deep breath and the alternation recurs. Damage to the respiratory center by brain tumor, encephalitis and brain injury can cause Cheyne-Stokes respiration.

Table 3.9. Herbal prescriptions for Cheyne-Stokes respiration

Cheyne-Stokes Respiration: https://meshb.nlm.nih.gov/record/ui?ui=D002639.	
Common prescriptions:	
Sìnìtāng 5g bànxià 1g dàhuáng 0g Sìnìtāng 5g guìzhī 1g máhuáng 1g xìxīn 1g Sìnìtāng 5g shēngjiāng 1g guìzhī 1g Sìnìtāng 5g rénshēn 1g bànxià 1g dàhuáng 0g	
Alternative prescriptions:	
Sìnìtāng 5g dàhuáng 0g Sìnìtāng 5g rénshēn 1g dàhuáng 0g Sìnìtāng 5g bànxià 1g Sìnìtāng 5g bànxià 1g yánhúsuǒ 1g dàhuáng 0g	
Indicated diseases:	
Congestive heart failure, unspecified 428.0 (Right heart failure due to left heart failure I50814, Heart failure, unspecified I509); Heart disease, unspecified 429.9 (Heart disease, unspecified I519); Cardiovascular disease, unspecified 429.2 (Atherosclerotic heart disease of native coronary artery without angina pectoris I2510); Secondary cardiomyopathy, unspecified 425.9 (Cardiomyopathy due to drug and external agent I427); Cardiac arrest 427.5 (Cardiac arrest, cause unspecified I469); Unspecified condition of brain 348.9 (Disorder of brain, unspecified G939); Unspecified disorders of nervous system 349.9 (Disorder of central nervous system, unspecified G969)	
Congestive heart failure, unspecified 428.0/I50814,I509 with Cheyne-Stokes respiration D002639:	
Shēngmàiyǐn 5g to ♀	Shēngmàiyǐn 5g zhēnwǔtāng 5g dānshēn 1g to ♂
Secondary cardiomyopathy, unspecified 425.9/I427 with Cheyne-Stokes respiration D002639:	
Xuèfǔzhúyūtāng 5g dānshēn 2g chuānqī 1g guìzhī 1g guālóurén 1g xièbái 1g to ♀	Xuèfǔzhúyūtāng 5g dānshēn 2g chuānqī 1g guìzhī 1g guālóurén 1g xièbái 1g to ♂
Cardiac arrest 427.5/I469 with Cheyne-Stokes respiration D002639:	
Zhēnwǔtāng 5g fùzǐ 1g xìxīn 1g to ♀	Zhēnwǔtāng 5g fùzǐ 1g gānjiāng 1g to ♂
Heart disease, unspecified 429.9/I519 with Cheyne-Stokes respiration D002639:	
Sìnìtāng 5g gānlùyǐn 5g mǔdānpí 1g zhīzǐ 1g huánglián 0g to ♀	Sìnìtāng 5g gānlùyǐn 5g to ♂
Unspecified condition of brain 348.9/G939 with Cheyne-Stokes respiration D002639:	
Xiǎoxùmìngtāng 5g bǔyánghuánwǔtāng 5g to ♀	Bǔyánghuánwǔtāng 5g chuānqī 1g dānshēn 1g shíchāngpú 1g yuǎnzhì 1g + acupuncture to ♂

Dying people take Cheyne-Stokes breathing and use of Sìnìtāng here is believed to try to resuscitate the ‘collapsing Yang.’ People with congestive heart failure have low cardiac output and recurrent hypoxia which can cause instability in the respiratory feedback control, leading to Cheyne-Stokes respiration.

3.10. Sneezing

Sneezing is a sudden and forceful expulsion of air or liquid droplets from the lungs through the nose and mouth. It is an involuntary reaction of the body to remove airborne irritants and pathogens from the nose and throat. Pollutants, pollen, perfume, allergens, cold air and pungent food can trigger a sneeze.

Table 3.10. Herbal prescriptions for sneezing

Sneezing: https://meshb.nlm.nih.gov/record/ui?ui=D012912.	
Common prescriptions:	
Jiégěngtāng 5g xuánshēn 2g mǔlì 2g bèimǔ 2g liánqiáo 2g zhīzǐ 1g dàhuáng 0g Jiégěngtāng 5g xuánshēn 2g mǔlì 2g bèimǔ 2g liánqiáo 2g zhīzǐ 1g Guìzhītāng 5g shēngjiāng 1g báisháo 1g dàhuáng 0g Jiégěngtāng 5g xuánshēn 2g mǔlì 2g bèimǔ 2g dàzǎo 2g shēngjiāng 2g zhīzǐ 1g liánqiáo 1g dàhuáng 0g Jiégěngtāng 5g xuánshēn 2g mǔlì 2g bèimǔ 2g liánqiáo 2g dàzǎo 1g shēngjiāng 1g zhīzǐ 1g	
Alternative prescriptions:	
Guìzhītāng 5g shēngjiāng 1g guìzhī 1g dàhuáng 0g Jiégěngtāng 5g xuánshēn 2g mǔlì 2g bèimǔ 2g liánqiáo 2g dàzǎo 2g shēngjiāng 2g zhīzǐ 1g Jiégěngtāng 5g xuánshēn 2g mǔlì 2g bèimǔ 2g liánqiáo 2g shānzhīzǐ 1g Guìzhītāng 5g bànxià 1g báisháo 1g dàhuáng 0g Jiégěngtāng 5g xuánshēn 2g mǔlì 2g bèimǔ 2g dàhuáng 0g	
Indicated and associated diseases:	
Unspecified cerebrovascular disease 437.9 (Cerebrovascular disease, unspecified I679); Unspecified condition of brain 348.9 (Disorder of brain, unspecified G939); Cardiovascular disease, unspecified 429.2 (Atherosclerotic heart disease of native coronary artery without angina pectoris I2510); Unspecified disorders of nervous system 349.9 (Disorder of central nervous system, unspecified G969); Unspecified disorder of orbit 376.9 (Unspecified disorder of orbit H059); Disorder of eye, unspecified 379.90 (Unspecified disorder of eye and adnexa H579); Heart disease, unspecified 429.9 (Heart disease, unspecified I519); Neoplasm of unspecified nature of brain 239.6 (Neoplasm of unspecified behavior of brain D496)	
Unspecified cerebrovascular disease 437.9/I679 with sneezing D012912:	
Bǔyánghuánwǔtāng 5g sānqī 1g dānshēn 1g shíchāngpú 1g yuǎnzhì 1g + acupuncture to ♀	Bǔyánghuánwǔtāng 5g chuānqī 1g dānshēn 1g shíchāngpú 1g yuǎnzhì 1g + acupuncture to ♂
Unspecified condition of brain 348.9/G939 with sneezing D012912:	
Bǔyánghuánwǔtāng 5g chuānqī 1g dānshēn 1g shíchāngpú 1g yuǎnzhì 1g + acupuncture to ♀	Bǔyánghuánwǔtāng 5g + acupuncture to ♂
Unspecified disorder of orbit 376.9/H059 with sneezing D012912:	
Qǐjúdìhuángwán 5g xǐgānmíngmùtāng 5g zīshènmíngmùtāng 5g to ♀	Qǐjúdìhuángwán 5g xǐgānmíngmùtāng 5g zīshènmíngmùtāng 5g to ♂
Heart disease, unspecified 429.9/I519 with sneezing D012912:	
Sìnìtāng 5g gānlùyǐn 5g mǔdānpí 1g zhīzǐ 1g huánglián 0g to ♀	Sìnìtāng 5g gānlùyǐn 5g mǔdānpí 1g zhīzǐ 1g huánglián 0g to ♂

As people with allergic rhinitis sneeze a lot, we see here the use of Jiégěngtāng, whose modern use is for allergic rhinitis (Wang, 2019). Sneezing transiently increases blood pressure, driving blood flow into the brain. Induction of sneeze shortly after embolic stroke may therefore improve its recovery (Vanaie et al., 2018). About one in five people in the world sneeze when moving from a dark to a bright space. The mechanism of photic sneeze reflex is not known but connection between the eyes and nose through the fifth cranial nerve is hypothesized. As inflammation stiffens arteries, common allergies including rhinitis and rhinoconjunctivitis and heart disease are linked.

3.11. Hypocapnia

Hypocapnia is low levels of carbon dioxide in the blood. Irritation or disease of the respiratory system can stimulate ventilation, causing hypocapnia. Excessive use of mechanical ventilation in intensive care unit can also cause hypocapnia.

Sìnìtāng is used in Section 3.7 for hypercapnia and is also used here for hypocapnia, which is the opposite of hypercapnia. It is not uncommon for herbal medicines to have bidirectional effects (Peng et al., 2022). It is thought that a disturbance to normocapnia can lead to either hypercapnia or hypocapnia, and the use of Sìnìtāng helps to restore homeostasis by *rebooting* the complex system which self organizes. Comparing the two tables however finds minute differences in the prescriptions in that tranquilizing Rénshēn is used for hypocapnia whereas digestion-aiding Lǐzhōngtāng, Fúlíng and Chuānqī are used for hypercapnia. The difference may reflect the fact that hypocapnia can result from panic derived hyperventilation and hypercapnia from debilitating sleep apnea.

Table 3.11. Herbal prescriptions for hypocapnia

<table>
<tr><td colspan="2">Hypocapnia: https://meshb.nlm.nih.gov/record/ui?ui=D016857.</td></tr>
<tr><td colspan="2">Common prescriptions:</td></tr>
<tr><td colspan="2">Sìnìtāng 5g rénshēn 1g bànxià 1g dàhuáng 0g
Sìnìtāng 5g rénshēn 2g bànxià 2g dàhuáng 0g
Sìnìtāng 5g rénshēn 1g wúzhūyú 1g
Sìnìtāng 5g rénshēn 1g
Sìnìtāng 5g rénshēn 1g bànxià 1g</td></tr>
<tr><td colspan="2">Alternative prescriptions:</td></tr>
<tr><td colspan="2">Sìnìtāng 5g rénshēn 1g dàhuáng 0g
Dāngguīsìnìtāng 5g shēngjiāng 1g wúzhūyú 1g
Sìnìtāng 5g rénshēn 1g bànxià 1g gānjiāng 1g dàhuáng 0g
Sìnìtāng 5g bànxià 1g dàhuáng 0g</td></tr>
<tr><td colspan="2">Indicated and associated diseases:</td></tr>
<tr><td colspan="2">Unspecified cerebrovascular disease 437.9 (Cerebrovascular disease, unspecified I679); Unspecified condition of brain 348.9 (Disorder of brain, unspecified G939); Cardiovascular disease, unspecified 429.2 (Atherosclerotic heart disease of native coronary artery without angina pectoris I2510); Unspecified disorders of nervous system 349.9 (Disorder of central nervous system, unspecified G969); Unspecified severity of birth asphyxia in liveborn infant 768.9 (Other problems with newborn P84); Neoplasm of unspecified nature of brain 239.6 (Neoplasm of unspecified behavior of brain D496); Heart disease, unspecified 429.9 (Heart disease, unspecified I519); Unspecified congenital anomaly of heart 746.9 (Congenital malformation of cardiac chambers and connections, unspecified Q209, Congenital malformation of heart, unspecified Q249)</td></tr>
<tr><td colspan="2">Unspecified cerebrovascular disease 437.9/I679 with hypocapnia D016857:</td></tr>
<tr><td>Bǔyánghuánwǔtāng 5g dānshēn 1g shíchāngpú 1g yuǎnzhì 1g + acupuncture to ♀</td><td>Bǔyánghuánwǔtāng 5g dānshēn 1g shíchāngpú 1g yuǎnzhì 1g + acupuncture to ♂</td></tr>
<tr><td colspan="2">Unspecified condition of brain 348.9/G939 with hypocapnia D016857:</td></tr>
<tr><td>Bǔyánghuánwǔtāng 5g dānshēn 1g shíchāngpú 1g yuǎnzhì 1g + acupuncture to ♀</td><td>Bǔyánghuánwǔtāng 5g chuānqī 1g dānshēn 1g shíchāngpú 1g yuǎnzhì 1g + acupuncture to ♂</td></tr>
<tr><td colspan="2">Heart disease, unspecified 429.9/I519 with hypocapnia D016857:</td></tr>
<tr><td>Sìnìtāng 5g gānlùyǐn 5g mǔdānpí 1g zhīzǐ 1g huánglián 0g to ♀</td><td>Sìnìtāng 5g gānlùyǐn 5g mǔdānpí 1g zhīzǐ 1g huánglián 0g to ♂</td></tr>
</table>

3.12. Fetal Hypoxia

Fetal hypoxia, also known as intrauterine hypoxia, occurs when the fetus is short of adequate supply of oxygen. Placental deficiency due to e.g., umbilical cord occlusion can cause fetal hypoxia. Conditions of the mother such as maternal cardiovascular disease, diabetes, anemia, and smoking can also cause fetal hypoxia.

Table 3.12. Herbal prescriptions for fetal hypoxia

Fetal Hypoxia: https://meshb.nlm.nih.gov/record/ui?ui=D005311.
Common prescriptions:
Gānlùyǐn 5g qīngwèisǎn 5g Gānlùyǐn 5g qīngwèisǎn 5g lóngdǎnxiègāntāng 5g Gānlùyǐn 5g zhībódìhuángwán 5g Gānlùyǐn 5g qīngwèisǎn 5g tiānhuā 1g xuánshēn 1g shíhú 1g
Alternative prescriptions:
Gānlùyǐn 5g jiāwèixiāoyáosǎn 2g bànxiàbáizhútiānmátāng 2g xuèfǔzhúyūtāng 2g dúhuójìshēngtāng 2g yúxīngcǎo 1g dānshēn 0g zhǐqiào 0g gégēn 0g chēqiánzǐ 0g Gānlùyǐn 5g qīngwèisǎn 3g shígāo 1g zhīmǔ 1g Gānlùyǐn 5g zhībódìhuángwán 2g lóngdǎnxiègāntāng 2g Gānlùyǐn 5g zhībódìhuángwán 5g qīngwèisǎn 5g lóngdǎnxiègāntāng 5g Gānlùyǐn 5g xiǎocháihútāng 2g shēngmàiyǐn 2g
Indicated diseases:
Unspecified cerebrovascular disease 437.9 (Cerebrovascular disease, unspecified I679); Unspecified condition of brain 348.9 (Disorder of brain, unspecified G939); Unspecified severity of birth asphyxia in liveborn infant 768.9 (Other problems with newborn P84); Cardiovascular disease, unspecified 429.2 (Atherosclerotic heart disease of native coronary artery without angina pectoris I2510); Unspecified disorders of nervous system 349.9 (Disorder of central nervous system, unspecified G969); Unspecified disorder of metabolism 277.9 (Metabolic disorder, unspecified E889); Unspecified diseases of blood and blood-forming organs 289.9 (Disease of blood and blood-forming organs, unspecified D759); Hemolytic disease of fetus or newborn, due to isoimmunization 773
Unspecified cerebrovascular disease 437.9/I679 with fetal hypoxia D005311:
Bǔyánghuánwǔtāng 5g dānshēn 1g shíchāngpú 1g yuǎnzhì 1g + acupuncture to ♀
Unspecified condition of brain 348.9/G939 with fetal hypoxia D005311:
Bǔyánghuánwǔtāng 5g + acupuncture to ♀

As both Gānlùyǐn and Qīngwèisǎn are these days used for peptic ulcer (Wang, 2019), their use here is thought to address the fetal hypoxia due to maternal anemia, which can result from the bleeding ulcers. Notice that hypoxia and liver fibrosis interact to exacerbate each other (Cai et al., 2021), so do hypoxia and diabetes (Catrina and Zheng, 2021). Modern uses of Lóngdǎnxiègāntāng and Zhībódìhuángwán are respectively for hepatitis and diabetes (Wang, 2019). Herbal prescription composition should focus on the underlying causes of the sign and symptom.

3.13. Anoxia

Anoxia is a state of oxygen depletion in tissues. It is an extreme form of hypoxia. Causes of anoxia include cardiac or respiratory arrest, loss of blood, blockage of blood flow, carbon monoxide or smoke inhalation, and drowning.

Table 3.13. Herbal prescriptions for anoxia

Anoxia: https://meshb.nlm.nih.gov/record/ui?ui=D000860.	
Common prescriptions:	
Sìnìtāng 5g bànxià 1g dàhuáng 0g Sìnìtāng 5g rénshēn 1g dàhuáng 0g Sìnìtāng 5g rénshēn 1g bànxià 1g dàhuáng 0g Sìnìtāng 5g rénshēn 1g bànxià 1g Sìnìtāng 5g rénshēn 1g	
Alternative prescriptions:	
Sìnìtāng 5g bànxià 1g fúlíng 1g dàhuáng 0g Sìnìtāng 5g bànxià 1g yánhúsuǒ 1g dàhuáng 0g Sìnìtāng 5g bànxià 1g rénshēn 1g dàhuáng 0g	
Indicated and associated diseases:	
Cardiovascular disease, unspecified 429.2 (Atherosclerotic heart disease of native coronary artery without angina pectoris I2510); Diabetic retinopathy 362.0; Diabetes with peripheral circulatory disorders 250.7; Unspecified retinal disorder 362.9 (Unspecified retinal disorder H359); Disorder of eye, unspecified 379.90 (Unspecified disorder of eye and adnexa H579); Diabetes mellitus 250; Unspecified endocrine disorder 259.9 (Endocrine disorder, unspecified E349); Unspecified disorder of metabolism 277.9 (Metabolic disorder, unspecified E889); Unspecified diseases of blood and blood-forming organs 289.9 (Disease of blood and blood-forming organs, unspecified D759)	
Cardiovascular disease, unspecified 429.2/I2510 with anoxia D000860:	
Sìnìtāng 5g gānlùyǐn 5g mǔdānpí 1g zhīzǐ 1g huánglián 0g to ♀	Sìnìtāng 5g gānlùyǐn 5g to ♂

Sìnìtāng is prescribed for obstructive sleep apnea and Chenye-Stokes respiration in previous sections. As it 'lifts Yang,' it can be imagined that Sìnìtāng is used to relieve and reverse the dire conditions that require emergent cardiopulmonary resuscitation including anoxia. A case was reported where patients with anoxic coma had cyclic, downward dipping motions of the eye (Ropper, 1981).

3.14. Mouth Breathing

Mouth breathing is breathing through the mouth. People breathe through their mouths when their noses are congested by, for example, colds and flu.

Table 3.14. Herbal prescriptions for mouth breathing

Mouth Breathing: https://meshb.nlm.nih.gov/record/ui?ui=D009058.
Common prescriptions:
Guìzhītāng 5g shēngjiāng 1g báisháo 1g dàhuáng 0g Guìzhītāng 5g wúzhūyútāng 3g fùzǐ 1g gānjiāng 1g Guìzhītāng 5g shēngjiāng 1g guìzhī 1g Guìzhītāng 5g wúzhūyútāng 3g fùzǐ 1g Guìzhītāng 5g shēngjiāng 1g báisháo 1g
Alternative prescriptions:
Guìzhītāng 5g shēngjiāng 0g guìzhī 0g Jiégěngtāng 5g xuánshēn 2g mǔlì 2g bèimǔ 2g zhīzǐ 1g liánqiáo 1g dàhuáng 0g Guìzhītāng 5g gégēn 2g dàhuáng 0g Guìzhītāng 5g bànxià 1g dàhuáng 0g + acupuncture

Mouth Breathing: https://meshb.nlm.nih.gov/record/ui?ui=D009058.	
Indicated and associated diseases:	
Unspecified disease of pharynx 478.20 (Other diseases of pharynx J392); Unspecified disorder of esophagus 530.9 (Disease of esophagus, unspecified K229); Diseases of the jaws 526; Myopathy, unspecified 359.9 (Myopathy, unspecified G729); Myoneural disorders 358; Unspecified disorders of nervous system 349.9 (Disorder of central nervous system, unspecified G969); Dental caries of smooth surface 521.07 (Dental caries on smooth surface limited to enamel K0261, Dental caries on smooth surface penetrating into dentin K0262, Dental caries on smooth surface penetrating into pulp K0263); Unspecified disorder of joint, site unspecified 719.90 (Joint disorder, unspecified M259)	
Unspecified disease of pharynx 478.20/J392 with mouth breathing D009058:	
Guìzhītāng 5g bànxià 1g dàhuáng 0g to ♀	Bànxiàhòupòtāng 5g màiméndōngtāng 5g to ♂
Myopathy, unspecified 359.9/G729 with mouth breathing D009058:	
Huángqíwǔwùtāng 5g dāngguīsìnìtāng 5g dānshēn 1g zhúrú 1g sāngzhī 1g jiānghuáng 1g to ♀	Guīlùèrxiānjiāo 5g to ♂
Dental caries of smooth surface 521.07/K0261,K0262,K0263 with mouth breathing D009058:	
Yùnǚjiān 5g qīngwèisǎn 5g to ♀	Yùnǚjiān 5g qīngwèisǎn 5g to ♂

Guìzhītāng is used in previous sections for snoring and hypoventilation where obstructions of the airways occur. Constant mouth breathing causes a dry mouth which in turn leads to problems with the gums, teeth, jaw joints, throat and esophagus.

3.15. Hyperoxia

Hyperoxia is excessive supply of oxygen to the tissue. As hypoxic tissues and organs are harmful, oxygen therapy is widely used for patients with hypoxemic respiratory failure in intensive care units and emergency rooms.

Table 3.15. Herbal prescriptions for hyperoxia

Hyperoxia: https://meshb.nlm.nih.gov/record/ui?ui=D018496.	
Common prescriptions:	
Sìnìtāng 5g rénshēn 1g bànxià 1g dàhuáng 0g Sìnìtāng 5g rénshēn 1g wúzhūyú 1g Sìnìtāng 5g rénshēn 1g Sìnìtāng 5g rénshēn 1g bànxià 1g gānjiāng 1g Sìnìtāng 5g rénshēn 1g bànxià 1g	
Alternative prescriptions:	
Sìnìtāng 5g bànxià 1g dàhuáng 0g Sìnìtāng 5g rénshēn 2g bànxià 2g dàhuáng 0g Zhēnwǔtāng 5g fùzǐ 1g xìxīn 1g tiáowèichéngqìtāng 0g Sìnìtāng 5g bànxià 1g guìzhī 1g dàhuáng 0g	
Indicated and associated diseases:	
Retrolental fibroplasia 362.21 (Retrolental fibroplasia, unspecified eye H35179); Unspecified retinal disorder 362.9 (Unspecified retinal disorder H359); Disorder of eye, unspecified 379.90 (Unspecified disorder of eye and adnexa H579); Cardiovascular disease, unspecified 429.2 (Atherosclerotic heart disease of native coronary artery without angina pectoris I2510); Diabetic retinopathy 362.0; Diabetes with peripheral circulatory disorders 250.7; Diabetes mellitus 250; Unspecified endocrine disorder 259.9 (Endocrine disorder, unspecified E349); Unspecified disorder of metabolism 277.9 (Metabolic disorder, unspecified E889)	
Retrolental fibroplasia 362.21/H35179 with hyperoxia D018496:	
Qǐjúdìhuángwán 5g zīshènmíngmùtāng 5g to ♀	Qǐjúdìhuángwán 5g zīshènmíngmùtāng 5g to ♂

Table 3.15. (Continued)

Hyperoxia: https://meshb.nlm.nih.gov/record/ui?ui=D018496.	
Cardiovascular disease, unspecified 429.2/I2510 with hyperoxia D018496:	
Sìnìtāng 5g gānlùyǐn 5g mǔdānpí 1g zhīzǐ 1g huánglián 0g to ♀	Sìnìtāng 5g gānlùyǐn 5g mǔdānpí 1g zhīzǐ 1g huánglián 0g to ♂
Unspecified retinal disorder 362.9/H359 with hyperoxia D018496:	
Qǐjúdìhuángwán 5g to ♀	Qǐjúdìhuángwán 5g yìqìcōngmíngtāng 5g xuèfǔzhúyūtāng 2g to ♂

Patients receiving oxygen therapy experience respiratory deficiencies such as sleep apnea, Cheyne-Stokes respiration and hypercapnia where Sìnìtāng is prescribed. This may explain the use of Sìnìtāng for hyperoxia here. Sustained oxygenation was shown to accelerate diabetic wound healing (Guan et al., 2021).

3.16. Dyspnea

Dyspnea, also known as shortness of breath, is a condition characterized by difficulty or labored breathing. Respiratory tract infections such as COVID-19, asthma, chronic obstructive pulmonary disease, and lung cancer can cause dyspnea.

Table 3.16. Herbal prescriptions for dyspnea

Dyspnea: https://meshb.nlm.nih.gov/record/ui?ui=D004417.	
Common prescriptions:	
Máxìnggānshítāng 5g níngsòuwán 5g dōngguāzǐ 1g táorén 1g yìyǐrén 1g lúgēn 1g gégēnhuángqínhuángliántāng 1g dàhuáng 0g fùzǐ 0g xìxīn 0g gégēnhuángqínhuángliántāng 1g dàhuáng 0g fùzǐ 0g	
Alternative prescriptions:	
Xìngsūyǐnyòukē 5g sāngjúyǐn 4g bèimǔ 1g pípáyè 1g púgōngyīng 1g Qīngfèitāng 5g níngsòuwán 5g Màiméndōngtāng 5g zhǐsòusǎn 2g xìngrén 1g bèimǔ 1g Dìngchuǎntāng 5g máxìnggānshítāng 5g bèimǔ 1g sāngbáipí 1g guālóurén 1g huángqín 1g Máxìnggānshítāng 5g níngsòuwán 2g dōngguāzǐ 1g táorén 1g yìyǐrén 1g lúgēn 1g xiǎoqīnglóngtāng 1g gégēnhuángqínhuángliántāng 1g	
Indicated diseases:	
Heart disease, unspecified 429.9 (Heart disease, unspecified I519); Malignant neoplasm of heart 164.1 (Malignant neoplasm of heart C380); Cardiovascular disease, unspecified 429.2 (Atherosclerotic heart disease of native coronary artery without angina pectoris I2510); Reticulosarcoma 200.0; Malignant neoplasm of thorax 195.1 (Malignant neoplasm of thorax C761); Unspecified disease of pharynx 478.20 (Other diseases of pharynx J392); Unspecified disorder of esophagus 530.9 (Disease of esophagus, unspecified K229); Diseases of the jaws 526	
Heart disease, unspecified 429.9/I519 with dyspnea D004417:	
Sìnìtāng 5g gānlùyǐn 5g mǔdānpí 1g zhīzǐ 1g huánglián 0g to ♀	Sìnìtāng 5g gānlùyǐn 5g mǔdānpí 1g zhīzǐ 1g huánglián 0g to ♂
Unspecified disease of pharynx 478.20/J392 with dyspnea D004417:	
Bànxiàhòupòtāng 5g màiméndōngtāng 5g jiégěng 1g to ♀	Bànxiàhòupòtāng 5g màiméndōngtāng 5g jiégěng 1g to ♂

Máxìnggānshítāng 'soothes the Lung, clears Heat, stops cough, quells asthma' and is at this time used for unspecified chronic bronchitis (Wang, 2019). Níngsòuwán literally reads 'quieting cough powder.' Combination of the two formulas is supposed to ease labored breathing.

3.17. Paroxysmal Dyspnea

Paroxysmal dyspnea is sudden feeling of severe shortness of breath when one is sleeping at night. The feeling wakes one up and the breathlessness relieves after one gets up to an upright from a reclining position. Heart and lung diseases can cause dyspnea and paroxysmal nocturnal dyspnea. In particular, when one lies down, redistribution of blood to the chest overloads the heart and congests the lung, causing paroxysmal dyspnea.

Table 3.17. Herbal prescriptions for paroxysmal dyspnea

Paroxysmal Dyspnea: https://meshb.nlm.nih.gov/record/ui?ui=D004418.	
Common prescriptions:	
Sìnìtāng 5g bànxià 1g dàhuáng 0g Guìzhītāng 5g shēngjiāng 1g guìzhī 1g Máhuángfùzǐxìxīntāng 5g shēngjiāng 2g guìzhī 2g zhìgāncǎo 1g Máhuángfùzǐxìxīntāng 5g shēngjiāng 1g guìzhī 1g Guìzhītāng 5g shēngjiāng 1g báisháo 1g	
Alternative prescriptions:	
Guìzhītāng 5g shēngjiāng 1g báisháo 1g dàhuáng 0g Sìnìtāng 5g shēngjiāng 1g guìzhī 1g Sìnìtāng 5g guìzhī 1g máhuáng 1g xìxīn 0g Guìzhītāng 5g gégēn 1g dàhuáng 0g Sìnìtāng 5g rénshēn 1g bànxià 1g	
Indicated diseases:	
Congestive heart failure, unspecified 428.0 (Right heart failure due to left heart failure I50814, Heart failure, unspecified I509); End stage renal disease 585.6 (End stage renal disease N186); Heart disease, unspecified 429.9 (Heart disease, unspecified I519); Cardiovascular disease, unspecified 429.2 (Atherosclerotic heart disease of native coronary artery without angina pectoris I2510); Renal failure, unspecified 586 (Unspecified kidney failure N19); Unspecified congenital anomaly of heart 746.9 (Congenital malformation of cardiac chambers and connections, unspecified Q209, Congenital malformation of heart, unspecified Q249); Atrial fibrillation 427.31 (Unspecified atrial fibrillation I4891)	
Congestive heart failure, unspecified 428.0/I50814,I509 with dyspnea, paroxysmal D004418:	
Shēngmàiyǐn 5g zhēnwǔtāng 5g dānshēn 1g to ♀	Shēngmàiyǐn 5g xuèfǔzhúyūtāng 5g dānshēn 1g yùjīn 1g to ♂
Atrial fibrillation 427.31/I4891 with dyspnea, paroxysmal D004418:	
Zhìgāncǎotāng 5g zhēnwǔtāng 5g to ♀	Zhìgāncǎotāng 5g xuèfǔzhúyūtāng 4g dānshēn 1g xiāngfù 1g yùjīn 1g to ♂

Máhuángfùzǐxìxīntāng has traditionally been used for 'Yang deficient' people who suffer from cold damages. Its modern uses are for chronic sinusitis, and allergic rhinitis (Wang, 2019). We can therefore say that it is used for 'Yang deficient' patients with difficulty breathing. Note that kidney failure leads to building up of fluids in the lungs, exacerbating paroxysmal dyspnea. A comparison of the prescriptions in the two tables suggests that paroxysmal dyspnea is a more serious or terminal condition than dyspnea as Sìnìtāng is also used for such urgencies as apnea and anoxia.

3.18. Tachypnea

Tachypnea is shallow and rapid breathing, at a rate higher than twenty breaths per minute, when one has too little oxygen or too much carbon dioxide in the body. Causes of tachypnea include asthma, pulmonary embolism, pneumonia, carbon monoxide poisoning, anemia, heart failure and sepsis.

Table 3.18. Herbal prescriptions for tachypnea

Tachypnea: https://meshb.nlm.nih.gov/record/ui?ui=D059246.	
Common prescriptions:	
Sìnìtāng 5g shēngjiāng 1g guìzhī 1g Sìnìtāng 5g rénshēn 1g bànxià 1g dàhuáng 0g Sìnìtāng 5g rénshēn 1g wúzhūyú 1g Sìnìtāng 5g rénshēn 1g Sìnìtāng 5g shēngjiāng 1g guìzhī 1g xìxīn 1g	
Alternative prescriptions:	
Sìnìtāng 5g shēngjiāng 1g guìzhī 1g dàhuáng 0g Sìnìtāng 5g guìzhī 1g máhuáng 1g xìxīn 0g Sìnìtāng 5g bànxià 1g Sìnìtāng 5g rénshēn 1g bànxià 1g yánhúsuǒ 1g dàhuáng 0g Sìnìtāng 5g rénshēn 2g yìzhìrén 2g fùpénzǐ 2g dàhuáng 0g	
Indicated diseases:	
Unspecified cerebrovascular disease 437.9 (Cerebrovascular disease, unspecified I679); Unspecified condition of brain 348.9 (Disorder of brain, unspecified G939); Cardiovascular disease, unspecified 429.2 (Atherosclerotic heart disease of native coronary artery without angina pectoris I2510); Unspecified disorders of nervous system 349.9 (Disorder of central nervous system, unspecified G969); Epilepsy, unspecified 345.9; Heart disease, unspecified 429.9 (Heart disease, unspecified I519); Unspecified congenital anomaly of heart 746.9 (Congenital malformation of cardiac chambers and connections, unspecified Q209, Congenital malformation of heart, unspecified Q249); Unspecified disorder of metabolism 277.9 (Metabolic disorder, unspecified E889); Neoplasm of unspecified nature of brain 239.6 (Neoplasm of unspecified behavior of brain D496)	
Unspecified cerebrovascular disease 437.9/I679 with tachypnea D059246:	
Bǔyánghuánwǔtāng 5g chuānqī 2g dānshēn 1g shíchāngpú 1g yuǎnzhì 1g + acupuncture to ♀	Bǔyánghuánwǔtāng 5g chuānqī 2g dānshēn 1g shíchāngpú 1g yuǎnzhì 1g + acupuncture to ♂
Epilepsy, unspecified 345.9 with tachypnea D059246:	
Yìgānsǎn 5g guìzhījiālónggǔmǔlìtāng 5g xiōngqiōng 1g dāngguī 1g to ♀	Yìgānsǎn 5g cháihújiālónggǔmǔlìtāng 5g shíchāngpú 1g yuǎnzhì 1g to ♂
Heart disease, unspecified 429.9/I519 with tachypnea D059246:	
Sìnìtāng 5g gānlùyǐn 5g mǔdānpí 1g zhīzǐ 1g huánglián 0g to ♀	Sìnìtāng 5g gānlùyǐn 5g mǔdānpí 1g zhīzǐ 1g huánglián 0g to ♂
Unspecified condition of brain 348.9/G939 with tachypnea D059246:	
Bǔyánghuánwǔtāng 5g chuānqī 1g dānshēn 1g shíchāngpú 1g yuǎnzhì 1g + acupuncture to ♀	Bǔyánghuánwǔtāng 5g tiānmá 1g shíchāngpú 1g yuǎnzhì 1g gōuténg 1g + acupuncture to ♂

Sìnìtāng is seen in previous sections for signs and symptoms including obstructive sleep apnea, Cheyne-Stokes respiration, anoxia and hyperoxia, any of which involves oxygen deprivation. Sìnìtāng is presumably used here again to help kick-start the body's self-healing process and restore homeostasis. Irregular breathing, including tachypnea, is associated with lesions in the medulla of the brain (North and Jennett, 1974).

3.19. Infantile Apparent Life-Threatening Event

Infantile apparent life-threatening event describes an episode of the infant displaying a certain combination of apnea, skin color change, muscle tone change, and choking, gagging and coughing. Although the event looks frightening and can recur, most infants return to normal after the episode. Causes of infantile apparent life-threatening event are unknown but convulsion and gastroesophageal reflux are frequently suspected.

Sháoyàogāncǎotāng is used in the first chapter to treat a myriad of neuromuscular conditions. It is therefore supposed to be prescribed here with respect to the neuromuscular abnormalities in infants presenting with an apparent life-threatening event.

Table 3.19. Herbal prescriptions for infantile apparent life-threatening event

Infantile Apparent Life-Threatening Event: https://meshb.nlm.nih.gov/record/ui?ui=D057768.	
Common prescriptions:	
Sháoyàogāncǎotāng 5g shūjīnghuóxuètāng 5g dāngguīniāntòngtāng 5g + acupuncture Sháoyàogāncǎotāng 5g shūjīnghuóxuètāng 5g + acupuncture	
Alternative prescriptions:	
Zhènggǔzǐjīndān 5g sháoyàogāncǎotāng 5g dāngguīniāntòngtāng 5g sānqī 2g yánhúsuǒ 2g sūmù 2g xùduàn 2g mòyào 1g rǔxiāng 1g + acupuncture Zhènggǔzǐjīndān 5g Jiāwèixiāoyáosǎn 5g zhībódìhuángwán 4g nǚzhēnzǐ 1g niúxī 1g gǒuqǐzǐ 1g màiméndōng 1g dìhuáng 0g Jiāwèixiāoyáosǎn 5g gāncǎoxiǎomàidàzǎotāng 5g sháoyàogāncǎotāng 5g Jiāwèixiāoyáosǎn 5g cháihúshūgāntāng 5g héhuānpí 4g yuǎnzhì 1g suānzǎorén 1g	
Indicated diseases:	
Cardiovascular disease, unspecified 429.2 (Atherosclerotic heart disease of native coronary artery without angina pectoris I2510); Unspecified disorder of metabolism 277.9 (Metabolic disorder, unspecified E889); Unspecified condition of brain 348.9 (Disorder of brain, unspecified G939); Unspecified disorders of nervous system 349.9 (Disorder of central nervous system, unspecified G969)	
Cardiovascular disease, unspecified 429.2/I2510 with infantile apparent life-threatening event D057768:	
Sìnìtāng 5g gānlùyǐn 5g mǔdānpí 1g zhīzǐ 1g huánglián 0g to ♀	Xuèfǔzhúyūtāng 5g zhìgāncǎotāng 5g to ♂
Unspecified disorder of metabolism 277.9/E889 with infantile apparent life-threatening event D057768:	
Rénshēnbàidúsǎn 5g xiǎocháihútāngqùrénshēn 5g yīnchénhāotāng 2g mùxiāng 1g yùjīn 1g to ♀	Dānshēn 5g tiānmágōuténgyǐn 5g sǎnzhǒngkuìjiāntāng 5g bǔyánghuánwǔtāng 5g to ♂
Unspecified condition of brain 348.9/G939 with infantile apparent life-threatening event D057768:	
Bǔyánghuánwǔtāng 5g + acupuncture to ♀	Bǔyánghuánwǔtāng 5g shíchāngpú 1g yuǎnzhì 1g + acupuncture to ♂

References

Cai, J., Hu, M., Chen, Z., & Ling, Z. (2021). The roles and mechanisms of hypoxia in liver fibrosis. *Journal of Translational Medicine*, *19*, 186. https://doi.org/10.1186/s12967-021-02854-x.

Catrina, S. B., & Zheng, X. (2021). Hypoxia and hypoxia-inducible factors in diabetes and its complications. *Diabetologia*, *64*(4), 709–716. https://doi.org/10.1007/s00125-021-05380-z.

Egea-Santaolalla, C., & Javaheri, S. (2016). Obesity Hypoventilation Syndrome. *Current Sleep Medicine Reports*, *2*, 12–19. https://doi.org/10.1007/s40675-016-0035-2.

Fabre, M., Fehlmann, C. A., Gartner, B., Zimmermann-Ivoll, C. G., Rey, F., Sarasin, F., & Suppan, L. (2021). Prehospital arterial hypercapnia in acute heart failure is associated with admission to acute care units and emergency room length of stay: a retrospective cohort study. *BMC Emergency Medicine*, *21*, 14. https://doi.org/10.1186/s12873-021-00411-9.

Godoy, D. A., Seifi, A., Garza, D., Lubillo-Montenegro, S., & Murillo-Cabezas, F. (2017). Hyperventilation Therapy for Control of Posttraumatic Intracranial Hypertension. *Frontiers in Neurology*, *8*, 250. https://doi.org/10.3389/fneur.2017.00250.

Grabczak, E., Stec, S., Dąbrowska, M., Plevkova, J., & Krenke, R. (2020). Cough as a Cause and Consequence of Heart Dysfunction - Current State of Art. *Physiological Research*, *69* (Suppl 1), S105–S121. https://doi.org/10.33549/physiolres.934408.

Guan, Y., Niu, H., Liu, Z., Dang, Y., Shen, J., Zayed, M., Ma, L., & Guan, J. (2021). Sustained oxygenation accelerates diabetic wound healing by promoting epithelialization and angiogenesis and decreasing inflammation. *Science Advances*, *7*(35), eabj0153. https://doi.org/10.1126/sciadv.abj0153.

Kawata, N., Tatsumi, K., Terada, J., Tada, Y., Tanabe, N., Takiguchi, Y., & Kuriyama, T. (2007). Daytime Hypercapnia in Obstructive Sleep Apnea Syndrome. *Chest*, *132*(6), 1832–1838. https://doi.org/10.1378/chest.07-0673.

Misery, L., Shourick, J., Reychler, G., & Taieb, C. (2021). Association between chronic idiopathic cough and sensitive skin syndromes is a new argument in favor of common neuropathic pathways: results from a survey on 4050 subjects. *Scientific Reports*, *11*, 16976. https://doi.org/10.1038/s41598-021-96608-w.

North, J. B., & Jennett, S. (1974). Abnormal Breathing Patterns Associated with Acute Brain Damage. *Archives of Neurology*, *31*(5), 338–344. https://doi.org/10.1001/archneur.1974.00490410086010.

Partinen, M., & Palomaki, H. (1985). Snoring and Cerebral Infarction. *The Lancet*, *326*(8468), 1325–1326. https://doi.org/10.1016/s0140-6736(85)92625-x.

Peng, X., Tang, F., Yang, Y., Li, T., Hu, X., Li, S., Wu, W., & He, K. (2022). Bidirectional effects and mechanisms of traditional Chinese medicine. *Journal of Ethnopharmacology*, *298*, 115578. https://doi.org/10.1016/j.jep.2022.115578.

Ropper, A. H. (1981). Ocular Dipping in Anoxic Coma. *Archives of Neurology*, *38*(5), 297–299. https://doi.org/10.1001/archneur.1981.00510050063010.

Salem, I., Kimak, M., Conic, R., Bragazzi, N. L., Watad, A., Adawi, M., Bridgewood, C., Pacifico, A., Santus, P., Rizzi, M., Petrou, S., Colombo, D., Fiore, M., Pigatto, P. D. M., & Damiani, G. (2019). Neutrophilic Dermatoses and Their Implication in Pathophysiology of Asthma and Other Respiratory Comorbidities: A Narrative Review. *BioMed Research International*, *2019*, 7315274, 1–17. https://doi.org/10.1155/2019/7315274.

Salvati, K. A., & Beenhakker, M. P. (2019). Out of thin air: Hyperventilation-triggered seizures. *Brain Research*, *1703*, 41–52. https://doi.org/10.1016/j.brainres.2017.12.037.

Tiruvoipati, R., Pilcher, D., Botha, J., Buscher, H., Simister, R., & Bailey, M. (2018). Association of Hypercapnia and Hypercapnic Acidosis With Clinical Outcomes in Mechanically Ventilated Patients With Cerebral Injury. *JAMA Neurology*, *75*(7), 818–826. https://doi.org/10.1001/jamaneurol.2018.0123.

Tsou, Y. A., Cheng, Y. K., Lin, C. D., Chang, W. C., & Tsai, M. H. (2004). Small B cell lymphocytic lymphoma presenting as obstructive sleep apnea. *World Journal of Surgical Oncology*, *2*(1), 26. https://doi.org/10.1186/1477-7819-2-26.

Vanaie, M., Boroujeni, M. V., Abarghuie, H. M., Pourshanazari, A. A, & Rezazadeh, H. (2018). The Effect of Sneezing on the Reduction of Infarct Volume and the Improvement of Neurological Deficits in Male Rats. *Advanced Biomedical Research*, *7*, 142. https://doi.org/10.4103/abr.abr_119_18.

Wang, S. C. (2019). *Clinical Herbal Prescriptions: Principles and Practices of Herbal Formulations from Deep Learning Health Insurance Herbal Prescription Big Data*. WSPC. https://doi.org/10.1142/11211.

Chapter 4

Signs and Symptoms, Digestive

Organisms consume food and water for their growth, survival and reproduction. The process of food ingestion, breakdown, nutrient absorption and waste elimination is called digestion. The human digestive system consists of a series of hollow organs including the mouth, esophagus, stomach, small intestine, large intestine, rectum and anus, all connected together to form the gastrointestinal tract. Additionally, solid organs including the salivary glands, liver, gallbladder and pancreas secrete digestive enzymes into the tract to help breaking down of large food into smaller molecules including amino acids, fatty acids, sugars, minerals and vitamins for better absorption.

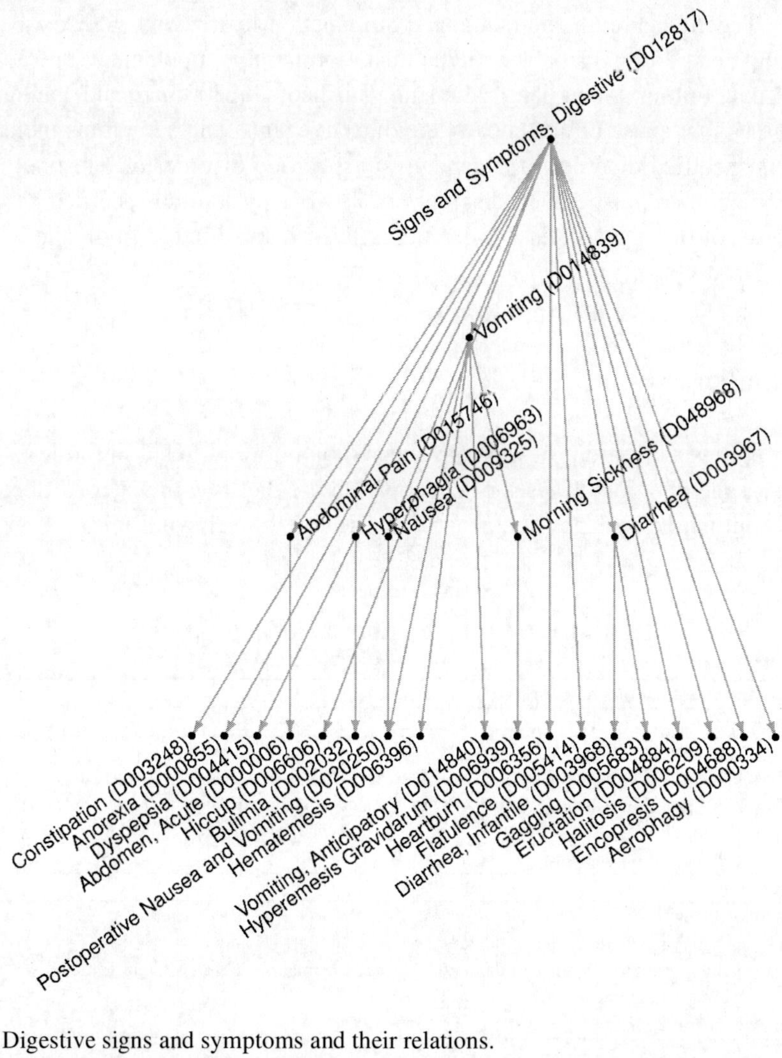

Figure 4.1. Digestive signs and symptoms and their relations.

The digestive process becomes involuntary after the food has been chewed and has passed through the larynx. Our enteric nervous system, a division of the autonomic nervous system, coordinates the wave-like contraction and relaxation motion of the gastrointestinal muscles to propel the food along the tract. Production and secretion of digestive enzymes in the stomach, liver and pancreas are triggered by hormones from the endocrine cells in the walls of the stomach and small intestine. Circulation of blood carries away the nutrients to where they are needed.

Finally, as food is foreign to the body, immune cells abound in the walls of the gastrointestinal tract. Immune responses from the immune inductive sites in the digestive system called gut-associated lymphoid tissues help maintain homeostasis between immune defense against foreign antigens and pathogens and immune tolerance for dietary antigens and commensal microbiome. Therefore, the digestive system works together with the nervous system, endocrine system, cardiovascular system and immune system to complete its tasks. Problems with any of the systems and their collaboration can lead to digestive signs and symptoms shown in Figure 4.1.

The formulas commonly used for the digestive signs and symptoms of Figure 4.1 are Guìzhītāng, Gégēnhuángqínhuángliántāng, Sìnìtāng, Mázǐrénwán, Sháoyàogāncǎotāng, Rùnchángwán, and Wǔlíngsǎn. The herbs that commonly supplement the formulas are Dàhuáng, Bànxià, Fúlíng, Shēngjiāng, Mùxiāng, Báisháo, Guìzhī, Fùzǐ, and Yánhúsuǒ.

The diseases that cause or accompany the digestive signs and symptoms include diseases of the jaws, unspecified disorder of esophagus, unspecified disorder of intestine, unspecified disorder of metabolism, unspecified disorders of nervous system, unspecified cardiovascular disease, diseases of the oral soft tissues excluding lesions specific for gingiva and tongue, and unspecified heart disease.

4.1. Constipation

Constipation is fewer or harder bowel movements than normal, resulting in less, difficult or incomplete passage of stools. Causes of constipation are diet low in water or fiber, change in diet or daily routine, lack of physical activities, irritable bowel syndrome, cancer, stress and medications.

Table 4.1. Herbal prescriptions for constipation

Constipation: https://meshb.nlm.nih.gov/record/ui?ui=D003248.
Common prescriptions:
Mázǐrénwán 5g rùnchángwán 5g dàhuáng 1g hòupò 1g zhǐshí 1g Mázǐrénwán 5g rùnchángwán 5g dàhuáng 1g Mázǐrénwán 5g rùnchángwán 5g dàhuáng 1g xuánshēn 1g dìhuáng 1g màiméndōng 1g Mázǐrénwán 5g rùnchángwán 5g Mázǐrénwán 5g rùnchángwán 4g dàhuáng 1g
Alternative prescriptions:
Rùnchángwán 5g dàhuáng 0g Mázǐrénwán 5g rùnchángwán 5g xuánshēn 1g dìhuáng 1g màiméndōng 1g + acupuncture Mázǐrénwán 5g rùnchángwán 5g xuánshēn 1g dìhuáng 1g bózǐrén 1g màiméndōng 1g zǐwǎn 1g Mázǐrénwán 5g bǔzhōngyìqìtāng 5g Rùnchángwán 5g dàhuáng 2g hòupò 1g zhǐshí 1g

Constipation: https://meshb.nlm.nih.gov/record/ui?ui=D003248.	
Indicated diseases:	
Constipation 564.0; Myoneural disorders 358; Neurofibromatosis, type 1 [von recklinghausen's disease] 237.71 (Neurofibromatosis, type 1 Q8501); Unspecified disorders of nervous system 349.9 (Disorder of central nervous system, unspecified G969); Neurofibromatosis 237.7; Malignant neoplasm of nervous system, part unspecified 192.9 (Malignant neoplasm of central nervous system, unspecified C729); Unspecified endocrine disorder 259.9 (Endocrine disorder, unspecified E349); Malignant neoplasm of ovary 183.0 (Malignant neoplasm of unspecified ovary C569); Unspecified disorder of female genital organs 629.9 (Unspecified condition associated with female genital organs and menstrual cycle N949); Malignant neoplasm of other and unspecified female genital organs 184; Malignant neoplasm of endocrine gland, site unspecified 194.9 (Malignant neoplasm of endocrine gland, unspecified C759); Perforation of intestine 569.83 (Perforation of intestine (nontraumatic) K631); Unspecified disorder of intestine 569.9 (Disease of intestine, unspecified K639); Unspecified intestinal obstruction 560.9 (Partial intestinal obstruction, unspecified as to cause K56600, Complete intestinal obstruction, unspecified as to cause K56601, Unspecified intestinal obstruction, unspecified as to partial versus complete obstruction K56609)	
Constipation 564.0 with constipation D003248:	
Mázǐrénwán 5g rùnchángwán 5g xuánshēn 1g dìhuáng 1g màiméndōng 1g to ♀	Mázǐrénwán 5g rùnchángwán 5g xuánshēn 1g dìhuáng 1g màiméndōng 1g to ♂
Perforation of intestine 569.83/K631 with constipation D003248:	
Tiáowèichéngqìtāng 5g to ♀	Tiáowèichéngqìtāng 5g dǐdāngtāng 2g to ♂

Mázǐrénwán has traditionally been used for dry and hard stools while Rùnchángwán for infrequent bowel movements. They are combined here to enhance the effect of the prescriptions for constipation. Neurofibromatosis type 1, a rare condition caused by mutations in a tumor suppressor gene, can be considered a generalized gastrointestinal motility disorder due to the high prevalence of constipation in adult patients with neurofibromatosis type 1 (Ejerskov et al., 2017).

4.2. Anorexia

People with anorexia, a serious eating disorder, try to keep their weights as low as possible by food restriction and excessive exercising, leading to a body mass index lower than what is considered healthy of their age. The exact causes of anorexia are unknown. Malnutrition in the patients with anorexia can lead to anemia, bone loss, muscle loss, fatigue, dysfunction of organs including the heart, kidney and liver, and digestive symptoms such as constipation.

Table 4.2. Herbal prescriptions for anorexia

Anorexia: https://meshb.nlm.nih.gov/record/ui?ui=D000855.
Common prescriptions:
Guìzhītāng 5g báisháo 1g dàhuáng 0g Guìzhītāng 5g dàhuáng 0g Guìzhītāng 5g bànxià 1g dàhuáng 0g Guìzhītāng 5g báizhú 1g fúlíng 1g Guìzhītāng 5g báisháo 1g
Alternative prescriptions:
Guìzhītāng 5g báisháo 2g dàhuáng 0g Guìzhītāng 5g gégēn 1g dàhuáng 0g Guìzhītāng 5g màiyá 2g huángqín 1g xiāngfù 1g dàhuáng 0g Guìzhītāng 5g bànxià 1g shēngjiāng 1g guìzhī 1g dàhuáng 0g

Table 4.2. (Continued)

Anorexia: https://meshb.nlm.nih.gov/record/ui?ui=D000855.	
Indicated and associated diseases:	
Cardiovascular disease, unspecified 429.2 (Atherosclerotic heart disease of native coronary artery without angina pectoris I2510); Multiple myeloma 203.0; Unspecified hemorrhagic conditions 287.9 (Hemorrhagic condition, unspecified D699); Unspecified diseases of blood and blood-forming organs 289.9 (Disease of blood and blood-forming organs, unspecified D759); Unspecified disorder of liver 573.9 (Liver disease, unspecified K769); Malignant neoplasm of liver, not specified as primary or secondary 155.2 (Malignant neoplasm of liver, not specified as primary or secondary C229); Diseases of the jaws 526; Heart disease, unspecified 429.9 (Heart disease, unspecified I519); Eating disorder, unspecified 307.50 (Eating disorder, unspecified F509)	
Cardiovascular disease, unspecified 429.2/I2510 with anorexia D000855:	
Yùzhú 5g sìnìtāng 5g mǔdānpí 1g zhīzǐ 1g huánglián 0g to ♀	Yùzhú 5g sìnìtāng 5g zhìgāncǎotāng 5g to ♂
Unspecified disorder of liver 573.9/K769 with anorexia D000855:	
Jiāwèixiāoyáosǎn 5g cháihúshūgāntāng 5g to ♀	Xuèfǔzhúyūtāng 5g cháihúshūgāntāng 5g to ♂
Heart disease, unspecified 429.9/I519 with anorexia D000855:	
Sìnìtāng 5g gānlùyǐn 5g mǔdānpí 1g zhīzǐ 1g huánglián 0g to ♀	Sìnìtāng 5g gānlùyǐn 5g mǔdānpí 1g zhīzǐ 1g huánglián 0g to ♂

Although Guìzhītāng is originally designed for symptoms of the common cold, according to classical Chinese medical sources, it also aids in digestion and promotes defense (i.e., immunity). Moreover, the modern uses of Guìzhī, which is the dominant herb in Guìzhītāng, are for allergic rhinitis and chronic pharyngitis and nasopharyngitis (Wang, 2019). A case was reported that a patient presenting with a two-week history of anorexia, weight loss, and fatigue was diagnosed with multiple myeloma (Andersen and Godwin, 1996).

4.3. Dyspepsia

Dyspepsia, or indigestion, is the feeling of fullness, discomfort or pain in the upper abdomen during or after a meal. Causes of dyspepsia include alcohol or caffeine overconsumption, acid reflux, and gastric ulcers.

Table 4.3. Herbal prescriptions for dyspepsia

Dyspepsia: https://meshb.nlm.nih.gov/record/ui?ui=D004415.
Common prescriptions:
Gégēnhuángqínhuángliántāng 5g bànxià 1g dàhuáng 0g Gégēnhuángqínhuángliántāng 5g mùxiāng 1g bànxià 1g dàhuáng 0g Gégēnhuángqínhuángliántāng 5g bànxià 1g fúlíng 1g dàhuáng 0g Gégēnhuángqínhuángliántāng 5g mùxiāng 1g bànxià 1g fúlíng 1g dàhuáng 0g Gégēnhuángqínhuángliántāng 5g mùxiāng 1g bànxià 1g fúlíng 1g
Alternative prescriptions:
Gégēnhuángqínhuángliántāng 5g mùxiāng 1g bànxià 1g Gégēnhuángqínhuángliántāng 5g bànxià 0g dàhuáng 0g
Indicated diseases:
Esophageal reflux 530.81 (Gastro-esophageal reflux disease without esophagitis K219); Dyskinesia of esophagus 530.5 (Dyskinesia of esophagus K224); Unspecified disorder of esophagus 530.9 (Disease of esophagus, unspecified K229); Unspecified disorder of gallbladder 575.9 (Disease of gallbladder, unspecified K829); Unspecified disorder of biliary tract 576.9 (Disease of biliary tract, unspecified K839); Diseases of the jaws 526; Unspecified disorder of intestine 569.9 (Disease of intestine, unspecified K639); Unspecified disorder of metabolism 277.9 (Metabolic disorder, unspecified E889); Amyloidosis 277.3

Dyspepsia: https://meshb.nlm.nih.gov/record/ui?ui=D004415.	
Esophageal reflux 530.81/K219 with dyspepsia D004415:	
Sìnìtāng 5g huòxiāngzhèngqìsǎn 5g yèjiāoténg 3g hǎipiāoxiāo 3g bózǐrén 2g cāngzhú 2g chántuì 2g to ♀	Sìnìtāng 5g huòxiāngzhèngqìsǎn 5g yèjiāoténg 3g hǎipiāoxiāo 3g bózǐrén 2g cāngzhú 2g chántuì 2g to ♂
Unspecified disorder of gallbladder 575.9/K829 with dyspepsia D004415:	
Dàcháihútāng 5g shānzhīzǐ 1g jīnqiáncǎo 1g yīnchén 1g to ♀	Dàcháihútāng 5g jīnqiáncǎo 1g jīnèijīn 1g yùjīn 1g to ♂
Unspecified disorder of intestine 569.9/K639 with dyspepsia D004415:	
Gégēnhuángqínhuángliántāng 5g bànxià 1g fúlíng 1g dàhuáng 0g to ♀	Gégēnhuángqínhuángliántāng 5g mùxiāng 1g bànxià 1g fúlíng 1g to ♂

Traditional uses of Gégēnhuángqínhuángliántāng are for 'upper body fever and diarrhea,' whereas its modern uses include functional disorder of stomach and non-infectious gastroenteritis and colitis (Wang, 2019). We will see its further uses for signs and symptoms of the digestive tract in later sections of the chapter.

4.4. Abdominal Pain

Abdominal pain is a dull ache anywhere between the chest and groin. Causes of abdominal pain include indigestion, constipation, lactose intolerance, food allergies or poisoning, irritable bowel syndrome, appendicitis, gastroenteritis, and so on.

Table 4.4. Herbal prescriptions for abdominal pain

Abdominal Pain: https://meshb.nlm.nih.gov/record/ui?ui=D015746.	
Common prescriptions:	
Yǐzìtāng 5g huáihuāsǎn 5g Yǐzìtāng 5g huáihuāsǎn 5g xiānhècǎo 1g báimáogēn 1g ǒujiē 1g Yǐzìtāng 5g huáihuāsǎn 5g xiānhècǎo 1g báimáogēn 1g Yǐzìtāng 5g huáihuāsǎn 5g xiānhècǎo 1g dìyú 1g	
Alternative prescriptions:	
Xiāozhìwán 5g huáihuāsǎn 5g lóngdǎnxiègāntāng 5g Yǐzìtāng 5g huáihuāsǎn 4g Yǐzìtāng 5g huáihuāsǎn 5g xiānhècǎo 1g dìyú 1g mǔdānpí 1g	
Yǐzìtāng 5g jiāwèixiāoyáosǎn 5g zhībódìhuángwán 5g Jiāwèixiāoyáosǎn 5g yǐzìtāng 4g huáihuāsǎn 4g xiānhècǎo 1g báimáogēn 1g ǒujiē 1g	
Indicated diseases:	
Unspecified disorder of liver 573.9 (Liver disease, unspecified K769); Malignant neoplasm of liver, not specified as primary or secondary 155.2 (Malignant neoplasm of liver, not specified as primary or secondary C229); Unspecified disorder of intestine 569.9 (Disease of intestine, unspecified K639); Malignant neoplasm of appendix vermiformis 153.5 (Malignant neoplasm of appendix C181); Unspecified disorder of metabolism 277.9 (Metabolic disorder, unspecified E889)	
Unspecified disorder of liver 573.9/K769 with abdominal pain D015746:	
Jiāwèixiāoyáosǎn 5g cháihúshūgāntāng 5g to ♀	Cháihúshūgāntāng 5g lóngdǎnxiègāntāng 5g to ♂
Unspecified disorder of intestine 569.9/K639 with abdominal pain D015746:	
Lǐzhōngtāng 5g báisháo 1g guìzhī 1g to ♀	Gégēnhuángqínhuángliántāng 5g mùxiāng 1g bànxià 1g dàhuáng 0g to ♂

Yǐzìtāng 'clears Heat and loosens congestion,' while Huáihuāsǎn 'cleans bowels and stops bleeding.' Their concurrent use in the prescriptions looks to relieve dyspepsia-related abdominal pain.

4.5. Hiccup

A hiccup is an involuntary contraction of the diaphragm and its resulting sound. One can get hiccups after taking in too much air or drinking carbonated beverages. Eating/drinking too much or too quickly can also cause hiccups.

Table 4.5. Herbal prescriptions for hiccup

<table>
<tr><td colspan="2">Hiccup: https://meshb.nlm.nih.gov/record/ui?ui=D006606.</td></tr>
<tr><td colspan="2">Common prescriptions:</td></tr>
<tr><td colspan="2">Sìnìtāng 5g bànxià 1g dàhuáng 0g
Sìnìtāng 5g shēngjiāng 1g guìzhī 1g
Zhēnwǔtāng 5g fùzǐ 1g xìxīn 1g
Zhēnwǔtāng 5g fùzǐ 1g xìxīn 1g tiáowèichéngqìtāng 1g
Zhēnwǔtāng 5g fùzǐ 1g gānjiāng 1g</td></tr>
<tr><td colspan="2">Alternative prescriptions:</td></tr>
<tr><td colspan="2">Sìnìtāng 5g shēngjiāng 0g guìzhī 0g
Máhuángfùzǐxìxīntāng 5g shēngjiāng 1g guìzhī 1g
Máhuángfùzǐxìxīntāng 5g fùzǐ 3g guìzhī 3g dàzǎo 2g wēilíngxiān 2g gānjiāng 2g zhìgāncǎotāng 2g
Máhuángfùzǐxìxīntāng 5g fùzǐ 2g guìzhī 2g gānjiāng 2g dàzǎo 2g zhìgāncǎotāng 2g</td></tr>
<tr><td colspan="2">Indicated diseases:</td></tr>
<tr><td colspan="2">Unspecified cerebrovascular disease 437.9 (Cerebrovascular disease, unspecified I679); Unspecified condition of brain 348.9 (Disorder of brain, unspecified G939); Cardiovascular disease, unspecified 429.2 (Atherosclerotic heart disease of native coronary artery without angina pectoris I2510); Unspecified disorders of nervous system 349.9 (Disorder of central nervous system, unspecified G969); Unspecified disorder of esophagus 530.9 (Disease of esophagus, unspecified K229); Diseases of the jaws 526; Diseases of the oral soft tissues, excluding lesions specific for gingiva and tongue 528; Neoplasm of unspecified nature of brain 239.6 (Neoplasm of unspecified behavior of brain D496); Malignant neoplasm of nervous system, part unspecified 192.9 (Malignant neoplasm of central nervous system, unspecified C729)</td></tr>
<tr><td colspan="2">Unspecified cerebrovascular disease 437.9/I679 with hiccup D006606:</td></tr>
<tr><td>Bǔyánghuánwǔtāng 5g sānqī 1g dānshēn 1g shíchāngpú 1g yuǎnzhì 1g + acupuncture to ♀</td><td>Bǔyánghuánwǔtāng 5g sānqī 1g dānshēn 1g shíchāngpú 1g yuǎnzhì 1g + acupuncture to ♂</td></tr>
<tr><td colspan="2">Unspecified disorder of esophagus 530.9/K229 with hiccup D006606:</td></tr>
<tr><td>Jiāwèixiāoyáosǎn 5g xiāngshāliùjūnzǐtāng 5g bànxiàxièxīntāng 3g zhǐqiào 2g hǎipiāoxiāo 2g to ♀</td><td>Jiāwèixiāoyáosǎn 5g xuánfùdàizhěshítāng 5g xuánfùdàizhěshítāng 5g dúhuójìshēngtāng 5g hǎipiāoxiāo 2g chuānliànzǐ 1g dānshēn 1g xiāngfù 0g to ♂</td></tr>
<tr><td colspan="2">Unspecified condition of brain 348.9/G939 with hiccup D006606:</td></tr>
<tr><td>Bǔyánghuánwǔtāng 5g dānshēn 1g tiānmá 1g shíchāngpú 1g yuǎnzhì 1g gōuténg 1g + acupuncture to ♀</td><td>Bǔyánghuánwǔtāng 5g dānshēn 1g shíchāngpú 1g yuǎnzhì 1g + acupuncture to ♂</td></tr>
</table>

Zhēnwǔtāng 'warms Yang up, drains water off,' and is used here to relieve hiccups. Lateral medullary infarction can lead to hiccups (Park et al., 2005). Esophagitis is also associated with hiccups (Levy et al., 2012).

4.6. Hyperphagia

Hyperphagia is a strong and constant feeling of hunger despite eating regularly. Causes of hyperphagia include hypoglycemia, hyperthyroidism, diabetes, sleep disturbances, stress and Prader-Willi syndrome.

The modern use of Xuèfǔzhúyūtāng includes hypercholesterolemia and hyper-glyceridemia and that of Cháihúshūgāntāng includes chronic hepatitis (Wang, 2019). The hypothalamus is a region of the brain that regulates food intake and energy expenditure and storage. Hypothalamic dysfunction usually leads to increased food intake and decreased energy burning and is associated with nonalcoholic fatty liver disease (Adams et al., 2004). Combining Xuèfǔzhúyūtāng and Cháihúshūgāntāng in the prescriptions in the table seems to target the complications or consequences of hyperphagia.

Table 4.6. Herbal prescriptions for hyperphagia

<table>
<tr><td colspan="2">Hyperphagia: https://meshb.nlm.nih.gov/record/ui?ui=D006963.</td></tr>
<tr><td colspan="2">Common prescriptions:</td></tr>
<tr><td colspan="2">Xuèfǔzhúyūtāng 5g cháihúshūgāntāng 5g chuānliànzǐ 1g yánhúsuǒ 1g
Xuèfǔzhúyūtāng 5g cháihúshūgāntāng 5g chuānliànzǐ 1g yánhúsuǒ 1g + acupuncture
Xuèfǔzhúyūtāng 5g cháihúshūgāntāng 5g chuānliànzǐ 1g yánhúsuǒ 1g yùjīn 1g
Xuèfǔzhúyūtāng 5g cháihúshūgāntāng 5g chuānliànzǐ 1g dānshēn 1g yánhúsuǒ 1g yùjīn 1g
Xuèfǔzhúyūtāng 5g cháihúshūgāntāng 5g chuānliànzǐ 1g dānshēn 1g yánhúsuǒ 1g</td></tr>
<tr><td colspan="2">Alternative prescriptions:</td></tr>
<tr><td colspan="2">Xuèfǔzhúyūtāng 5g cháihúshūgāntāng 5g chuānliànzǐ 1g mùxiāng 1g yùjīn 1g
Guìzhītāng 5g bànxià 1g báisháo 1g xiāngfù 1g màiyá 1g dàhuáng 0g
Guìzhītāng 5g bànxià 1g báisháo 1g dàhuáng 0g
Bāwèidìhuángwán 5g bājǐtiān 1g ròucōngróng 1g yínyánghuò 1g + acupuncture</td></tr>
<tr><td colspan="2">Indicated diseases:</td></tr>
<tr><td colspan="2">Anorexia nervosa 307.1 (Anorexia nervosa, unspecified F5000); Eating disorder, unspecified 307.50 (Eating disorder, unspecified F509); Unspecified disorder of metabolism 277.9 (Metabolic disorder, unspecified E889); Diabetes mellitus 250; Unspecified endocrine disorder 259.9 (Endocrine disorder, unspecified E349); Schizoaffective disorder 295.7; Schizophreniform disorder 295.4</td></tr>
<tr><td colspan="2">Anorexia nervosa 307.1/F5000 with Hyperphagia D006963:</td></tr>
<tr><td>Lǐzhōngtāng 5g bànxià 1g shārén 1g fúlíng 1g to ♀</td><td>Lǐzhōngtāng 5g bànxià 1g shārén 1g fúlíng 1g to ♂</td></tr>
<tr><td colspan="2">Eating disorder, unspecified 307.50/F509 with hyperphagia D006963:</td></tr>
<tr><td>Jiāwèixiāoyáosǎn 5g suānzǎoréntāng 5g to ♀</td><td>Jiāwèixiāoyáosǎn 5g suānzǎoréntāng 5g to ♂</td></tr>
<tr><td colspan="2">Unspecified disorder of metabolism 277.9/E889 with hyperphagia D006963:</td></tr>
<tr><td>Huángqíwǔwùtāng 5g dāngguīsìnìtāng 5g dānshēn 1g zhúrú 1g sāngzhī 1g jiānghuáng 1g to ♀</td><td>Liùwèidìhuángwán 5g xuèfǔzhúyūtāng 5g shānzhā 1g dānshēn 1g to ♂</td></tr>
<tr><td colspan="2">Diabetes mellitus 250 with hyperphagia D006963:</td></tr>
<tr><td>Bāwèidìhuángwán 5g báihǔjiārénshēntāng 5g to ♀</td><td>Bāwèidìhuángwán 5g yùquánwán 5g to ♂</td></tr>
</table>

4.7. Bulimia

Bulimia, an eating disorder, is overeating in one meal followed by excessive fasting, exercising, or self-induced vomiting to get rid of the extra calorie intake, in order to keep an ideal body weight and shape. Biological causes of bulimia are unknown although dysregulation of sex hormone is suspected.

Table 4.7. Herbal prescriptions for bulimia

Bulimia: https://meshb.nlm.nih.gov/record/ui?ui=D002032.	
Common prescriptions:	
Sháoyàogāncǎotāng 5g shūjīnghuóxuètāng 5g dāngguīniāntòngtāng 5g + acupuncture Sháoyàogāncǎotāng 5g shūjīnghuóxuètāng 5g + acupuncture Sháoyàogāncǎotāng 5g gégēntāng 5g + acupuncture	
Alternative prescriptions:	
Sháoyàogāncǎotāng 5g gégēntāng 5g qínjiāo 1g gōuténg 1g Sháoyàogāncǎotāng 5g cháihúguìzhītāng 5g yánhúsuǒ 1g qínjiāo 1g gōuténg 1g + acupuncture Sháoyàogāncǎotāng 5g cháihúguìzhītāng 5g gégēn 1g jīxuèténg 1g + acupuncture Sháoyàogāncǎotāng 5g gégēntāng 5g yánhúsuǒ 2g jīxuèténg 2g	
Indicated and associated diseases:	
Anorexia nervosa 307.1 (Anorexia nervosa, unspecified F5000); Eating disorder, unspecified 307.50 (Eating disorder, unspecified F509); Erosion 521.3; Somatization disorder 300.81 (Somatization disorder F450); Phobia, unspecified 300.20 (Phobic anxiety disorder, unspecified F409)	
Anorexia nervosa 307.1/F5000 with bulimia D002032:	
Lǐzhōngtāng 5g bànxià 1g shārén 1g fúlíng 1g to ♀	Lǐzhōngtāng 5g bànxià 1g shārén 1g fúlíng 1g to ♂
Erosion 521.3 with Bulimia D002032:	
Gānlùyǐn 5g qīngwèisǎn 5g to ♀	Gānlùyǐn 5g qīngwèisǎn 5g to ♂
Phobia, unspecified 300.20/F409 with bulimia D002032:	
Zhēnwǔtāng 5g fùzǐ 1g gānjiāng 1g to ♀	Jiāwèixiāoyáosǎn 5g gāncǎoxiǎomàidàzǎotāng 5g héhuānpí 1g xiāngfù 1g yùjīn 1g to ♂

Sháoyàogāncǎotāng is used for pains (Wang, 2019) and both Gégēntāng and Cháihúguìzhītāng are for migraine (Wang, 2019). There are reported associations between migraine and a predisposition to bulimia (Brewerton and George, 1933; Ostuzzi et al., 2008). It is therefore assumed that the herbal prescriptions aim to address the comorbidity of bulimia.

4.8. Nausea and Vomiting

Nausea is the feeling of an urge to vomit. Vomiting is forcible expulsion of the contents of the stomach through the mouth. Nausea and vomiting can occur alone, or nausea precedes vomiting. Causes of nausea and vomiting include motion sickness, food poisoning, gastritis and appendicitis. We show in Table 4.8.1 the herbal prescriptions for nausea and Table 4.8.2 for vomiting.

Nausea usually accompanies anorexia. Guìzhītāng is used for anorexia in Section 4.2. We therefore see its use for nausea here. Bǎohéwán 'digests food, guides stagnation,' and is used here for vomiting. Note that high levels of calcium in the blood of patients with multiple myeloma can cause nausea, so can the side effects of anti-myeloma medications. In addition to chest pain of patients with heart disease, women are more likely than men to experience nausea and vomiting.

Table 4.8.1. Herbal prescriptions for nausea

Nausea: https://meshb.nlm.nih.gov/record/ui?ui=D009325.	
Common prescriptions:	
Guìzhītāng 5g dàhuáng 0g Guìzhītāng 5g báisháo 1g dàhuáng 0g Guìzhītāng 5g bànxià 1g dàhuáng 0g Guìzhītāng 5g báisháo 1g	
Alternative prescriptions:	
Guìzhītāng 5g màiyá 2g xiāngfù 1g huángqín 1g dàhuáng 0g Guìzhītāng 5g màiyá 1g huángqín 1g xiāngfù 1g dàhuáng 0g Guìzhītāng 5g báisháo 2g dàhuáng 0g Guìzhītāng 5g huángqín 2g bànxià 1g xiāngfù 1g màiyá 1g dàhuáng 0g	
Indicated diseases:	
Unspecified disorder of liver 573.9 (Liver disease, unspecified K769); Malignant neoplasm of liver, not specified as primary or secondary 155.2 (Malignant neoplasm of liver, not specified as primary or secondary C229); Diseases of the jaws 526; Cardiovascular disease, unspecified 429.2 (Atherosclerotic heart disease of native coronary artery without angina pectoris I2510); Multiple myeloma 203.0; Unspecified hemorrhagic conditions 287.9 (Hemorrhagic condition, unspecified D699); Unspecified diseases of blood and blood-forming organs 289.9 (Disease of blood and blood-forming organs, unspecified D759); Unspecified disorder of intestine 569.9 (Disease of intestine, unspecified K639); Malignant neoplasm of intestinal tract, part unspecified 159.0 (Malignant neoplasm of intestinal tract, part unspecified C260); Malignant neoplasm of rectum 154.1 (Malignant neoplasm of rectum C20); Unspecified endocrine disorder 259.9 (Endocrine disorder, unspecified E349); Malignant neoplasm of pancreatic duct 157.3 (Malignant neoplasm of pancreatic duct C253)	
Unspecified disorder of liver 573.9/K769 with nausea D009325:	
Jiāwèixiāoyáosǎn 5g cháihúshūgāntāng 5g to ♀	Xuèfǔzhúyūtāng 5g cháihúshūgāntāng 5g lóngdǎnxiègāntāng 5g to ♂
Cardiovascular disease, unspecified 429.2/I2510 with nausea D009325:	
Sìnìtāng 5g gānlùyǐn 5g mǔdānpí 1g zhīzǐ 1g huánglián 0g to ♀	Sìnìtāng 5g gānlùyǐn 5g mǔdānpí 1g zhīzǐ 1g huánglián 0g to ♂
Unspecified disorder of intestine 569.9/K639 with nausea D009325:	
Lǐzhōngtāng 5g báisháo 1g guìzhī 1g to ♀	Lǐzhōngtāng 5g bànxià 1g shārén 1g fúlíng 1g to ♂
Diseases of the jaws 526 with Nausea D009325:	
Guìzhītāng 5g dàhuáng 0g to ♀	Gégēnhuángqínhuángliántāng 5g bànxià 1g dàhuáng 0g to ♂

Table 4.8.2. Herbal prescriptions for vomiting

Vomiting: https://meshb.nlm.nih.gov/record/ui?ui=D014839.
Common prescriptions:
Bǎohéwán 5g xiāngshāliùjūnzǐtāng 5g shānzhā 1g shénqū 1g màiyá 1g jīnèijīn 1g Bǎohéwán 5g xiāngshāliùjūnzǐtāng 5g shānzhā 1g shénqū 1g màiyá 1g Bǎohéwán 5g xiāngshāliùjūnzǐtāng 5g
Alternative prescriptions:
Bǎohéwán 5g xiāngshāliùjūnzǐtāng 5g shénqū 1g màiyá 1g Bǎohéwán 5g xiāngshāliùjūnzǐtāng 5g shānzhā 1g màiyá 1g jīnèijīn 1g Xiǎojiànzhōngtāng 5g cānlíngbáizhúsǎn 5g shānzhā 1g shénqū 1g màiyá 1g Bǎohéwán 5g xiāngshāliùjūnzǐtāng 5g shénqū 1g Jiāwèipíngwèisǎn 5g xiāngshāliùjūnzǐtāng 5g
Indicated diseases:
Unspecified disorder of esophagus 530.9 (Disease of esophagus, unspecified K229); Diseases of the jaws 526; Diseases of the oral soft tissues, excluding lesions specific for gingiva and tongue 528; Unspecified disorder of intestine 569.9 (Disease of intestine, unspecified K639); Gastric ulcer 531; Esophageal reflux 530.81 (Gastro-esophageal reflux disease without esophagitis K219); Eating disorder, unspecified 307.50 (Eating disorder, unspecified F509); Dyskinesia of esophagus 530.5 (Dyskinesia of esophagus K224); Heart disease, unspecified 429.9 (Heart disease, unspecified I519); Cardiovascular disease, unspecified 429.2 (Atherosclerotic heart disease of native coronary artery without angina pectoris I2510); Malignant neoplasm of sigmoid colon 153.3 (Malignant neoplasm of sigmoid colon C187)

Table 4.8.2. (Continued)

Vomiting: https://meshb.nlm.nih.gov/record/ui?ui=D014839.	
Unspecified disorder of esophagus 530.9/K229 with vomiting D014839:	
Jiāwèixiāoyáosǎn 5g xiāngshāliùjūnzǐtāng 5g huòxiāngzhèngqìsǎn 5g bànxiàxièxīntāng 3g zhǐqiào 2g hǎipiāoxiāo 2g to ♀	Xiāngshāliùjūnzǐtāng 5g cānlíngbáizhúsǎn 5g huòxiāngzhèngqìsǎn 5g bànxiàxièxīntāng 3g zhǐqiào 2g to ♂
Unspecified disorder of intestine 569.9/K639 with vomiting D014839:	
Gégēnhuángqínhuángliántāng 5g mùxiāng 1g bànxià 1g fúlíng 1g dàhuáng 0g to ♀	Xiāngshāliùjūnzǐtāng 5g cānlíngbáizhúsǎn 5g huòxiāngzhèngqìsǎn 5g to ♂
Esophageal reflux 530.81/K219 with vomiting D014839:	
Sìnìtāng 5g huòxiāngzhèngqìsǎn 5g yèjiāoténg 3g hǎipiāoxiāo 3g bózǐrén 2g cāngzhú 2g chántuì 2g to ♀	Sìnìtāng 5g huòxiāngzhèngqìsǎn 5g yèjiāoténg 3g hǎipiāoxiāo 3g bózǐrén 2g cāngzhú 2g chántuì 2g to ♂
Heart disease, unspecified 429.9/I519 with vomiting D014839:	
Sìnìtāng 5g gānlùyǐn 5g mǔdānpí 1g zhīzǐ 1g huánglián 0g to ♀	Sìnìtāng 5g gānlùyǐn 5g mǔdānpí 1g zhīzǐ 1g huánglián 0g to ♂

4.9. Anticipatory Vomiting

Anticipatory vomiting is vomiting caused by expectation of discomfort or unpleasantness. Classical conditioning can explain the development of anticipatory vomiting in that, for example, sights or smells of chemotherapy drugs become associated with the side effects of the treatment in such a way that, later on, smelling of the drugs alone can elicit the side effects.

Table 4.9. Herbal prescriptions for anticipatory vomiting

Anticipatory Vomiting: https://meshb.nlm.nih.gov/record/ui?ui=D014840.
Common prescriptions:
Sháoyàogāncǎotāng 5g shūjīnghuóxuètāng 5g dāngguīniāntòngtāng 5g + acupuncture Sháoyàogāncǎotāng 5g shūjīnghuóxuètāng 5g + acupuncture
Alternative prescriptions:
Jiāwèixiāoyáosǎn 5g xiāngshāliùjūnzǐtāng 5g gāncǎoxiǎomàidàzǎotāng 2g héhuānpí 1g yánhúsuǒ 1g Zhènggǔzǐjīndān 5g sháoyàogāncǎotāng 2g mòyào 1g rǔxiāng 1g + acupuncture Shūjīnghuóxuètāng 5g sháoyàogāncǎotāng 2g + acupuncture Xuèfǔzhúyūtāng 5g shūjīnghuóxuètāng 5g mòyào 1g rǔxiāng 1g + acupuncture Zhènggǔzǐjīndān 5g sháoyàogāncǎotāng 2g chuānqī 1g mòyào 1g rǔxiāng 1g + acupuncture
Indicated diseases:
Secondary cardiomyopathy, unspecified 425.9 (Cardiomyopathy due to drug and external agent I427); Unspecified disorders of nervous system 349.9 (Disorder of central nervous system, unspecified G969); Glycogenosis 271.0 (Glycogen storage disease, unspecified E7400, von Gierke disease E7401, McArdle disease E7404, Other glycogen storage disease E7409, Disorders of pyruvate metabolism and gluconeogenesis E744); Congenital stenosis of aortic valve 746.3 (Congenital stenosis of aortic valve Q230); Heart disease, unspecified 429.9 (Heart disease, unspecified I519); Cardiovascular disease, unspecified 429.2 (Atherosclerotic heart disease of native coronary artery without angina pectoris I2510); Unspecified disorder of metabolism 277.9 (Metabolic disorder, unspecified E889); Unspecified condition of brain 348.9 (Disorder of brain, unspecified G939); Peroxisomal disorders 277.86 (Peroxisomal disorder, unspecified E7150, Zellweger syndrome E71510, Neonatal adrenoleukodystrophy E71511, Adrenomyeloneuropathy E71522, X-linked adrenoleukodystrophy, unspecified type E71529, Other peroxisomal disorders E71548); Unspecified diseases of blood and blood-forming organs 289.9 (Disease of blood and blood-forming organs, unspecified D759); Congestive heart failure, unspecified 428.0 (Right heart failure due to left heart failure I50814, Heart failure, unspecified I509)

Anticipatory Vomiting: https://meshb.nlm.nih.gov/record/ui?ui=D014840.	
Secondary cardiomyopathy, unspecified 425.9/I427 with vomiting, anticipatory D014840:	
Xuèfǔzhúyūtāng 5g dānshēn 2g chuānqī 1g báijí 1g rénshēn 1g guìzhī 1g guālóurén 1g xièbái 1g to ♀	Xuèfǔzhúyūtāng 5g dānshēn 2g chuānqī 1g báijí 1g rénshēn 1g guìzhī 1g guālóurén 1g xièbái 1g to ♂
Unspecified condition of brain 348.9/G939 with vomiting, anticipatory D014840:	
Cháihújiālónggǔmǔlìtāng 5g wēndǎntāng 5g zhúrú 1g yèjiāoténg 1g yuǎnzhì 1g to ♀	Bǔyánghuánwǔtāng 5g dānshēn 1g tiānmá 1g shíchāngpú 1g yuǎnzhì 1g + acupuncture to ♂

Pain can be the extreme discomfort or unpleasantness that one tries to avoid. Sháoyàogāncǎotāng, Shūjīnghuóxuètāng and Dāngguīniāntòngtāng are used in the first chapter for a variety of pains. It is likely that they are used here to diminish the negative expectation by relieving the discomfort. Note that vomiting is among the adverse effects of many medications including cancer and heart disease medications.

4.10. Postoperative Nausea and Vomiting

Postoperative nausea and vomiting is the second most common complaint of patients after generalized anesthesia, next to postoperative pain. Postoperative nausea and vomiting is caused by the complex neural, chemical and mechanical interactions between the brain, anesthetics and gastrointestinal tract.

Table 4.10. Herbal prescriptions for postoperative nausea and vomiting

Postoperative Nausea and Vomiting: https://meshb.nlm.nih.gov/record/ui?ui=D020250.	
Common prescriptions:	
Sìnìtāng 5g bànxià 1g dàhuáng 0g Sìnìtāng 5g yánhúsuǒ 1g guìzhī 1g Sìnìtāng 5g báizhú 2g fúlíng 2g niúxī 1g guìzhī 1g	
Alternative prescriptions:	
Sìnìtāng 5g bànxià 1g yánhúsuǒ 1g dàhuáng 0g Sìnìtāng 5g niúxī 1g chēqiánzǐ 1g dàhuáng 0g Zhēnwǔtāng 5g Sìnìtāng 5g báizhú 2g fùzǐ 2g báisháo 2g fúlíng 2g dǎngshēn 1g wúzhūyú 1g gānjiāng 1g huánglián 0g	
Indicated diseases:	
Unspecified condition of brain 348.9 (Disorder of brain, unspecified G939); Neoplasm of unspecified nature of brain 239.6 (Neoplasm of unspecified behavior of brain D496); Unspecified disorders of nervous system 349.9 (Disorder of central nervous system, unspecified G969); Diseases of the jaws 526; Diseases of the oral soft tissues, excluding lesions specific for gingiva and tongue 528; Gastric ulcer 531; Unspecified disorder of intestine 569.9 (Disease of intestine, unspecified K639); Malignant neoplasm of intestinal tract, part unspecified 159.0 (Malignant neoplasm of intestinal tract, part unspecified C260); Heart disease, unspecified 429.9 (Heart disease, unspecified I519); Cardiovascular disease, unspecified 429.2 (Atherosclerotic heart disease of native coronary artery without angina pectoris I2510)	
Unspecified condition of brain 348.9/G939 with postoperative nausea and vomiting D020250:	
Xiǎoxùmìngtāng 5g bǔyánghuánwǔtāng 5g + acupuncture to ♀	Xiǎoxùmìngtāng 5g bǔyánghuánwǔtāng 5g + acupuncture to ♂
Diseases of the jaws 526 with postoperative nausea and vomiting D020250:	
Guìzhītāng 5g báisháo 1g dàhuáng 0g to ♀	Gégēnhuángqínhuángliántāng 5g bànxià 1g dàhuáng 0g to ♂
Unspecified disorder of intestine 569.9/K639 with postoperative nausea and vomiting D020250:	
Lǐzhōngtāng 5g báisháo 1g guìzhī 1g to ♀	Xiāngshāliùjūnzǐtāng 5g cānlíngbáizhúsǎn 5g to ♂
Heart disease, unspecified 429.9/I519 with postoperative nausea and vomiting D020250:	
Sìnìtāng 5g gānlùyǐn 5g mǔdānpí 1g zhīzǐ 1g huánglián 0g to ♀	Sìnìtāng 5g gānlùyǐn 5g mǔdānpí 1g zhīzǐ 1g huánglián 0g to ♂

Sìnìtāng's modern uses include irritable bowel syndrome (Wang, 2019) and its use here is believed to alleviate postoperative nausea and vomiting. Note again that prescriptions to female patients can differ from those to male with the same disease.

4.11. Hematemesis

Hematemesis is vomiting of bright red blood from the upper gastrointestinal tract including the esophagus, stomach and parts of the small intestine. Causes of hematemesis include peptic ulcers, gastroesophageal varices and liver failure.

Table 4.11. Herbal prescriptions for hematemesis

Hematemesis: https://meshb.nlm.nih.gov/record/ui?ui=D006396.	
Common prescriptions:	
Gégēnhuángqínhuángliántāng 5g mùxiāng 1g bànxià 1g dàhuáng 0g Gégēnhuángqínhuángliántāng 5g bànxià 1g dàhuáng 0g Gégēnhuángqínhuángliántāng 5g mùxiāng 1g bànxià 1g fúlíng 1g dàhuáng 0g Gégēnhuángqínhuángliántāng 5g mùxiāng 1g bànxià 1g fúlíng 1g	
Alternative prescriptions:	
Gégēnhuángqínhuángliántāng 5g fúlíng 1g bànxià 1g dàhuáng 0g	
Indicated and associated diseases:	
Portal hypertension 572.3 (Portal hypertension K766); Unspecified disorder of esophagus 530.9 (Disease of esophagus, unspecified K229); Unspecified disorder of liver 573.9 (Liver disease, unspecified K769); Cardiovascular disease, unspecified 429.2 (Atherosclerotic heart disease of native coronary artery without angina pectoris I2510); Fasciolopsiasis 121.4 (Fasciolopsiasis B665); Unspecified disorder of metabolism 277.9 (Metabolic disorder, unspecified E889); Amyloidosis 277.3	
Portal hypertension 572.3/K766 with hematemesis D006396:	
Jiāwèixiāoyáosǎn 5g bànxiàxièxīntāng 5g xīnyíqīngfèitāng 5g gégēntāng 5g chuānxiōngchádiàosǎn 4g to ♀	Xiǎocháihútāng 5g wǔlíngsǎn 5g to ♂
Cardiovascular disease, unspecified 429.2/I2510 with hematemesis D006396:	
Yùzhú 5g sìnìtāng 5g mǔdānpí 1g zhīzǐ 1g huánglián 0g to ♀	Yùzhú 5g sìnìtāng 5g zhìgāncǎotāng 5g to ♂

A modern use of Jiāwèixiāoyáosǎn and Xiǎocháihútāng is for chronic hepatitis (Wang, 2019). Jiāwèixiāoyáosǎn also takes care of symptomatic menopausal state of female (Wang, 2019). The multi-indication property of Jiāwèixiāoyáosǎn may explain its prescription to women with portal hypertension in the table. Patients with gastric amyloidosis can present with massive hematemesis (Singh et al., 2019).

4.12. Morning Sickness

Morning sickness is nausea and vomiting in early pregnancy. Causes of morning sickness are unknown but changes in estrogen of the mother and release of hormone from the embryo are suspected. Generally, morning sickness affects only the quality of life of the mother and does no physical harm to the mother and fetus.

Table 4.12. Herbal prescriptions for morning sickness

Morning Sickness: https://meshb.nlm.nih.gov/record/ui?ui=D048968.
Common prescriptions:
Sháoyàogāncǎotāng 5g shūjīnghuóxuètāng 5g dāngguīniāntòngtāng 5g + acupuncture Sháoyàogāncǎotāng 5g shūjīnghuóxuètāng 5g + acupuncture
Alternative prescriptions:
Jiāwèixiāoyáosǎn 5g cháihúshūgāntāng 5g dānshēn 1g yùjīn 1g Jiāwèixiāoyáosǎn 5g xiāngshāliùjūnzǐtāng 5g gāncǎoxiǎomàidàzǎotāng 3g héhuānpí 1g yánhúsuǒ 1g Sháoyàogāncǎotāng 5g shūjīnghuóxuètāng 5g yánhúsuǒ 1g + acupuncture Dāngguīsìnìtāng 5g niúxī 1g shēngjiāng 1g wúzhūyú 1g
Indicated diseases:
Cardiovascular disease, unspecified 429.2 (Atherosclerotic heart disease of native coronary artery without angina pectoris I2510); Multiple myeloma 203.0; Unspecified hemorrhagic conditions 287.9 (Hemorrhagic condition, unspecified D699); Unspecified diseases of blood and blood-forming organs 289.9 (Disease of blood and blood-forming organs, unspecified D759); Unspecified condition of brain 348.9 (Disorder of brain, unspecified G939); Unspecified disorders of nervous system 349.9 (Disorder of central nervous system, unspecified G969); Unspecified disorder of metabolism 277.9 (Metabolic disorder, unspecified E889)
Cardiovascular disease, unspecified 429.2/I2510 with morning sickness D048968:
Sìnìtāng 5g gānlùyǐn 5g mǔdānpí 1g zhīzǐ 1g huánglián 0g to ♀
Unspecified condition of brain 348.9/G939 with morning sickness D048968:
Bǔyánghuánwǔtāng 5g + acupuncture to ♀
Unspecified disorder of metabolism 277.9/E889 with morning sickness D048968:
Rénshēnbàidúsǎn 5g xiǎocháihútāngqùrénshēn 5g yīnchénhāotāng 2g mùxiāng 1g yùjīn 1g to ♀

We have seen Sháoyàogāncǎotāng's use for pains, which may accompany such signs and symptoms as nausea and vomiting in the previous section. The other reason for its use for morning sickness here is that modern uses of Zhìgāncǎo, a predominant herb in Sháoyàogāncǎotāng, are for disorders of the function of stomach and functional digestive disorders (Wang, 2019).

4.13. Hyperemesis Gravidarum

Hyperemesis gravidarum is severe nausea and vomiting during pregnancy. Causes of hyperemesis gravidarum are unknown but some hormones from the placenta are suspected. Its complications include weight loss, dehydration and electrolyte imbalance, and can harm the mother and fetus.

Table 4.13. Herbal prescriptions for hyperemesis gravidarum

Hyperemesis Gravidarum: https://meshb.nlm.nih.gov/record/ui?ui=D006939.
Common prescriptions:
Sìnìtāng 5g lǐzhōngtāng 5g ròuguì 1g yánhúsuǒ 1g zhìgāncǎotāng 1g Sìnìtāng 5g lǐzhōngtāng 5g ròuguì 1g zhìgāncǎotāng 1g Sìnìtāng 5g lǐzhōngtāng 5g ròuguì 1g yánhúsuǒ 1g zhìgāncǎotāng 1g + acupuncture Sìnìtāng 5g lǐzhōngtāng 5g ròuguì 1g yánhúsuǒ 1g
Alternative prescriptions:
Sìnìtāng 5g dāngguīsìnìtāng 5g shēngjiāng 1g wúzhūyú 1g Sìnìtāng 5g lǐzhōngtāng 5g wúzhūyú 1g Sìnìtāng 5g ròuguì 1g yánhúsuǒ 1g Sìnìtāng 5g máhuángfùzǐxìxīntāng 2g Sìnìtāng 5g niúxī 2g huángbò 2g cāngzhú 2g

Table 4.13. (Continued)

Hyperemesis Gravidarum: https://meshb.nlm.nih.gov/record/ui?ui=D006939.
Indicated diseases:
Unspecified disorder of liver 573.9 (Liver disease, unspecified K769); Diseases of the jaws 526; Diseases of the oral soft tissues, excluding lesions specific for gingiva and tongue 528; Unspecified endocrine disorder 259.9 (Endocrine disorder, unspecified E349); Malignant neoplasm of ovary 183.0 (Malignant neoplasm of unspecified ovary C569); Unspecified disorder of female genital organs 629.9 (Unspecified condition associated with female genital organs and menstrual cycle N949); Malignant neoplasm of other and unspecified female genital organs 184; Malignant neoplasm of endocrine gland, site unspecified 194.9 (Malignant neoplasm of endocrine gland, unspecified C759); Malignant neoplasm of liver, not specified as primary or secondary 155.2 (Malignant neoplasm of liver, not specified as primary or secondary C229)
Unspecified disorder of liver 573.9/K769 with hyperemesis gravidarum D006939:
Jiāwèixiāoyáosǎn 5g cháihúshūgāntāng 5g to ♀
Unspecified endocrine disorder 259.9/E349 with hyperemesis gravidarum D006939:
Jiāwèixiāoyáosǎn 5g wēnjīngtāng 4g nǚzhēnzǐ 1g hànliáncǎo 1g tùsīzǐ 1g to ♀

Lǐzhōngtāng 'warms up the middle, regulates Qi' and is used for dyspepsia, functional disorder of stomach and irritable bowel syndrome (Wang, 2019). The starvation associated with hyperemesis gravidarum can cause liver dysfunction (Conchillo et al., 2002), as we also see in the table.

4.14. Heartburn

Heartburn is the burning and uncomfortable feeling in the central chest or throat, caused by refluxing back of the acid from the stomach to the esophagus. Acidic, spicy or fatty foods can cause heartburn, so can overeating, smoking and medications.

Table 4.14. Herbal prescriptions for heartburn

Heartburn: https://meshb.nlm.nih.gov/record/ui?ui=D006356	
Common prescriptions:	
Gégēnhuángqínhuángliántāng 5g bànxià 1g dàhuáng 0g Gégēnhuángqínhuángliántāng 5g mùxiāng 1g bànxià 1g dàhuáng 0g Gégēnhuángqínhuángliántāng 5g bànxià 1g fúlíng 1g dàhuáng 0g Gégēnhuángqínhuángliántāng 5g mùxiāng 1g bànxià 1g fúlíng 1g dàhuáng 0g Gégēnhuángqínhuángliántāng 5g mùxiāng 1g bànxià 1g fúlíng 1g	
Alternative prescriptions:	
Gégēnhuángqínhuángliántāng 5g bànxià 1g fúlíng 1g Gégēnhuángqínhuángliántāng 5g bànxià 0g fúlíng 0g	
Indicated diseases:	
Reflux esophagitis 530.11 (Gastro-esophageal reflux disease with esophagitis K210); Esophagitis 530.1; Unspecified disorder of esophagus 530.9 (Disease of esophagus, unspecified K229); Vaginal enterocele, congenital or acquired 618.6 (Vaginal enterocele N815); Barrett's esophagus 530.85 (Barrett's esophagus without dysplasia K2270); Malignant neoplasm of other specified part of esophagus 150.8 (Malignant neoplasm of overlapping sites of esophagus C158); Esophageal reflux 530.81 (Gastro-esophageal reflux disease without esophagitis K219)	
Reflux esophagitis 530.11/K210 with heartburn D006356:	
Wǔlíngsǎn 5g báisháo 1g huángqín 1g to ♀	Wǔlíngsǎn 5g báisháo 1g huángqín 1g to ♂
Barrett's esophagus 530.85/K2270 with heartburn D006356:	
Bànxiàxièxīntāng 5g xiāngshāliùjūnzǐtāng 5g cháihúshūgāntāng 5g báijí 2g bèimǔ 2g hǎipiāoxiāo 2g to ♀	Bànxiàxièxīntāng 5g xiāngshāliùjūnzǐtāng 5g cháihúshūgāntāng 5g báijí 2g bèimǔ 2g hǎipiāoxiāo 2g to ♂

Here, heartburn is added to the use of Gégēnhuángqínhuángliántāng, in addition to dyspepsia and hematemesis in previous sections. The modern uses of Bànxiàxièxīntāng and Xiāngshāliùjūnzǐtāng, both of which 'regulate the Stomach Qi,' are for gastritis, gastroduodenitis, and functional disorder of stomach (Wang, 2019).

4.15. Flatulence

Flatulence, also known as farting, is passing of intestinal gas through the anus. Flatulence can be caused by gas producing foods such as whole grains, high-fiber plants, and dairy products. Swallowed air can also cause flatulence. Lactose intolerance and irritable bowel syndrome can cause excessive flatulence.

Table 4.15. Herbal prescriptions for flatulence

<table>
<tr><td colspan="2">Flatulence: https://meshb.nlm.nih.gov/record/ui?ui=D005414.</td></tr>
<tr><td colspan="2">Common prescriptions:</td></tr>
<tr><td colspan="2">Wǔlíngsǎn 5g fùzǐ 1g huángqín 1g
Wǔlíngsǎn 5g fùzǐ 1g huángqín 1g dǐdāngtāng 0g
Wǔlíngsǎn 5g báisháo 1g huángqín 1g
Wǔlíngsǎn 5g fùzǐ 1g huángqín 1g tiáowèichéngqìtāng 1g
Wǔlíngsǎn 5g fùzǐ 1g huángqín 1g tiáowèichéngqìtāng 0g</td></tr>
<tr><td colspan="2">Alternative prescriptions:</td></tr>
<tr><td colspan="2">Wǔlíngsǎn 5g gāncǎo 0g
Wǔlíngsǎn 5g gāncǎo 1g báisháo 1g tiáowèichéngqìtāng 1g dàhuáng 0g
Zhēnwǔtāng 5g báisháo 1g fùzǐ 1g mázǐrénwán 1g dàhuáng 0g</td></tr>
<tr><td colspan="2">Indicated diseases:</td></tr>
<tr><td colspan="2">Unspecified disorder of intestine 569.9 (Disease of intestine, unspecified K639); Unspecified disorder of metabolism 277.9 (Metabolic disorder, unspecified E889); Diseases of the jaws 526; Perforation of intestine 569.83 (Perforation of intestine (nontraumatic) K631); Malignant neoplasm of rectum 154.1 (Malignant neoplasm of rectum C20); Esophageal reflux 530.81 (Gastro-esophageal reflux disease without esophagitis K219); Dyskinesia of esophagus 530.5 (Dyskinesia of esophagus K224); Unspecified disorder of esophagus 530.9 (Disease of esophagus, unspecified K229); Malignant neoplasm of colon 153</td></tr>
<tr><td colspan="2">Unspecified disorder of intestine 569.9/K639 with flatulence D005414:</td></tr>
<tr><td>Lǐzhōngtāng 5g báisháo 1g guìzhī 1g to ♀</td><td>Lǐzhōngtāng 5g báisháo 1g guìzhī 1g to ♂</td></tr>
<tr><td colspan="2">Perforation of intestine 569.83/K631 with flatulence D005414:</td></tr>
<tr><td>Tiáowèichéngqìtāng 5g dǐdāngtāng 4g to ♀</td><td>Lǐzhōngtāng 5g fúlíng 2g bànxià 1g shārén 1g to ♂</td></tr>
<tr><td colspan="2">Esophageal reflux 530.81/K219 with flatulence D005414:</td></tr>
<tr><td>Sìnìtāng 5g huòxiāngzhèngqìsǎn 5g yèjiāoténg 3g hǎipiāoxiāo 3g bózǐrén 2g cāngzhú 2g chántuì 2g to ♀</td><td>Sìnìtāng 5g huòxiāngzhèngqìsǎn 5g yèjiāoténg 3g hǎipiāoxiāo 3g bózǐrén 2g cāngzhú 2g chántuì 2g to ♂</td></tr>
</table>

Traditional Chinese medicine believes that frequent flatulence is attributed to 'deficiency of the Spleen,' which governs digestion. A prominent manifestation in patients with deficient Spleen is 'Dampness of the body.' Wǔlíngsǎn 'promotes urination, drains Dampness' and is believed to be used here for people with 'deficient Spleen' and flatulence.

4.16. Diarrhea

Diarrhea is passing loose and watery stools more than three times a day. A common cause of diarrhea is viral, bacterial or parasitic infections of the intestines by ingesting contaminated foods or water.

Table 4.16. Herbal prescriptions for diarrhea

Diarrhea: https://meshb.nlm.nih.gov/record/ui?ui=D003967.	
Common prescriptions:	
Gégēnhuángqínhuángliántāng 5g bànxià 1g dàhuáng 0g Gégēnhuángqínhuángliántāng 5g mùxiāng 1g bànxià 1g dàhuáng 0g Gégēnhuángqínhuángliántāng 5g bànxià 1g fúlíng 1g dàhuáng 0g Gégēnhuángqínhuángliántāng 5g mùxiāng 1g bànxià 1g fúlíng 1g dàhuáng 0g Gégēnhuángqínhuángliántāng 5g mùxiāng 1g bànxià 1g fúlíng 1g	
Alternative prescriptions:	
Gégēnhuángqínhuángliántāng 5g bànxià 1g fúlíng 1g Gégēnhuángqínhuángliántāng 5g bànxià 0g fúlíng 0g dàhuáng 0g Gégēnhuángqínhuángliántāng 5g fúlíng 2g bànxià 1g dàhuáng 0g Gégēnhuángqínhuángliántāng 5g fúlíng 2g mùxiāng 1g bànxià 1g dàhuáng 0g	
Indicated diseases:	
Unspecified disorder of intestine 569.9 (Disease of intestine, unspecified K639); Amyloidosis 277.3; Diseases of the jaws 526; Tropical sprue 579.1 (Tropical sprue K901); Unspecified disorder of metabolism 277.9 (Metabolic disorder, unspecified E889); Celiac disease 579.0 (Celiac disease K900); Malignant neoplasm of intestinal tract, part unspecified 159.0 (Malignant neoplasm of intestinal tract, part unspecified C260)	
Unspecified disorder of intestine 569.9/K639 with diarrhea D003967:	
Gégēnhuángqínhuángliántāng 5g bànxià 1g fúlíng 1g dàhuáng 0g to ♀	Gégēnhuángqínhuángliántāng 5g mùxiāng 1g bànxià 1g fúlíng 1g to ♂
Tropical sprue 579.1/K901 with diarrhea D003967:	
Wèilíngtāng 5g xiāngshāliùjūnzǐtāng 5g gégēnhuángqínhuángliántāng 5g to ♀	Wèilíngtāng 5g cānlíngbáizhúsǎn 5g lǐzhōngtāng 5g to ♂
Celiac disease 579.0/K900 with diarrhea D003967:	
Wèilíngtāng 5g gégēnhuángqínhuángliántāng 5g huòxiāngzhèngqìsǎn 5g to ♀	Wèilíngtāng 5g xiāngshāliùjūnzǐtāng 5g gégēnhuángqínhuángliántāng 5g to ♂

Gégēnhuángqínhuángliántāng is used for dyspepsia, hematemesis and heartburn in previous sections, though its traditional use is for diarrhea, as we pointed out in Section 4.3. Modern uses of Wèilíngtāng include irritable bowel syndrome, functional diarrhea, non-infectious gastroenteritis and colitis (Wang, 2019).

4.17. Gagging

Gagging, i.e., pharyngeal reflex, is contraction of the pharyngeal muscle to prevent from swallowing something that is potentially harmful or unpleasant. Gagging can be elicited by either a physical stimulation of the tonsils or psychological thought of disgust.

Guìzhītāng is used for anorexia in Section 4.2. Shared psychological factors behind anorexia and gagging may explain the use of Guìzhītāng for anorexia and gagging.

Table 4.17. Herbal prescriptions for gagging

Gagging https://meshb.nlm.nih.gov/record/ui?ui=D005683	
Common prescriptions:	
Guìzhītāng 5g shēngjiāng 1g báisháo 1g dàhuáng 0g Guìzhītāng 5g shēngjiāng 1g guìzhī 1g Guìzhītāng 5g bànxià 1g dàhuáng 0g Guìzhītāng 5g shēngjiāng 1g guìzhī 1g dàhuáng 0g Guìzhītāng 5g shēngjiāng 1g báisháo 1g	
Alternative prescriptions:	
Guìzhītāng 5g jiégěng 1g dàhuáng 0g Guìzhītāng 5g xìngrén 1g hòupò 1g dàhuáng 0g Guìzhītāng 5g báisháo 1g dàhuáng 0g Guìzhītāng 5g shēngjiāng 1g báisháo 1g guìzhī 1g dàhuáng 0g	
Indicated diseases:	
Esophageal reflux 530.81 (Gastro-esophageal reflux disease without esophagitis K219); Dyskinesia of esophagus 530.5 (Dyskinesia of esophagus K224); Unspecified disorder of esophagus 530.9 (Disease of esophagus, unspecified K229); Diseases of the jaws 526; Diseases of the oral soft tissues, excluding lesions specific for gingiva and tongue 528; Unspecified disease of pharynx 478.20 (Other diseases of pharynx J392)	
Esophageal reflux 530.81/K219 with gagging D005683:	
Sìnìtāng 5g huòxiāngzhèngqìsǎn 5g yèjiāoténg 3g hǎipiāoxiāo 3g bózǐrén 2g cāngzhú 2g chántuì 2g to ♀	Sìnìtāng 5g huòxiāngzhèngqìsǎn 5g yèjiāoténg 3g hǎipiāoxiāo 3g bózǐrén 2g cāngzhú 2g chántuì 2g to ♂
Unspecified disorder of esophagus 530.9/K229 with gagging D005683:	
Jiāwèixiāoyáosǎn 5g xiāngshāliùjūnzǐtāng 5g bànxiàxièxīntāng 3g zhǐqiào 2g hǎipiāoxiāo 2g to ♀	Bànxiàxièxīntāng 5g xiāngshāliùjūnzǐtāng 5g cháihúshūgāntāng 5g huòxiāngzhèngqìsǎn 5g zhǐqiào 2g hǎipiāoxiāo 2g to ♂
Unspecified disease of pharynx 478.20/J392 with gagging D005683:	
Bànxiàhòupòtāng 5g màiméndōngtāng 5g to ♀	Èrchéntāng 5g bànxiàhòupòtāng 5g to ♂

4.18. Eructation

Eructation, also known as belching or burping, is expelling of swallowed gas from the esophagus or stomach through the mouth. Eating too fast, chatting while eating, chewing gum or drinking carbonated beverages can cause belching. Excessive belching can be caused by gastroesophageal reflux disease or stomach ulcers.

Table 4.18. Herbal prescriptions for eructation

Eructation: https://meshb.nlm.nih.gov/record/ui?ui=D004884.
Common prescriptions:
Guìzhītāng 5g báisháo 1g dàhuáng 0g Guìzhītāng 5g shēngjiāng 1g báisháo 1g dàhuáng 0g Guìzhītāng 5g shēngjiāng 1g guìzhī 1g Guìzhītāng 5g wúzhūyútāng 3g fùzǐ 1g gānjiāng 1g Guìzhītāng 5g shēngjiāng 1g báisháo 1g
Alternative prescriptions:
Guìzhītāng 5g shēngjiāng 1g guìzhī 1g dàhuáng 0g Sìnìtāng 5g bànxià 1g dàhuáng 0g Guìzhītāng 5g wúzhūyútāng 3g fùzǐ 1g

Table 4.18. (Continued)

Eructation: https://meshb.nlm.nih.gov/record/ui?ui=D004884.	
Indicated diseases:	
Esophageal reflux 530.81 (Gastro-esophageal reflux disease without esophagitis K219); Dyskinesia of esophagus 530.5 (Dyskinesia of esophagus K224); Unspecified disorder of esophagus 530.9 (Disease of esophagus, unspecified K229); Reflux esophagitis 530.11 (Gastro-esophageal reflux disease with esophagitis K210); Esophagitis 530.1; Diseases of the jaws 526; Diseases of the oral soft tissues, excluding lesions specific for gingiva and tongue 528	
Esophageal reflux 530.81/K219 with eructation D004884:	
Sìnìtāng 5g huòxiāngzhèngqìsǎn 5g yèjiāoténg 3g hǎipiāoxiāo 3g bózǐrén 2g cāngzhú 2g chántuì 2g to ♀	Sìnìtāng 5g huòxiāngzhèngqìsǎn 5g yèjiāoténg 3g hǎipiāoxiāo 3g bózǐrén 2g cāngzhú 2g chántuì 2g to ♂
Reflux esophagitis 530.11/K210 with eructation D004884:	
Lǐzhōngtāng 5g báisháo 1g fùzǐ 1g to ♀	Lǐzhōngtāng 5g báisháo 1g fùzǐ 1g to ♂
Unspecified disorder of esophagus 530.9/K229 with eructation D004884:	
Jiāwèixiāoyáosǎn 5g xiāngshāliùjūnzǐtāng 5g huòxiāngzhèngqìsǎn 5g bànxiàxièxīntāng 3g zhǐqiào 2g hǎipiāoxiāo 2g to ♀	Bànxiàxièxīntāng 5g xiāngshāliùjūnzǐtāng 5g cháihúshūgāntāng 5g huòxiāngzhèngqìsǎn 5g zhǐqiào 2g hǎipiāoxiāo 2g to ♂

Huòxiāngzhèngqìsǎn 'regulates Qi, harmonizes interior' and is used in these days for gastritis and gastroduodenitis (Wang, 2019).

4.19. Halitosis

Halitosis is bad smelling breath, a common source of embarrassment. Buildup of sulphur-producing bacteria inside the mouth due to poor oral hygiene, tobacco use, gum disease or upper digestive tract infections can cause halitosis.

Table 4.19. Herbal prescriptions for halitosis

Halitosis: https://meshb.nlm.nih.gov/record/ui?ui=D006209	
Common prescriptions:	
Yùnǚjiān 5g qīngwèisǎn 5g Yùnǚjiān 5g gānlùyǐn 5g qīngwèisǎn 5g	
Alternative prescriptions:	
Qīngwèisǎn 5g yùnǚjiān 2g Qīngwèisǎn 5g lóngdǎnxiègāntāng 4g Yùnǚjiān 5g sháoyàogāncǎotāng 5g yánhúsuǒ 1g Qīngwèisǎn 5g liánggésǎn 3g	
Indicated diseases:	
Diseases of the jaws 526; Diseases of the oral soft tissues, excluding lesions specific for gingiva and tongue 528; Gastric ulcer 531; Dental caries of smooth surface 521.07 (Dental caries on smooth surface limited to enamel K0261, Dental caries on smooth surface penetrating into dentin K0262, Dental caries on smooth surface penetrating into pulp K0263); Diabetes mellitus 250; Unspecified endocrine disorder 259.9 (Endocrine disorder, unspecified E349); Unspecified disorder of metabolism 277.9 (Metabolic disorder, unspecified E889); Chronic gingivitis 523.1	
Diseases of the jaws 526 with halitosis D006209:	
Guìzhītāng 5g báisháo 1g dàhuáng 0g to ♀	Gégēnhuángqínhuángliántāng 5g bànxià 1g dàhuáng 0g to ♂
Dental caries of smooth surface 521.07/K0261,K0262,K0263 with halitosis D006209:	
Yùnǚjiān 5g qīngwèisǎn 5g to ♀	Yùnǚjiān 5g qīngwèisǎn 5g to ♂
Chronic gingivitis 523.1 with halitosis D006209:	
Yùnǚjiān 5g gānlùyǐn 5g qīngwèisǎn 5g to ♀	Yùnǚjiān 5g gānlùyǐn 5g qīngwèisǎn 5g to ♂

Yùnǚjiān, Gānlùyǐn and Qīngwèisǎn are used in Section 1.9 for toothache. Their use here for halitosis is understandable. Elevated glucose levels in the saliva of diabetic patients increase forming of dental plaques, causing halitosis in diabetics.

4.20. Encopresis

Encopresis is functional fecal incontinence. Encopresis occurs in children past their toilet training age. Diarrhea, constipation, anxiety and depression can cause encopresis.

Table 4.20. Herbal prescriptions for encopresis

Encopresis: https://meshb.nlm.nih.gov/record/ui?ui=D004688.	
Common prescriptions:	
Bǔzhōngyìqìtāng 5g Guìzhītāng 5g huángqí 1g gégēn 1g Guìzhītāng 5g huángqí 1g Guìzhītāng 5g huángqí 2g gégēn 2g	
Alternative prescriptions:	
Guìzhītāng 5g bànxià 1g jiégěng 1g dàhuáng 0g Guìzhītāng 5g báisháo 1g Guìzhītāng 5g shēngjiāng 0g guìzhī 0g Bǔzhōngyìqìtāng 5g shēngmàiyǐn 4g Guìzhītāng 5g shēngjiāng 1g báisháo 1g dàhuáng 0g	
Indicated diseases:	
Epilepsy, unspecified 345.9; Unspecified condition of brain 348.9 (Disorder of brain, unspecified G939); Unspecified disorders of nervous system 349.9 (Disorder of central nervous system, unspecified G969); Heart disease, unspecified 429.9 (Heart disease, unspecified I519); Unspecified congenital anomaly of heart 746.9 (Congenital malformation of cardiac chambers and connections, unspecified Q209, Congenital malformation of heart, unspecified Q249); Cardiovascular disease, unspecified 429.2 (Atherosclerotic heart disease of native coronary artery without angina pectoris I2510); Neoplasm of unspecified nature of brain 239.6 (Neoplasm of unspecified behavior of brain D496)	
Epilepsy, unspecified 345.9 with encopresis D004688:	
Yìgānsǎn 5g cháihújiālónggǔmǔlìtāng 5g shíchāngpú 1g yuǎnzhì 1g to ♀	Yìgānsǎn 5g cháihújiālónggǔmǔlìtāng 5g shíchāngpú 1g yuǎnzhì 1g to ♂
Heart disease, unspecified 429.9/I519 with encopresis D004688:	
Sìnìtāng 5g gānlùyǐn 5g mǔdānpí 1g zhīzǐ 1g huánglián 0g to ♀	Sìnìtāng 5g gānlùyǐn 5g mǔdānpí 1g zhīzǐ 1g huánglián 0g to ♂
Unspecified condition of brain 348.9/G939 with encopresis D004688:	
Bǔyánghuánwǔtāng 5g tiānmá 1g shíchāngpú 1g yuǎnzhì 1g gōuténg 1g + acupuncture to ♀	Bǔyánghuánwǔtāng 5g tiānmá 1g shíchāngpú 1g yuǎnzhì 1g gōuténg 1g + acupuncture to ♂
Unspecified disorders of nervous system 349.9/G969 with encopresis D004688:	
Huángqíwǔwùtāng 5g chuānxiōng 1g dānshēn 1g zhúrú 1g sāngzhī 1g dāngguī 1g jiānghuáng 1g to ♀	Huángqíwǔwùtāng 5g chuānxiōng 1g dānshēn 1g zhúrú 1g sāngzhī 1g dāngguī 1g jiānghuáng 1g to ♂

We have seen Guìzhītāng's use for anorexia, gagging and eructation in this chapter. Its use in this section is supposed to take care of the emotional cause of encopresis. Bǔzhōngyìqìtāng has traditionally been used for archoptosis, hysteroptosia, gastroptosis and chronic diarrhea, through its effect of upholding things in their anatomic positions via 'elevating Yang and lifting collapse.' Note that constipation shares many of the risk factors with cardiovascular diseases (Sundboll et al., 2020).

4.21. Aerophagy

Aerophagy is excessive swallowing of air into the stomach. Causes of eructation also cause aerophagy.

Table 4.21. Herbal prescriptions for aerophagy

Aerophagy: https://meshb.nlm.nih.gov/record/ui?ui=D000334.	
Common prescriptions:	
Guìzhītāng 5g báisháo 1g dàhuáng 0g Guìzhītāng 5g shēngjiāng 1g báisháo 1g dàhuáng 0g Guìzhītāng 5g shēngjiāng 1g guìzhī 1g Guìzhītāng 5g shēngjiāng 1g báisháo 1g	
Alternative prescriptions:	
Guìzhītāng 5g báisháo 1g màiyá 1g xiāngfù 1g huángqín 1g dàhuáng 0g Guìzhītāng 5g fùzǐ 0g Guìzhītāng 5g bànxià 1g dàhuáng 0g Guìzhītāng 5g shēngjiāng 0g báisháo 0g Gégēnhuángqínhuángliántāng 5g mùxiāng 1g bànxià 1g dàhuáng 0g	
Indicated diseases:	
Esophageal reflux 530.81 (Gastro-esophageal reflux disease without esophagitis K219); Dyskinesia of esophagus 530.5 (Dyskinesia of esophagus K224); Unspecified disorder of esophagus 530.9 (Disease of esophagus, unspecified K229); Diseases of the jaws 526; Diseases of the oral soft tissues, excluding lesions specific for gingiva and tongue 528; Gastric ulcer 531; Unspecified disorder of intestine 569.9 (Disease of intestine, unspecified K639)	
Esophageal reflux 530.81/K219 with aerophagy D000334:	
Sìnìtāng 5g huòxiāngzhèngqìsǎn 5g yèjiāoténg 3g hǎipiāoxiāo 3g bózǐrén 2g cāngzhú 2g chántuì 2g to ♀	Sìnìtāng 5g huòxiāngzhèngqìsǎn 5g yèjiāoténg 3g hǎipiāoxiāo 3g bózǐrén 2g cāngzhú 2g chántuì 2g to ♂
Diseases of the jaws 526 with aerophagy D000334:	
Guìzhītāng 5g báisháo 1g dàhuáng 0g to ♀	Gégēnhuángqínhuángliántāng 5g bànxià 1g fúlíng 1g dàhuáng 0g to ♂
Unspecified disorder of intestine 569.9/K639 with aerophagy D000334:	
Xiāngshāliùjūnzǐtāng 5g cānlíngbáizhúsǎn 5g huòxiāngzhèngqìsǎn 5g to ♀	Xiāngshāliùjūnzǐtāng 5g cānlíngbáizhúsǎn 5g huòxiāngzhèngqìsǎn 5g to ♂
Unspecified disorder of esophagus 530.9/K229 with aerophagy D000334:	
Jiāwèixiāoyáosǎn 5g xiāngshāliùjūnzǐtāng 5g huòxiāngzhèngqìsǎn 5g bànxiàxièxīntāng 3g zhǐqiào 2g hǎipiāoxiāo 2g to ♀	Xiāngshāliùjūnzǐtāng 5g cānlíngbáizhúsǎn 5g huòxiāngzhèngqìsǎn 5g bànxiàxièxīntāng 3g hǎipiāoxiāo 2g to ♂

Aerophagy is most likely followed by eructation. We therefore see that Guìzhītāng is used for both symptoms.

References

Adams, L. A., Feldstein, A., Lindor, K. D., & Angulo, P. (2004). Nonalcoholic fatty liver disease among patients with hypothalamic and pituitary dysfunction. *Hepatology*, *39*(4), 909–914. https://doi.org/10.1002/hep.20140.

Andersen, H. S., & Godwin, J. H. (1996). Multiple Myeloma. *New England Journal of Medicine*, *334*(8), 513–513. https://doi.org/10.1056/nejm199602223340806.

Brewerton, T. D., & George, M. S. (1993). Is migraine related to the eating disorders? *International Journal of Eating Disorders*, *14*(1), 75–79. https://doi.org/10.1002/1098-108x(199307)14:1.

Conchillo, J. M., Pijnenborg, J. M., Peeters, P., Stockbrügger, R. W., Fevery, J., & Koek, G. H. (2002). Liver enzyme elevation induced by hyperemesis gravidarum: aetiology, diagnosis and treatment. *The Netherlands Journal of Medicine*, *60*(9), 374-378.

Ejerskov, C., Krogh, K., Ostergaard, J. R., Fassov, J. L., & Haagerup, A. (2017). Constipation in adults with neurofibromatosis type 1. *Orphanet Journal of Rare Diseases*, *12*, 139. https://doi.org/10.1186/s13023-017-0691-4.

Levy, A. N., Rahaman, S. M., Bonis, P. A., Javid, G., & Leung, J. (2012). Hiccups as a Presenting Symptom of Eosinophilic Esophagitis. *Case Reports in Gastroenterology*, *6*(2), 340–343. https://doi.org/10.1159/000338739.

Ostuzzi, R., D'Andrea, G., Francesconi, F., & Musco, F. (2008). Eating disorders and headache: coincidence or consequence? *Neurological Sciences*, *29*(S1), 83–87. https://doi.org/10.1007/s10072-008-0894-5.

Park, M. H., Kim, B. J., Koh, S. B., Park, M. K., Park, K. W., & Lee, D. H. (2005). Lesional location of lateral medullary infarction presenting hiccups (singultus). *Journal of Neurology, Neurosurgery and Psychiatry*, *76*(1), 95–98. https://doi.org/10.1136/jnnp.2004.039362.

Singh, V., Singla, S., Singh, H., Sharma, V., & Das, A. (2019). Massive hematemesis in a case of gastric amyloidosis masquerading as gastric carcinoma. *Autopsy and Case Reports*, *9*(1), e2018074. https://doi.org/10.4322/acr.2018.074.

Sundbøll, J., Szépligeti, S. K., Adelborg, K., Szentkúti, P., Gregersen, H., & Sørensen, H. T. (2020). Constipation and risk of cardiovascular diseases: a Danish population-based matched cohort study. *BMJ Open*, *10*(9), e037080. https://doi.org/10.1136/bmjopen-2020-037080.

Wang, S. C. (2019). *Clinical Herbal Prescriptions: Principles and Practices of Herbal Formulations from Deep Learning Health Insurance Herbal Prescription Big Data*. WSPC. https://doi.org/10.1142/11211.

Chapter 5

Dyskinesias

Dyskinesias are characterized by increased involuntary and decreased voluntary movements of one or multiple parts of the body. The types of uncontrolled movements can range from continuous, slow, and dance-like motion of the entire body to discrete, rapid, and shock-like twitching of a single leg. Figure 5.1 shows the specific dyskinesias discussed in this chapter. As dyskinesias are movement disorders, they are signs and symptoms of central nervous system diseases. However, many dyskinesias are caused by anti-Parkinsonian and antipsychotic medications.

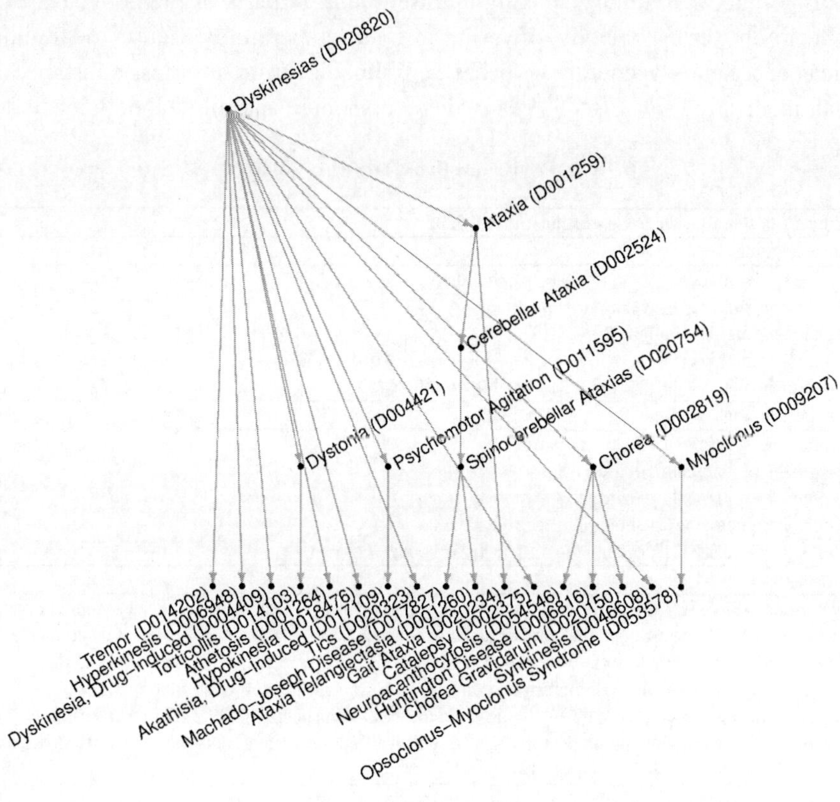

Figure 5.1. Different types and affected body parts of uncontrolled muscle movements.

The herbal formulas that are commonly prescribed for dyskinesias are Sháoyàogāncǎotāng, Dāngguīsìnìtāng, Dāngguīniāntòngtāng, Shūjīnghuóxuètāng, Máhuángfùzǐxìxīntāng, Sìnìtāng, Huángqíwǔwùtāng, and Dàzhēnjiāotāng, many of which have to do with Qi and Blood. The single herbs that are commonly added to support the formulas include Guìzhī, Shēngjiāng, Fùzǐ, Wúzhūyú, Niúxī, Gānjiāng, Dàzǎo, Yánhúsuǒ, and Zhìgāncǎo.

The diseases that commonly underlie or accompany the dyskinesia signs and symptoms are unspecified disorders of nervous system, orofacial dyskinesia, unspecified condition of brain, unspecified disorder of metabolism, unspecified disorder of cranial nerves, unspecified disorder of eye, Brown's (tendon) sheath syndrome, internuclear ophthalmoplegia, unspecified disorder of eye movements, unspecified disease of spinal cord, and unspecified cardiovascular disease. Note that a disease diagnosis such as cerebrovascular disease can manifest different signs and symptoms in patients depending on the location and severity of the injury. Herbal prescriptions should ideally be tailored to the individual patient and their specific symptoms. We see many such examples of *precision* herbal medicine in the tables throughout the book.

5.1. Tremor

Tremor is rhythmic, involuntary shaking and trembling in parts of the body. An example of tremor is teeth chattering or body shivering in cold temperatures. Causes of tremor include neurological and neurodegenerative diseases, traumatic brain injuries, substance abuse or withdrawal, medication side effects, heavy metal poisoning and mineral deficiencies.

Table 5.1. Herbal prescriptions for tremor

<table>
<tr><td colspan="2">Tremor: https://meshb.nlm.nih.gov/record/ui?ui=D014202.</td></tr>
<tr><td colspan="2">Common prescriptions:</td></tr>
<tr><td colspan="2">Dāngguīsìnìtāng 5g sìnìtāng 4g shēngjiāng 1g wúzhūyú 1g
Dāngguīsìnìtāng 5g sìnìtāng 4g wúzhūyú 1g gānjiāng 1g
Dāngguīsìnìtāng 5g fùzǐ 1g gānjiāng 1g
Dāngguīsìnìtāng 5g fùzǐ 1g
Dāngguīsìnìtāng 5g sìnìtāng 4g shēngjiāng 1g wúzhūyú 1g fùzǐ 1g</td></tr>
<tr><td colspan="2">Alternative prescriptions:</td></tr>
<tr><td colspan="2">Dāngguīsìnìtāng 5g shēngjiāng 1g wúzhūyú 1g
Sìnìtāng 5g guìzhī 1g máhuáng 1g xìxīn 0g
Dāngguīsìnìtāng 5g sìnìtāng 4g wúzhūyú 1g jīxuèténg 1g
Dāngguīsìnìtāng 5g jīxuèténg 2g shēngjiāng 1g wúzhūyú 0g
Dāngguīsìnìtāng 5g chuānwū 1g shēngjiāng 1g wúzhūyú 1g fùzǐ 1g</td></tr>
<tr><td colspan="2">Indicated diseases:</td></tr>
<tr><td colspan="2">Secondary parkinsonism 332.1 (Neuroleptic induced parkinsonism G2111, Other drug induced secondary parkinsonism G2119, Other secondary parkinsonism G218); Orofacial dyskinesia 333.82 (Idiopathic orofacial dystonia G244); Unspecified condition of brain 348.9 (Disorder of brain, unspecified G939); Unspecified disorders of nervous system 349.9 (Disorder of central nervous system, unspecified G969); Unspecified cerebrovascular disease 437.9 (Cerebrovascular disease, unspecified I679); Cardiovascular disease, unspecified 429.2 (Atherosclerotic heart disease of native coronary artery without angina pectoris I2510); Unspecified disorder of metabolism 277.9 (Metabolic disorder, unspecified E889); Alcohol abuse 305.0</td></tr>
<tr><td colspan="2">Secondary parkinsonism 332.1/G2111,G2119,G218 with tremor D014202:</td></tr>
<tr><td>Xiǎoxùmìngtāng 5g bǔyánghuánwǔtāng 5g dānshēn 1g shíchāngpú 1g yuǎnzhì 1g to ♀</td><td>Yìgānsǎn 5g bǔyánghuánwǔtāng 5g tiānmá 1g shíchāngpú 1g yuǎnzhì 1g to ♂</td></tr>
<tr><td colspan="2">Unspecified cerebrovascular disease 437.9/I679 with tremor D014202:</td></tr>
<tr><td>Bǔyánghuánwǔtāng 5g bànxiàbáizhútiānmátāng 3g xuèfǔzhúyūtāng 3g chuānxiōng 1g dānshēn 1g dìlóng 1g jiāngcán 1g to ♀</td><td>Bǔyánghuánwǔtāng 5g xuèfǔzhúyūtāng 3g huángqíwǔwùtāng 3g dānshēn 1g dìlóng 1g fùzǐ 1g jiāngcán 1g to ♂</td></tr>
<tr><td colspan="2">Orofacial dyskinesia 333.82/G244 with tremor D014202:</td></tr>
<tr><td>Sháoyàogāncǎotāng 5g mùguā 1g niúxī 1g qínjiāo 1g gōuténg 1g to ♀</td><td>Sháoyàogāncǎotāng 5g mùguā 1g niúxī 1g qínjiāo 1g gōuténg 1g to ♂</td></tr>
</table>

Dāngguīsìnìtāng 'nourishes Blood, expels chills,' and 'warms up meridians, interlinks collaterals.' The meridian-collateral system in traditional Chinese medicine is a network of channels inside the body where Qi, a form of life-energy, flows (Wang, 2013). As tremor is a type of muscle movement problems, restoring erratic or obstructed Qi flow by Dāngguīsìnìtāng is believed to improve the condition.

5.2. Hyperkinesis

Hyperkinesis is abnormally heightened activity of the muscles in the body as a whole. Metabolic disorders, endocrine disorders, autoimmune disorders, brain diseases, infections and injuries can cause hyperkinesis.

Table 5.2. Herbal prescriptions for hyperkinesis

Hyperkinesis: https://meshb.nlm.nih.gov/record/ui?ui=D006948.	
Common prescriptions:	
Dāngguīsìnìtāng 5g fùzǐ 1g shēngjiāng 1g wúzhūyú 1g Dāngguīsìnìtāng 5g sìnìtāng 4g shēngjiāng 1g wúzhūyú 1g Dāngguīsìnìtāng 5g fùzǐ 1g Dāngguīsìnìtāng 5g sìnìtāng 4g shēngjiāng 1g wúzhūyú 1g fùzǐ 1g	
Alternative prescriptions:	
Sìnìtāng 5g dāngguīsìnìtāng 5g shēngjiāng 1g wúzhūyú 1g Máhuángfùzǐxìxīntāng 5g fùzǐ 3g guìzhī 3g gānjiāng 3g dàzǎo 2g zhìgāncǎotāng 2g Máhuángfùzǐxìxīntāng 5g shēngjiāng 1g zhìgāncǎo 1g guìzhī 1g Sìnìtāng 5g dāngguīsìnìtāng 5g shēngjiāng 0g wúzhūyú 0g	
Indicated diseases:	
Epilepsy, unspecified 345.9; Orofacial dyskinesia 333.82 (Idiopathic orofacial dystonia G244); Unspecified condition of brain 348.9 (Disorder of brain, unspecified G939); Unspecified disorders of nervous system 349.9 (Disorder of central nervous system, unspecified G969); Schizoaffective disorder 295.7; Schizophreniform disorder 295.4; Unspecified disorder of metabolism 277.9 (Metabolic disorder, unspecified E889); Tourette's disorder 307.23 (Tourette's disorder F952); Chronic motor or vocal tic disorder 307.22 (Chronic motor or vocal tic disorder F951); Transient tic disorder 307.21 (Transient tic disorder F950); Tic disorder, unspecified 307.20 (Tic disorder, unspecified F959)	
Epilepsy, unspecified 345.9 with hyperkinesis D006948:	
Tiānmágōuténgyǐn 5g jiāwèixiāoyáosǎn 5g cháihújiālónggǔmǔlìtāng 5g dúhuójìshēngtāng 5g shēntòngzhúyūtāng 4g dǎngshēn 2g to ♀	Tiānmágōuténgyǐn 5g jiāwèixiāoyáosǎn 5g cháihújiālónggǔmǔlìtāng 5g xuánfùdàizhěshítāng 5g dúhuójìshēngtāng 5g dǎngshēn 2g to ♂
Orofacial dyskinesia 333.82/G244 with hyperkinesis D006948:	
Sháoyàogāncǎotāng 5g mùguā 1g niúxī 1g qínjiāo 1g gōuténg 1g to ♀	Sháoyàogāncǎotāng 5g mùguā 1g niúxī 1g qínjiāo 1g gōuténg 1g to ♂

Máhuángfùzǐxìxīntāng 'warms up meridians and releases exterior.' If hyperkinesis can be understood as a manifestation of a stray Yang, then as Máhuángfùzǐxìxīntāng thaws Yin, reunion of Yin and Yang resolves hyperkinesis.

5.3. Drug-Induced Dyskinesia

Drug-induced dyskinesia is involuntary, repetitive movements of the mouth, face, limbs or torso induced by drugs. Antipsychotic drugs and anti-Parkinson's drugs are known to caused drug-induced dyskinesia.

Table 5.3. Herbal prescriptions for drug-induced dyskinesia

Drug-Induced Dyskinesia: https://meshb.nlm.nih.gov/record/ui?ui=D004409.	
Common prescriptions:	
Wūyàoshùnqìsǎn 5g huángqíwǔwùtāng 5g + acupuncture Xiǎoxùmìngtāng 5g wūyàoshùnqìsǎn 5g bǔyánghuánwǔtāng 5g Wūyàoshùnqìsǎn 5g huángqíwǔwùtāng 5g	
Alternative prescriptions:	
Sháoyàogāncǎotāng 5g máhuángfùzǐxìxīntāng 4g fùzǐ 1g Huángqíwǔwùtāng 5g dānshēn 1g niúxī 1g zhúrú 1g sāngzhī 1g jīxuèténg 1g Dāngguīsìnìtāng 5g fùzǐ 0g Dāngguīsìnìtāng 5g wúzhūyú 1g fùzǐ 1g gānjiāng 1g cāngzhú 1g Máhuángfùzǐxìxīntāng 5g dāngguīsìnìtāng 4g fùzǐ 2g guìzhī 2g gānjiāng 2g dàzǎo 1g zhìgāncǎo 1g	
Indicated diseases:	
Secondary parkinsonism 332.1 (Neuroleptic induced parkinsonism G2111, Other drug induced secondary parkinsonism G2119, Other secondary parkinsonism G218); Schizophreniform disorder 295.4; Orofacial dyskinesia 333.82 (Idiopathic orofacial dystonia G244); Unspecified condition of brain 348.9 (Disorder of brain, unspecified G939); Unspecified disorders of nervous system 349.9 (Disorder of central nervous system, unspecified G969); Schizoaffective disorder 295.7; Tourette's disorder 307.23 (Tourette's disorder F952); Tic disorder, unspecified 307.20 (Tic disorder, unspecified F959); Transient tic disorder 307.21 (Transient tic disorder F950); Chronic motor or vocal tic disorder 307.22 (Chronic motor or vocal tic disorder F951)	
Secondary parkinsonism 332.1/G2111,G2119,G218 with dyskinesia, drug-induced D004409:	
Yìgānsǎn 5g bǔyánghuánwǔtāng 5g tiānmá 1g shíchāngpú 1g yuǎnzhì 1g to ♀	Yìgānsǎn 5g bǔyánghuánwǔtāng 5g tiānmá 1g shíchāngpú 1g yuǎnzhì 1g to ♂
Orofacial dyskinesia 333.82/G244 with dyskinesia, drug-induced D004409:	
Sháoyàogāncǎotāng 5g mùguā 1g niúxī 1g qínjiāo 1g gōuténg 1g to ♀	Sháoyàogāncǎotāng 5g mùguā 1g niúxī 1g qínjiāo 1g gōuténg 1g to ♂

Wūyàoshùnqìsǎn 'rectifies Qi, expels Wind,' and 'unties knots, moves stagnation.' Again, restoration of Qi circulation is involved in the herbal prescriptions for dyskinesia. Note that one of the modern uses of Yìgānsǎn is for unspecified nonpsychotic mental disorder (Wang, 2019).

5.4. Dystonia

Dystonia is uncontrolled contractions or spasms of the muscles in some part of the body. Damages, by trauma, tumor, stroke, infection, poisoning or genetic mutations, to the brain regions, such as the basal ganglia, that control movement cause dystonia.

Table 5.4. Herbal prescriptions for dystonia

Dystonia: https://meshb.nlm.nih.gov/record/ui?ui=D004421.
Common prescriptions:
Huángqíwǔwùtāng 5g dānshēn 1g zhúrú 1g sāngzhī 1g jiānghuáng 1g Huángqíwǔwùtāng 5g dānshēn 1g zhúrú 1g sāngzhī 1g dāngguī 1g jiānghuáng 1g Huángqíwǔwùtāng 5g dānshēn 1g zhúrú 1g sāngzhī 1g jiānghuáng 1g + acupuncture Huángqíwǔwùtāng 5g dānshēn 1g zhúrú 1g sāngzhī 1g qínjiāo 1g jiānghuáng 1g
Alternative prescriptions:
Huángqíwǔwùtāng 5g dānshēn 0g jīxuèténg 0g Dāngguīsìnìtāng 5g fùzǐ 1g wúzhūyú 0g Dāngguīsìnìtāng 5g chuānwū 0g shēngjiāng 0g wúzhūyú 0g Dāngguīsìnìtāng 5g wúzhūyú 1g gānjiāng 1g Dāngguīsìnìtāng 5g fùzǐ 1g shēngjiāng 1g wúzhūyú 1g + acupuncture

<table>
<tr><td colspan="2">Dystonia: https://meshb.nlm.nih.gov/record/ui?ui=D004421.</td></tr>
<tr><td colspan="2">Indicated diseases:</td></tr>
<tr><td colspan="2">Unspecified cerebrovascular disease 437.9 (Cerebrovascular disease, unspecified I679); Orofacial dyskinesia 333.82 (Idiopathic orofacial dystonia G244); Cardiovascular disease, unspecified 429.2 (Atherosclerotic heart disease of native coronary artery without angina pectoris I2510); Unspecified condition of brain 348.9 (Disorder of brain, unspecified G939); Unspecified disorders of nervous system 349.9 (Disorder of central nervous system, unspecified G969); Unspecified disorder of metabolism 277.9 (Metabolic disorder, unspecified E889); Obsessive-compulsive disorders 300.3 (Mixed obsessional thoughts and acts F422, Hoarding disorder F423, Other obsessive-compulsive disorder F428, Obsessive-compulsive disorder, unspecified F429)</td></tr>
<tr><td colspan="2">Unspecified cerebrovascular disease 437.9/I679 with dystonia D004421:</td></tr>
<tr><td>Bǔyánghuánwǔtāng 5g sānqī 1g dānshēn 1g shíchāngpú 1g yuǎnzhì 1g + acupuncture to ♀</td><td>Bǔyánghuánwǔtāng 5g chuānqī 1g dānshēn 1g shíchāngpú 1g yuǎnzhì 1g + acupuncture to ♂</td></tr>
<tr><td colspan="2">Orofacial dyskinesia 333.82/G244 with dystonia D004421:</td></tr>
<tr><td>Sháoyàogāncǎotāng 5g mùguā 1g niúxī 1g qínjiāo 1g gōuténg 1g to ♀</td><td>Sháoyàogāncǎotāng 5g mùguā 1g niúxī 1g qínjiāo 1g gōuténg 1g to ♂</td></tr>
<tr><td colspan="2">Unspecified condition of brain 348.9/G939 with dystonia D004421:</td></tr>
<tr><td>Xiǎoxùmìngtāng 5g bǔyánghuánwǔtāng 5g to ♀</td><td>Bǔyánghuánwǔtāng 5g dānshēn 1g shíchāngpú 1g yuǎnzhì 1g + acupuncture to ♂</td></tr>
</table>

Huángqíwǔwùtāng 'nourishes Qi, Blood' and 'harmonizes nutrition and defense.' Alternating use of Huángqíwǔwùtāng and Dāngguīsìnìtāng in the herbal prescriptions is believed to reflect the diverse types, causes, and associated symptoms of dystonia.

5.5. Torticollis

Torticollis is a tilted or twisted neck. Injuries and spasms to the muscles and ligaments supporting the head can cause torticollis.

Table 5.5. Herbal prescriptions for torticollis

<table>
<tr><td colspan="2">Torticollis: https://meshb.nlm.nih.gov/record/ui?ui=D014103.</td></tr>
<tr><td colspan="2">Common prescriptions:</td></tr>
<tr><td colspan="2">Sháoyàogāncǎotāng 5g mùguā 1g niúxī 1g huángbò 1g cāngzhú 1g yìyǐrén 1g
Sháoyàogāncǎotāng 5g mùguā 1g niúxī 1g
Sháoyàogāncǎotāng 5g mùguā 1g niúxī 1g huángbò 1g cāngzhú 1g yìyǐrén 1g + acupuncture
Sháoyàogāncǎotāng 5g mùguā 1g niúxī 1g huángbò 1g cāngzhú 1g</td></tr>
<tr><td colspan="2">Alternative prescriptions:</td></tr>
<tr><td colspan="2">Sháoyàogāncǎotāng 5g mùguā 0g niúxī 0g
Sháoyàogāncǎotāng 5g mùguā 1g niúxī 1g jīxuèténg 1g
Sháoyàogāncǎotāng 5g shūjīnghuóxuètāng 5g mùguā 1g niúxī 1g mòyào 1g rǔxiāng 1g
Sháoyàogāncǎotāng 5g mùguā 1g niúxī 1g jīxuèténg 1g + acupuncture
Sháoyàogāncǎotāng 5g niúxī 1g xùduàn 1g + acupuncture</td></tr>
<tr><td colspan="2">Indicated and associated diseases:</td></tr>
<tr><td colspan="2">Hypertropia 378.31 (Vertical strabismus, right eye H5021, Vertical strabismus, left eye H5022); Mechanical strabismus 378.6; Brown's (tendon) sheath syndrome 378.61 (Brown's sheath syndrome, right eye H50611, Brown's sheath syndrome, left eye H50612); Internuclear ophthalmoplegia 378.86 (Internuclear ophthalmoplegia, unspecified eye H5120); Unspecified disorder of eye movements 378.9 (Unspecified disorder of binocular movement H519); Orofacial dyskinesia 333.82 (Idiopathic orofacial dystonia G244); Unspecified disorder of cranial nerves 352.9 (Cranial nerve disorder, unspecified G529); Disorder of eye, unspecified 379.90 (Unspecified disorder of eye and adnexa H579); Unspecified disorders of nervous system 349.9 (Disorder of central nervous system, unspecified G969)</td></tr>
<tr><td colspan="2">Hypertropia 378.31/H5021,H5022 with torticollis D014103:</td></tr>
<tr><td>Qǐjúdìhuángwán 5g zīshènmíngmùtāng 5g to ♀</td><td>Qǐjúdìhuángwán 5g zīshènmíngmùtāng 5g to ♂</td></tr>
<tr><td colspan="2">Brown's (tendon) sheath syndrome 378.61/H50611,H50612 with torticollis D014103:</td></tr>
<tr><td>Xiǎocháihútāng 5g liùwèidìhuángwán 5g gǒuqǐzǐ 2g júhuā 2g to ♀</td><td>Qǐjúdìhuángwán 5g zīshènmíngmùtāng 5g to ♂</td></tr>
</table>

Sháoyàogāncǎotāng has traditionally been used for spasms and cramps of the muscle. Children with strabismus may keep an abnormal head posture in order to optimally utilize both their eyes, leading to what is called ocular torticollis.

5.6. Athetosis

Athetosis is continuous, slow, involuntary writhing movements of the hands and feet. Damage to the part of the brain responsible for motor control causes athetosis.

Table 5.6. Herbal prescriptions for athetosis

Athetosis: https://meshb.nlm.nih.gov/record/ui?ui=D001264.	
Common prescriptions:	
Sháoyàogāncǎotāng 5g shūjīnghuóxuètāng 5g dāngguīniāntòngtāng 5g + acupuncture Shūjīnghuóxuètāng 5g dāngguīniāntòngtāng 5g dúhuójìshēngtāng 5g	
Alternative prescriptions:	
Huángqíwǔwùtāng 5g dānshēn 2g zhúrú 2g sāngzhī 2g qínjiāo 2g jiānghuáng 2g Guìzhīsháoyàozhīmǔtāng 5g huángqíwǔwùtāng 5g dānshēn 1g zhúrú 1g sāngzhī 1g dāngguī 1g jiānghuáng 1g Shūjīnghuóxuètāng 5g huángqíwǔwùtāng 5g dānshēn 2g zhúrú 2g yánhúsuǒ 2g sāngzhī 2g jiānghuáng 2g Bāxiāntāng 5g Dāngguīsìnìtāng 5g huángqíwǔwùtāng 4g sāngzhī 1g jiānghuáng 1g jīxuèténg 1g	
Indicated diseases:	
Congenital diplegia 343.0 (Spastic diplegic cerebral palsy G801); Congenital monoplegia 343.3 (Other cerebral palsy G808); Congenital quadriplegia 343.2 (Spastic quadriplegic cerebral palsy G800); Orofacial dyskinesia 333.82 (Idiopathic orofacial dystonia G244); Unspecified condition of brain 348.9 (Disorder of brain, unspecified G939); Unspecified disorders of nervous system 349.9 (Disorder of central nervous system, unspecified G969); Unspecified disorder of metabolism 277.9 (Metabolic disorder, unspecified E889)	
Congenital diplegia 343.0/G801 with athetosis D001264:	
Shūjīnghuóxuètāng 5g dúhuójìshēngtāng 5g mázǐrénwán 2g mùguā 1g niúxī 1g to ♀	Bǔyánghuánwǔtāng 5g mázǐrénwán 2g dānshēn 1g niúxī 1g sāngzhī 1g jīxuèténg 1g to ♂
Congenital quadriplegia 343.2/G800 with athetosis D001264:	
Dāngguīniāntòngtāng 5g dúhuójìshēngtāng 5g mùguā 1g hónghuā 1g qínjiāo 1g sūmù 1g to ♀	Dāngguīniāntòngtāng 5g dúhuójìshēngtāng 5g mùguā 1g hónghuā 1g qínjiāo 1g sūmù 1g to ♂
Orofacial dyskinesia 333.82/G244 with athetosis D001264:	
Sháoyàogāncǎotāng 5g mùguā 1g niúxī 1g qínjiāo 1g gōuténg 1g to ♀	Sháoyàogāncǎotāng 5g mùguā 1g niúxī 1g qínjiāo 1g gōuténg 1g to ♂

Shūjīnghuóxuètāng ‘dredges meridians and enlivens Blood.’ Its modern uses are for neuralgia, neuritis and radiculitis (Wang, 2019). The herbal prescriptions in the table look to alleviate the severity of the symptom.

5.7. Hypokinesia

Hypokinesia is decreased range and pace of bodily movements. Parkinson’s disease is characterized by hypokinesia.

Each of Sìnìtāng, Máhuángfùzǐxìxīntāng and Dāngguīsìnìtāng augments Yang Qi, which represents motions and activities in the concept of traditional Chinese medicine. Their use for hypokinesia is therefore conceivable.

Table 5.7. Herbal prescriptions for hypokinesia

Hypokinesia: https://meshb.nlm.nih.gov/record/ui?ui=D018476.	
Common prescriptions:	
Sìnìtāng 5g máhuángfùzǐxìxīntāng 5g shēngjiāng 1g guìzhī 1g Sìnìtāng 5g dāngguīsìnìtāng 5g wúzhūyú 1g gānjiāng 1g Sìnìtāng 5g dāngguīsìnìtāng 5g wúzhūyú 1g Sìnìtāng 5g wúzhūyútāng 5g máhuángfùzǐxìxīntāng 5g	
Alternative prescriptions:	
Máhuángfùzǐxìxīntāng 5g fùzǐ 3g guìzhī 3g gānjiāng 3g dàzǎo 2g zhìgāncǎo 2g Máhuángfùzǐxìxīntāng 5g fùzǐ 3g guìzhī 3g dàzǎo 2g niúxī 2g zhìgāncǎo 2g gānjiāng 2g Sìnìtāng 5g wúzhūyú 1g yánhúsuǒ 1g Máhuángfùzǐxìxīntāng 5g dāngguīsìnìtāng 5g wúzhūyú 2g fùzǐ 2g guìzhī 2g wūméi 2g gānjiāng 2g Máhuángfùzǐxìxīntāng 5g fùzǐ 3g guìzhī 3g dàzǎo 2g shēngjiāng 2g wúzhūyú 2g zhìgāncǎo 2g	
Indicated diseases:	
Unspecified cerebrovascular disease 437.9 (Cerebrovascular disease, unspecified I679); Orofacial dyskinesia 333.82 (Idiopathic orofacial dystonia G244); Cardiovascular disease, unspecified 429.2 (Atherosclerotic heart disease of native coronary artery without angina pectoris I2510); Unspecified condition of brain 348.9 (Disorder of brain, unspecified G939); Unspecified disorders of nervous system 349.9 (Disorder of central nervous system, unspecified G969); Secondary parkinsonism 332.1 (Neuroleptic induced parkinsonism G2111, Other drug induced secondary parkinsonism G2119, Other secondary parkinsonism G218); Unspecified disorder of joint, site unspecified 719.90 (Joint disorder, unspecified M259); Myopathy, unspecified 359.9 (Myopathy, unspecified G729); Unspecified disorder of metabolism 277.9 (Metabolic disorder, unspecified E889)	
Unspecified cerebrovascular disease 437.9/I679 with hypokinesia D018476:	
Xiǎoxùmìngtāng 5g bǔyánghuánwǔtāng 5g to ♀	Bǔyánghuánwǔtāng 5g dānshēn 1g tiānmá 1g shíchāngpú 1g yuǎnzhì 1g + acupuncture to ♂
Secondary parkinsonism 332.1/G2111,G2119,G218 with hypokinesia D018476:	
Wūyàoshùnqìsǎn 5g bǔyánghuánwǔtāng 5g dàhuáng 2g yuǎnzhì 2g to ♀	Xiǎoxùmìngtāng 5g bǔyánghuánwǔtāng 5g tiānmá 1g shíchāngpú 1g yuǎnzhì 1g + acupuncture to ♂
Orofacial dyskinesia 333.82/G244 with hypokinesia D018476:	
Sháoyàogāncǎotāng 5g mùguā 1g niúxī 1g qínjiāo 1g gōuténg 1g to ♀	Sháoyàogāncǎotāng 5g mùguā 1g niúxī 1g qínjiāo 1g gōuténg 1g to ♂

5.8. Psychomotor Agitation

Psychomotor agitation is a state of mental tension and motor restlessness that results in repetitive and meaningless movements. Examples of psychomotor agitation are hand wringing, nail biting and room pacing. Psychomotor agitation is associated with mood disorders such as bipolar disorder, depression and schizophrenia.

Table 5.8. Herbal prescriptions for psychomotor agitation

Psychomotor Agitation: https://meshb.nlm.nih.gov/record/ui?ui=D011595.
Common prescriptions:
Máhuángfùzǐxìxīntāng 5g fùzǐ 3g guìzhī 3g dàzǎo 2g zhìgāncǎo 2g gānjiāng 2g Máhuángfùzǐxìxīntāng 5g fùzǐ 3g guìzhī 3g gānjiāng 3g dàzǎo 2g zhìgāncǎotāng 2g Máhuángfùzǐxìxīntāng 5g fùzǐ 3g guìzhī 3g gānjiāng 3g dàzǎo 2g zhìgāncǎo 2g wēilíngxiān 2g
Alternative prescriptions:
Máhuángfùzǐxìxīntāng 5g fùzǐ 3g guìzhī 3g báizhú 2g wúzhūyú 2g gānjiāng 2g zhìgāncǎotāng 2g Sìnìtāng 5g guìzhī 1g máhuáng 1g xìxīn 0g Dāngguīsìnìtāng 5g wúzhūyú 1g fùzǐ 1g gānjiāng 1g Dāngguīsìnìtāng 5g shēngjiāng 1g wúzhūyú 1g

Table 5.8. (Continued)

Psychomotor Agitation: https://meshb.nlm.nih.gov/record/ui?ui=D011595.	
Indicated diseases:	
Neuroleptic malignant syndrome 333.92 (Malignant neuroleptic syndrome G210); Orofacial dyskinesia 333.82 (Idiopathic orofacial dystonia G244); Unspecified condition of brain 348.9 (Disorder of brain, unspecified G939); Unspecified disorders of nervous system 349.9 (Disorder of central nervous system, unspecified G969); Schizoaffective disorder 295.7; Schizophreniform disorder 295.4; Alcohol abuse 305.0	
Neuroleptic malignant syndrome 333.92/G210 with psychomotor agitation D011595:	
Yìgānsǎn 5g sháoyàogāncǎotāng 5g mùguā 1g niúxī 1g to ♀	Sháoyàogāncǎotāng 5g shūjīnghuóxuètāng 5g mùguā 1g niúxī 1g to ♂
Orofacial dyskinesia 333.82/G244 with psychomotor agitation D011595:	
Sháoyàogāncǎotāng 5g mùguā 1g niúxī 1g qínjiāo 1g gōuténg 1g to ♀	Sháoyàogāncǎotāng 5g mùguā 1g niúxī 1g qínjiāo 1g gōuténg 1g to ♂

If psychomotor agitation is considered a type of hyperkinesis, the idea of restoring Yin-Yang homeostasis behind Máhuángfùzǐxìxīntāng's use for hyperkinesis applies here.

5.9. Drug-Induced Akathisia

Akathisia is a subjective feeling of restlessness, making one unable to sit still. Akathisia is most often a side effect of antipsychotics.

As a subtype of psychomotor agitation, akathisia is prescribed Máhuángfùzǐxìxīntāng, which is used for psychomotor agitation.

Table 5.9. Herbal prescriptions for drug-induced akathisia

Drug-Induced Akathisia: https://meshb.nlm.nih.gov/record/ui?ui=D017109.	
Common prescriptions:	
Máhuángfùzǐxìxīntāng 5g shēngjiāng 2g guìzhī 2g zhìgāncǎo 1g Máhuángfùzǐxìxīntāng 5g shēngjiāng 2g zhìgāncǎo 2g guìzhī 2g dàzǎo 1g Máhuángfùzǐxìxīntāng 5g shēngjiāng 2g zhìgāncǎo 2g guìzhī 2g Máhuángfùzǐxìxīntāng 5g shēngjiāng 2g guìzhī 2g gāncǎo 1g	
Alternative prescriptions:	
Máhuángfùzǐxìxīntāng 5g shēngjiāng 3g fùzǐ 3g guìzhī 3g dàzǎo 2g zhìgāncǎo 2g gānjiāng 2g Huángqíwǔwùtāng 5g dānshēn 1g zhúrú 1g sāngzhī 1g jiānghuáng 1g Sháoyàogāncǎotāng 5g máhuángfùzǐxìxīntāng 4g dìlóng 1g sūmù 1g Sháoyàogāncǎotāng 5g shūjīnghuóxuètāng 5g gégēntāng 5g	
Indicated diseases:	
Orofacial dyskinesia 333.82 (Idiopathic orofacial dystonia G244); Schizoaffective disorder 295.7; Unspecified disorders of nervous system 349.9 (Disorder of central nervous system, unspecified G969); Schizophreniform disorder 295.4; Alcohol abuse 305.0; Bipolar disorder, unspecified 296.80 (Bipolar disorder, unspecified F319)	
Orofacial dyskinesia 333.82/G244 with akathisia, drug-induced D017109:	
Sháoyàogāncǎotāng 5g mùguā 1g niúxī 1g qínjiāo 1g gōuténg 1g to ♀	Sháoyàogāncǎotāng 5g mùguā 1g niúxī 1g qínjiāo 1g gōuténg 1g to ♂

5.10. Tics

Tics are semi-voluntary, repetitive yet non-rhythmic contraction of the muscle group, resulting in sudden movement or vocalization. Examples of tics are excessive eye blinking and throat clearing. Causes of tics are unknown but changes in the region of the brain controlling the affected muscle are suspected.

Table 5.10. Herbal prescriptions for tics

<table>
<tr><td colspan="2">Tics: https://meshb.nlm.nih.gov/record/ui?ui=D020323.</td></tr>
<tr><td colspan="2">Common prescriptions:</td></tr>
<tr><td colspan="2">Huángqíwǔwùtāng 5g dāngguīsìnìtāng 5g dānshēn 1g zhúrú 1g sāngzhī 1g jiānghuáng 1g
Dāngguīsìnìtāng 5g fùzǐ 1g shēngjiāng 1g wúzhūyú 1g
Huángqíwǔwùtāng 5g dāngguīsìnìtāng 5g dānshēn 2g zhúrú 2g sāngzhī 2g jiānghuáng 2g</td></tr>
<tr><td colspan="2">Alternative prescriptions:</td></tr>
<tr><td colspan="2">Dāngguīsìnìtāng 5g sìnìtāng 4g shēngjiāng 1g wúzhūyú 1g
Dāngguīsìnìtāng 5g sìnìtāng 3g shēngjiāng 1g wúzhūyú 1g
Dāngguīsìnìtāng 5g fùzǐ 1g
Dāngguīsìnìtāng 5g sìnìtāng 3g wúzhūyú 0g
Dāngguīsìnìtāng 5g shēngjiāng 1g wúzhūyú 1g</td></tr>
<tr><td colspan="2">Indicated diseases:</td></tr>
<tr><td colspan="2">Orofacial dyskinesia 333.82 (Idiopathic orofacial dystonia G244); Tourette's disorder 307.23 (Tourette's disorder F952); Unspecified condition of brain 348.9 (Disorder of brain, unspecified G939); Unspecified disorders of nervous system 349.9 (Disorder of central nervous system, unspecified G969); Chronic motor or vocal tic disorder 307.22 (Chronic motor or vocal tic disorder F951); Transient tic disorder 307.21 (Transient tic disorder F950); Tic disorder, unspecified 307.20 (Tic disorder, unspecified F959)</td></tr>
<tr><td colspan="2">Orofacial dyskinesia 333.82/G244 with tics D020323:</td></tr>
<tr><td>Sháoyàogāncǎotāng 5g gégēntāng 5g qínjiāo 1g gōuténg 1g to ♀</td><td>Sháoyàogāncǎotāng 5g gégēntāng 5g qínjiāo 1g gōuténg 1g to ♂</td></tr>
</table>

Either Huángqíwǔwùtāng or Dāngguīsìnìtāng improves the movements of Qi and Blood. Their concurrent use in the prescription is thought to enhance the effect of each other.

5.11. Cerebellar Ataxia

Ataxia is lack of voluntary coordination of muscle movements in one or both sides of the body, leading to abnormal patterns of gait, speech or eye movements. Damages, by stroke, alcohol, medications or inherited mutations, affecting the cerebellum and cerebellar pathways cause cerebellar ataxia.

Table 5.11. Herbal prescriptions for cerebellar ataxia

Cerebellar Ataxia: https://meshb.nlm.nih.gov/record/ui?ui=D002524.
Common prescriptions:
Dàzhēnjiāotāng 5g dāngguīniāntòngtāng 5g sháoyàogāncǎotāng 4g Dàzhēnjiāotāng 5g dāngguīniāntòngtāng 5g sháoyàogāncǎotāng 4g yánhúsuǒ 1g Máhuángfùzǐxìxīntāng 5g fùzǐ 3g guìzhī 3g dàzǎo 2g gānjiāng 2g zhìgāncǎotāng 2g Máhuángfùzǐxìxīntāng 5g fùzǐ 3g guìzhī 3g dàzǎo 2g zhìgāncǎo 2g gānjiāng 2g Máhuángfùzǐxìxīntāng 5g fùzǐ 3g guìzhī 3g gānjiāng 3g dàzǎo 2g zhìgāncǎo 2g wēilíngxiān 2g
Alternative prescriptions:
Dàzhēnjiāotāng 5g dāngguīniāntòngtāng 5g sháoyàogāncǎotāng 4g hòupò 1g Máhuángfùzǐxìxīntāng 5g fùzǐ 3g guìzhī 3g dàzǎo 2g wúzhūyú 2g gānjiāng 2g zhìgāncǎo 2g Dàzhēnjiāotāng 5g dāngguīniāntòngtāng 4g máxìngyìgāntāng 3g Dàzhēnjiāotāng 5g shàngzhōngxiàtōngyòngtòngfēngwán 4g dāngguīniāntòngtāng 4g

Table 5.11. (Continued)

Cerebellar Ataxia: https://meshb.nlm.nih.gov/record/ui?ui=D002524.	
Indicated diseases:	
Primary cerebellar degeneration 334.2 (Congenital nonprogressive ataxia G110, Late-onset cerebellar ataxia G112); Unspecified disease of spinal cord 336.9 (Disease of spinal cord, unspecified G959); Orofacial dyskinesia 333.82 (Idiopathic orofacial dystonia G244); Unspecified condition of brain 348.9 (Disorder of brain, unspecified G939); Unspecified disorders of nervous system 349.9 (Disorder of central nervous system, unspecified G969); Acute poliomyelitis 045; Myoneural disorders 358; Other dermatoses 702; Herpes simplex 054; Unspecified endocrine disorder 259.9 (Endocrine disorder, unspecified E349)	
Primary cerebellar degeneration 334.2/G110,G112 with cerebellar ataxia D002524:	
Xiǎoxùmìngtāng 5g + acupuncture to ♀	Bǔyánghuánwǔtāng 5g dānshēn 1g shíchāngpú 1g yuǎnzhì 1g + acupuncture to ♂
Unspecified disease of spinal cord 336.9/G959 with cerebellar ataxia D002524:	
Guīlùèrxiānjiāo 5g to ♀	Guīlùèrxiānjiāo 5g to ♂
Other dermatoses 702 with cerebellar ataxia D002524:	
Jiědúsìwùtāng 5g xiāofēngsǎn 4g zhēnrénhuómìngyǐnqùchuānshānjiǎ 4g huángliánjiědútāng 4g to ♀	Yùnǚjiān 5g xuèfǔzhúyūtāng 3g dāngguīsháoyàosǎn 3g báijiāngcán 1g to ♂
Orofacial dyskinesia 333.82/G244 with cerebellar ataxia D002524:	
Dāngguīsìnìtāng 5g sháoyàogāncǎotāng 3g fùzǐ 1g to ♀	Xiǎoxùmìngtāng 5g wūyàoshùnqìsǎn 5g to ♂

Dàzhēnjiāotāng contains Qínjiāo as its major herb. Qínjiāo's modern use is for other and unspecified disorder of joint (Wang, 2019). Dāngguīniāntòngtāng's modern uses are for gout, and rheumatoid arthritis (Wang, 2019). Their use in the prescriptions is thought to alleviate the mobility challenges associated with ataxia. A case of a child with rash and ataxia was reported (Helsing and Froen, 2007).

5.12. Gait Ataxia

Gait ataxia is when the poor coordination of muscles affects the lower limbs, making it difficult to walk steadily in a straight line. Damage to the cerebellum or spinal cord can cause gait ataxia.

Table 5.12. Herbal prescriptions for gait ataxia

Gait Ataxia: https://meshb.nlm.nih.gov/record/ui?ui=D020234.
Common prescriptions:
Máhuángfùzǐxìxīntāng 5g fùzǐ 3g guìzhī 3g gānjiāng 3g dàzǎo 2g zhìgāncǎotāng 2g Máhuángfùzǐxìxīntāng 5g fùzǐ 3g guìzhī 3g dàzǎo 2g zhìgāncǎo 2g gānjiāng 2g Máhuángfùzǐxìxīntāng 5g fùzǐ 3g guìzhī 3g gānjiāng 3g dàzǎo 2g zhìgāncǎo 2g wēilíngxiān 2g
Alternative prescriptions:
Dàzhēnjiāotāng 5g dāngguīniāntòngtāng 5g Dàzhēnjiāotāng 5g dāngguīniāntòngtāng 5g sháoyàogāncǎotāng 4g yánhúsuǒ 1g Máhuángfùzǐxìxīntāng 5g fùzǐ 2g guìzhī 2g gānjiāng 2g dàzǎo 1g zhìgāncǎotāng 1g
Máhuángfùzǐxìxīntāng 5g fùzǐ 3g guìzhī 3g gānjiāng 3g dàzǎo 2g zhìgāncǎotāng 1g
Indicated diseases:
Friedreich's ataxia 334.0 (Early-onset cerebellar ataxia G111); Unspecified disorder of metabolism 277.9 (Metabolic disorder, unspecified E889); Primary cerebellar degeneration 334.2 (Congenital nonprogressive ataxia G110, Late-onset cerebellar ataxia G112); Unspecified disease of spinal cord 336.9 (Disease of spinal cord, unspecified G959); Orofacial dyskinesia 333.82 (Idiopathic orofacial dystonia G244); Unspecified condition of brain 348.9 (Disorder of brain, unspecified G939); Unspecified disorders of nervous system 349.9 (Disorder of central nervous system, unspecified G969); Hereditary spastic paraplegia 334.1 (Hereditary spastic paraplegia G114); Critical illness polyneuropathy 357.82 (Critical illness polyneuropathy G6281); Myoneural disorders 358

Gait Ataxia: https://meshb.nlm.nih.gov/record/ui?ui=D020234.	
Friedreich's ataxia 334.0/G111 with gait ataxia D020234:	
Bǔyánghuánwǔtāng 5g dānshēn 1g tiānmá 1g shíchāngpú 1g yuǎnzhì 1g + acupuncture to ♀	Bǔyánghuánwǔtāng 5g dānshēn 1g tiānmá 1g shíchāngpú 1g yuǎnzhì 1g + acupuncture to ♂
Primary cerebellar degeneration 334.2/G110,G112 with gait ataxia D020234:	
Bǔyánghuánwǔtāng 5g dānshēn 1g tiānmá 1g shíchāngpú 1g yuǎnzhì 1g + acupuncture to ♀	Bǔyánghuánwǔtāng 5g dānshēn 1g tiānmá 1g shíchāngpú 1g yuǎnzhì 1g + acupuncture to ♂
Hereditary spastic paraplegia 334.1/G114 with gait ataxia D020234:	
Bǔyánghuánwǔtāng 5g mázǐrénwán 2g tiānmá 1g shíchāngpú 1g yuǎnzhì 1g + acupuncture to ♀	Bǔyánghuánwǔtāng 5g jishēngshènqìwán 5g dānshēn 1g shíchāngpú 1g yuǎnzhì 1g to ♂

Dàzhēnjiāotāng is used in the last section for cerebellar ataxia which encompasses gait ataxia. A modern use of Bǔyánghuánwǔtāng is for unspecified late effects of cerebrovascular disease (Wang, 2019) or stroke sequelae as we pointed out in previous chapters.

5.13. Machado-Joseph Disease

People with Machado-Joseph disease exhibit clumsy movements resembling those who are drunken or Parkinsonian. The cause of Machado-Joseph disease is an expansion of a repeat in the coding region of a gene on chromosome 14 of the human genome.

Table 5.13. Herbal prescriptions for Machado-Joseph disease

Machado-Joseph Disease: https://meshb.nlm.nih.gov/record/ui?ui=D017827.	
Common prescriptions:	
Sānbìtāng 5g Sānbìtāng 5g shūjīnghuóxuètāng 5g + acupuncture Sānbìtāng 5g huángqíwǔwùtāng 5g Sānbìtāng 5g shūjīnghuóxuètāng 5g	
Alternative prescriptions:	
Máhuángfùzǐxìxīntāng 5g sìnìtāng 4g sháoyàogāncǎotāng 4g chuānliànzǐ 1g yánhúsuǒ 1g Sānbìtāng 5g huángqíwǔwùtāng 3g jīxuèténg 1g Huángqíwǔwùtāng 5g Sānbìtāng 5g huángqíwǔwùtāng 3g	
Indicated diseases:	
Primary cerebellar degeneration 334.2 (Congenital nonprogressive ataxia G110, Late-onset cerebellar ataxia G112); Brown's (tendon) sheath syndrome 378.61 (Brown's sheath syndrome, right eye H50611, Brown's sheath syndrome, left eye H50612); Internuclear ophthalmoplegia 378.86 (Internuclear ophthalmoplegia, unspecified eye H5120); Unspecified disorder of eye movements 378.9 (Unspecified disorder of binocular movement H519); Unspecified disease of spinal cord 336.9 (Disease of spinal cord, unspecified G959); Orofacial dyskinesia 333.82 (Idiopathic orofacial dystonia G244); Unspecified disorder of cranial nerves 352.9 (Cranial nerve disorder, unspecified G529); Disorder of eye, unspecified 379.90 (Unspecified disorder of eye and adnexa H579); Unspecified condition of brain 348.9 (Disorder of brain, unspecified G939); Unspecified disorders of nervous system 349.9 (Disorder of central nervous system, unspecified G969); Unspecified retinal disorder 362.9 (Unspecified retinal disorder H359); Unspecified disorder of metabolism 277.9 (Metabolic disorder, unspecified E889)	
Primary cerebellar degeneration 334.2/G110,G112 with Machado-Joseph disease D017827:	
Bǔyánghuánwǔtāng 5g dānshēn 1g shíchāngpú 1g yuǎnzhì 1g + acupuncture to ♀	Bǔyánghuánwǔtāng 5g dānshēn 1g shíchāngpú 1g yuǎnzhì 1g + acupuncture to ♂

Sānbìtāng, which literally means 'three paralysis decoction,' has traditionally been used for paralysis due to 'Wind, Dampness and chills.' It is thought to relieve the muscle spasticity of the patients with Machado-Joseph disease. Note that a modern use of Sānbitāng is for lumbago (Wang, 2019).

5.14. Ataxia Telangiectasia

Ataxia-telangiectasia syndrome, a progressive cerebellar degeneration, shows poor muscle coordination, weakened immunity and impaired cellular repair. The cause of ataxia telangiectasia is mutations in a gene on chromosome 11 of the human genome.

A modern use of both Dāngguīniāntòngtāng and Dúhuójìshēngtāng is for rheumatoid arthritis (Wang, 2019). The mutated gene causing ataxia telangiectasia was linked to rheumatoid arthritis (Shao et al., 2009) and there was a report of juvenile idiopathic arthritis in a child with ataxia telangiectasia (Pasini et al., 2017). Use of the two herbal formulas here is therefore supposed to relieve the autoimmune phenomena in ataxia telangiectasia.

Table 5.14. Herbal prescriptions for ataxia telangiectasia

Ataxia Telangiectasia: https://meshb.nlm.nih.gov/record/ui?ui=D001260.	
Common prescriptions:	
Dāngguīniāntòngtāng 5g dúhuójìshēngtāng 5g sháoyàogāncǎotāng 3g shūjīnghuóxuètāng 3g gégēntāng 3g guīlùèrxiānjiāo 3g niúxī 2g yánhúsuǒ 2g Dāngguīniāntòngtāng 5g dúhuójìshēngtāng 5g sháoyàogāncǎotāng 3g shūjīnghuóxuètāng 3g gégēntāng 3g guīlùèrxiānjiāo 3g niúxī 2g Dāngguīniāntòngtāng 5g dúhuójìshēngtāng 5g sháoyàogāncǎotāng 3g shūjīnghuóxuètāng 3g gégēntāng 3g guīlùèrxiānjiāo 3g niúxī 2g gǔsuìbǔ 2g Dāngguīniāntòngtāng 5g dúhuójìshēngtāng 5g sháoyàogāncǎotāng 3g shūjīnghuóxuètāng 3g gégēntāng 3g guīlùèrxiānjiāo 3g niúxī 2g guìzhīsháoyàozhīmǔtāng 2g Dāngguīniāntòngtāng 5g dúhuójìshēngtāng 5g sháoyàogāncǎotāng 3g shūjīnghuóxuètāng 3g gégēntāng 3g guīlùèrxiānjiāo 3g niúxī 2g yánhúsuǒ 2g guìzhīsháoyàozhīmǔtāng 2g	
Alternative prescriptions:	
Dāngguīniāntòngtāng 5g jìshēngshènqìwán 4g shūjīnghuóxuètāng 3g fóshǒugān 1g Dāngguīniāntòngtāng 5g shūjīnghuóxuètāng 2g jìshēngshènqìwán 2g fóshǒugān 1g Dāngguīniāntòngtāng 5g dúhuójìshēngtāng 5g sháoyàogāncǎotāng 3g gégēntāng 3g shūjīnghuóxuètāng 2g guīlùèrxiānjiāo 2g niúxī 1g Dāngguīniāntòngtāng 5g shūjīnghuóxuètāng 3g jìshēngshènqìwán 2g fóshǒugān 1g Dāngguīniāntòngtāng 5g shàngzhōngxiàtōngyòngtòngfēngwán 3g niúxī 1g huángbò 1g cāngzhú 1g yìyǐrén 1g	
Indicated diseases:	
Cardiovascular disease, unspecified 429.2 (Atherosclerotic heart disease of native coronary artery without angina pectoris I2510); Orofacial dyskinesia 333.82 (Idiopathic orofacial dystonia G244); Unspecified disorder of metabolism 277.9 (Metabolic disorder, unspecified E889); Lymphoid leukemia 204; Unspecified condition of brain 348.9 (Disorder of brain, unspecified G939); Unspecified disorders of nervous system 349.9 (Disorder of central nervous system, unspecified G969); Leukemia of unspecified cell type 208; Reticulosarcoma 200.0; Mixed cellularity 201.6; Lymphocytic depletion 201.7; Lymphocytic-histiocytic predominance 201.4; Hodgkin's disease 201	
Cardiovascular disease, unspecified 429.2/I2510 with ataxia telangiectasia D001260:	
Yùzhú 5g sìnìtāng 5g gānlùyǐn 5g to ♀	Sìnìtāng 5g gānlùyǐn 5g mǔdānpí 1g zhīzǐ 1g huánglián 0g to ♂

5.15. Catalepsy

Catalepsy is a state of muscular rigidity, leaving the body in a fixed posture for a prolonged period of time, during which the patient also becomes less sensitive to pain. Parkinson's disease, epilepsy, and drug toxicity can cause catalepsy.

Table 5.15. Herbal prescriptions for catalepsy

Catalepsy: https://meshb.nlm.nih.gov/record/ui?ui=D002375.	
Common prescriptions:	
Sìnìtāng 5g shēngjiāng 1g guìzhī 1g Sìnìtāng 5g shēngjiāng 1g guìzhī 1g dàhuáng 0g Sìnìtāng 5g shēngjiāng 1g guìzhī 1g xìxīn 1g	
Alternative prescriptions:	
Sìnìtāng 5g shēngjiāng 0g guìzhī 0g Sìnìtāng 5g rénshēn 1g bànxià 1g yánhúsuǒ 1g dàhuáng 0g Sìnìtāng 5g bànxià 1g dàhuáng 0g Sìnìtāng 5g shēngjiāng 1g guìzhī 1g máhuáng 1g	
Indicated diseases:	
Orofacial dyskinesia 333.82 (Idiopathic orofacial dystonia G244); Schizoaffective disorder 295.7; Unspecified disorders of nervous system 349.9 (Disorder of central nervous system, unspecified G969); Schizophreniform disorder 295.4; Unspecified condition of brain 348.9 (Disorder of brain, unspecified G939)	
Orofacial dyskinesia 333.82/G244 with catalepsy D002375:	
Zhēnwǔtāng 5g fùzǐ 1g gānjiāng 1g to ♀	Xiǎoxùmìngtāng 5g wūyàoshùnqìsǎn 5g bǔyánghuánwǔtāng 5g to ♂
Unspecified condition of brain 348.9/G939 with catalepsy D002375:	
Xiǎoxùmìngtāng 5g bǔyánghuánwǔtāng 5g + acupuncture to ♀	Bǔyánghuánwǔtāng 5g dānshēn 1g shíchāngpú 1g yuǎnzhì 1g + acupuncture to ♂

Sìnìtāng was at first composed to reverse loss of sensation and motion of the four limbs. Its use here for catalepsy can be expected. Note that, from the tables, patients who have the same disease diagnosis, e.g., orofacial dyskinesia, but are presenting different signs and symptoms, e.g., tics, ataxia, and catalepsy can receive different herbal prescriptions.

5.16. Chorea

Chorea is involuntary, excessive, irregular and unpredictable bodily movements. Bacterial infections, antipsychotic medications, cerebrovascular diseases, metabolic derangements, autoimmune reactions and neurodegeneration such as Huntington's disease can cause chorea.

Dāngguīsìnìtāng is prescribed for tremor and hyperkinesis in the beginning of the chapter. Chorea, a form of hyperkinesis, is therefore prescribed Dāngguīsìnìtāng in the table.

Table 5.16. Herbal prescriptions for chorea

Chorea: https://meshb.nlm.nih.gov/record/ui?ui=D002819.
Common prescriptions:
Dāngguīsìnìtāng 5g shēngjiāng 1g wúzhūyú 1g Dāngguīsìnìtāng 5g shēngjiāng 1g wúzhūyú 1g fùzǐ 1g Dāngguīsìnìtāng 5g fùzǐ 1g shēngjiāng 1g wúzhūyú 1g Dāngguīsìnìtāng 5g shēngjiāng 1g wúzhūyú 1g jīxuèténg 1g
Alternative prescriptions:
Dāngguīsìnìtāng 5g shēngjiāng 0g wúzhūyú 0g Huángqíwǔwùtāng 5g chuānxiōng 2g dāngguī 2g dānshēn 1g zhúrú 1g yánhúsuǒ 1g sāngzhī 1g jiānghuáng 1g + acupuncture Huángqíwǔwùtāng 5g chuānxiōng 0g dāngguī 0g Máhuángfùzǐxìxīntāng 5g fùzǐ 3g guìzhī 3g gānjiāng 3g dàzǎo 2g zhìgāncǎotāng 2g

Table 5.16. (Continued)

Chorea: https://meshb.nlm.nih.gov/record/ui?ui=D002819.	
Indicated and associated diseases:	
Rheumatic fever with heart involvement 391; Orofacial dyskinesia 333.82 (Idiopathic orofacial dystonia G244); Unspecified disorder of joint, site unspecified 719.90 (Joint disorder, unspecified M259); Rheumatic chorea 392; Rheumatic fever without mention of heart involvement 390 (Rheumatic fever without heart involvement I00); Unspecified disorders of nervous system 349.9 (Disorder of central nervous system, unspecified G969); Unspecified cerebrovascular disease 437.9 (Cerebrovascular disease, unspecified I679); Cardiovascular disease, unspecified 429.2 (Atherosclerotic heart disease of native coronary artery without angina pectoris I2510); Unspecified condition of brain 348.9 (Disorder of brain, unspecified G939); Heart disease, unspecified 429.9 (Heart disease, unspecified I519); Obsessive-compulsive disorders 300.3 (Mixed obsessional thoughts and acts F422, Hoarding disorder F423, Other obsessive-compulsive disorder F428, Obsessive-compulsive disorder, unspecified F429); Unspecified disorder of metabolism 277.9 (Metabolic disorder, unspecified E889)	
Rheumatic fever with heart involvement 391 with chorea D002819:	
Zhēnwǔtāng 5g fùzǐ 1g gānjiāng 1g to ♀	Zhēnwǔtāng 5g fùzǐ 1g gānjiāng 1g to ♂
Unspecified cerebrovascular disease 437.9/I679 with chorea D002819:	
Xiǎoxùmìngtāng 5g bǔyánghuánwǔtāng 5g + acupuncture to ♀	Bǔyánghuánwǔtāng 5g dānshēn 1g niúxī 1g sāngzhī 1g jīxuèténg 1g + acupuncture to ♂
Orofacial dyskinesia 333.82/G244 with chorea D002819:	
Sháoyàogāncǎotāng 5g mùguā 1g niúxī 1g qínjiāo 1g gōuténg 1g to ♀	Xiǎoxùmìngtāng 5g wūyàoshùnqìsǎn 5g báijiāngcán 1g qínjiāo 1g chántuì 1g gōuténg 1g to ♂

5.17. Neuroacanthocytosis

Neuroacanthocytosis is a neurodegeneration of the brain characterized by chorea and deformed red blood cells, called acanthocytes, in the peripheral blood. Neuroacanthocytosis is caused by mutated genes on chromosome 9 or chromosome X.

Table 5.17. Herbal prescriptions for neuroacanthocytosis

Neuroacanthocytosis: https://meshb.nlm.nih.gov/record/ui?ui=D054546.	
Common prescriptions:	
Sháoyàogāncǎotāng 5g shūjīnghuóxuètāng 5g dāngguīniāntòngtāng 5g + acupuncture Sháoyàogāncǎotāng 5g shūjīnghuóxuètāng 5g + acupuncture	
Alternative prescriptions:	
Shūjīnghuóxuètāng 5g niúxī 1g mòyào 1g rǔxiāng 1g yánhúsuǒ 1g fùzǐ 1g guìzhī 1g jīxuèténg 1g + acupuncture Jiāwèixiāoyáosǎn 5g xiāngshāliùjūnzǐtāng 5g bànxiàxièxīntāng 3g héhuānpí 1g yánhúsuǒ 1g Sháoyàogāncǎotāng 5g shūjīnghuóxuètāng 5g mùguā 1g niúxī 1g + acupuncture Sháoyàogāncǎotāng 5g yánhúsuǒ 1g + acupuncture Jiāwèixiāoyáosǎn 5g gāncǎoxiǎomàidàzǎotāng 5g héhuānpí 1g bǎihé 1g yùjīn 1g	
Indicated and associated diseases:	
Unspecified condition of brain 348.9 (Disorder of brain, unspecified G939); Peroxisomal disorders 277.86 (Peroxisomal disorder, unspecified E7150, Zellweger syndrome E71510, Neonatal adrenoleukodystrophy E71511, Adrenomyeloneuropathy E71522, X-linked adrenoleukodystrophy, unspecified type E71529, Other peroxisomal disorders E71548); Unspecified diseases of blood and blood-forming organs 289.9 (Disease of blood and blood-forming organs, unspecified D759); Unspecified disorders of nervous system 349.9 (Disorder of central nervous system, unspecified G969); Unspecified disorder of metabolism 277.9 (Metabolic disorder, unspecified E889); Cardiovascular disease, unspecified 429.2 (Atherosclerotic heart disease of native coronary artery without angina pectoris I2510); Multiple myeloma 203.0; Unspecified hemorrhagic conditions 287.9 (Hemorrhagic condition, unspecified D699); Alcohol abuse 305.0	
Unspecified condition of brain 348.9/G939 with neuroacanthocytosis D054546:	
Bǔyánghuánwǔtāng 5g dānshēn 1g tiānmá 1g shíchāngpú 1g yuǎnzhì 1g + acupuncture to ♀	Bǔyánghuánwǔtāng 5g dānshēn 1g tiānmá 1g shíchāngpú 1g yuǎnzhì 1g + acupuncture to ♂

Neuroacanthocytosis: https://meshb.nlm.nih.gov/record/ui?ui=D054546.	
Cardiovascular disease, unspecified 429.2/I2510 with neuroacanthocytosis D054546:	
Sìnìtāng 5g gānlùyǐn 5g mǔdānpí 1g zhīzǐ 1g huánglián 0g to ♀	Shēngmàiyǐn 5g zhìgāncǎotāng 5g dānshēn 1g to ♂
Unspecified disorders of nervous system 349.9/G969 with neuroacanthocytosis D054546:	
Shūjīnghuóxuètāng 5g píngwèisǎn 2g mùguā 1g sāngzhī 1g jīxuèténg 1g to ♀	Shūjīnghuóxuètāng 5g píngwèisǎn 2g mùguā 1g sāngzhī 1g jīxuèténg 1g to ♂

As acanthocytosis can lead to hemolytic anemia and both Sháoyàogāncǎotāng and Shūjīnghuóxuètāng 'nourish Blood,' we see their use for neuroacanthocytosis. Note that the proteins encoded by the family of genes on chromosome 9 causing neuroacanthocytosis were shown in the laboratory to promote peroxisome biogenesis (Baldwin et al., 2021). Neuroacanthocytosis could therefore be associated with peroxisomal disorders as shown in the table. Also noted is that neuroacanthocytosis by gene mutations on chromosome X presents cardiomyopathy as one of its features.

5.18. Huntington's Disease

Huntington's disease is a progressive neurodegenerative disease of the brain. Major symptoms of Huntington's disease include uncontrolled motions, abnormal postures, changes in behavior, emotion and cognition. An increased number of the repeat in a gene on chromosome 4 causes Huntington's disease.

Table 5.18. Herbal prescriptions for Huntington's disease

Huntington's Disease: https://meshb.nlm.nih.gov/record/ui?ui=D006816.	
Common prescriptions:	
Dàzhēnjiāotāng 5g dāngguīniāntòngtāng 5g sháoyàogāncǎotāng 4g yánhúsuǒ 1g Dàzhēnjiāotāng 5g dāngguīniāntòngtāng 5g sháoyàogāncǎotāng 4g Sānbìtāng 5g dàzhēnjiāotāng 5g dāngguīniāntòngtāng 5g Dàzhēnjiāotāng 5g dāngguīniāntòngtāng 5g sháoyàogāncǎotāng 4g hòupò 1g Dàzhēnjiāotāng 5g dāngguīniāntòngtāng 5g sháoyàogāncǎotāng 4g dàhuáng 1g	
Alternative prescriptions:	
Dàzhēnjiāotāng 5g máxìngyìgāntāng 5g dāngguīniāntòngtāng 5g Dàzhēnjiāotāng 5g sháoyàogāncǎotāng 4g dāngguīniāntòngtāng 4g hòupò 1g	
Indicated diseases:	
Primary lateral sclerosis 335.24 (Primary lateral sclerosis G1223); Unspecified disorder of metabolism 277.9 (Metabolic disorder, unspecified E889); Motor neuron disease 335.2; Anterior horn cell disease 335; Unspecified disease of spinal cord 336.9 (Disease of spinal cord, unspecified G959); Orofacial dyskinesia 333.82 (Idiopathic orofacial dystonia G244); Myoneural disorders 358; Unspecified condition of brain 348.9 (Disorder of brain, unspecified G939); Unspecified disorders of nervous system 349.9 (Disorder of central nervous system, unspecified G969); Primary cerebellar degeneration 334.2 (Congenital nonprogressive ataxia G110, Late-onset cerebellar ataxia G112); Unspecified cerebrovascular disease 437.9 (Cerebrovascular disease, unspecified I679); Cardiovascular disease, unspecified 429.2 (Atherosclerotic heart disease of native coronary artery without angina pectoris I2510)	
Primary lateral sclerosis 335.24/G1223 with Huntington's disease D006816:	
Huángqíwǔwùtāng 5g bǔyánghuánwǔtāng 5g + acupuncture to ♀	Bǔyánghuánwǔtāng 5g dúhuójìshēngtāng 5g + acupuncture to ♂
Primary cerebellar degeneration 334.2/G110,G112 with Huntington's disease D006816:	
Bǔyánghuánwǔtāng 5g dānshēn 1g shíchāngpú 1g yuǎnzhì 1g + acupuncture to ♀	Bǔyánghuánwǔtāng 5g dānshēn 1g shíchāngpú 1g yuǎnzhì 1g + acupuncture to ♂
Unspecified cerebrovascular disease 437.9/I679 with Huntington's disease D006816:	
Xiǎoxùmìngtāng 5g bǔyánghuánwǔtāng 5g + acupuncture to ♀	Bǔyánghuánwǔtāng 5g chuānqī 2g dānshēn 1g shíchāngpú 1g yuǎnzhì 1g + acupuncture to ♂

Dàzhēnjiāotāng and Dāngguīniāntòngtāng are used for cerebellar ataxia in Section 5.11. Since cerebellar ataxia was suggested to be involved in Huntington's disease (Franklin et al., 2020), we see both formulas in the prescriptions for the motor condition of Huntington's disease.

5.19. Synkinesis

Synkinesis is an involuntary contraction of a facial muscle during voluntary contraction of the other facial muscles. An example of synkinesis is eye closure during smiling or chewing. Anomalous nerve regeneration after nerve injury can cause synkinesis.

Table 5.19. Herbal prescriptions for synkinesis

Synkinesis: https://meshb.nlm.nih.gov/record/ui?ui=D046608.	
Common prescriptions:	
Wūyàoshùnqìsǎn 5g huángqíwǔwùtāng 5g + acupuncture Xiǎoxùmìngtāng 5g wūyàoshùnqìsǎn 5g bǔyánghuánwǔtāng 5g Wūyàoshùnqìsǎn 5g huángqíwǔwùtāng 5g	
Alternative prescriptions:	
Dāngguīsìnìtāng 5g shēngjiāng 0g wúzhūyú 0g Xiǎoxùmìngtāng 5g huángqíwǔwùtāng 5g dānshēn 1g zhúrú 1g sāngzhī 1g jiānghuáng 1g Máhuángfùzǐxìxīntāng 5g gāncǎo 2g báizhú 2g fùzǐ 2g fúlíng 2g gānjiāng 2g dǎngshēn 2g Sháoyàogāncǎotāng 5g máhuángfùzǐxìxīntāng 5g fùzǐ 3g guìzhī 3g dàzǎo 2g gānjiāng 2g Dàzhēnjiāotāng 5g dāngguīniāntòngtāng 4g sháoyàogāncǎotāng 3g	
Indicated diseases:	
Brown's (tendon) sheath syndrome 378.61 (Brown's sheath syndrome, right eye H50611, Brown's sheath syndrome, left eye H50612); Internuclear ophthalmoplegia 378.86 (Internuclear ophthalmoplegia, unspecified eye H5120); Unspecified disorder of eye movements 378.9 (Unspecified disorder of binocular movement H519); Orofacial dyskinesia 333.82 (Idiopathic orofacial dystonia G244); Unspecified disorder of cranial nerves 352.9 (Cranial nerve disorder, unspecified G529); Disorder of eye, unspecified 379.90 (Unspecified disorder of eye and adnexa H579); Unspecified disorders of nervous system 349.9 (Disorder of central nervous system, unspecified G969); Bell's palsy 351.0 (Bell's palsy G510); Geniculate ganglionitis 351.1 (Geniculate ganglionitis G511); Facial nerve disorders 351; Neoplasm of unspecified nature of brain 239.6 (Neoplasm of unspecified behavior of brain D496); Unspecified condition of brain 348.9 (Disorder of brain, unspecified G939)	
Brown's (tendon) sheath syndrome 378.61/H50611,H50612 with synkinesis D046608:	
Wūyàoshùnqìsǎn 5g to ♀	Wūyàoshùnqìsǎn 5g bǔyánghuánwǔtāng 5g to ♂
Bell's palsy 351.0/G510 with synkinesis D046608:	
Wūyàoshùnqìsǎn 5g bǔyánghuánwǔtāng 5g + acupuncture to ♀	Wūyàoshùnqìsǎn 5g bǔyánghuánwǔtāng 5g báijiāngcán 1g dìlóng 1g + acupuncture to ♂
Geniculate ganglionitis 351.1/G511 with synkinesis D046608:	
Wūyàoshùnqìsǎn 5g bǔyánghuánwǔtāng 5g + acupuncture to ♀	Wūyàoshùnqìsǎn 5g bǔyánghuánwǔtāng 5g báijiāngcán 1g dìlóng 1g + acupuncture to ♂
Orofacial dyskinesia 333.82/G244 with synkinesis D046608:	
Sháoyàogāncǎotāng 5g gégēntāng 5g qínjiāo 1g gōuténg 1g to ♀	Sháoyàogāncǎotāng 5g gégēntāng 5g qínjiāo 1g gōuténg 1g to ♂

Wūyàoshùnqìsǎn and Huángqíwǔwùtāng 'regulate and supply Qi,' and we see here their use for synkinesis, which involves abnormal movements of muscles.

5.20. Myoclonus

Myoclonus is a sudden, brief, involuntary twitch or jerk of a muscle or a group of muscles. Body jerks before falling asleep are an example of myoclonus. Causes of myoclonus include head injury, spinal injury, tumor on the central nervous system, liver or kidney failure.

Table 5.20. Herbal prescriptions for myoclonus

<table>
<tr><td colspan="2">Myoclonus: https://meshb.nlm.nih.gov/record/ui?ui=D009207.</td></tr>
<tr><td colspan="2">Common prescriptions:</td></tr>
<tr><td colspan="2">Sānbìtāng 5g dúhuójìshēngtāng 5g
Sānbìtāng 5g
Sānbìtāng 5g shūjīnghuóxuètāng 5g</td></tr>
<tr><td colspan="2">Alternative prescriptions:</td></tr>
<tr><td colspan="2">Dàzhēnjiāotāng 5g dāngguīniāntòngtāng 5g sháoyàogāncǎotāng 4g hòupò 1g
Dàzhēnjiāotāng 5g sānbìtāng 2g
Dàzhēnjiāotāng 5g dāngguīniāntòngtāng 5g
Sānbìtāng 5g dàzhēnjiāotāng 2g
Dàzhēnjiāotāng 5g sānbìtāng 3g</td></tr>
<tr><td colspan="2">Indicated diseases:</td></tr>
<tr><td colspan="2">Primary cerebellar degeneration 334.2 (Congenital nonprogressive ataxia G110, Late onset cerebellar ataxia G112); Unspecified disease of spinal cord 336.9 (Disease of spinal cord, unspecified G959); Orofacial dyskinesia 333.82 (Idiopathic orofacial dystonia G244); Unspecified condition of brain 348.9 (Disorder of brain, unspecified G939); Unspecified disorders of nervous system 349.9 (Disorder of central nervous system, unspecified G969); Epilepsy, unspecified 345.9; Unspecified disorder of metabolism 277.9 (Metabolic disorder, unspecified E889)</td></tr>
<tr><td colspan="2">Primary cerebellar degeneration 334.2/G110,G112 with myoclonus D009207:</td></tr>
<tr><td>Bǔyánghuánwǔtāng 5g dānshēn 1g tiānmá 1g shíchāngpú 1g yuǎnzhì 1g + acupuncture to ♀</td><td>Bǔyánghuánwǔtāng 5g dānshēn 1g shíchāngpú 1g yuǎnzhì 1g + acupuncture to ♂</td></tr>
<tr><td colspan="2">Epilepsy, unspecified 345.9 with myoclonus D009207:</td></tr>
<tr><td>Tiānmágōuténgyǐn 5g jiāwèixiāoyáosǎn 5g cháihújiālónggǔmǔlìtāng 5g dúhuójìshēngtāng 5g shēntòngzhúyūtāng 4g dǎngshēn 2g to ♀</td><td>Tiānmágōuténgyǐn 5g jiāwèixiāoyáosǎn 5g cháihújiālónggǔmǔlìtāng 5g dúhuójìshēngtāng 5g shēntòngzhúyūtāng 4g dǎngshēn 2g to ♂</td></tr>
<tr><td colspan="2">Orofacial dyskinesia 333.82/G244 with myoclonus D009207:</td></tr>
<tr><td>Sháoyàogāncǎotāng 5g mùguā 1g niúxī 1g qínjiāo 1g gōuténg 1g to ♀</td><td>Sháoyàogāncǎotāng 5g mùguā 1g niúxī 1g qínjiāo 1g gōuténg 1g to ♂</td></tr>
</table>

Sānbìtāng and Dàzhēnjiāotāng are used for Huntington's disease. As juvenile Huntington's disease can present with myoclonic epilepsy (Gambardella et al., 2001), it is thought that the same combination is also used here for myoclonus. On the other hand, the characteristic of sudden and sporadic infliction is called 'Wind' in traditional Chinese medicine. Sānbitāng, Dàzhēnjiāotāng and Dāngguīniāntòngtāng all treat Wind syndromes, which explains their use for myoclonus.

References

Baldwin, H. A., Wang, C., Kanfer, G., Shah, H. V., Velayos-Baeza, A., Dulovic-Mahlow, M., Brüggemann, N., Anding, A., Baehrecke, E. H., Maric, D., Prinz, W. A., & Youle, R. J. (2021). VPS13D promotes peroxisome biogenesis. *Journal of Cell Biology*, *220*(5), e202001188. https://doi.org/10.1083/jcb.202001188.

Franklin, G. L., Camargo, C. H. F., Meira, A. T., Pavanelli, G. M., Milano, S. S., Germiniani, F. B., Lima, N. S. C., Raskin, S., Barsottini, O. G. P., Pedroso, J. L., Maggi, F. A., Tumas, V., de Carvalho, P. M., de

Oliveira, A. C., Braga, B., Souza, L. C., Guimarães, R. P., Piovesana, L. G., Lopes-Cendes, Í. T., & de Azevedo, P. C. (2020). Is Ataxia an Underestimated Symptom of Huntington's Disease? *Frontiers in Neurology*, *11*, 571843. https://doi.org/10.3389/fneur.2020.571843.

Gambardella, A., Muglia, M., Labate, A., Magariello, A., Gabriele, A. L., Mazzei, R., Pirritano, D., Conforti, F. L., Patitucci, A., Valentino, P., Zappia, M., & Quattrone, A. (2001). Juvenile Huntington's disease presenting as progressive myoclonic epilepsy. *Neurology*, *57*(4), 708–711. https://doi.org/10.1212/wnl.57.4.708.

Helsing, P., & Frøen, H. (2007). Dermatitis Herpetiformis Presenting as Ataxia in a Child. *Acta Dermato-Venereologica*, *87*(2), 163–165. https://doi.org/10.2340/00015555-0220.

Pasini, A. M., Gagro, A., Roić, G., Vrdoljak, O., Lujić, L., & Žutelija-Fattorini, M. (2017). Ataxia Telangiectasia and Juvenile Idiopathic Arthritis. *Pediatrics*, *139*(2), e20161279. https://doi.org/10.1542/peds.2016-1279.

Shao, L., Fujii, H., Colmegna, I., Oishi, H., Goronzy, J. J., & Weyand, C. M. (2009). Deficiency of the DNA repair enzyme ATM in rheumatoid arthritis. *Journal of Experimental Medicine*, *206*(6), 1435–1449. https://doi.org/10.1084/jem.20082251.

Wang, S. C. (2013). *Western Biomedicine and Eastern Therapeutics: An Integrative Strategy for Personalized and Preventive Healthcare*. WSPC. https://doi.org/10.1142/8533.

Wang, S. C. (2019). *Clinical Herbal Prescriptions: Principles and Practices of Herbal Formulations from Deep Learning Health Insurance Herbal Prescription Big Data*. WSPC. https://doi.org/10.1142/11211.

Chapter 6

Metabolic Diseases

Metabolism changes biochemicals from one to another. Changes can have two opposite directions: breaking down and building up. The former takes place when we take in food in order to gain energy and maintain our structures, and the latter when we grow and reproduce. At the cellular level, organic component compounds that are essential to organisms are amino acids, fatty acids, monosaccharides and nucleic acids. Amino acids make up enzymes and proteins which in turn constitute most parts of the cytoskeleton. Fatty acids make up cell membranes. Monosaccharides make up glycogen and cellulose. Nucleic acids make up DNA and RNA. Chemical energy in the form of ATP is released during the breakdown of digested food. ATP is then used in the assembly and transportation of components to form complex macromolecules during the cell cycle and DNA repair.

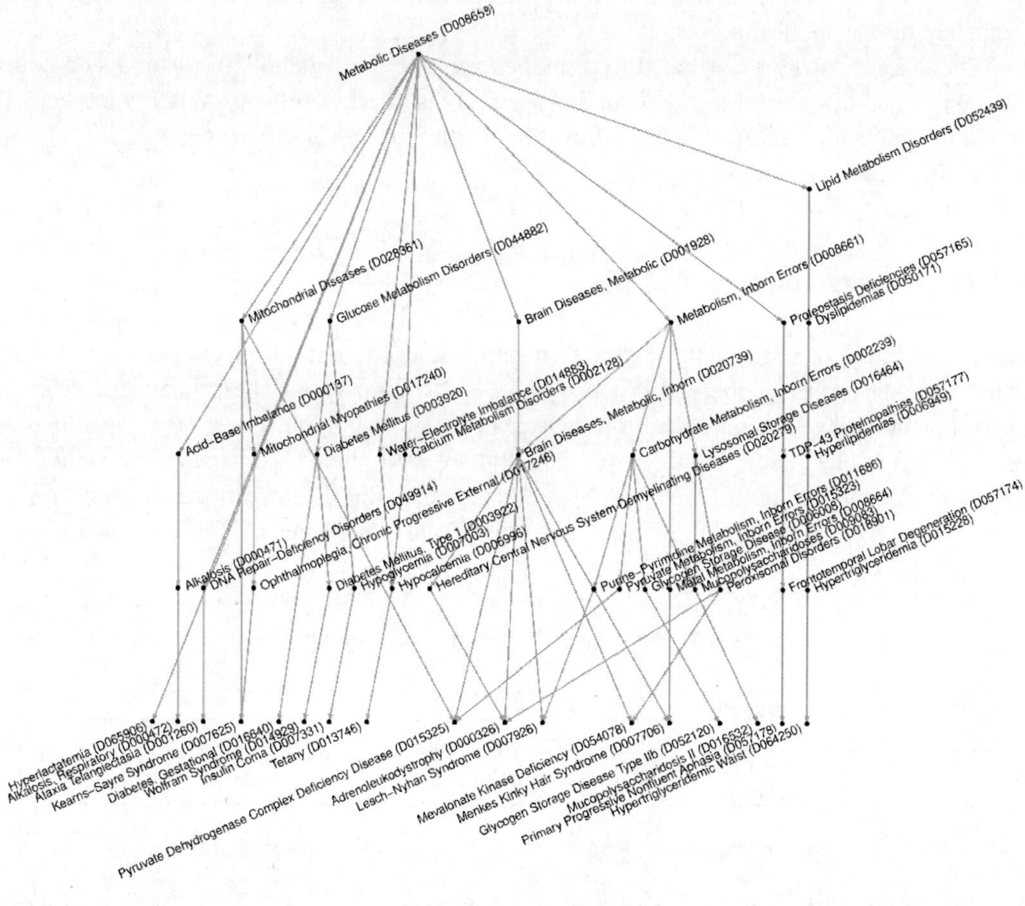

Figure 6.1. Physiological manifestations due to imbalances in the breakdown of large complex molecules into smaller ones and in the assembly of small simpler molecules into large complex ones.

The series of biochemical reactions that break down and build up biochemicals are known as metabolic pathways. An important discovery in biochemistry is that the core metabolic pathways in the cells of organisms across the three domains are similar, suggesting that extant metabolic pathways are optimized for their purpose. Deficiencies in human metabolism cause a cluster of diseases called metabolic diseases. The deficiencies can arise from genetic defects in enzymes that catalyze reactions in the metabolic pathways, or they can be acquired from damage to an endocrine organ such as pancreas, which secretes hormones that stimulate the metabolism of other cells. In addition to biochemicals, inorganic substances such as minerals and metals also play critical roles in human metabolism. Figure 6.1 shows various types and consequences of metabolic deficiencies.

The herbal formulas that are commonly used for the signs and symptoms of metabolic diseases include Shūjīnghuóxuètāng, Sháoyàogāncǎotāng, Dāngguīniāntòngtāng, Sìnìtāng, Xuèfǔzhúyūtāng, Bǔzhōngyìqìtāng, Dāngguīsìnìtāng, Jiāwèixiāoyáosǎn, and Bǔyánghuánwǔtāng. The single herbs that are commonly used to support the formulas in the prescriptions are Dānshēn, Shēngjiāng, Yánhúsuǒ, Guìzhī, Niúxī, Wúzhūyú, Héshǒuwū, Shānzhā, and Zéxiè. Many of the formulas and herbs help Qi and digestion. Moreover, Qi in traditional medicine is reminiscent of ATP resynthesis in metabolism. Needling at acupoints frees Qi flowing along the meridian. Acupuncture is therefore a common modality, along with herbal medicine, for metabolic diseases.

The diseases that are attributed to or associated with the metabolic signs and symptoms are unspecified disorder of metabolism, unspecified disorders of nervous system, unspecified condition of brain, unspecified cardiovascular disease, unspecified heart disease, and unspecified secondary cardiomyopathy.

6.1. Hyperlactatemia

Hyperlactatemia is abnormally elevated resting concentrations of lactate in the blood. Biochemically, lactate is the end product of anaerobic glycolysis. The principal production sites of lactate in the body are therefore muscle cells and red blood cells. Lactate is primarily removed from the blood by the liver and kidneys. An increased lactate production or decreased lactate clearance can cause hyperlactatemia. Specific conditions include tissue hypoperfusion, mitochondrial disorder, hypermetabolic state, liver dysfunction, alcoholism and malignancy.

Table 6.1. Herbal prescriptions for hyperlactatemia

Hyperlactatemia: https://meshb.nlm.nih.gov/record/ui?ui=D065906.
Common prescriptions:
Sháoyàogāncǎotāng 5g shūjīnghuóxuètāng 5g dāngguīniāntòngtāng 5g + acupuncture Sháoyàogāncǎotāng 5g shūjīnghuóxuètāng 5g + acupuncture
Alternative prescriptions:
Zhènggǔzǐjīndān 5g dāngguīniāntòngtāng 5g sānqī 1g dàdīnghuáng 1g gāncǎo 1g dǎodìwúgōng 1g sūmù 1g xùduàn 1g + acupuncture Sháoyàogāncǎotāng 5g yánhúsuǒ 1g mòyào 1g rǔxiāng 1g + acupuncture Shūjīnghuóxuètāng 5g sháoyàogāncǎotāng 2g mòyào 1g rǔxiāng 1g jiānghuáng 1g + acupuncture Jiāwèixiāoyáosǎn 5g sháoyàogāncǎotāng 5g shūjīnghuóxuètāng 5g Jiāwèixiāoyáosǎn 5g cháihúshūgāntāng 5g chuānliànzǐ 1g yánhúsuǒ 1g yùjīn 1g

Hyperlactatemia: https://meshb.nlm.nih.gov/record/ui?ui=D065906.	
Indicated diseases:	
Unspecified condition of brain 348.9 (Disorder of brain, unspecified G939); Peroxisomal disorders 277.86 (Peroxisomal disorder, unspecified E7150, Zellweger syndrome E71510, Neonatal adrenoleukodystrophy E71511, Adrenomyeloneuropathy E71522, X-linked adrenoleukodystrophy, unspecified type E71529, Other peroxisomal disorders E71548); Unspecified diseases of blood and blood-forming organs 289.9 (Disease of blood and blood-forming organs, unspecified D759); Unspecified disorders of nervous system 349.9 (Disorder of central nervous system, unspecified G969); Unspecified disorder of metabolism 277.9 (Metabolic disorder, unspecified E889); Cardiovascular disease, unspecified 429.2 (Atherosclerotic heart disease of native coronary artery without angina pectoris I2510); Multiple myeloma 203.0; Unspecified hemorrhagic conditions 287.9 (Hemorrhagic condition, unspecified D699); Alexia 315.01 (Dyslexia and alexia R480)	
Unspecified condition of brain 348.9/G939 with hyperlactatemia D065906:	
Bǔyánghuánwǔtāng 5g dānshēn 1g tiānmá 1g shíchāngpú 1g yuǎnzhì 1g + acupuncture to ♀	Bǔyánghuánwǔtāng 5g dānshēn 1g tiānmá 1g shíchāngpú 1g yuǎnzhì 1g + acupuncture to ♂
Cardiovascular disease, unspecified 429.2/I2510 with hyperlactatemia D065906:	
Sìnìtāng 5g gānlùyǐn 5g mǔdānpí 1g zhīzǐ 1g huánglián 0g to ♀	Xuèfǔzhúyūtāng 5g zhìgāncǎotāng 5g dānshēn 1g to ♂

Many of the formulas in the prescriptions for hyperlactatemia are known to improve blood circulation. On the other hand, Jiāwèixiāoyáosǎn promotes Liver health. Herbalists therefore target the causes of hyperlactatemia. Hyperlactatemia is common in patients following brain tumor surgery (de Smalen et al., 2020) and cardiac surgery (Minton and Sidebotham, 2017). Hyperlactatemia can lead to lactic acidosis which was reported to serve as biomarker for multiple myeloma progression (Ziegler et al., 2021). A child with dyslexia was reported to develop hyperlactatemia (Buda et al., 2013).

6.2. Respiratory Alkalosis

Too many bases or alkalis in the body fluids is called alkalosis. Since carbon dioxide is acidic, breathing away too much carbon dioxide in a process called hyperventilation can cause respiratory alkalosis. Hyperventilation can in turn be caused by stress, fever, hypoxemia, hypoxia, anemia, high altitude, heart attack and such pulmonary disorders as asthma and chronic obstructive pulmonary disease.

Table 6.2. Herbal prescriptions for respiratory alkalosis

Respiratory Alkalosis: https://meshb.nlm.nih.gov/record/ui?ui=D000472.
Common prescriptions:
Sìnìtāng 5g dāngguīsìnìtāng 5g shēngjiāng 1g wúzhūyú 1g Sìnìtāng 5g rénshēn 1g bànxià 1g dàhuáng 0g Sìnìtāng 5g rénshēn 1g wúzhūyú 1g Sìnìtāng 5g dāngguīsìnìtāng 5g shēngjiāng 1g wúzhūyú 1g fùzǐ 1g Sìnìtāng 5g rénshēn 1g
Alternative prescriptions:
Sìnìtāng 5g bànxià 1g fúlíng 1g dàhuáng 0g Sìnìtāng 5g dāngguīsìnìtāng 4g shēngjiāng 1g wúzhūyú 1g Sìnìtāng 5g rénshēn 1g bànxià 1g Sìnìtāng 5g rénshēn 2g rénshēn 2g

Table 6.2. (Continued)

Respiratory Alkalosis: https://meshb.nlm.nih.gov/record/ui?ui=D000472.	
Indicated diseases:	
Unspecified cerebrovascular disease 437.9 (Cerebrovascular disease, unspecified I679); Unspecified condition of brain 348.9 (Disorder of brain, unspecified G939); Unspecified disorder of metabolism 277.9 (Metabolic disorder, unspecified E889); Cardiovascular disease, unspecified 429.2 (Atherosclerotic heart disease of native coronary artery without angina pectoris I2510); Unspecified disorders of nervous system 349.9 (Disorder of central nervous system, unspecified G969); Heart disease, unspecified 429.9 (Heart disease, unspecified I519)	
Unspecified cerebrovascular disease 437.9/I679 with alkalosis, respiratory D000472:	
Bǔyánghuánwǔtāng 5g dānshēn 1g shíchāngpú 1g yuǎnzhì 1g + acupuncture to ♀	Bǔyánghuánwǔtāng 5g dānshēn 1g shíchāngpú 1g yuǎnzhì 1g + acupuncture to ♂
Heart disease, unspecified 429.9/I519 with alkalosis, respiratory D000472:	
Sìnìtāng 5g gānlùyǐn 5g mǔdānpí 1g zhīzǐ 1g huánglián 0g to ♀	Sìnìtāng 5g gānlùyǐn 5g mǔdānpí 1g zhīzǐ 1g huánglián 0g to ♂
Unspecified disorder of metabolism 277.9/E889 with alkalosis, respiratory D000472:	
Huángqíwǔwùtāng 5g dāngguīsìnìtāng 5g dānshēn 1g sāngzhī 1g jiānghuáng 1g to ♀	Liùwèidìhuángwán 5g bǔzhōngyìqìtāng 5g dānshēn 1g to ♂
Unspecified condition of brain 348.9/G939 with alkalosis, respiratory D000472:	
Bǔyánghuánwǔtāng 5g chuānqī 1g dānshēn 1g shíchāngpú 1g yuǎnzhì 1g + acupuncture to ♀	Bǔyánghuánwǔtāng 5g chuānqī 1g dānshēn 1g shíchāngpú 1g yuǎnzhì 1g + acupuncture to ♂

Sìnìtāng 'lifts Yang Qi' and one of its modern uses is for chronic bronchitis (Wang, 2019). We see that herbalists aim to relieve the pulmonary conditions behind respiratory alkalosis.

6.3. Kearns-Sayre Syndrome

Kearns-Sayre syndrome is characterized by limited eye mobility, skeletal muscle weakness, impaired cognition, deafness and cardiac conduction defects. Kearns-Sayre Syndrome is rare and caused by large deletions in mitochondrial DNA.

Table 6.3. Herbal prescriptions for Kearns-Sayre syndrome

Kearns-Sayre Syndrome: https://meshb.nlm.nih.gov/record/ui?ui=D007625.
Common prescriptions:
Xuèfǔzhúyūtāng 5g bǔyánghuánwǔtāng 5g dānshēn 2g chuānqī 1g guìzhī 1g Xuèfǔzhúyūtāng 5g bǔyánghuánwǔtāng 5g dānshēn 2g chuānqī 1g báijí 1g guìzhī 1g Xuèfǔzhúyūtāng 5g bǔyánghuánwǔtāng 5g chuānqī 1g dānshēn 1g guìzhī 1g Xuèfǔzhúyūtāng 5g bǔyánghuánwǔtāng 5g dānshēn 2g chuānqī 1g guìzhī 1g guālóurén 1g xièbái 1g Xuèfǔzhúyūtāng 5g bǔyánghuánwǔtāng 5g chuānqī 1g dānshēn 1g
Alternative prescriptions:
Bǔyánghuánwǔtāng 5g xuèfǔzhúyūtāng 4g huángqí 3g dāngguī 3g guālóurén 2g púhuáng 2g xièbái 1g Xuèfǔzhúyūtāng 5g bǔyánghuánwǔtāng 5g dānshēn 2g chuānqī 1g báijí 1g hòupò 1g guìzhī 1g chénpí 1g huánglián 1g Xuèfǔzhúyūtāng 5g bǔyánghuánwǔtāng 5g dānshēn 2g báijí 1g guìzhī 1g huánglián 1g dàhuáng 0g Xuèfǔzhúyūtāng 5g bǔyánghuánwǔtāng 5g dānshēn 2g chuānqī 1g Xuèfǔzhúyūtāng 5g qǐjúdìhuángwán 5g cháihúshūgāntāng 5g

Kearns-Sayre Syndrome: https://meshb.nlm.nih.gov/record/ui?ui=D007625.	
Indicated diseases:	
Secondary cardiomyopathy, unspecified 425.9 (Cardiomyopathy due to drug and external agent I427); Progressive external ophthalmoplegia 378.72 (Other specified strabismus H5089); Unspecified disorder of metabolism 277.9 (Metabolic disorder, unspecified E889); Heart disease, unspecified 429.9 (Heart disease, unspecified I519); Cardiovascular disease, unspecified 429.2 (Atherosclerotic heart disease of native coronary artery without angina pectoris I2510); Total ophthalmoplegia 378.56 (Total (external) ophthalmoplegia, unspecified eye H4930); Brown's (tendon) sheath syndrome 378.61 (Brown's sheath syndrome, right eye H50611, Brown's sheath syndrome, left eye H50612); Internuclear ophthalmoplegia 378.86 (Internuclear ophthalmoplegia, unspecified eye H5120); Unspecified disorder of eye movements 378.9 (Unspecified disorder of binocular movement H519); Unspecified retinal disorder 362.9 (Unspecified retinal disorder H359); Myopathy, unspecified 359.9 (Myopathy, unspecified G729); Unspecified disorder of cranial nerves 352.9 (Cranial nerve disorder, unspecified G529); Myoneural disorders 358; Disorder of eye, unspecified 379.90 (Unspecified disorder of eye and adnexa H579); Unspecified disorders of nervous system 349.9 (Disorder of central nervous system, unspecified G969); Epilepsy, unspecified 345.9; Unspecified condition of brain 348.9 (Disorder of brain, unspecified G939); Ptosis of eyelid 374.3; Unspecified disorder of eyelid 374.9 (Unspecified disorder of eyelid H029); Unspecified cerebrovascular disease 437.9 (Cerebrovascular disease, unspecified I679)	
Secondary cardiomyopathy, unspecified 425.9/I427 with Kearns-Sayre syndrome D007625:	
Xuèfǔzhúyūtāng 5g dānshēn 2g chuānqī 1g báijí 1g rénshēn 1g guìzhī 1g guālóurén 1g xièbái 1g to ♀	Xuèfǔzhúyūtāng 5g dānshēn 2g chuānqī 1g báijí 1g rénshēn 1g guìzhī 1g guālóurén 1g xièbái 1g to ♂

Both Xuèfǔzhúyūtāng and Bǔyánghuánwǔtāng ‘invigorate Blood and move Qi.’ As mitochondria are powerhouses of cells, combining both formulas in the prescriptions is believed to help ameliorate mitochondrial deficiency.

6.4. Insulin Coma

Insulin coma is loss of consciousness due to extremely low sugar levels in the blood induced by an exogenous insulin shot. Insulin coma is life-threatening, so medical treatment in a hospital emergency room is needed to awaken the patient going into insulin coma.

Table 6.4. Herbal prescriptions for insulin coma

Insulin Coma: https://meshb.nlm.nih.gov/record/ui?ui=D007331.
Common prescriptions:
Sìnìtāng 5g dāngguīsìnìtāng 5g shēngjiāng 1g wúzhūyú 1g Sìnìtāng 5g lǐzhōngtāng 5g ròuguì 1g yánhúsuǒ 1g zhìgāncǎotāng 1g Sìnìtāng 5g dāngguīsìnìtāng 5g wúzhūyú 1g gānjiāng 1g Sìnìtāng 5g dāngguīsìnìtāng 5g shēngjiāng 1g wúzhūyú 1g fùzǐ 1g Sìnìtāng 5g lǐzhōngtāng 5g ròuguì 1g yánhúsuǒ 1g
Alternative prescriptions:
Dāngguīsìnìtāng 5g shēngjiāng 1g wúzhūyú 1g Zhēnwǔtāng 5g wúzhūyútāng 4g fùzǐ 1g Sìnìtāng 5g máhuángfùzǐxìxīntāng 4g ròuguì 1g gānjiāng 1g zhìgāncǎotāng 1g
Guìzhītāng 5g huángqí 1g dāngguī 1g dàhuáng 0g Dāngguīsìnìtāng 5g wúzhūyú 1g gānjiāng 1g fùzǐ 1g
Indicated diseases:
Unspecified disorders of nervous system 349.9 (Disorder of central nervous system, unspecified G969); Hypoglycemia, unspecified 251.2 (Hypoglycemia, unspecified E162); Schizophreniform disorder 295.4; Unspecified disorder of metabolism 277.9 (Metabolic disorder, unspecified E889); Schizoaffective disorder 295.7; Schizophrenic disorders 295; Unspecified condition of brain 348.9 (Disorder of brain, unspecified G939)

Table 6.4. Herbal prescriptions for insulin coma

Insulin Coma: https://meshb.nlm.nih.gov/record/ui?ui=D007331.	
Unspecified disorders of nervous system 349.9/G969 with insulin coma D007331:	
Huángqíwǔwùtāng 5g chuānxiōng 1g dānshēn 1g zhúrú 1g sāngzhī 1g dāngguī 1g jiānghuáng 1g to ♀	Huángqíwǔwùtāng 5g chuānxiōng 1g dānshēn 1g zhúrú 1g sāngzhī 1g dāngguī 1g jiānghuáng 1g to ♂
Unspecified condition of brain 348.9/G939 with insulin coma D007331:	
Bǔyánghuánwǔtāng 5g + acupuncture to ♀	Bǔyánghuánwǔtāng 5g + acupuncture to ♂

Both Sìnìtāng and Dāngguīsìnìtāng are believed to reverse the passing out as they 'fortify Yang.' Note that insulin coma was used as a therapy for schizophrenia before the introduction of antipsychotics (Doroshow, 2006).

6.5. Tetany

Tetany is involuntary, rhythmic contraction of the muscles of the hands and feet. Tetany is caused by electrolyte imbalances in the blood such as hypocalcemia, hypomagnesemia and hypokalemia.

Table 6.5. Herbal prescriptions for tetany

Tetany: https://meshb.nlm.nih.gov/record/ui?ui=D013746.	
Common prescriptions:	
Bǔzhōngyìqìtāng 5g guīpítāng 5g Bǔzhōngyìqìtāng 5g shēngmàiyǐn 2g Bǔzhōngyìqìtāng 5g shēngmàiyǐn 3g Bǔzhōngyìqìtāng 5g guīpítāng 5g dānshēn 1g	
Alternative prescriptions:	
Bǔzhōngyìqìtāng 5g guīpítāng 4g Bǔzhōngyìqìtāng 5g guīpítāng 5g shēngmàiyǐn 2g Shēngmàiyǐn 5g bǔzhōngyìqìtāng 5g Bǔzhōngyìqìtāng 5g guīpítāng 2g	
Indicated diseases:	
Unspecified disorders of nervous system 349.9 (Disorder of central nervous system, unspecified G969); Hypoparathyroidism 252.1 (Hypoparathyroidism, unspecified E209); Unspecified disorder of parathyroid gland 252.9 (Disorder of parathyroid gland, unspecified E215); Disorders of calcium metabolism 275.4; Unspecified endocrine disorder 259.9 (Endocrine disorder, unspecified E349); Unspecified disorder of metabolism 277.9 (Metabolic disorder, unspecified E889); Rickets, active 268.0 (Rickets, active E550); Hyperparathyroidism 252.0; Tetanus 037 (Other tetanus A35)	
Unspecified disorders of nervous system 349.9/G969 with tetany D013746:	
Huángqíwǔwùtāng 5g chuānxiōng 1g dānshēn 1g zhúrú 1g sāngzhī 1g dāngguī 1g jiānghuáng 1g to ♀	Huángqíwǔwùtāng 5g chuānxiōng 1g dānshēn 1g zhúrú 1g sāngzhī 1g dāngguī 1g jiānghuáng 1g to ♂

Bǔzhōngyìqìtāng literally reads 'nourishing viscera and tonifying Qi decoction.' Guīpítāng 'tonifies Qi, Blood and benefits the Spleen,' which in traditional Chinese medicine is responsible for digestion and metabolism. Their use in the prescriptions is believed to correct the metabolic imbalances through improved digestion.

6.6. Pyruvate Dehydrogenase Complex Deficiency Disease

Pyruvate dehydrogenase complex deficiency disease is caused by mutations in the family of genes encoding pyruvate dehydrogenase complex, which are enzymes converting pyruvate into acetyl-CoA in mitochondria. Signs and symptoms of pyruvate dehydrogenase complex deficiency disease are related to lactic acidosis and include tiredness, respiratory infections and distress, mental retardation, microcephaly, poor muscle coordination and tone.

Sìnìtāng is thought to help the cellular energetics and Máhuángfùzǐxìxīntāng to relieve the respiratory infection and distress in patients with pyruvate dehydrogenase complex deficiency.

Table 6.6. Herbal prescriptions for pyruvate dehydrogenase complex deficiency disease

<table>
<tr><td colspan="2">Pyruvate Dehydrogenase Complex Deficiency Disease: https://meshb.nlm.nih.gov/record/ui?ui=D015325.</td></tr>
<tr><td colspan="2">Common prescriptions:</td></tr>
<tr><td colspan="2">Sìnìtāng 5g shēngjiāng 1g guìzhī 1g
Máhuángfùzǐxìxīntāng 5g shēngjiāng 2g guìzhī 2g zhìgāncǎo 1g
Máhuángfùzǐxìxīntāng 5g shēngjiāng 1g guìzhī 1g
Máhuángfùzǐxìxīntāng 5g shēngjiāng 1g guìzhī 1g zhìgāncǎo 1g
Máhuángfùzǐxìxīntāng 5g shēngjiāng 2g zhìgāncǎo 2g guìzhī 2g</td></tr>
<tr><td colspan="2">Alternative prescriptions:</td></tr>
<tr><td colspan="2">Sìnìtāng 5g rénshēn 2g dàhuáng 0g
Sìnìtāng 5g shēngjiāng 1g guìzhī 1g xìxīn 1g
Sìnìtāng 5g shēngjiāng 0g guìzhī 0g</td></tr>
<tr><td colspan="2">Indicated diseases:</td></tr>
<tr><td colspan="2">Unspecified condition of brain 348.9 (Disorder of brain, unspecified G939); Unspecified disorder of metabolism 277.9 (Metabolic disorder, unspecified E889); Autistic disorder 299.0; Unspecified disorders of nervous system 349.9 (Disorder of central nervous system, unspecified G969); Schizoaffective disorder 295.7; Schizophreniform disorder 295.4; Renal failure, unspecified 586 (Unspecified kidney failure N19)</td></tr>
<tr><td colspan="2">Unspecified condition of brain 348.9/G939 with pyruvate dehydrogenase complex deficiency disease D015325:</td></tr>
<tr><td>Bǔyánghuánwǔtāng 5g chuānqī 1g dānshēn 1g shíchāngpú 1g yuǎnzhì 1g + acupuncture to ♀</td><td>Bǔyánghuánwǔtāng 5g chuānqī 1g dānshēn 1g shíchāngpú 1g yuǎnzhì 1g + acupuncture to ♂</td></tr>
</table>

6.7. Adrenoleukodystrophy

Adrenoleukodystrophy is a metabolic condition affecting the white matter of the brain, spinal cord and adrenal cortex. Signs and symptoms of adrenoleukodystrophy include learning disabilities, trouble swallowing, visual impairment, poor muscle coordination, seizures, deafness and urinary tract problems. Mutations in a gene, whose products break down very long-chain fatty acids, on chromosome X cause adrenoleukodystrophy.

A modern use of Shānzhā and Héshǒuwū is for disorders of lipoid metabolism (Wang, 2019). A modern use of Cǎojuémíng is for glaucoma and that of Juémíngzǐ is for disorders of lacrimal system (Wang, 2019). Zéxiè's modern uses include vertiginous syndromes and other disorders of vestibular system (Wang, 2019). Adult patients with adrenoleukodystrophy were demonstrated to manifest balance difficulty (Godbole et al., 2021). Herbal prescriptions are therefore composed to relieve many of the signs and symptoms of adrenoleukodystrophy.

Table 6.7. Herbal prescriptions for adrenoleukodystrophy

Adrenoleukodystrophy: https://meshb.nlm.nih.gov/record/ui?ui=D000326.	
Common prescriptions:	
Xuèfǔzhúyūtāng 5g shānzhā 1g dānshēn 1g héshǒuwū 1g cǎojuémíng 1g héyè 1g zéxiè 1g Xuèfǔzhúyūtāng 5g shānzhā 1g dānshēn 1g héshǒuwū 1g cǎojuémíng 1g zéxiè 1g Xuèfǔzhúyūtāng 5g shānzhā 1g dānshēn 1g héshǒuwū 1g juémíngzǐ 1g zéxiè 1g Xuèfǔzhúyūtāng 5g shānzhā 1g dānshēn 1g héshǒuwū 1g juémíngzǐ 1g héyè 1g zéxiè 1g Xuèfǔzhúyūtāng 5g shānzhā 1g dānshēn 1g héshǒuwū 1g zéxiè 1g	
Alternative prescriptions:	
Xuèfǔzhúyūtāng 5g shānzhā 1g héshǒuwū 1g cǎojuémíng 1g zéxiè 1g Xuèfǔzhúyūtāng 5g shānzhā 1g héshǒuwū 1g zéxiè 1g Dāngguīsinìtāng 5g dānshēn 1g jīxuèténg 1g Xuèfǔzhúyūtāng 5g dāngguīniāntòngtāng 5g shānzhā 2g dānshēn 2g héshǒuwū 2g zéxiè 2g	
Indicated diseases:	
Schilder's disease 341.1 (Diffuse sclerosis of central nervous system G370, Concentric sclerosis [Balo] of central nervous system G375); Peroxisomal disorders 277.86 (Peroxisomal disorder, unspecified E7150, Zellweger syndrome E71510, Neonatal adrenoleukodystrophy E71511, Adrenomyeloneuropathy E71522, X-linked adrenoleukodystrophy, unspecified type E71529, Other peroxisomal disorders E71548); Unspecified disease of spinal cord 336.9 (Disease of spinal cord, unspecified G959); Unspecified condition of brain 348.9 (Disorder of brain, unspecified G939); Unspecified disorders of nervous system 349.9 (Disorder of central nervous system, unspecified G969); Unspecified disorder of adrenal glands 255.9 (Disorder of adrenal gland, unspecified E279); Unspecified endocrine disorder 259.9 (Endocrine disorder, unspecified E349); Unspecified disorder of metabolism 277.9 (Metabolic disorder, unspecified E889); Primary cerebellar degeneration 334.2 (Congenital nonprogressive ataxia G110, Late-onset cerebellar ataxia G112)	
Schilder's disease 341.1/G370,G375 with adrenoleukodystrophy D000326:	
Huángqíwǔwùtāng 5g bǔyánghuánwǔtāng 5g dānshēn 1g sāngzhī 1g jīxuèténg 1g to ♀	Xuèfǔzhúyūtāng 5g bǔyánghuánwǔtāng 5g dānshēn 1g niúxī 1g to ♂
Unspecified condition of brain 348.9/G939 with adrenoleukodystrophy D000326:	
Huángqíwǔwùtāng 5g bǔyánghuánwǔtāng 5g dānshēn 1g zhúrú 1g sāngzhī 1g jiānghuáng 1g to ♀	Bǔyánghuánwǔtāng 5g dānshēn 1g shíchāngpú 1g yuǎnzhì 1g + acupuncture to ♂

6.8. Lesch-Nyhan Syndrome

Lesch-Nyhan syndrome is caused by mutations in a gene that plays a central role in purine metabolism, which result in a buildup of uric acid in the blood and urine. Other signs and symptoms of Lesch-Nyhan syndrome include problems with the kidneys, joints, muscles, brain and behaviors.

Both Guìzhīfúlíngwán and Wēnjīngtāng 'invigorate Blood and dissolve stasis.' Their use in the prescriptions is therefore believed to relieve the formation and deposition of tophi from uric acid overproduction.

Table 6.8. Herbal prescriptions for Lesch-Nyhan syndrome

Lesch-Nyhan Syndrome: https://meshb.nlm.nih.gov/record/ui?ui=D007926.
Common prescriptions:
Guìzhīfúlíngwán 5g wēnjīngtāng 5g Guìzhīfúlíngwán 5g dāngguīsháoyàosǎn 5g dānshēn 1g xiāngfù 1g yìmǔcǎo 1g zélán 1g Guìzhīfúlíngwán 5g dāngguīsháoyàosǎn 5g dānshēn 1g xiāngfù 1g yìmǔcǎo 1g Guìzhīfúlíngwán 5g wēnjīngtāng 5g dāngguīsháoyàosǎn 5g Guìzhīfúlíngwán 5g dāngguīsháoyàosǎn 5g dānshēn 1g yánhúsuǒ 1g xiāngfù 1g yìmǔcǎo 1g

<table>
<tr><td colspan="2">Lesch-Nyhan Syndrome: https://meshb.nlm.nih.gov/record/ui?ui=D007926.</td></tr>
<tr><td colspan="2">Alternative prescriptions:</td></tr>
<tr><td colspan="2">Xiāoyáosǎn 5g guìzhīfúlíngwán 3g dānshēn 2g yìmǔcǎo 2g niúxī 1g xiāngfù 1g
Dāngguīsinitāng 5g wúzhūyú 1g fùzǐ 1g gānjiāng 1g yìyǐrén 1g
Guìzhīfúlíngwán 5g wēnjīngtāng 5g yìmǔcǎo 2g hónghuā 1g táorén 1g
Guìzhīfúlíngwán 5g wēnjīngtāng 5g sānléng 1g éshù 1g
Táohóngsìwùtāng 5g guìzhīfúlíngwán 4g yìmǔcǎo 1g</td></tr>
<tr><td colspan="2">Indicated diseases:</td></tr>
<tr><td colspan="2">Unspecified condition of brain 348.9 (Disorder of brain, unspecified G939); Unspecified disorder of metabolism 277.9 (Metabolic disorder, unspecified E889); Renal failure, unspecified 586 (Unspecified kidney failure N19); Unspecified disorders of nervous system 349.9 (Disorder of central nervous system, unspecified G969); Unspecified cerebrovascular disease 437.9 (Cerebrovascular disease, unspecified I679); Cardiovascular disease, unspecified 429.2 (Atherosclerotic heart disease of native coronary artery without angina pectoris I2510); Tourette's disorder 307.23 (Tourette's disorder F952); Transient tic disorder 307.21 (Transient tic disorder F950); Tic disorder, unspecified 307.20 (Tic disorder, unspecified F959); Chronic motor or vocal tic disorder 307.22 (Chronic motor or vocal tic disorder F951)</td></tr>
<tr><td colspan="2">Unspecified condition of brain 348.9/G939 with Lesch-Nyhan syndrome D007926:</td></tr>
<tr><td>Bǔyánghuánwǔtāng 5g dānshēn 1g tiānmá 1g shíchāngpú 1g yuǎnzhì 1g gōuténg 1g + acupuncture to ♀</td><td>Bǔyánghuánwǔtāng 5g + acupuncture to ♂</td></tr>
<tr><td colspan="2">Unspecified cerebrovascular disease 437.9/I679 with Lesch-Nyhan syndrome D007926:</td></tr>
<tr><td>Bǔyánghuánwǔtāng 5g sānqī 1g dānshēn 1g shíchāngpú 1g yuǎnzhì 1g + acupuncture to ♀</td><td>Bǔyánghuánwǔtāng 5g dānshēn 1g shíchāngpú 1g yuǎnzhì 1g + acupuncture to ♂</td></tr>
</table>

6.9. Mevalonate Kinase Deficiency

Mevalonate kinase deficiency is caused by mutations in the gene coding for mevalonate kinase, deficiency of which leads to innate immune activation and systemic hyper-inflammation. The signs and symptoms of mevalonate kinase deficiency therefore include recurrent fever, abnormal enlargement of the liver and spleen, oral ulcers, abdominal pain, arthralgia, myalgia and skin rash.

Table 6.9. Herbal prescriptions for mevalonate kinase deficiency

Mevalonate Kinase Deficiency: https://meshb.nlm.nih.gov/record/ui?ui=D054078.
Common prescriptions:
Sháoyàogāncǎotāng 5g shūjīnghuóxuètāng 5g dāngguīniāntòngtāng 5g + acupuncture Sháoyàogāncǎotāng 5g shūjīnghuóxuètāng 5g + acupuncture
Alternative prescriptions:
Zhènggǔzǐjīndān 5g Zhènggǔzǐjīndān 5g sháoyàogāncǎotāng 5g dāngguīniāntòngtāng 5g sānqī 1g mòyào 1g rǔxiāng 1g yánhúsuǒ 1g sūmù 1g xùduàn 1g Sǎnzhǒngkuìjiāntāng 5g + acupuncture Shūjīnghuóxuètāng 5g sháoyàogāncǎotāng 2g mùguā 1g Shūjīnghuóxuètāng 5g sháoyàogāncǎotāng 4g dāngguīniāntòngtāng 4g mùguā 1g yánhúsuǒ 1g
Indicated diseases:
Secondary cardiomyopathy, unspecified 425.9 (Cardiomyopathy due to drug and external agent I427); Unspecified disorders of nervous system 349.9 (Disorder of central nervous system, unspecified G969); Glycogenosis 271.0 (Glycogen storage disease, unspecified E7400, von Gierke disease E7401, McArdle disease E7404, Other glycogen storage disease E7409, Disorders of pyruvate metabolism and gluconeogenesis E744); Congenital stenosis of aortic valve 746.3 (Congenital stenosis of aortic valve Q230); Heart disease, unspecified 429.9 (Heart disease, unspecified I519); Cardiovascular disease, unspecified 429.2 (Atherosclerotic heart disease of native coronary artery without angina pectoris I2510); Unspecified disorder of metabolism 277.9 (Metabolic disorder, unspecified E889);

Table 6.9. (Continued)

Mevalonate Kinase Deficiency: https://meshb.nlm.nih.gov/record/ui?ui=D054078.	
Congestive heart failure, unspecified 428.0 (Right heart failure due to left heart failure I50814, Heart failure, unspecified I509); Unspecified condition of brain 348.9 (Disorder of brain, unspecified G939); Peroxisomal disorders 277.86 (Peroxisomal disorder, unspecified E7150, Zellweger syndrome E71510, Neonatal adrenoleukodystrophy E71511, Adrenomyeloneuropathy E71522, X-linked adrenoleukodystrophy, unspecified type E71529, Other peroxisomal disorders E71548); Unspecified diseases of blood and blood-forming organs 289.9 (Disease of blood and blood-forming organs, unspecified D759)	
Secondary cardiomyopathy, unspecified 425.9/I427 with mevalonate kinase deficiency D054078:	
Xuèfǔzhúyūtāng 5g dānshēn 2g chuānqī 1g báijí 1g rénshēn 1g guìzhī 1g guālóurén 1g xièbái 1g to ♀	Xuèfǔzhúyūtāng 5g dānshēn 2g chuānqī 1g báijí 1g rénshēn 1g guìzhī 1g guālóurén 1g xièbái 1g to ♂
Unspecified condition of brain 348.9/G939 with mevalonate kinase deficiency D054078:	
Cháihújiālónggǔmǔlìtāng 5g wēndǎntāng 5g zhúrú 1g yèjiāoténg 1g yuǎnzhì 1g to ♀	Bǔyánghuánwǔtāng 5g dānshēn 1g tiānmá 1g shíchāngpú 1g yuǎnzhì 1g + acupuncture to ♂

Zhènggǔzǐjīndān is used today for rheumatoid arthritis (Wang, 2019). Sǎnzhǒngkuìjiāntāng reads literally 'dispersing swelling, crushing hardening decoction,' and is used nowadays for dermatitis, eczema, goiter and internal hemorrhoids (Wang, 2019). The herbal prescriptions therefore relieve many of the autoinflammatory manifestations of mevalonate kinase deficiency. Note that cardiomyopathy was also found to be associated with mevalonate kinase deficiency (Brennenstuhl et al., 2021).

6.10. Menkes Kinky Hair Syndrome

Menkes kinky hair syndrome, also known as Menkes syndrome, is caused by mutations in gene encoding proteins for copper transport across cell membranes. Copper-dependent enzymes control development of the hair, brain, bones, liver and arteries. Reduced activities of these enzymes due to abnormal distribution of copper in the body lead to dry skin, steely or kinky hair, jaundice, seizures, osteoporosis, slow growth and cognitive disability.

Guìzhītāng and Gégēn are used for headache as shown at the end of Chapter 1. Copper deficiency is associated with acute migraine headache (Gonullu et al., 2015).

Table 6.10. Herbal prescriptions for Menkes kinky hair syndrome

Menkes Kinky Hair Syndrome: https://meshb.nlm.nih.gov/record/ui?ui=D007706.
Common prescriptions:
Guìzhītāng 5g gégēn 2g bànxià 1g dàhuáng 0g Guìzhītāng 5g gégēn 1g Guìzhītāng 5g huángqí 2g dāngguī 1g Guìzhītāng 5g gégēn 2g bànxià 1g
Alternative prescriptions:
Guìzhītāng 5g gégēn 1g dàhuáng 0g Guìzhītāng 5g báisháo 1g dàhuáng 0g Dāngguīsìnìtāng 5g máhuángfùzǐxìxīntāng 2g shēngjiāng 0g wúzhūyú 0g Guìzhītāng 5g shēngjiāng 1g báisháo 1g Jiāwèixiāoyáosǎn 5g cháihúshūgāntāng 5g dānshēn 1g shíchāngpú 1g yuǎnzhì 1g suānzǎorén 1g

Menkes Kinky Hair Syndrome: https://meshb.nlm.nih.gov/record/ui?ui=D007706.	
Indicated diseases:	
Cardiovascular disease, unspecified 429.2 (Atherosclerotic heart disease of native coronary artery without angina pectoris I2510); Other dermatoses 702; Unspecified condition of brain 348.9 (Disorder of brain, unspecified G939); Unspecified disorder of metabolism 277.9 (Metabolic disorder, unspecified E889); Ehlers-Danlos syndrome 756.83 (Ehlers-Danlos syndrome Q796); Unspecified hemorrhagic conditions 287.9 (Hemorrhagic condition, unspecified D699); Unspecified disorders of nervous system 349.9 (Disorder of central nervous system, unspecified G969); Unspecified diseases of blood and blood-forming organs 289.9 (Disease of blood and blood-forming organs, unspecified D759); Unspecified cerebrovascular disease 437.9 (Cerebrovascular disease, unspecified I679); Unspecified disorder of liver 573.9 (Liver disease, unspecified K769)	
Cardiovascular disease, unspecified 429.2/I2510 with Menkes kinky hair syndrome D007706:	
Yùzhú 5g sìnìtāng 5g mǔdānpí 1g zhīzǐ 1g huánglián 1g to ♀	Yùzhú 5g sìnìtāng 5g zhìgāncǎotāng 5g to ♂
Unspecified cerebrovascular disease 437.9/I679 with Menkes kinky hair syndrome D007706:	
Bǔyánghuánwǔtāng 5g dānshēn 1g shíchāngpú 1g yuǎnzhì 1g + acupuncture to ♀	Bǔyánghuánwǔtāng 5g dānshēn 1g shíchāngpú 1g yuǎnzhì 1g + acupuncture to ♂
Other dermatoses 702 with Menkes kinky hair syndrome D007706:	
Wǔwèixiāodúyǐn 5g huángliánjiědútāng 5g to ♀	Qīngshàngfángfēngtāng 5g huángliánjiědútāng 5g jīnyínhuā 1g liánqiáo 1g to ♂
Unspecified disorder of liver 573.9/K769 with Menkes kinky hair syndrome D007706:	
Jiāwèixiāoyáosǎn 5g cháihúshūgāntāng 5g to ♀	Xuèfǔzhúyūtāng 5g cháihúshūgāntāng 5g to ♂

6.11. Glycogen Storage Disease Type IIb

Glycogen storage disease affects the synthesis and breakdown of glycogen in the muscles, nerves, heart and liver. Mutational defects in enzymes responsible for glycogen metabolism can cause the disease. The major signs and symptoms of the disease are muscle weakness and breathing difficulties. Table 6.11 shows the prescriptions for glycogen storage disease type IIb, also called Pompe disease, which is the first identified glycogen storage disease.

Table 6.11. Herbal prescriptions for glycogen storage disease type IIb

Glycogen Storage Disease Type IIb: https://meshb.nlm.nih.gov/record/ui?ui=D052120.
Common prescriptions:
Sháoyàogāncǎotāng 5g shūjīnghuóxuètāng 5g + acupuncture Bǔzhōngyìqìtāng 5g + acupuncture
Alternative prescriptions:
Shūjīnghuóxuètāng 5g Jiāwèixiāoyáosǎn 5g xiāngshāliùjūnzǐtāng 5g gāncǎoxiǎomàidàzǎotāng 3g héhuānpí 1g yánhúsuǒ 1g Shūjīnghuóxuètāng 5g sháoyàogāncǎotāng 2g guìzhī 1g + acupuncture Sháoyàogāncǎotāng 5g huángqíwǔwùtāng 5g dānshēn 1g zhúrú 1g sāngzhī 1g qínjiāo 1g gōuténg 1g + acupuncture Bǔyánghuánwǔtāng 5g
Indicated diseases:
Secondary cardiomyopathy, unspecified 425.9 (Cardiomyopathy due to drug and external agent I427); Unspecified disorders of nervous system 349.9 (Disorder of central nervous system, unspecified G969); Glycogenosis 271.0 (Glycogen storage disease, unspecified E7400, von Gierke disease E7401, McArdle disease E7404, Other glycogen storage disease E7409, Disorders of pyruvate metabolism and gluconeogenesis E744); Congenital stenosis of aortic valve 746.3 (Congenital stenosis of aortic valve Q230); Heart disease, unspecified 429.9 (Heart disease, unspecified I519); Cardiovascular disease, unspecified 429.2 (Atherosclerotic heart disease of native coronary artery without angina pectoris I2510); Unspecified disorder of metabolism 277.9 (Metabolic disorder, unspecified E889); Recurrent hypersomnia 327.13 (Recurrent hypersomnia G4713); Unspecified condition of brain 348.9 (Disorder of brain,

Table 6.11. (Continued)

Glycogen Storage Disease Type IIb: https://meshb.nlm.nih.gov/record/ui?ui=D052120.	
unspecified G939); Peroxisomal disorders 277.86 (Peroxisomal disorder, unspecified E7150, Zellweger syndrome E71510, Neonatal adrenoleukodystrophy E71511, Adrenomyeloneuropathy E71522, X-linked adrenoleukodystrophy, unspecified type E71529, Other peroxisomal disorders E71548); Unspecified diseases of blood and blood-forming organs 289.9 (Disease of blood and blood-forming organs, unspecified D759)	
Secondary cardiomyopathy, unspecified 425.9/I427 with glycogen storage disease type IIb D052120:	
Xuèfǔzhúyūtāng 5g dānshēn 2g chuānqī 1g báijí 1g rénshēn 1g guìzhī 1g guālóurén 1g xièbái 1g to ♀	Xuèfǔzhúyūtāng 5g dānshēn 2g chuānqī 1g báijí 1g rénshēn 1g guìzhī 1g guālóurén 1g xièbái 1g to ♂
Recurrent hypersomnia 327.13/G4713 with glycogen storage disease type IIb D052120:	
Sháoyàogāncǎotāng 5g shūjīnghuóxuètāng 5g dāngguīniāntòngtāng 5g + acupuncture to ♀	Xuèfǔzhúyūtāng 5g sháoyàogāncǎotāng 5g shūjīnghuóxuètāng 5g + acupuncture to ♂
Unspecified condition of brain 348.9/G939 with glycogen storage disease type IIb D052120:	
Bǔyánghuánwǔtāng 5g tiānmá 1g shíchāngpú 1g yuǎnzhì 1g gōuténg 1g + acupuncture to ♀	Bǔyánghuánwǔtāng 5g tiānmá 1g shíchāngpú 1g yuǎnzhì 1g + acupuncture to ♂

Sháoyàogāncǎotāng and Shūjīnghuóxuètāng are frequently used for myopathy-related movement problems in the last chapter. Hypersomnia is associated with glycogen storage disease (Smith et al., 2017) and both Zhúrú and Gōuténg are used today for such general symptoms as sleep disturbances (Wang, 2019).

6.12. Mucopolysaccharidosis II

Instead of glycogen in Pompe disease, deficiency in the breakdown of mucopolysaccharides is involved in mucopolysaccharidoses. Accumulation of mucopolysaccharides can damage nerves, connective tissues and organs including the skeleton and heart. Mutations in the genes encoding lysosomal enzymes that degrade mucopolysaccharides cause the disease. Table 6.12 shows the herbal prescriptions for mucopolysaccharidosis II, also called Hunter syndrome, which is the only mucopolysaccharidosis that is X-linked.

Table 6.12. Herbal prescriptions for mucopolysaccharidosis II

Mucopolysaccharidosis II: https://meshb.nlm.nih.gov/record/ui?ui=D016532.
Common prescriptions:
Sháoyàogāncǎotāng 5g shūjīnghuóxuètāng 5g dāngguīniāntòngtāng 5g + acupuncture Sháoyàogāncǎotāng 5g shūjīnghuóxuètāng 5g dāngguīniāntòngtāng 5g Sháoyàogāncǎotāng 5g shūjīnghuóxuètāng 5g + acupuncture
Alternative prescriptions:
Huángqíwǔwùtāng 5g chuānxiōng 1g dānshēn 1g zhúrú 1g sāngzhī 1g dāngguī 1g jiānghuáng 1g gōuténg 1g Huángqíwǔwùtāng 5g dānshēn 1g zhúrú 1g sāngzhī 1g jiānghuáng 1g Huángqíwǔwùtāng 5g dānshēn 1g jīxuèténg 1g
Dāngguīniāntòngtāng 5g shūjīnghuóxuètāng 4g dānshēn 2g niúxī 2g yánhúsuǒ 2g yùjīn 2g Shūjīnghuóxuètāng 5g dāngguīniāntòngtāng 4g niúxī 1g mòyào 1g rǔxiāng 1g yánhúsuǒ 1g fùzǐ 1g guìzhī 1g jīxuèténg 1g + acupuncture
Indicated diseases:
Unspecified retinal disorder 362.9 (Unspecified retinal disorder H359); Mucopolysaccharidosis 277.5 (Hurler's syndrome E7601, Scheie's syndrome E7603, Mucopolysaccharidosis, type II E761, Morquio mucopolysaccharidoses, unspecified E76219, Sanfilippo mucopolysaccharidoses E7622, Other mucopolysaccharidoses E7629,

Mucopolysaccharidosis II: https://meshb.nlm.nih.gov/record/ui?ui=D016532.	
Mucopolysaccharidosis, unspecified E763); Disorder of eye, unspecified 379.90 (Unspecified disorder of eye and adnexa H579); Unspecified disorders of nervous system 349.9 (Disorder of central nervous system, unspecified G969); Unspecified disorder of metabolism 277.9 (Metabolic disorder, unspecified E889); Heart disease, unspecified 429.9 (Heart disease, unspecified I519); Cardiovascular disease, unspecified 429.2 (Atherosclerotic heart disease of native coronary artery without angina pectoris I2510); Unspecified condition of brain 348.9 (Disorder of brain, unspecified G939); Unspecified diseases of blood and blood-forming organs 289.9 (Disease of blood and blood-forming organs, unspecified D759)	
Unspecified retinal disorder 362.9/H359 with mucopolysaccharidosis II D016532:	
Qǐjúdìhuángwán 5g yìqìcōngmíngtāng 3g xuèfǔzhúyūtāng 2g to ♀	Qǐjúdìhuángwán 5g yìqìcōngmíngtāng 3g xuèfǔzhúyūtāng 2g to ♂
Unspecified disorders of nervous system 349.9/G969 with mucopolysaccharidosis II D016532:	
Huángqíwǔwùtāng 5g chuānxiōng 1g dānshēn 1g zhúrú 1g sāngzhī 1g dāngguī 1g jiānghuáng 1g to ♀	Huángqíwǔwùtāng 5g chuānxiōng 1g dānshēn 1g zhúrú 1g sāngzhī 1g dāngguī 1g jiānghuáng 1g to ♂
Heart disease, unspecified 429.9/I519 with mucopolysaccharidosis II D016532:	
Xuèfǔzhúyūtāng 5g zhìgāncǎotāng 5g dānshēn 2g chuānqī 1g huángqí 1g guìzhī 1g guālóurén 1g xièbái 1g to ♀	Shēngmàiyǐn 5g xuèfǔzhúyūtāng 5g chuānqī 1g dānshēn 1g wǔlíngzhī 1g púhuáng 1g to ♂
Unspecified condition of brain 348.9/G939 with mucopolysaccharidosis II D016532:	
Bǔyánghuánwǔtāng 5g + acupuncture to ♀	Bǔyánghuánwǔtāng 5g + acupuncture to ♂

Nasal, throaty and respiratory signs and symptoms are among the first signs and symptoms to appear in mucopolysaccharidoses (Berger et al., 2013) and Huángqíwǔwùtāng's contemporary uses include chronic sinusitis and chronic bronchitis (Wang, 2019).

6.13. Primary Progressive Nonfluent Aphasia

Proteostasis refers to regulation of the concentration, folding, interactions and localization of each of the proteins that make up the proteome, the integrity of which also includes their post-translational modifications and degradation and clearance of misfolded proteins. Proteostasis deficiencies not only make proteins to lose their functions but also make misfolded proteins to aggregate, leading to many of the age-related neurodegenerative diseases such as primary progressive nonfluent aphasia, in which the frontotemporal lobes of the brain are affected.

Progressive motor decline is a common complication of frontotemporal lobar degeneration, and we see here the use of Sháoyàogāncǎotāng, Shūjīnghuóxuètāng and Dāngguīniāntòngtāng in the prescriptions.

Table 6.13. Herbal prescriptions for primary progressive nonfluent aphasia

Primary Progressive Nonfluent Aphasia: https://meshb.nlm.nih.gov/record/ui?ui=D057178.
Common prescriptions:
Sháoyàogāncǎotāng 5g shūjīnghuóxuètāng 5g dāngguīniāntòngtāng 5g + acupuncture Sháoyàogāncǎotāng 5g shūjīnghuóxuètāng 5g + acupuncture
Alternative prescriptions:
Shēntòngzhúyūtāng 5g shūjīnghuóxuètāng 4g huángqí 1g + acupuncture Jiāwèixiāoyáosǎn 5g cháihúshūgāntāng 5g héhuānpí 2g dānshēn 1g shíchāngpú 1g yuǎnzhì 1g Zhènggǔzǐjīndān 5g dāngguīniāntòngtāng 5g sānqī 2g mòyào 2g rǔxiāng 2g yánhúsuǒ 2g sūmù 2g xùduàn 2g + acupuncture Jiāwèixiāoyáosǎn 5g xiāngshāliùjūnzǐtāng 4g gāncǎoxiǎomàidàzǎotāng 2g héhuānpí 1g yánhúsuǒ 1g Shūjīnghuóxuètāng 5g sháoyàogāncǎotāng 3g yánhúsuǒ 1g + acupuncture

Table 6.13. (Continued)

Primary Progressive Nonfluent Aphasia: https://meshb.nlm.nih.gov/record/ui?ui=D057178.	
Indicated and associated diseases:	
Unspecified condition of brain 348.9 (Disorder of brain, unspecified G939); Peroxisomal disorders 277.86 (Peroxisomal disorder, unspecified E7150, Zellweger syndrome E71510, Neonatal adrenoleukodystrophy E71511, Adrenomyeloneuropathy E71522, X-linked adrenoleukodystrophy, unspecified type E71529, Other peroxisomal disorders E71548); Unspecified diseases of blood and blood-forming organs 289.9 (Disease of blood and blood-forming organs, unspecified D759); Unspecified disorders of nervous system 349.9 (Disorder of central nervous system, unspecified G969); Unspecified disorder of metabolism 277.9 (Metabolic disorder, unspecified E889); Cardiovascular disease, unspecified 429.2 (Atherosclerotic heart disease of native coronary artery without angina pectoris I2510); Unspecified hemorrhagic conditions 287.9 (Hemorrhagic condition, unspecified D699); Alexia 315.01 (Dyslexia and alexia R480)	
Unspecified condition of brain 348.9/G939 with primary progressive nonfluent aphasia D057178:	
Bǔyánghuánwǔtāng 5g dānshēn 1g tiānmá 1g shíchāngpú 1g yuǎnzhì 1g + acupuncture to ♀	Bǔyánghuánwǔtāng 5g dānshēn 1g tiānmá 1g shíchāngpú 1g yuǎnzhì 1g + acupuncture to ♂
Cardiovascular disease, unspecified 429.2/I2510 with primary progressive nonfluent aphasia D057178:	
Sìnìtāng 5g gānlùyǐn 5g mǔdānpí 1g zhīzǐ 1g huánglián 0g to ♀	Xuèfǔzhúyūtāng 5g zhìgāncǎotāng 5g dānshēn 1g to ♂

6.14. Hypertriglyceridemic Waist

Triglycerides, the most abundant fatty molecule in organisms, are the main constituent of body fat in vertebrates. Hypertriglyceridemia means high levels of triglycerides in the blood. Hypertriglyceridemia greatly increases the risk of atherosclerosis, cardiovascular diseases, nonalcoholic fatty liver disease, and acute pancreatitis. Overeating can cause hypertriglyceridemia. Hypertriglyceridemic waist is defined as an increased waist circumference along with hypertriglyceridemia. Hypertriglyceridemic waist phenotype has been proposed as a simple and practical screening marker for visceral obesity, lipid metabolic disorder, coronary artery disease, and type 2 diabetes.

Table 6.14. Herbal prescriptions for hypertriglyceridemic waist

Hypertriglyceridemic Waist: https://meshb.nlm.nih.gov/record/ui?ui=D064250.
Common prescriptions:
Sháoyàogāncǎotāng 5g shūjīnghuóxuètāng 5g dāngguīniāntòngtāng 5g + acupuncture Sháoyàogāncǎotāng 5g shūjīnghuóxuètāng 5g + acupuncture
Alternative prescriptions:
Jiāwèixiāoyáosǎn 5g zhībódìhuángwán 5g nǚzhēnzǐ 1g wǔwèizǐ 1g héhuānpí 1g xiāngfù 1g huángqí 1g Sháoyàogāncǎotāng 5g zhībódìhuángwán 5g shūjīnghuóxuètāng 5g Shūjīnghuóxuètāng 5g gégēntāng 5g mùguā 1g niúxī 1g yánhúsuǒ 1g + acupuncture Shūjīnghuóxuètāng 5g sháoyàogāncǎotāng 3g mùguā 1g niúxī 1g + acupuncture Sháoyàogāncǎotāng 5g mùguā 1g niúxī 1g jīxuèténg 1g + acupuncture
Indicated diseases:
Cardiovascular disease, unspecified 429.2 (Atherosclerotic heart disease of native coronary artery without angina pectoris I2510); Multiple myeloma 203.0; Unspecified hemorrhagic conditions 287.9 (Hemorrhagic condition, unspecified D699); Unspecified diseases of blood and blood-forming organs 289.9 (Disease of blood and blood-forming organs, unspecified D759); Unspecified condition of brain 348.9 (Disorder of brain, unspecified G939); Unspecified disorders of nervous system 349.9 (Disorder of central nervous system, unspecified G969); Unspecified disorder of metabolism 277.9 (Metabolic disorder, unspecified E889)

Hypertriglyceridemic Waist: https://meshb.nlm.nih.gov/record/ui?ui=D064250.	
Cardiovascular disease, unspecified 429.2/I2510 with hypertriglyceridemic waist D064250:	
Sìnìtāng 5g gānlùyǐn 5g mǔdānpí 1g zhīzǐ 1g huánglián 0g to ♀	Xuèfǔzhúyūtāng 5g zhìgāncǎotāng 5g to ♂
Unspecified condition of brain 348.9/G939 with hypertriglyceridemic waist D064250:	
Bǔyánghuánwǔtāng 5g + acupuncture to ♀	Bǔyánghuánwǔtāng 5g shíchāngpú 1g yuǎnzhì 1g + acupuncture to ♂
Unspecified disorder of metabolism 277.9/E889 with hypertriglyceridemic waist D064250:	
Rénshēnbàidúsǎn 5g xiǎocháihútāngqùrénshēn 5g yīnchénhāotāng 2g mùxiāng 1g yùjīn 1g to ♀	Dānshēn 5g tiānmágōuténgyǐn 5g sǎnzhǒngkuìjiāntāng 5g bǔyánghuánwǔtāng 5g to ♂

Báisháo, one of the only two herbs in Sháoyàogāncǎotāng, is said to 'soften the Liver,' and indeed one of the modern uses of Báisháo is for pure hypercholesterolemia (Wang, 2020). Also, as bile produced by the liver breaks down lipids in the small intestine during digestion, these could be the reason why Sháoyàogāncǎotāng or Jiāwèixiāoyáosǎn are used here for hypertriglyceridemia, a type of hyperlipidemias. Note that acupuncture is used for hyperlipidemias (Liang, 2005; Wang et al., 2020).

References

Berger, K. I., Fagondes, S. C., Giugliani, R., Hardy, K. A., Lee, K. S., McArdle, C., Scarpa, M., Tobin, M. J., Ward, S. A., & Rapoport, D. M. (2012). Respiratory and sleep disorders in mucopolysaccharidosis. *Journal of Inherited Metabolic Disease*, *36*(2), 201–210. https://doi.org/10.1007/s10545-012-9555-1.

Brennenstuhl, H., Nashawi, M., Schröter, J., Baronio, F., Beedgen, L., Gleich, F., Jeltsch, K., Landenberg, C., Martini, S., Simon, A., Thiel, C., Tsiakas, K., Opladen, T., Kölker, S., Hoffmann, G. F., & Haas, D. (2021). Phenotypic diversity, disease progression, and pathogenicity of *MVK* missense variants in mevalonic aciduria. *Journal of Inherited Metabolic Disease*, *44*(5), 1272–1287. https://doi.org/10.1002/jimd.12412.

Buda, P., Piekutowska-Abramczuk, D., Karkucińska-Więckowska, A., Jurkiewicz, E., Chełstowska, S., Pajdowska, M., Migdał, M., Książyk, J., Kotulska, K., & Pronicka, E. (2013). "Drop attacks" as first clinical symptoms in a child carrying MTTK m.8344A>G mutation. *Folia Neuropathologica*, *4*, 347–354. https://doi.org/10.5114/fn.2013.39726.

de Smalen, P. P., van Ark, T. J., Stolker, R. J., Vincent, A. J. P. E., & Klimek, M. (2020). Hyperlactatemia After Intracranial Tumor Surgery Does Not Affect 6-Month Survival: A Retrospective Case Series. *Journal of Neurosurgical Anesthesiology*, *32*(1), 48–56. https://doi.org/10.1097/ana.0000000000000594.

Doroshow, D. B. (2006). Performing a Cure for Schizophrenia: Insulin Coma Therapy on the Wards. *Journal of the History of Medicine and Allied Sciences*, *62*(2), 213–243. https://doi.org/10.1093/jhmas/jrl044.

Godbole, N. P., Sadjadi, R., DeBono, M. A., Grant, N. R., Kelly, D. C., James, P. F., Stephen, C. D., Balkwill, M. D., Lewis, R. F., & Eichler, F. S. (2021). Gait Difficulties and Postural Instability in Adrenoleukodystrophy. *Frontiers in Neurology*, *12*, 684102. https://doi.org/10.3389/fneur.2021.684102.

Gonullu, H., Gonullu, E., Karadas, S., Arslan, M., Kalemci, O., Aycan, A., Sayin, R., & Demir, H. (2015). The levels of trace elements and heavy metals in patients with acute migraine headache. *J Pak Med Assoc.*, *65*(7), 694–697. PMID: 26160074.

Liang, F. Y. (2005). Effects of acupuncture on hyperlipidemia and hyperviscosity in old people. *Journal of Acupuncture and Tuina Science*, *3*(1), 4–6. https://doi.org/10.1007/bf02900007.

Minton, J., & Sidebotham, D. A. (2017). Hyperlactatemia and Cardiac Surgery. *The Journal ExtraCorporeal Technology*, *49*(1), 7–15.

Smith, P., Nicotra, A., Williams, S., & Robertson, B. (2017). 1231 Hypersomnia in a patient with a glycogen storage disease. *Sleep*, *40*(suppl_1), A459–A459. https://doi.org/10.1093/sleepj/zsx052.022.

Wang, S. C. (2019). *Clinical Herbal Prescriptions: Principles and Practices of Herbal Formulations from Deep Learning Health Insurance Herbal Prescription Big Data*. WSPC. https://doi.org/10.1142/11211.

Wang, S. C. (2020). *Veterinary Herbal Pharmacopoeia*. Nova Science Publishers. https://doi.org/10.52305/GHTR1903.

Wang, X. S., Wang, Y. S., Li, J. J., Yu, C. C., Wu, M., & Kong, L. H. (2020). Acupuncture and Related Therapies for Hyperlipidemia: A Network Meta-Analysis. *Digital Chinese Medicine*, *3*(4), 309–326. https://doi.org/10.1016/j.dcmed.2020.12.002.

Ziegler, C., Volkov, L., Marnai, R., Courte, G., Cravoisy, A., Conrad, M., Nace, L., Melone, A., Perrot, A., & Gibot, S. (2021). Lactic acidosis and hypoglycemia as markers of disease progression of multiple myeloma: A case report. *EJHaem*, *2*(3), 539–544. https://doi.org/10.1002/jha2.176.

Chapter 7

Skin Manifestations

The skin makes up most of our integumentary system which also contains the hair, nails and glands. The integumentary system forms the outermost surface of our body and serves as the interface between the internal tissues and external environment. The skin plays a crucial role in maintaining homeostasis for our optimal living. Its functions include defending against foreign pathogens, regulating body temperature through mechanisms such as perspiration to rapidly lower body temperature, sensing touch, pain, pleasure, heat and cold, protecting against ultraviolet rays, producing vitamin D, and defining the boundary of self. Many diagnoses of skin diseases are based on skin lesions' morphology, local organization and global distribution. Figure 7.1 shows the characteristic displays of many skin-related disorders.

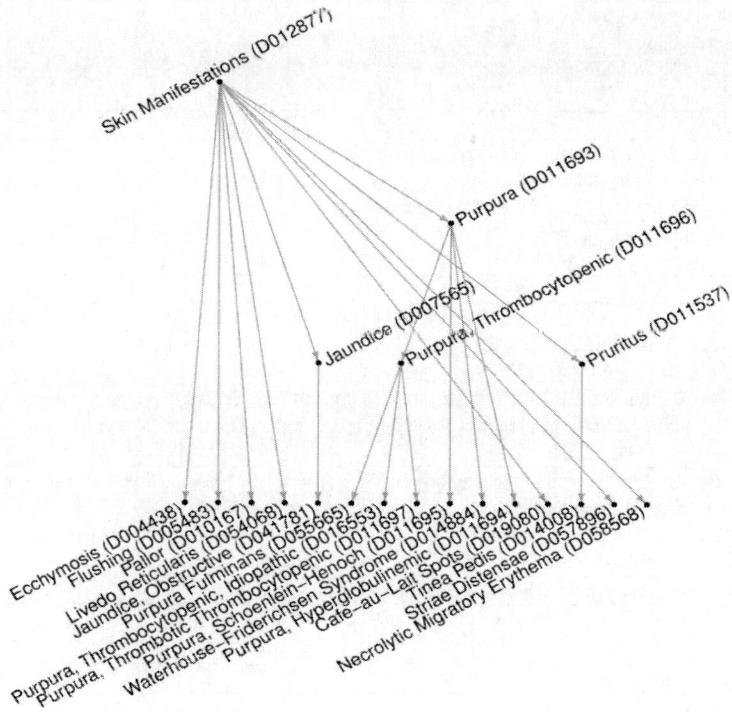

Figure 7.1. Skin signs and symptoms accompanying or following results of non-skin diseases or injuries.

The herbal formulas that are commonly prescribed for the skin manifestations are Xiāofēngsǎn, Bǔzhōngyìqìtāng, Jīngfángbàidúsǎn, Yùnǚjiān, Guìzhītāng, Sháoyàogāncǎotāng, Shūjīnghuóxuètāng, and Xiǎocháihútāng. Many of them have traditionally been used for cutaneous conditions. The supportive single herbs are Huángqín, Shēngjiāng, Dàhuáng, Báixiānpí, Dìfūzǐ, Tiānhuā, Yánhúsuǒ, and Xìxīn.

The diseases that cause or relate to the skin manifestations are unspecified diseases of blood and blood-forming organs, coagulation defects, unspecified disorders of nervous system, unspecified cardiovascular disease, unspecified hemorrhagic conditions, other dermatoses, unspecified condition of brain, and unspecified endocrine disorder.

7.1. Ecchymosis

Ecchymosis is leakage of blood from the blood vessels into the surrounding tissues under the skin, resulting in a non-elevated, rounded or irregularly shaped, bluish or purplish patch larger than 1 centimeter. Common causes of ecchymosis are blunt traumas such as a punch or a fall which rupture the vessels. However, medications such as blood thinners, cancers such as leukemia, and infections such as meningitis can cause ecchymosis.

Table 7.1. Herbal prescriptions for ecchymosis

<table>
<tr><td colspan="2">Ecchymosis: https://meshb.nlm.nih.gov/record/ui?ui=D004438.</td></tr>
<tr><td colspan="2">Common prescriptions:</td></tr>
<tr><td colspan="2">Yùnǚjiān 5g gānlùyǐn 5g qīngwèisǎn 5g
Yùnǚjiān 5g qīngwèisǎn 5g
Yùnǚjiān 5g gānlùyǐn 5g zhībódìhuángwán 5g
Yùnǚjiān 5g gānlùyǐn 5g</td></tr>
<tr><td colspan="2">Alternative prescriptions:</td></tr>
<tr><td colspan="2">Yùnǚjiān 5g gānlùyǐn 5g zhībódìhuángwán 5g qīngwèisǎn 5g
Yùnǚjiān 5g qīngwèisǎn 3g lóngdǎnxiègāntāng 3g
Yùnǚjiān 5g gānlùyǐn 5g xuánshēn 2g dìhuáng 2g màiméndōng 2g
Yùnǚjiān 5g zhībódìhuángwán 3g
Yùnǚjiān 5g zhībódìhuángwán 3g xuánshēn 1g</td></tr>
<tr><td colspan="2">Indicated diseases:</td></tr>
<tr><td colspan="2">Unspecified disorder of orbit 376.9 (Unspecified disorder of orbit H059); Malignant neoplasm of orbit 190.1 (Malignant neoplasm of unspecified orbit C6960); Coagulation defects 286; Disorder of eye, unspecified 379.90 (Unspecified disorder of eye and adnexa H579);
Malignant neoplasm of other specified sites of eye 190.8 (Malignant neoplasm of overlapping sites of unspecified eye and adnexa C6980); Malignant neoplasm of nervous system, part unspecified 192.9 (Malignant neoplasm of central nervous system, unspecified C729);</td></tr>
<tr><td colspan="2">Unspecified diseases of blood and blood-forming organs 289.9 (Disease of blood and blood-forming organs, unspecified D759); Cardiovascular disease, unspecified 429.2 (Atherosclerotic heart disease of native coronary artery without angina pectoris I2510); Other dermatoses 702; Ehlers-Danlos syndrome 756.83 (Ehlers-Danlos syndrome Q796); Unspecified hemorrhagic conditions 287.9 (Hemorrhagic condition, unspecified D699)</td></tr>
<tr><td colspan="2">Unspecified disorder of orbit 376.9/H059 with ecchymosis D004438:</td></tr>
<tr><td>Xǐgānmíngmùtāng 5g zīshènmíngmùtāng 5g to ♀</td><td>Qǐjúdìhuángwán 5g xǐgānmíngmùtāng 5g zīshènmíngmùtāng 5g to ♂</td></tr>
<tr><td colspan="2">Coagulation defects 286 with ecchymosis D004438:</td></tr>
<tr><td>Dāngguīsìnìtāng 5g to ♀</td><td>Xuèfǔzhúyūtāng 5g bǔyánghuánwǔtāng 5g to ♂</td></tr>
<tr><td colspan="2">Cardiovascular disease, unspecified 429.2/I2510 with ecchymosis D004438:</td></tr>
<tr><td>Yùzhú 5g sìnìtāng 5g mǔdānpí 1g zhīzǐ 1g huánglián 0g to ♀</td><td>Yùzhú 5g sìnìtāng 5g mǔdānpí 1g zhīzǐ 1g huánglián 1g to ♂</td></tr>
</table>

Both Yùnǚjiān and Gānlùyǐn 'nourish Yin.' Gānlùyǐn additionally 'clears Heat.' They are presumably used here to promote healing after the bruising. Note that Yùnǚjiān and Gānlùyǐn are used in the next chapter for gingival hemorrhage, which is bleeding of the mucous membranes in the mouth. Similarity between the gingival and cutaneous bleeding may be behind the use of Yùnǚjiān and Gānlùyǐn here. Note also that injury to the face easily leads to a black eye as the blood quickly pools in the area around the eye, where the skin is loose.

7.2. Flushing

Flushing is involuntary widening of the tiny blood vessels under the skin, leading to redness of the involved skin. Flushing usually occurs in the cheeks or neck. Excitement, embarrassment, exercise, heat, fever, alcohol and medications can cause flushes.

Table 7.2. Herbal prescriptions for flushing

Flushing: https://meshb.nlm.nih.gov/record/ui?ui=D005483.	
Common prescriptions:	
Bǔzhōngyìqìtāng 5g Guìzhītāng 5g huángqí 2g báizhú 1g fùzǐ 1g Guìzhītāng 5g huángqí 2g báizhú 1g fúlíng 1g Guìzhītāng 5g huángqí 2g báizhú 1g fùzǐ 1g fúlíng 1g Bǔzhōngyìqìtāng 5g huángqí 1g	
Alternative prescriptions:	
Huángqíwǔwùtāng 5g dānshēn 1g zhúrú 1g sāngzhī 1g jiānghuáng 1g Máhuángfùzǐxìxīntāng 5g dāngguīsìnìtāng 4g shēngjiāng 1g wúzhūyú 1g	
Guìzhītāng 5g báizhú 0g fúlíng 0g Bǔzhōngyìqìtāng 5g huángqí 1g dāngguī 0g Máhuángfùzǐxìxīntāng 5g shēngjiāng 2g zhìgāncǎo 2g guìzhī 2g	
Indicated or associated diseases:	
Anhidrosis 705.0 (Anhidrosis L744); Unspecified disorders of nervous system 349.9 (Disorder of central nervous system, unspecified G969); Unspecified disorder of sweat glands 705.9 (Eccrine sweat disorder, unspecified L749, Apocrine sweat disorder, unspecified L759); Other dermatoses 702; Malignant neoplasm of mediastinum, part unspecified 164.9 (Malignant neoplasm of mediastinum, part unspecified C383); Malignant neoplasm of thorax 195.1 (Malignant neoplasm of thorax C761); Malignant neoplasm of nervous system, part unspecified 192.9 (Malignant neoplasm of central nervous system, unspecified C729); Hypertensive heart and chronic kidney disease 404; Secondary hypertension 405; Essential hypertension 401; Hypertensive chronic kidney disease 403; Hypertensive heart disease 402; Cardiovascular disease, unspecified 429.2 (Atherosclerotic heart disease of native coronary artery without angina pectoris I2510)	
Anhidrosis 705.0/L744 with flushing D005483:	
Yùpíngfēngsǎn 5g guìzhītāng 5g to ♀	Yùpíngfēngsǎn 5g bǔzhōngyìqìtāng 5g to ♂
Hypertensive heart and chronic kidney disease 404 with flushing D005483:	
Tiānmágōuténgyǐn 5g jiāwèixiāoyáosǎn 5g zhībódìhuángwán 5g to ♀	Tiānmágōuténgyǐn 5g xuèfǔzhúyūtāng 5g zhībódìhuángwán 5g to ♂

Guìzhītāng is for the common cold and is used here for fever induced flushing. Niacin, i.e., vitamin B3, is used as a drug for hypertensive heart and chronic kidney disease as it lowers the lipid and phosphorous levels in the blood. However, a well-known side-effect of niacin is flushing.

7.3. Pallor

Pallor, or paleness, is the lightness of the color of the skin over the body such as the face or palms. Severe pallor turns the color of the mucous membranes of the lips, tongue and mouth into paleness. Panic, malnutrition, anemia, poisoning and hypoglycemia can cause pallor.

Table 7.3. Herbal prescriptions for pallor

Pallor: https://meshb.nlm.nih.gov/record/ui?ui=D010167.	
Common prescriptions:	
Bāwèidìhuángwán 5g bǔzhōngyìqìtāng 5g Bǔzhōngyìqìtāng 5g Sìnìtāng 5g bǔzhōngyìqìtāng 5g ròuguì 1g zhìgāncǎotāng 1g Sìnìtāng 5g lǐzhōngtāng 5g ròuguì 1g yánhúsuǒ 1g zhìgāncǎotāng 1g	
Alternative prescriptions:	
Sìnìtāng 5g dāngguīsìnìtāng 5g shēngjiāng 1g wúzhūyú 1g Sìnìtāng 5g ròuguì 1g wúzhūyú 1g Sìnìtāng 5g lǐzhōngtāng 5g ròuguì 1g zhìgāncǎotāng 1g Sìnìtāng 5g shēngjiāng 1g guìzhī 1g rénshēn 1g Sìnìtāng 5g fùzǐ 2g ròuguì 1g	
Indicated diseases:	
Unspecified disorder of metabolism 277.9 (Metabolic disorder, unspecified E889); Hereditary hemolytic anemias 282; Anemia, unspecified 285.9 (Anemia, unspecified D649); Unspecified diseases of blood and blood-forming organs 289.9 (Disease of blood and blood-forming organs, unspecified D759); Falciparum malaria [malignant tertian] 084.0 (Other severe and complicated Plasmodium falciparum malaria B508, Plasmodium falciparum malaria, unspecified B509); Malaria 084	
Unspecified disorder of metabolism 277.9/E889 with pallor D010167:	
Liùwèidìhuángwán 5g bǔzhōngyìqìtāng 5g to ♀	Liùwèidìhuángwán 5g bǔzhōngyìqìtāng 5g to ♂
Anemia, unspecified 285.9/D649 with pallor D010167:	
Shèngyùtāng 5g bǔzhōngyìqìtāng 5g guīpítāng 5g to ♀	Rénshēnyǎngróngtāng 5g bǔzhōngyìqìtāng 5g guīpítāng 5g to ♂
Falciparum malaria [malignant tertian] 084.0/B508,B509 with pallor D010167:	
Chuānxiōngchádiàosǎn 5g to ♀	Xiǎocháihútāng 5g chuānxiōng 1g báizhǐ 1g to ♂

Pallor is one of the initial signs and symptoms of diabetic hypoglycemia. Bāwèidìhuángwán and Liùwèidìhuángwán are nowadays used for diabetes, and Shèngyùtāng, Bǔzhōngyìqìtāng and Guīpítāng for unspecified anemia (Wang, 2019).

7.4. Livedo Reticularis

Livedo reticularis refers to a reddish-purplish discoloration and net-like pattern of the skin, due to reduced flow of blood and oxygen to the surface of the affected skin. Spasms of the blood vessels and exposure to low temperatures can cause livedo reticularis.

Table 7.4. Herbal prescriptions for livedo reticularis

Livedo Reticularis: https://meshb.nlm.nih.gov/record/ui?ui=D054068.
Common prescriptions:
Guìzhītāng 5g shēngjiāng 1g báisháo 1g dàhuáng 0g Guìzhītāng 5g shēngjiāng 1g guìzhī 1g Máhuángfùzǐxìxīntāng 5g shēngjiāng 2g guìzhī 2g zhìgāncǎo 1g Guìzhītāng 5g shēngjiāng 1g báisháo 1g Máhuángfùzǐxìxīntāng 5g shēngjiāng 2g zhìgāncǎo 2g guìzhī 2g dàzǎo 1g
Alternative prescriptions:
Guìzhītāng 5g shēngjiāng 0g guìzhī 0g Guìzhītāng 5g shēngjiāng 1g guìzhī 1g dàhuáng 0g Guìzhītāng 5g báisháo 1g dàhuáng 0g Guìzhītāng 5g shēngjiāng 2g báisháo 2g dàhuáng 0g Guìzhītāng 5g shēngjiāng 0g báisháo 0g

Livedo Reticularis: https://meshb.nlm.nih.gov/record/ui?ui=D054068.	
Indicated and associated diseases:	
Unspecified cerebrovascular disease 437.9 (Cerebrovascular disease, unspecified I679); Vascular disorders of skin 709.1 (Vasculitis limited to the skin, unspecified L959); Unspecified condition of brain 348.9 (Disorder of brain, unspecified G939); Cardiovascular disease, unspecified 429.2 (Atherosclerotic heart disease of native coronary artery without angina pectoris I2510); Other dermatoses 702; Unspecified disorders of nervous system 349.9 (Disorder of central nervous system, unspecified G969); Unspecified diseases of blood and blood-forming organs 289.9 (Disease of blood and blood-forming organs, unspecified D759); Unspecified hemorrhagic conditions 287.9 (Hemorrhagic condition, unspecified D699)	
Unspecified cerebrovascular disease 437.9/I679 with livedo reticularis D054068:	
Bǔyánghuánwǔtāng 5g chuānqī 1g dānshēn 1g shíchāngpú 1g yuǎnzhì 1g + acupuncture to ♀	Bǔyánghuánwǔtāng 5g chuānqī 1g dānshēn 1g shíchāngpú 1g yuǎnzhì 1g + acupuncture to ♂
Cardiovascular disease, unspecified 429.2/I2510 with livedo reticularis D054068:	
Sìnìtāng 5g gānlùyǐn 5g mǔdānpí 1g zhīzǐ 1g huánglián 0g to ♀	Sìnìtāng 5g gānlùyǐn 5g mǔdānpí 1g zhīzǐ 1g huánglián 1g to ♂

Any of Guìzhītāng, Shēngjiāng and Máhuángfùzǐxìxīntāng warms up the body via promoting circulation. They are thus used here for livedo reticularis. Note that a rare, occlusive arterial condition that causes a reduction of blood flow to the brain and skin is called Sneddon syndrome (Wu et al., 2014).

7.5. Jaundice

Jaundice is yellowish discoloration of the skin, whites of the eyes and mucous membranes due to high levels of bilirubin in the blood. Bilirubin is a product of the biochemical pathway that breaks down aged or abnormal red blood cells. As the liver filters bilirubin out of the blood stream, damage of the liver by infection or alcohol can cause jaundice.

Table 7.5. Herbal prescriptions for jaundice

Jaundice: https://meshb.nlm.nih.gov/record/ui?ui=D007565.
Common prescriptions:
Cháihúshūgāntāng 5g lóngdǎnxiègāntāng 5g Jiāwèixiāoyáosǎn 5g cháihúshūgāntāng 5g dānshēn 1g shíchāngpú 1g yuǎnzhì 1g suānzǎorén 1g Jiāwèixiāoyáosǎn 5g cháihúshūgāntāng 5g lóngdǎnxiègāntāng 5g Jiāwèixiāoyáosǎn 5g cháihúshūgāntāng 5g dānshēn 1g shíchāngpú 1g yuǎnzhì 1g Jiāwèixiāoyáosǎn 5g cháihúshūgāntāng 5g dānshēn 1g yīnchén 1g huángqín 1g
Alternative prescriptions:
Jiāwèixiāoyáosǎn 5g cháihúshūgāntāng 5g héhuānpí 2g dānshēn 1g shíchāngpú 1g yuǎnzhì 1g Xiǎocháihútāng 5g xiāngshāliùjūnzǐtāng 5g huòxiāngzhèngqìsǎn 5g báisháo 1g cháihú 1g zéxiè 1g Xiǎocháihútāng 5g lóngdǎnxiègāntāng 5g Jiāwèixiāoyáosǎn 5g yīnchénwǔlíngsǎn 5g dānshēn 2g niúxī 2g xiāngfù 2g yùjīn 2g Xiǎocháihútāng 5g gānlùxiāodúdān 5g cháihúshūgāntāng 5g báizhú 1g fúlíng 1g dǎngshēn 1g
Indicated diseases:
Unspecified disorder of liver 573.9 (Liver disease, unspecified K769); Malignant neoplasm of liver, not specified as primary or secondary 155.2 (Malignant neoplasm of liver, not specified as primary or secondary C229); Diseases of the jaws 526; Unspecified disorder of biliary tract 576.9 (Disease of biliary tract, unspecified K839); Malignant neoplasm of extrahepatic bile ducts 156.1 (Malignant neoplasm of extrahepatic bile duct C240); Unspecified disorder of gallbladder 575.9 (Disease of gallbladder, unspecified K829); Unspecified endocrine disorder 259.9 (Endocrine disorder, unspecified E349); Malignant neoplasm of gallbladder 156.0 (Malignant neoplasm of gallbladder C23); Unspecified disorder of metabolism 277.9 (Metabolic disorder, unspecified E889); Cardiovascular disease, unspecified 429.2 (Atherosclerotic heart disease of native coronary artery without angina pectoris I2510)

Table 7.5. (Continued)

Jaundice: https://meshb.nlm.nih.gov/record/ui?ui=D007565.	
Unspecified disorder of liver 573.9/K769 with jaundice D007565:	
Jiāwèixiāoyáosǎn 5g cháihúshūgāntāng 5g lóngdǎnxiègāntāng 5g to ♀	Cháihúshūgāntāng 5g lóngdǎnxiègāntāng 5g to ♂
Unspecified disorder of biliary tract 576.9/K839 with jaundice D007565:	
Jiāwèixiāoyáosǎn 5g xiāngshāliùjūnzǐtāng 5g bànxiàxièxīntāng 2g shānzhā 1g héhuānpí 1g to ♀	Jiāwèixiāoyáosǎn 5g xiāngshāliùjūnzǐtāng 5g bànxiàxièxīntāng 2g shānzhā 1g héhuānpí 1g to ♂
Unspecified disorder of gallbladder 575.9/K829 with jaundice D007565:	
Dàcháihútāng 5g jīnqiáncǎo 1g jīnèijīn 1g yùjīn 1g to ♀	Lóngdǎnxiègāntāng 5g jiāwèixiāoyáosǎn 3g wèilíngtāng 3g dānshēn 1g bǎnlángēn 1g yīnchén 1g huángshuǐqié 1g to ♂
Cardiovascular disease, unspecified 429.2/I2510 with jaundice D007565:	
Yùzhú 5g sìnìtāng 5g mǔdānpí 1g zhīzǐ 1g huánglián 0g to ♀	Sìnìtāng 5g gānlùyǐn 5g lóngdǎnxiègāntāng 5g to ♂

Cháihúshūgāntāng, Lóngdǎnxiègāntāng and Jiāwèixiāoyáosǎn are all used today to treat chronic hepatitis (Wang, 2019). Xiǎocháihútāng is used for obstructive jaundice as we see below.

7.6. Obstructive Jaundice

The liver produces bile, which contains bilirubin, and drains bile into the small intestine. If the drainage is obstructed by e.g., gallstones, bilirubin builds up in the liver and spills over to the blood stream, causing obstructive jaundice. Obstruction can also be caused by bile duct cancer and pancreatic cancer.

Table 7.6. Herbal prescriptions for obstructive jaundice

Obstructive Jaundice: https://meshb.nlm.nih.gov/record/ui?ui=D041781.	
Common prescriptions:	
Xiǎocháihútāng 5g píngwèisǎn 5g Xiǎocháihútāng 5g píngwèisǎn 5g xiāngshāliùjūnzǐtāng 5g Xiǎocháihútāng 5g píngwèisǎn 5g mùxiāng 1g yánhúsuǒ 1g shārén 1g Xiǎocháihútāng 5g píngwèisǎn 5g mùxiāng 1g yánhúsuǒ 1g shārén 1g xiāngfù 1g	
Alternative prescriptions:	
Xiǎocháihútāng 5g píngwèisǎn 5g shānzhā 1g shénqū 1g màiyá 1g jīnèijīn 1g Xiǎocháihútāng 5g píngwèisǎn 2g mùxiāng 0g huánglián 0g Xiǎocháihútāng 5g píngwèisǎn 5g shānzhā 1g shénqū 1g màiyá 1g + acupuncture Xiǎocháihútāng 5g sháoyàogāncǎotāng 2g yánhúsuǒ 1g jīnèijīn 1g	
Indicated diseases:	
Unspecified disorder of biliary tract 576.9 (Disease of biliary tract, unspecified K839); Diseases of the jaws 526; Diseases of the oral soft tissues, excluding lesions specific for gingiva and tongue 528; Unspecified disorder of gallbladder 575.9 (Disease of gallbladder, unspecified K829); Unspecified endocrine disorder 259.9 (Endocrine disorder, unspecified E349); Malignant neoplasm of gallbladder 156.0 (Malignant neoplasm of gallbladder C23); Malignant neoplasm of extrahepatic bile ducts 156.1 (Malignant neoplasm of extrahepatic bile duct C240); Malignant neoplasm of biliary tract, part unspecified site 156.9 (Malignant neoplasm of biliary tract, unspecified C249)	
Unspecified disorder of biliary tract 576.9/K839 with jaundice, obstructive D041781:	
Xiǎocháihútāng 5g báisháo 1g guìzhī 1g to ♀	Dàcháihútāng 5g jīnqiáncǎo 1g jīnèijīn 1g yùjīn 1g to ♂
Unspecified disorder of gallbladder 575.9/K829 with jaundice, obstructive D041781:	
Dàcháihútāng 5g shānzhīzǐ 1g jīnqiáncǎo 1g yīnchén 1g to ♀	Dàcháihútāng 5g shānzhīzǐ 1g jīnqiáncǎo 1g yīnchén 1g to ♂

Both Xiǎocháihútāng and Dàcháihútāng are also used for chronic hepatitis (Wang, 2019). However, according to traditional Chinese medical texts, Dàcháihútāng is used after Xiǎocháihútāng fails to contain the illness.

7.7. Purpura

Purpura is purplish-reddish dots or patches of the skin or mucous membranes resulting from pooling of blood leaked from burst small blood vessels under the affected tissues. They usually are within 1 centimeter in size. Problems with platelet, coagulation and micro-vasculature can all cause purpura.

Table 7.7. Herbal prescriptions for purpura

Purpura: https://meshb.nlm.nih.gov/record/ui?ui=D011693.	
Common prescriptions:	
Xiāofēngsǎn 5g jīngfángbàidúsǎn 5g Xiāofēngsǎn 5g huángliánjiědútāng 5g Xiāofēngsǎn 5g jīngfángbàidúsǎn 5g báixiānpí 1g dìfūzǐ 1g	
Alternative prescriptions:	
Xiāofēngsǎn 5g báixiānpí 0g dìfūzǐ 0g Xiāofēngsǎn 5g báixiānpí 1g dìfūzǐ 1g shéchuángzǐ 1g Xiāofēngsǎn 5g jīngfángbàidúsǎn 5g yínqiàosǎn 5g Xiāofēngsǎn 5g jīngfángbàidúsǎn 5g yínqiàosǎn 5g lóngdǎnxiègāntāng 5g Xiāofēngsǎn 5g huángliánjiědútāng 4g báixiānpí 1g dìfūzǐ 1g	
Indicated diseases:	
Cardiovascular disease, unspecified 429.2 (Atherosclerotic heart disease of native coronary artery without angina pectoris I2510); Other dermatoses 702; Unspecified hemorrhagic conditions 287.9 (Hemorrhagic condition, unspecified D699); Coagulation defects 286; Unspecified diseases of blood and blood-forming organs 289.9 (Disease of blood and blood-forming organs, unspecified D759); Ehlers-Danlos syndrome 756.83 (Ehlers-Danlos syndrome Q796); Multiple myeloma 203.0; Vascular disorders of skin 709.1 (Vasculitis limited to the skin, unspecified L959); Eosinophilia 288.3 (Eosinophilia D721); Diseases of white blood cells 288	
Cardiovascular disease, unspecified 429.2/I2510 with purpura D011693:	
Yùzhú 5g sìnìtāng 5g mǔdānpí 1g zhīzǐ 1g huánglián 0g to ♀	Yùzhú 5g sìnìtāng 5g mǔdānpí 1g zhīzǐ 1g huánglián 1g to ♂

Xiāofēngsǎn 'nourishes Blood, expels Wind' and 'clears Heat, drains Dampness.' Jīngfángbàidúsǎn 'excretes sweat, resolves exterior' and 'disperses Wind, expels Dampness.' Their present-day uses include contact dermatitis and other eczema (Wang, 2019).

7.8. Purpura Fulminans

Purpura fulminans is sudden and severe purpura that can lead to death of skin cells. Common causes of purpura fulminans are bacterial infections such as meningococcal meningitis.

Both Xiāofēngsǎn and Jīngfángbàidúsǎn have traditionally been used for Dampness due to acute infections.

Table 7.8. Herbal prescriptions for purpura fulminans

Purpura Fulminans: https://meshb.nlm.nih.gov/record/ui?ui=D055665.	
Common prescriptions:	
Xiāofēngsǎn 5g jīngfángbàidúsǎn 5g Xiāofēngsǎn 5g jīngfángbàidúsǎn 5g báixiānpí 1g dìfūzǐ 1g Yùnǚjiān 5g xiāofēngsǎn 5g jīngfángbàidúsǎn 5g	
Alternative prescriptions:	
Xiāofēngsǎn 5g tǔfúlíng 1g jīnyínhuā 1g dǎodìwúgōng 1g liánqiáo 1g Xiāofēngsǎn 5g jīngfángbàidúsǎn 5g yínqiàosǎn 5g Xiāofēngsǎn 5g jiědúsìwùtāng 5g Yùnǚjiān 5g xiāofēngsǎn 5g dāngguīyǐnzǐ 5g báixiānpí 1g dìfūzǐ 1g yìyǐrén 1g Xiāofēngsǎn 5g huángliánjiědútāng 2g báixiānpí 1g dìfūzǐ 1g shéchuángzǐ 1g	
Indicated diseases:	
Unspecified cerebrovascular disease 437.9 (Cerebrovascular disease, unspecified I679); Unspecified condition of brain 348.9 (Disorder of brain, unspecified G939); Coagulation defects 286; Cardiovascular disease, unspecified 429.2 (Atherosclerotic heart disease of native coronary artery without angina pectoris I2510); Unspecified disorders of nervous system 349.9 (Disorder of central nervous system, unspecified G969); Unspecified diseases of blood and blood-forming organs 289.9 (Disease of blood and blood-forming organs, unspecified D759); Bacterial meningitis 320; Meningococcal meningitis 036.0 (Meningococcal meningitis A390); Meningitis, unspecified 322.9 (Meningitis, unspecified G039); Other dermatoses 702; Rash and other nonspecific skin eruption 782.1 (Rash and other nonspecific skin eruption R21)	
Unspecified cerebrovascular disease 437.9/I679 with purpura fulminans D055665:	
Bǔyánghuánwǔtāng 5g dānshēn 1g shíchāngpú 1g yuǎnzhì 1g + acupuncture to ♀	Bǔyánghuánwǔtāng 5g dānshēn 1g shíchāngpú 1g yuǎnzhì 1g + acupuncture to ♂
Bacterial meningitis 320 with purpura fulminans D055665:	
Huángqíwǔwùtāng 5g dāngguīsìnìtāng 5g dānshēn 1g zhúrú 1g sāngzhī 1g jiānghuáng 1g to ♀	Shūjīnghuóxuètāng 5g dāngguīniāntòngtāng 5g dúhuójìshēngtāng 5g + acupuncture to ♂
Other dermatoses 702 with purpura fulminans D055665:	
Yùnǚjiān 5g xuèfǔzhúyūtāng 3g dāngguīsháoyàosǎn 3g báijiāngcán 1g to ♀	Xiāofēngsǎn 5g bàidúsǎn 5g zhēnrénhuómìngyǐnqùchuānshānjiǎ 4g huángliánjiědútāng 4g to ♂

7.9. Idiopathic Thrombocytopenic Purpura

Idiopathic thrombocytopenic purpura is purpura due to low counts of thrombocytes, also called platelets, which clot broken vessels in order to stop bleeding. Although the cause of idiopathic thrombocytopenic purpura is unknown, viral infection or allergy produced antibodies that cross react with platelets are suspected.

Table 7.9. Herbal prescriptions for idiopathic thrombocytopenic purpura

Idiopathic Thrombocytopenic Purpura: https://meshb.nlm.nih.gov/record/ui?ui=D016553.
Common prescriptions:
Xiāofēngsǎn 5g jīngfángbàidúsǎn 5g Xiāofēngsǎn 5g huángqín 1g tiānhuā 1g xìxīn 0g Xiāofēngsǎn 5g huángqín 1g tiānhuā 1g xìxīn 1g Xiāofēngsǎn 5g huángqín 1g tiānhuā 1g xìxīn 1g dàhuáng 0g
Alternative prescriptions:
Xiāofēngsǎn 5g huángqín 2g tiānhuā 1g xìxīn 1g dàhuáng 0g Xiāofēngsǎn 5g huángqín 1g tiānhuā 1g xìxīn 0g dàhuáng 0g Xiāofēngsǎn 5g huángqín 1g Xiāofēngsǎn 5g huángqín 1g tiānhuā 1g Xiāofēngsǎn 5g jīngfángbàidúsǎn 5g báixiānpí 1g dìfūzǐ 1g

Idiopathic Thrombocytopenic Purpura: https://meshb.nlm.nih.gov/record/ui?ui=D016553.	
Indicated and associated diseases:	
Heart disease, unspecified 429.9 (Heart disease, unspecified I519); Digeorge's syndrome 279.11 (Di George's syndrome D821); Velo-cardio-facial syndrome 758.32 (Velo-cardio-facial syndrome Q9381); Immune thrombocytopenic purpura 287.31 (Immune thrombocytopenic purpura D693); Cardiovascular disease, unspecified 429.2 (Atherosclerotic heart disease of native coronary artery without angina pectoris I2510); Hypoparathyroidism 252.1 (Hypoparathyroidism, unspecified E209); Unspecified disorder of parathyroid gland 252.9 (Disorder of parathyroid gland, unspecified E215); Unspecified endocrine disorder 259.9 (Endocrine disorder, unspecified E349); Unspecified congenital anomaly of heart 746.9 (Congenital malformation of cardiac chambers and connections, unspecified Q209, Congenital malformation of heart, unspecified Q249); Thrombocytopenia, unspecified 287.5 (Thrombocytopenia, unspecified D696); Unspecified hemorrhagic conditions 287.9 (Hemorrhagic condition, unspecified D699); Coagulation defects 286; Unspecified diseases of blood and blood-forming organs 289.9 (Disease of blood and blood-forming organs, unspecified D759); Multiple myeloma 203.0; Common variable immunodeficiency 279.06 (Common variable immunodeficiency with predominant immunoregulatory T-cell disorders D831)	
Heart disease, unspecified 429.9/I519 with purpura, thrombocytopenic, idiopathic D016553:	
Shēngmàiyǐn 5g xuèfǔzhúyūtāng 5g dānshēn 2g chuānqī 1g guìzhī 1g guālóurén 1g xièbái 1g to ♀	Shēngmàiyǐn 5g xuèfǔzhúyūtāng 5g dānshēn 2g chuānqī 1g guìzhī 1g guālóurén 1g xièbái 1g to ♂
Cardiovascular disease, unspecified 429.2/I2510 with purpura, thrombocytopenic, idiopathic D016553:	
Yùzhú 5g sìnìtāng 5g mǔdānpí 1g zhīzǐ 1g huánglián 0g to ♀	Sìnìtāng 5g gānlùyǐn 5g mǔdānpí 1g zhīzǐ 1g huánglián 1g to ♂
Common variable immunodeficiency 279.06/D831 with purpura, thrombocytopenic, idiopathic D016553:	
Dāngguīsìnìtāng 5g shēngjiāng 1g wúzhūyú 1g to ♀	Dāngguīsìnìtāng 5g shēngjiāng 1g wúzhūyú 1g to ♂

The modern uses of Tiānhuā and Xìxīn include allergic rhinitis, while those of Huángqín and Dàhuáng include functional digestive disorders (Wang, 2019). Idiopathic thrombocytopenic purpura was found to be associated with cardiovascular disease (Chandan et al., 2018).

7.10. Thrombotic Thrombocytopenic Purpura

Thrombotic thrombocytopenic purpura is blood clots that form in small blood vessels, resulting in purpura throughout the body. It is caused by a faulty enzyme that controls blood clotting. The enzyme does not work properly because of mutations or autoantibodies. Thrombotic thrombocytopenic purpura can therefore be inherited or acquired. The blood clots can limit blood flow to vital organs such as the brain, kidneys and heart. Thrombotic thrombocytopenic purpura is therefore life-threatening if left untreated.

Table 7.10. Herbal prescriptions for thrombotic thrombocytopenic purpura

Thrombotic Thrombocytopenic Purpura: https://meshb.nlm.nih.gov/record/ui?ui=D011697.
Common prescriptions:
Xiāofēngsǎn 5g jīngfángbàidúsǎn 5g Xiāofēngsǎn 5g báixiānpí 1g dìfūzǐ 1g shéchuángzǐ 1g Xiāofēngsǎn 5g jīngfángbàidúsǎn 5g báixiānpí 1g dìfūzǐ 1g Xiāofēngsǎn 5g jīngfángbàidúsǎn 5g lóngdǎnxiègāntāng 5g Xiāofēngsǎn 5g báixiānpí 1g dìfūzǐ 1g mǔdānpí 1g chìsháo 1g
Alternative prescriptions:
Xiāofēngsǎn 5g huángqín 2g tiānhuā 1g xìxīn 1g dàhuáng 0g Xiāofēngsǎn 5g huángqín 1g huánglián 1g dàhuáng 0g Xiāofēngsǎn 5g huángqín 2g tiānhuā 1g xìxīn 0g dàhuáng 0g Xiāofēngsǎn 5g huángqín 2g gāncǎo 1g shārén 1g dàhuáng 0g Xiāofēngsǎn 5g huángqín 1g tiānhuā 1g xìxīn 1g

Table 7.10. (Continued)

Thrombotic Thrombocytopenic Purpura: https://meshb.nlm.nih.gov/record/ui?ui=D011697.	
Indicated diseases:	
Unspecified cerebrovascular disease 437.9 (Cerebrovascular disease, unspecified I679); Unspecified condition of brain 348.9 (Disorder of brain, unspecified G939); Thrombocytopenia, unspecified 287.5 (Thrombocytopenia, unspecified D696); Cardiovascular disease, unspecified 429.2 (Atherosclerotic heart disease of native coronary artery without angina pectoris I2510); Unspecified disorders of nervous system 349.9 (Disorder of central nervous system, unspecified G969); Coagulation defects 286; Unspecified diseases of blood and blood-forming organs 289.9 (Disease of blood and blood-forming organs, unspecified D759); Renal failure, unspecified 586 (Unspecified kidney failure N19); Hemolytic-uremic syndrome 283.11 (Hemolytic-uremic syndrome D593); Anemia, unspecified 285.9 (Anemia, unspecified D649); Multiple myeloma 203.0; Unspecified hemorrhagic conditions 287.9 (Hemorrhagic condition, unspecified D699);	
Human immunodeficiency virus [HIV] disease 042 (Human immunodeficiency virus [HIV] disease B20)	
Unspecified cerebrovascular disease 437.9/I679 with purpura, thrombotic thrombocytopenic D011697:	
Bǔyánghuánwǔtāng 5g dānshēn 1g niúxī 1g sāngzhī 1g huángqín 1g jīxuèténg 1g + acupuncture to ♀	Bǔyánghuánwǔtāng 5g dānshēn 1g shíchāngpú 1g yuǎnzhì 1g + acupuncture to ♂
Renal failure, unspecified 586/N19 with purpura, thrombotic thrombocytopenic D011697:	
Wǔlíngsǎn 5g jìshēngshènqìwán 5g to ♀	Zhūlíngtāng 5g jìshēngshènqìwán 5g dānshēn 1g dōngguāzǐ 1g báimáogēn 1g zélán 1g to ♂
Cardiovascular disease, unspecified 429.2/I2510 with purpura, thrombotic thrombocytopenic D011697:	
Sìnìtāng 5g gānlùyǐn 5g mǔdānpí 1g zhīzǐ 1g huánglián 1g to ♀	Sìnìtāng 5g gānlùyǐn 5g mǔdānpí 1g zhīzǐ 1g huánglián 1g to ♂
Human immunodeficiency virus [HIV] disease 042/B20 with purpura, thrombotic thrombocytopenic D011697:	
Xiāofēngsǎn 5g jīngfángbàidúsǎn 5g to ♀	Xiāofēngsǎn 5g jīngfángbàidúsǎn 5g to ♂

The modern uses of Báixiānpí and Dìfūzǐ are contact dermatitis and other eczema, and urticaria (Wang, 2019). Shéchuángzǐ is today used for contact dermatitis and other eczema, and hemorrhoids (Wang, 2019). They are used here to support the remedy for skin lesions.

7.11. Schoenlein-Henoch Purpura

Schoenlein-Henoch purpura is characterized by purpura, arthritis and abdominal pain, due to inflammation of small blood vessels. As Schoenlein-Henoch purpura usually follows an upper respiratory tract infection, immune system dysfunction is suspected to cause it.

Table 7.11. Herbal prescriptions for Schoenlein-Henoch purpura

Schoenlein-Henoch Purpura: https://meshb.nlm.nih.gov/record/ui?ui=D011695.
Common prescriptions:
Xiāofēngsǎn 5g jīngfángbàidúsǎn 5g Xiāofēngsǎn 5g jīngfángbàidúsǎn 5g yínqiàosǎn 5g Xiāofēngsǎn 5g jīngfángbàidúsǎn 5g lóngdǎnxiègāntāng 5g Xiāofēngsǎn 5g jīngfángbàidúsǎn 5g báixiānpí 1g dìfūzǐ 1g
Alternative prescriptions:
Xiāofēngsǎn 5g huángqín 1g Xiāofēngsǎn 5g huángqín 1g tiānhuā 1g xìxīn 1g Xiāofēngsǎn 5g jīngfángbàidúsǎn 5g jīnyínhuā 1g liánqiáo 1g Xiāofēngsǎn 5g tǔfúlíng 1g báixiānpí 1g Jīngfángbàidúsǎn 5g xiāofēngsǎn 4g tǔfúlíng 1g jīnyínhuā 1g liánqiáo 1g

Schoenlein-Henoch Purpura: https://meshb.nlm.nih.gov/record/ui?ui=D011695.	
Indicated diseases:	
Cardiovascular disease, unspecified 429.2 (Atherosclerotic heart disease of native coronary artery without angina pectoris I2510); Allergic purpura 287.0 (Allergic purpura D690); Unspecified hemorrhagic conditions 287.9 (Hemorrhagic condition, unspecified D699); Coagulation defects 286; Unspecified diseases of blood and blood-forming organs 289.9 (Disease of blood and blood-forming organs, unspecified D759); Vascular disorders of skin 709.1 (Vasculitis limited to the skin, unspecified L959); Panuveitis 360.12	
(Panuveitis, unspecified eye H44119); Behcet's syndrome 136.1 (Behcet's disease M352); Other dermatoses 702; Disorder of eye, unspecified 379.90 (Unspecified disorder of eye and adnexa H579)	
Cardiovascular disease, unspecified 429.2/I2510 with purpura, Schoenlein-Henoch D011695:	
Yùzhú 5g sìnìtāng 5g mǔdānpí 1g zhīzǐ 1g huánglián 0g to ♀	Sìnìtāng 5g gānlùyǐn 5g mǔdānpí 1g zhīzǐ 1g huánglián 1g to ♂

Yínqiàosǎn is used for allergic rhinitis, unspecified chronic sinusitis, and throat pain in these days (Wang, 2019). On the other hand, Lóngdǎnxiègāntāng is nowadays used for chronic hepatitis (Wang, 2019) and is supposedly used here for the abdominal pain associated with Schoenlein-Henoch purpura.

7.12. Waterhouse-Friderichsen Syndrome

Waterhouse-Friderichsen syndrome occurs when the adrenal glands bleed, resulting in acute adrenal insufficiency. The signs and symptoms of Waterhouse-Friderichsen syndrome include fever, headache, dizziness, joint and muscle pain, weakness, vomiting, purpura, septic shock and coma. The root cause of Waterhouse-Friderichsen syndrome is severe bacterial infection.

Table 7.12. Herbal prescriptions for Waterhouse-Friderichsen syndrome

Waterhouse-Friderichsen Syndrome: https://meshb.nlm.nih.gov/record/ui?ui=D014884.	
Common prescriptions:	
Bǔzhōngyìqìtāng 5g huánshǎodān 5g Huánshǎodān 5g Liùwèidìhuángwán 5g bǔzhōngyìqìtāng 5g	
Alternative prescriptions:	
Huánshǎodān 5g yínyánghuò 1g Qībǎoměirándān 5g huánshǎodān 5g bājǐtiān 1g ròucōngróng 1g yínyánghuò 1g Bāwèidìhuángwán 5g zuǒguīwán 5g yínyánghuò 1g tùsīzǐ 1g Liùwèidìhuángwán 5g sìwùtāng 5g bǔzhōngyìqìtāng 5g Zuǒguīwán 5g bǔzhōngyìqìtāng 5g yínyánghuò 1g	
Indicated diseases:	
Bacterial meningitis 320; Unspecified disorder of adrenal glands 255.9 (Disorder of adrenal gland, unspecified E279); Meningococcal meningitis 036.0 (Meningococcal meningitis A390); Unspecified hemorrhagic conditions 287.9 (Hemorrhagic condition, unspecified D699); Meningitis, unspecified 322.9 (Meningitis, unspecified G039); Unspecified disorders of nervous system 349.9 (Disorder of central nervous system, unspecified G969); Unspecified endocrine disorder 259.9 (Endocrine disorder, unspecified E349); Coagulation defects 286; Unspecified diseases of blood and blood-forming organs 289.9 (Disease of blood and blood-forming organs, unspecified D759); Cardiovascular disease, unspecified 429.2 (Atherosclerotic heart disease of native coronary artery without angina pectoris I2510); Defibrination syndrome 286.6 (Disseminated intravascular coagulation [defibrination syndrome] D65); Toxic shock syndrome 040.82 (Toxic shock syndrome A483); Other dermatoses 702	
Bacterial meningitis 320 with Waterhouse-Friderichsen syndrome D014884:	
Jiāwèixiāoyáosǎn 5g dāngguīsháoyàosǎn 5g dùzhòng 1g xùduàn 1g to ♀	Shūjīnghuóxuètāng 5g dúhuójìshēngtāng 5g + acupuncture to ♂

Table 7.12. (Continued)

Waterhouse-Friderichsen Syndrome: https://meshb.nlm.nih.gov/record/ui?ui=D014884.	
Cardiovascular disease, unspecified 429.2/I2510 with Waterhouse-Friderichsen syndrome D014884:	
Sìnìtāng 5g gānlùyǐn 5g mǔdānpí 1g zhīzǐ 1g huánglián 0g to ♀	Xuèfǔzhúyūtāng 5g zhìgāncǎotāng 5g dānshēn 1g guālóurén 1g xièbái 1g to ♂
Other dermatoses 702 with Waterhouse-Friderichsen syndrome D014884:	
Yùnǚjiān 5g xuèfǔzhúyūtāng 3g dāngguīsháoyàosǎn 3g mǔdānpí 1g liánqiáo 1g to ♀	Yùnǚjiān 5g xuèfǔzhúyūtāng 3g dāngguīsháoyàosǎn 3g báijiāngcán 1g to ♂

Modern uses of Bǔzhōngyìqìtāng and Qībǎoměirándān include anemia (Wang, 2019) and they are supposedly used here for the bleeding. Huánshǎodān and Zuǒguīwán are today used for osteoporosis (Wang, 2019) and they are supposedly used here for the joint and muscle pain. Both Liùwèidìhuángwán and Bāwèidìhuángwán protect the kidneys as their use today is for diabetes (Wang, 2019). Yínyánghuò has traditionally been used for male impotence and indeed its main use these-days is for impotence of organic origin (Wang, 2020). As the adrenal cortex produces androgens, incorporating Yínyánghuò into the prescriptions is believed to compensate compromised adrenal glands.

7.13. Hyperglobulinemic Purpura

Hyperglobulinemic purpura is characterized by recurrent purpura on the lower extremities along with high levels of polyclonal globulins in blood circulation. Tight-fitting clothing and prolonged standing or walking can bring on hyperglobulinemic purpura. Its cause is unknown but immune system dysfunction is suspected as it is significantly associated with autoimmune diseases.

Table 7.13. Herbal prescriptions for hyperglobulinemic purpura

Hyperglobulinemic Purpura: https://meshb.nlm.nih.gov/record/ui?ui=D011694.
Common prescriptions:
Xiāofēngsǎn 5g jīngfángbàidúsǎn 5g Yùnǚjiān 5g xiāofēngsǎn 5g jīngfángbàidúsǎn 5g Yùnǚjiān 5g xiāofēngsǎn 5g Yùnǚjiān 5g xiāofēngsǎn 5g lóngdǎnxiègāntāng 5g
Alternative prescriptions:
Xiāofēngsǎn 5g jīngfángbàidúsǎn 5g báixiānpí 1g dìfūzǐ 1g jīnchán 1g Xiāofēngsǎn 5g huángliánjiědútāng 5g jīnyínhuā 1g liánqiáo 1g púgōngyīng 1g Yùnǚjiān 5g máxìnggānshítāng 4g jīnyínhuā 1g liánqiáo 1g yìyǐrén 1g Yùnǚjiān 5g jīngfángbàidúsǎn 5g huángliánjiědútāng 5g gāncǎo 1g Xiāofēngsǎn 5g tǔfúlíng 2g báixiānpí 2g dìfūzǐ 2g chántuì 2g
Indicated and associated diseases:
Cardiovascular disease, unspecified 429.2 (Atherosclerotic heart disease of native coronary artery without angina pectoris I2510); Epiphora 375.2; Sicca syndrome 710.2 (Sicca syndrome, unspecified M3500, Sicca syndrome with keratoconjunctivitis M3501); Unspecified hemorrhagic conditions 287.9 (Hemorrhagic condition, unspecified D699); Disorders of lacrimal system 375; Disorder of eye, unspecified 379.90 (Unspecified disorder of eye and adnexa H579); Unspecified disorder of joint, site unspecified 719.90 (Joint disorder, unspecified M259); Coagulation defects 286; Unspecified diseases of blood and blood-forming organs 289.9 (Disease of blood and blood-forming organs, unspecified D759); Other dermatoses 702; Multiple myeloma 203.0

Hyperglobulinemic Purpura: https://meshb.nlm.nih.gov/record/ui?ui=D011694.	
Cardiovascular disease, unspecified 429.2/I2510 with purpura, hyperglobulinemic D011694:	
Sìnìtāng 5g gānlùyǐn 5g mǔdānpí 1g zhīzǐ 1g huánglián 1g to ♀	Sìnìtāng 5g gānlùyǐn 5g mǔdānpí 1g zhīzǐ 1g huánglián 0g to ♂

Huángliánjiědútāng 'quenches Fire, neutralizes pathogens,' and is in these days used for contact dermatitis and other eczema (Wang, 2019). A case of a multiple myeloma patient who developed hyperglobulinemic purpura was reported (Shalit et al., 1980).

7.14. Café-au-Lait Spots

Café-au-lait spots are darkened, flat patches of skin in the trunk or extremities that start appearing at birth. The size of the spot varies from a few millimeters to tens of centimeters. They are benign however multiple and segmental café-au-lait spots are associated with mutations in a tumor suppressor gene on chromosome 17, predisposing one to such malignancy as leukemia.

Table 7.14. Herbal prescriptions for café-au-lait spots

Café-au-Lait Spots: https://meshb.nlm.nih.gov/record/ui?ui=D019080.	
Common prescriptions:	
Bǔzhōngyìqìtāng 5g	
Alternative prescriptions:	
Sìnìtāng 5g shēngjiāng 1g guìzhī 1g Guìzhītāng 5g huángqí 3g chuānxiōng 1g dāngguī 1g Bǔzhōngyìqìtāng 5g gǒuqǐzǐ 1g júhuā 1g Guìzhītāng 5g báisháo 1g yánhúsuǒ 1g huángqín 1g dàhuáng 0g Bǔzhōngyìqìtāng 5g fùzǐ 1g	
Indicated diseases:	
Other dermatoses 702; Myoneural disorders 358; Neurofibromatosis, type 1 [von recklinghausen's disease] 237.71 (Neurofibromatosis, type 1 Q8501); Unspecified disorders of nervous system 349.9 (Disorder of central nervous system, unspecified G969); Neurofibromatosis 237.7; Malignant neoplasm of nervous system, part unspecified 192.9 (Malignant neoplasm of central nervous system, unspecified C729); Unspecified condition of brain 348.9 (Disorder of brain, unspecified G939); Neoplasm of unspecified nature of brain 239.6 (Neoplasm of unspecified behavior of brain D496)	
Other dermatoses 702 with café-au-lait spots D019080:	
Dāngguīsìnìtāng 5g shēngjiāng 1g wúzhūyú 1g to ♀	Zhēnrénhuómìngyǐn 5g huángliánjiědútāng 5g to ♂
Myoneural disorders 358 with café-au-lait spots D019080:	
Huángqíwǔwùtāng 5g dāngguīsìnìtāng 5g dānshēn 1g zhúrú 1g sāngzhī 1g jiānghuáng 1g + acupuncture to ♀	Huángqíwǔwùtāng 5g dāngguīsìnìtāng 5g dānshēn 1g zhúrú 1g sāngzhī 1g jiānghuáng 1g to ♂

Bǔzhōngyìqìtāng is today used for chronic bronchitis and anemia; Guìzhītāng for allergic rhinitis; and Sìnìtāng for chronic hepatitis and chronic bronchitis (Wang, 2019). They are thought to antagonize the various symptoms of leukemia.

7.15. Pruritus

Pruritus is itchy skin. Causes of localized and generalized itching include allergies, dry skin, insect bites, infection, neuropathy, renal failure, liver disease, anemia and diabetes.

Qīngshàngfángfēngtāng 'quenches Fire in the upper body,' and has traditionally been used for 'Wind-Heat pathogens,' and furuncles and carbuncles on the face and scalp. It is nowadays used for acne varioliformis, and contact dermatitis and other eczema (Wang, 2019).

Table 7.15. Herbal prescriptions for pruritus

Pruritus: https://meshb.nlm.nih.gov/record/ui?ui=D011537.	
Common prescriptions:	
Qīngshàngfángfēngtāng 5g huángliánjiědútāng 5g jīnyínhuā 1g liánqiáo 1g Qīngshàngfángfēngtāng 5g huángliánjiědútāng 5g jīnyínhuā 1g liánqiáo 1g púgōngyīng 1g Qīngshàngfángfēngtāng 5g huángliánjiědútāng 5g Qīngshàngfángfēngtāng 5g huángliánjiědútāng 5g jīnyínhuā 1g liánqiáo 1g zǐhuādìdīng 1g púgōngyīng 1g	
Alternative prescriptions:	
Qīngshàngfángfēngtāng 5g jīnyínhuā 0g zǐhuādìdīng 0g púgōngyīng 0g Qīngshàngfángfēngtāng 5g huángliánjiědútāng 3g jīnyínhuā 1g zǐhuādìdīng 1g púgōngyīng 1g Qīngshàngfángfēngtāng 5g jīnyínhuā 1g liánqiáo 1g púgōngyīng 1g Qīngshàngfángfēngtāng 5g jīnyínhuā 1g Qīngshàngfángfēngtāng 5g zhēnrénhuómìngyǐn 2g liánqiáo 1g zǐhuādìdīng 1g púgōngyīng 1g gāncǎo 0g	
Indicated diseases:	
Obstruction of bile duct 576.2 (Obstruction of bile duct K831); Other dermatoses 702; Unspecified disorder of biliary tract 576.9 (Disease of biliary tract, unspecified K839); Cardiovascular disease, unspecified 429.2 (Atherosclerotic heart disease of native coronary artery without angina pectoris I2510); Multiple myeloma 203.0; Unspecified hemorrhagic conditions 287.9 (Hemorrhagic condition, unspecified D699); Unspecified diseases of blood and blood-forming organs 289.9 (Disease of blood and blood-forming organs, unspecified D759); Unspecified disorder of metabolism 277.9 (Metabolic disorder, unspecified E889); Amyloidosis 277.3	
Obstruction of bile duct 576.2/K831 with pruritus D011537:	
Xiǎocháihútāng 5g jīnyínhuā 1g liánqiáo 1g to ♀	Xiǎocháihútāng 5g lóngdǎnxiègāntāng 5g to ♂
Cardiovascular disease, unspecified 429.2/I2510 with pruritus D011537:	
Sìnìtāng 5g gānlùyǐn 5g mǔdānpí 1g zhīzǐ 1g huánglián 0g to ♀	Sìnìtāng 5g gānlùyǐn 5g lóngdǎnxiègāntāng 5g to ♂
Other dermatoses 702 with pruritus D011537:	
Qīngshàngfángfēngtāng 5g jīnyínhuā 1g liánqiáo 1g to ♀	Xiāofēngsǎn 5g zhēnrénhuómìngyǐnqùchuānshānjiǎ 5g bàidúsǎn 5g huángliánjiědútāng 4g to ♂

7.16. Pruritus Vulvae

Pruritus vulvae are itchiness of the vulval skin. Fungal infections, inflammation, vaginal sweat, menopause, urinary incontinence, diabetes, and stress can cause an itchy vulva.

Guìzhītāng is today used for allergic rhinitis (Wang, 2019). It is used here for pruritus vulvae presumably because it is anti-inflammatory.

Table 7.16. Herbal prescriptions for pruritus vulvae

Pruritus Vulvae: https://meshb.nlm.nih.gov/record/ui?ui=D011539.
Common prescriptions:
Guìzhītāng 5g shēngjiāng 1g báisháo 1g dàhuáng 0g Guìzhītāng 5g shēngjiāng 1g guìzhī 1g Guìzhītāng 5g shēngjiāng 1g guìzhī 1g dàhuáng 0g Guìzhītāng 5g shēngjiāng 1g báisháo 1g Guìzhītāng 5g shēngjiāng 1g báisháo 1g guìzhī 1g
Alternative prescriptions:
Guìzhītāng 5g shēngjiāng 0g guìzhī 0g Sháoyàogāncǎotāng 5g tiānhuā 0g xuánshēn 0g mǔlì 0g màiméndōng 0g fùzǐ 0g Guìzhītāng 5g gégēn 3g bànxià 1g dàhuáng 0g Guìzhītāng 5g bànxià 1g
Indicated diseases:
Other dermatoses 702; Vaginitis and vulvovaginitis 616.1; Candidiasis of vulva and vagina 112.1 (Candidiasis of vulva and vagina B373); Unspecified disorder of female genital organs 629.9 (Unspecified condition associated with female genital organs and menstrual cycle N949); Candidiasis 112; Coccidioidomycosis 114; Histoplasmosis 115; Blastomycotic infection 116; Other mycoses 117; Opportunistic mycoses 118 (Other specified mycoses B488); Dermatophytosis 110; Dermatomycosis, other and unspecified 111; Human immunodeficiency virus [HIV] disease 042 (Human immunodeficiency virus [HIV] disease B20); Unspecified disorder of sweat glands 705.9 (Eccrine sweat disorder, unspecified L749, Apocrine sweat disorder, unspecified L759)
Other dermatoses 702 with pruritus vulvae D011539:
Yùnǚjiān 5g xuèfǔzhúyūtāng 3g dāngguīsháoyàosǎn 3g báijiāngcán 1g to ♀
Vaginitis and vulvovaginitis 616.1 with pruritus vulvae D011539:
Wándàitāng 5g tǔfúlíng 1g báixiānpí 1g dìfūzǐ 1g shéchuángzǐ 1g to ♀
Unspecified disorder of sweat glands 705.9/L749,L759 with pruritus vulvae D011539:
Yùpíngfēngsǎn 5g bǔzhōngyìqìtāng 5g to ♀

7.17. Pruritus Ani

Pruritus ani is itchiness of the perianal skin. Causes of anal itchiness include fungal infection, anal sweat, fecal incontinence, diarrhea, hemorrhoids, and diabetes.

Table 7.17. Herbal prescriptions for pruritus ani

Pruritus Ani: https://meshb.nlm.nih.gov/record/ui?ui=D011538.
Common prescriptions:
Yǐzìtāng 5g huáihuāsǎn 5g Yǐzìtāng 5g huángliánjiědútāng 5g huáihuāsǎn 5g Yǐzìtāng 5g huáihuāsǎn 5g xiānhècǎo 1g báimáogēn 1g ǒujiē 1g Yǐzìtāng 5g huáihuāsǎn 5g xiānhècǎo 1g báimáogēn 1g Yǐzìtāng 5g huáihuāsǎn 5g xiānhècǎo 1g dìyú 1g
Alternative prescriptions:
Huáihuāsǎn 5g xiānhècǎo 1g Yǐzìtāng 5g huáihuāsǎn 5g lóngdǎnxiègāntāng 5g xiānhècǎo 1g báimáogēn 1g Huáihuāsǎn 5g xiānhècǎo 1g báimáogēn 1g dìyú 1g ǒujiē 1g
Indicated diseases:
Other dermatoses 702; Dermatomycosis, unspecified 111.9 (Superficial mycosis, unspecified B369); Candidiasis 112; Coccidioidomycosis 114; Histoplasmosis 115; Blastomycotic infection 116; Other mycoses 117; Opportunistic mycoses 118 (Other specified mycoses B488); Dermatophytosis 110; Dermatomycosis, other and unspecified 111; Human immunodeficiency virus [HIV] disease 042 (Human immunodeficiency virus [HIV] disease B20); Hemorrhoids 455; Unspecified disorder of intestine 569.9 (Disease of intestine, unspecified K639)

Table 7.17. (Continued)

Pruritus Ani: https://meshb.nlm.nih.gov/record/ui?ui=D011538.	
Other dermatoses 702 with pruritus ani D011538:	
Huángliánjiědútāng 5g zhúyèshígāotāng 3g fángjǐhuángqítāng 2g fángfēngtōngshèngsǎn 2g xiàkūcǎo 2g máhuáng 2g shānzhā 1g hónghuā 1g héyè 1g chénpí 1g huánglián 1g huáshí 1g to ♀	Huángliánjiědútāng 5g zhúyèshígāotāng 3g fángjǐhuángqítāng 2g fángfēngtōngshèngsǎn 2g xiàkūcǎo 2g máhuáng 2g shānzhā 1g hónghuā 1g héyè 1g chénpí 1g huánglián 1g huáshí 1g to ♂
Hemorrhoids 455 with pruritus ani D011538:	
Yǐzìtāng 5g huáihuāsǎn 5g to ♀	Yǐzìtāng 5g huángliánjiědútāng 5g huáihuāsǎn 5g to ♂

Yǐzìtāng has traditionally been used for problems with the anus. Indeed, its modern uses are for unspecified hemorrhoids, and internal hemorrhoids (Wang, 2019).

7.18. Tinea Pedis

Tinea pedis, or athlete's foot, is dermatophyte infection of the foot. The fungal infection usually starts between the toes and can spread to the nails and sole. The signs and symptoms are itching, burning, scaling and cracking of the affected skin. People with diabetes mellitus and weakened immunity who easily sweat are susceptible to athlete's foot.

Table 7.18. Herbal prescriptions for tinea pedis

Tinea Pedis: https://meshb.nlm.nih.gov/record/ui?ui=D014008.	
Common prescriptions:	
Bǔzhōngyìqìtāng 5g + acupuncture Bǔzhōngyìqìtāng 5g	
Alternative prescriptions:	
Bǔzhōngyìqìtāng 5g xiǎoqīnglóngtāng 4g Bǔzhōngyìqìtāng 5g xìngrén 1g jiégěng 1g Xiǎoqīnglóngtāng 5g bǔzhōngyìqìtāng 5g	
Indicated diseases:	
Other dermatoses 702; Dermatophytosis of foot 110.4 (tinea pedis B353); Dermatomycosis, unspecified 111.9 (Superficial mycosis, unspecified B369); Candidiasis 112; Coccidioidomycosis 114; Histoplasmosis 115; Blastomycotic infection 116; Other mycoses 117; Opportunistic mycoses 118 (Other specified mycoses B488); Dermatophytosis 110; Dermatomycosis, other and unspecified 111; Cardiovascular disease, unspecified 429.2 (Atherosclerotic heart disease of native coronary artery without angina pectoris I2510); Pityriasis versicolor 111.0 (Pityriasis versicolor B360); Diseases of nail 703	
Other dermatoses 702 with tinea pedis D014008:	
Xiāofēngsǎn 5g zhēnrénhuómìngyǐnqùchuānshānjiǎ 5g báixiānpí 1g yúxīngcǎo 1g to ♀	Xiāofēngsǎn 5g zhēnrénhuómìngyǐnqùchuānshānjiǎ 5g báixiānpí 1g yúxīngcǎo 1g to ♂
Cardiovascular disease, unspecified 429.2/I2510 with tinea pedis D014008:	
Sìnìtāng 5g gānlùyǐn 5g mǔdānpí 1g zhīzǐ 1g huánglián 0g to ♀	Sìnìtāng 5g gānlùyǐn 5g mǔdānpí 1g zhīzǐ 1g huánglián 1g to ♂
Diseases of nail 703 with tinea pedis D014008:	
Dāngguīsìnìtāng 5g wúzhūyú 1g fùzǐ 1g gānjiāng 1g to ♀	Dāngguīsìnìtāng 5g wúzhūyú 1g fùzǐ 1g gānjiāng 1g to ♂

Xiǎoqīnglóngtāng is thought to improve the immunity as its modern uses are for such respiratory tract infections as rhinitis, sinusitis and bronchitis (Wang, 2019). Zhēnrénhuómìngyǐnqùchuānshānjiǎ has traditionally been used for swelling and ulcer on the body surface. Its current uses are for dermatitis, eczema and internal hemorrhoids (Wang, 2019). Cardiovascular disease is associated with tinea pedis (Ogasawara, 2003).

7.19. Striae Distensae

Striae distensae, or stretch marks, are hypopigmented linear scarring of the skin, caused by tearing of the skin when the part of the body beneath the skin grows rapidly. Examples of rapid weight gain periods include puberty, pregnancy and body building by weightlifting. Stretch marks therefore commonly appear in breasts, hips, buttocks, navel, abdomen, thighs and upper arms. Although stretch marks are not harmful, they inflict psychological distress to the bearer.

Sháoyàogāncǎotāng, Shūjīnghuóxuètāng or Dāngguīniāntòngtāng help blood circulation and therefore are believed to relieve tearing and atrophy of the affected connective tissues.

Table 7.19. Herbal prescriptions for striae distensae

<table>
<tr><td colspan="2">Striae Distensae: https://meshb.nlm.nih.gov/record/ui?ui=D057896.</td></tr>
<tr><td colspan="2">Common prescriptions:</td></tr>
<tr><td colspan="2">Sháoyàogāncǎotāng 5g shūjīnghuóxuètāng 5g dāngguīniāntòngtāng 5g + acupuncture
Sháoyàogāncǎotāng 5g shūjīnghuóxuètāng 5g + acupuncture</td></tr>
<tr><td colspan="2">Alternative prescriptions:</td></tr>
<tr><td colspan="2">Shūjīnghuóxuètāng 5g dāngguīniāntòngtāng 5g sháoyàogāncǎotāng 2g + acupuncture
Shūjīnghuóxuètāng 5g sháoyàogāncǎotāng 4g yánhúsuǒ 2g mòyào 1g rǔxiāng 1g + acupuncture
Shūjīnghuóxuètāng 5g dāngguīniāntòngtāng 5g sháoyàogāncǎotāng 3g + acupuncture
Sháoyàogāncǎotāng 5g guìzhīfúlíngwán 5g chuānqī 2g dìlóng 2g biējiǎ 2g dānshēn 2g
Shēntòngzhúyūtāng 5g dāngguīniāntòngtāng 5g niúxī 1g huángbò 1g cāngzhú 1g + acupuncture</td></tr>
<tr><td colspan="2">Indicated and associated diseases:</td></tr>
<tr><td colspan="2">Unspecified condition of brain 348.9 (Disorder of brain, unspecified G939); Unspecified disorder of metabolism 277.9 (Metabolic disorder, unspecified E889); Alexia 315.01 (Dyslexia and alexia R480); Unspecified disorders of nervous system 349.9 (Disorder of central nervous system, unspecified G969)</td></tr>
<tr><td colspan="2">Unspecified condition of brain 348.9/G939 with striae distensae D057896:</td></tr>
<tr><td>Bǔyánghuánwǔtāng 5g + acupuncture to ♀</td><td>Bǔyánghuánwǔtāng 5g dānshēn 1g tiānmá 1g shíchāngpú 1g yuǎnzhì 1g + acupuncture to ♂</td></tr>
</table>

7.20. Necrolytic Migratory Erythema

Necrolytic migratory erythema is an irregularly shaped skin rash that blisters, heals with hyperpigmentation, and migrates. Causes of necrolytic migratory erythema are unknown but it is strongly associated with alpha-cell tumor of the pancreatic islets, liver disease and intestinal malabsorption.

Table 7.20. Herbal prescriptions for necrolytic migratory erythema

Necrolytic Migratory Erythema: https://meshb.nlm.nih.gov/record/ui?ui=D058568.	
Common prescriptions:	
Sháoyàogāncǎotāng 5g shūjīnghuóxuètāng 5g dāngguīniāntòngtāng 5g + acupuncture Sháoyàogāncǎotāng 5g shūjīnghuóxuètāng 5g + acupuncture	
Alternative prescriptions:	
Jiāwèixiāoyáosǎn 5g xiāngshāliùjūnzǐtāng 4g bànxiàxièxīntāng 2g héhuānpí 1g yánhúsuǒ 1g Sháoyàogāncǎotāng 5g shūjīnghuóxuètāng 5g dāngguīniāntòngtāng 5g Sháoyàogāncǎotāng 5g shūjīnghuóxuètāng 5g Sháoyàogāncǎotāng 5g shūjīnghuóxuètāng 4g niúxī 1g yánhúsuǒ 1g + acupuncture Sháoyàogāncǎotāng 5g gégēntāng 5g yánhúsuǒ 2g	
Indicated diseases:	
Unspecified condition of brain 348.9 (Disorder of brain, unspecified G939); Unspecified disorders of nervous system 349.9 (Disorder of central nervous system, unspecified G969); Unspecified disorder of metabolism 277.9 (Metabolic disorder, unspecified E889)	
Unspecified condition of brain 348.9/G939 with necrolytic migratory erythema D058568:	
Bǔyánghuánwǔtāng 5g + acupuncture to ♀	Bǔyánghuánwǔtāng 5g shíchāngpú 1g yuǎnzhì 1g + acupuncture to ♂
Unspecified disorder of metabolism 277.9/E889 with necrolytic migratory erythema D058568:	
Rénshēnbàidúsǎn 5g xiǎocháihútāngqùrénshēn 5g yīnchénhāotāng 2g mùxiāng 1g yùjīn 1g to ♀	Dānshēn 5g tiānmágōuténgyǐn 5g sǎnzhǒngkuìjiāntāng 5g bǔyánghuánwǔtāng 5g to ♂

Jiāwèixiāoyáosǎn treats chronic hepatitis; Xiāngshāliùjūnzǐtāng dyspepsia and other specified disorders of function of stomach; and Bànxiàxièxīntāng functional disorder of stomach and gastritis and gastroduodenitis (Wang, 2019). We therefore see that the prescription targets the conditions that are associated with necrolytic migratory erythema. Note that high levels of glucagon in the blood from pancreatic tumor can impact the central nervous system (Khandekar et al., 1979).

References

Chandan, J. S., Thomas, T., Lee, S., Marshall, T., Willis, B., Nirantharakumar, K., & Gill, P. (2018). The association between idiopathic thrombocytopenic purpura and cardiovascular disease: a retrospective cohort study. *Journal of Thrombosis and Haemostasis*, *16*(3), 474–480. https://doi.org/10.1111/jth.13940.

Khandekar, J. D., Oyer, D., Miller, H. J., & Vick, N. A. (1979). Neurologic involvement in glucagonoma syndrome: Response to combination chemotherapy with 5-fluorouracil and streptozotocin. *Cancer*, *44*(6), 2014–2016. PMID: 228832.

Ogasawara, Y. (2003). Prevalence and patient's consciousness of tinea pedis and onychomycosis. *Nihon Ishinkin Gakkai Zasshi*, *44*(4), 253–260. https://doi.org/10.33 14/jjmm.44.253.

Shalit, M., Bar-Sela, S., Leviatan, A., & Naparstek, Y. (1980). Hyperglobulinemic Purpura in the Course of Multiple Myeloma. *Acta Haematologica*, *64*(6), 331–334. https://doi.org/10.1159/000207313.

Wang, S. C. (2019). *Clinical Herbal Prescriptions: Principles and Practices of Herbal Formulations from Deep Learning Health Insurance Herbal Prescription Big Data*. WSPC. https://doi.org/10.1142/11211.

Wang, S. C. (2020). *Veterinary Herbal Pharmacopoeia*. Nova Science Publishers. https://doi.org/10.52305/GHTR1903.

Wu, S., Xu, Z., & Liang, H. (2014). Sneddon's syndrome: a comprehensive review of the literature. *Orphanet Journal of Rare Diseases*, *9*, 215. https://doi.org/10.1186/s13023-014-0215-4.

Chapter 8

Hemorrhage

A hemorrhage is the escape of blood from the circulation system through damaged blood vessels. As a pathological process, hemorrhage involves abnormal mechanisms or forms of dysfunctional tissues or organs. Abnormalities such as the rupture of weakened blood vessel wall, where the blood vessel has bulged out due to high blood pressure, and deficiencies of coagulation factors due to gene mutations that thicken blood to cease blood flow are examples of such conditions. Figure 8.1 lists other examples, among which purpuras are discussed in the previous chapter. Note that traumatic injuries such as a cut or contusion over the skin can also cause bleeding. Ideally, the treatment for hemorrhage should not only stop the bleeding but also target the underlying cause, such as high blood pressure or blood vessel inflammation.

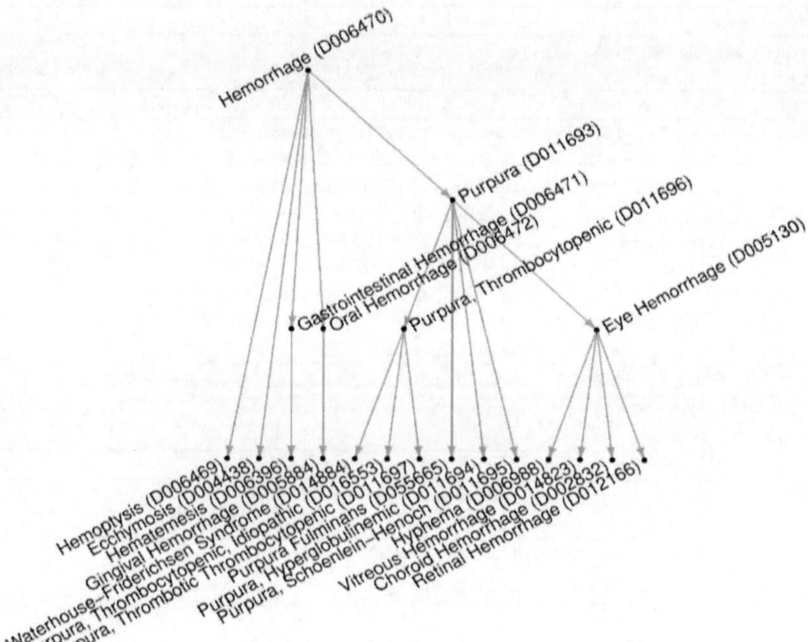

Figure 8.1. Leakage of blood out of blood vessels to the respiratory tract, skin, digestive tract, mouth and eye.

The herbal formulas frequently prescribed for the hemorrhagic signs and symptoms in Figure 8.1 are Xiāofēngsǎn, Yùnǚjiān, Qǐjúdìhuángwán, Xǐgānmíngmùtāng, Zīshènmíngmùtāng, Jīngfángbàidúsǎn, Qīngwèisǎn, and Gégēnhuángqínhuángliántāng, while the supportive single herbs are Dàhuáng, Bànxià, Liánqiáo, Báixiānpí, Huángqín, Dìfūzǐ, Tiānhuā, Mùzéicǎo, Tǔfúlíng, and Jīnyínhuā.

The disease diagnoses that most likely cause or accompany hemorrhage are unspecified diseases of blood and blood-forming organs, unspecified cardiovascular disease, coagulation defects, unspecified hemorrhagic conditions, unspecified disorder of eye, unspecified endocrine disorder, and unspecified retinal disorder.

8.1. Oral Hemorrhage

Oral hemorrhage is bleeding from the blood vessels in the mouth. Causes of oral hemorrhage include oral surgery, anticoagulant medication, infection, tumor, and trauma to the mouth.

Table 8.1. Herbal prescriptions for oral hemorrhage

<table>
<tr><td colspan="2">Oral Hemorrhage: https://meshb.nlm.nih.gov/record/ui?ui=D006472.</td></tr>
<tr><td colspan="2">Common prescriptions:</td></tr>
<tr><td colspan="2">Yùnǚjiān 5g qīngwèisǎn 5g
Yùnǚjiān 5g gānlùyǐn 5g qīngwèisǎn 5g
Yùnǚjiān 5g zhībódìhuángwán 5g qīngwèisǎn 5g
Yùnǚjiān 5g qīngwèisǎn 3g</td></tr>
<tr><td colspan="2">Alternative prescriptions:</td></tr>
<tr><td colspan="2">Yùnǚjiān 5g qīngwèisǎn 4g liánggésǎn 2g
Yùnǚjiān 5g gānlùyǐn 4g qīngwèisǎn 4g xuánshēn 1g</td></tr>
<tr><td colspan="2">Indicated diseases:</td></tr>
<tr><td colspan="2">Congenital factor VIII disorder 286.0 (Hereditary factor VIII deficiency D66);
Unspecified hemorrhagic conditions 287.9 (Hemorrhagic condition, unspecified D699); Coagulation defects 286;
Unspecified diseases of blood and blood-forming organs 289.9 (Disease of blood and blood-forming organs, unspecified D759); Cardiovascular disease, unspecified 429.2 (Atherosclerotic heart disease of native coronary artery without angina pectoris I2510); Hemangioma of unspecified site 228.00 (Hemangioma unspecified site D1800);
Multiple myeloma 203.0; Unspecified condition of the tongue 529.9
(Disease of tongue, unspecified K149); Malignant neoplasm of lingual tonsil 141.6
(Malignant neoplasm of lingual tonsil C024)</td></tr>
<tr><td colspan="2">Congenital factor VIII disorder 286.0/D66 with oral hemorrhage D006472:</td></tr>
<tr><td>Xuèfǔzhúyūtāng 5g huángqíwǔwùtāng 5g
dānshēn 1g sāngzhī 1g jiānghuáng 1g
jīxuèténg 1g to ♀</td><td>Xuèfǔzhúyūtāng 5g bǔyánghuánwǔtāng 5g to ♂</td></tr>
<tr><td colspan="2">Cardiovascular disease, unspecified 429.2/I2510 with oral hemorrhage D006472:</td></tr>
<tr><td>Yùzhú 5g sìnìtāng 5g zhìgāncǎotāng 2g
to ♀</td><td>Sìnìtāng 5g gānlùyǐn 5g lóngdǎnxiègāntāng 5g
to ♂</td></tr>
<tr><td colspan="2">Unspecified condition of the tongue 529.9/K149 with oral hemorrhage D006472:</td></tr>
<tr><td>Yùnǚjiān 5g gānlùyǐn 5g qīngwèisǎn 5g
to ♀</td><td>Yùnǚjiān 5g gānlùyǐn 5g qīngwèisǎn 5g to ♂</td></tr>
</table>

Zhībódìhuángwán 'nourishes Yin, lowers Fire,' and has traditionally been used for Yin deficient patients manifesting such symptoms as dry mouth, sore throat and burning bones. Liánggésǎn 'clears Heat accumulated in the upper and middle body' and has traditionally been used for sores and ulcers in the mouth.

8.2. Gingival Hemorrhage

Gingival hemorrhage is bleeding of the gums. The common cause of gingival hemorrhage is gum inflammation due to deposit, at the gum line, of dental plaque, which is an adherent biofilm laden with bacteria. Medication such as blood thinner and vitamin C deficiency can also cause gingival hemorrhage. If gum infection is not eradicated, the infection can advance to jaw bone, leading to periodontitis, which is the main cause of tooth loss in adults.

Table 8.2. Herbal prescriptions for gingival hemorrhage

Gingival Hemorrhage: https://meshb.nlm.nih.gov/record/ui?ui=D005884.	
Common prescriptions:	
Yùnǚjiān 5g qīngwèisǎn 5g Yùnǚjiān 5g gānlùyǐn 5g qīngwèisǎn 5g Yùnǚjiān 5g zhībódìhuángwán 5g qīngwèisǎn 5g Yùnǚjiān 5g qīngwèisǎn 3g	
Alternative prescriptions:	
Yùnǚjiān 5g gānlùyǐn 5g qīngwèisǎn 4g Yùnǚjiān 5g zhībódìhuángwán 5g xuánshēn 1g Yùnǚjiān 5g liánggésǎn 5g xuánshēn 1g	
Indicated and associated diseases:	
Cardiovascular disease, unspecified 429.2 (Atherosclerotic heart disease of native coronary artery without angina pectoris I2510); Multiple myeloma 203.0; Unspecified hemorrhagic conditions 287.9 (Hemorrhagic condition, unspecified D699); Unspecified diseases of blood and blood-forming organs 289.9 (Disease of blood and blood-forming organs, unspecified D759); Chronic gingivitis 523.1; Dental caries of smooth surface 521.07 (Dental caries on smooth surface limited to enamel K0261, Dental caries on smooth surface penetrating into dentin	
K0262, Dental caries on smooth surface penetrating into pulp K0263); Reticulosarcoma 200.0	
Cardiovascular disease, unspecified 429.2/I2510 with gingival hemorrhage D005884:	
Yùzhú 5g sìnìtāng 5g mǔdānpí 1g zhīzǐ 1g huánglián 0g to ♀	Yùzhú 5g sìnìtāng 5g mǔdānpí 1g zhīzǐ 1g huánglián 1g to ♂
Dental caries of smooth surface 521.07/K0261,K0262,K0263 with gingival hemorrhage D005884:	
Yùnǚjiān 5g gānlùyǐn 5g qīngwèisǎn 5g to ♀	Yùnǚjiān 5g gānlùyǐn 5g qīngwèisǎn 5g to ♂

The prescriptions that treat oral hemorrhage are also used for gingival hemorrhage. Note that shared mechanisms in dental and arterial plaque induced chronic inflammation may be behind the association between periodontitis and cardiovascular disease.

8.3. Hyphema

Hyphema is accumulation of blood in the space between the iris and cornea in the front eye called the annular chamber, which is normally filled with mostly water and also nutrients to the ocular tissue. Blunt trauma that compresses and shears the eyeball is the main cause of hyphema. Other causes include intraocular surgery, blood disease, and vascular disease.

We have become familiar with the use of Qǐjúdìhuángwán, Xǐgānmíngmùtāng and Zīshènmíngmùtāng for eye problems since Chapters 1 and 2. Both Mùzéicǎo and Gǔjīngcǎo are used these-days for disorders of lacrimal system (Wang, 2019).

Table 8.3. Herbal prescriptions for hyphema

Hyphema: https://meshb.nlm.nih.gov/record/ui?ui=D006988.	
Common prescriptions:	
Xǐgānmíngmùtāng 5g zīshènmíngmùtāng 5g Qǐjúdìhuángwán 5g xǐgānmíngmùtāng 5g zīshènmíngmùtāng 5g Qǐjúdìhuángwán 5g xǐgānmíngmùtāng 5g Xǐgānmíngmùtāng 5g qǐjúdìhuángwán 4g	
Alternative prescriptions:	
Qǐjúdìhuángwán 5g xǐgānmíngmùtāng 5g mùzéicǎo 1g juémíngzǐ 1g mìmēnghuā 1g gǔjīngcǎo 1g Zīshènmíngmùtāng 5g gǒuqǐzǐ 1g júhuā 1g Xǐgānmíngmùtāng 5g qiānlǐguāng 1g xiàkūcǎo 1g	
Xǐgānmíngmùtāng 5g qǐjúdìhuángwán 4g mùzéicǎo 1g mìmēnghuā 1g Xǐgānmíngmùtāng 5g mìmēnghuā 1g + acupuncture	
Indicated diseases:	
Disorder of eye, unspecified 379.90 (Unspecified disorder of eye and adnexa H579); Malignant neoplasm of other specified sites of eye 190.8 (Malignant neoplasm of overlapping sites of unspecified eye and adnexa C6980); Neuroendocrine tumors 209; Malignant neoplasm of nervous system, part unspecified 192.9 (Malignant neoplasm of central nervous system, unspecified C729); Primary open angle glaucoma 365.11 (Primary open-angle glaucoma, right eye, stage unspecified H401110, Primary open-angle glaucoma, right eye, mild stage H401111, Primary open-angle glaucoma, right eye, moderate stage H401112, Primary open-angle glaucoma, right eye, severe stage H401113, Primary open-angle glaucoma, right eye, indeterminate stage H401114, Primary open-angle glaucoma, left eye, stage unspecified H401120, Primary open-angle glaucoma, left eye, mild stage H401121, Primary open-angle glaucoma, left eye, moderate stage H401122, Primary open-angle glaucoma, left eye, severe stage H401123, Primary open-angle glaucoma, left eye, indeterminate stage H401124, Primary open-angle glaucoma, bilateral, stage unspecified H401130, Primary open-angle glaucoma, bilateral, mild stage H401131, Primary open-angle glaucoma, bilateral, moderate stage H401132, Primary open-angle glaucoma, bilateral, severe stage H401133, Primary open-angle glaucoma, bilateral, indeterminate stage H401134, Primary open-angle glaucoma, unspecified eye, stage unspecified H401190, Primary open-angle glaucoma, unspecified eye, mild stage H401191, Primary open-angle glaucoma, unspecified eye, moderate stage H401192, Primary open-angle glaucoma, unspecified eye, severe stage H401193, Primary open-angle glaucoma, unspecified eye, indeterminate stage H401194); Open-angle glaucoma 365.1; Glaucoma 365; Ocular hypertension 365.04 (Ocular hypertension, unspecified eye H40059); Cardiovascular disease, unspecified 429.2 (Atherosclerotic heart disease of native coronary artery without angina pectoris I2510); Diabetic retinopathy 362.0; Diabetes with peripheral circulatory disorders 250.7; Unspecified retinal disorder 362.9 (Unspecified retinal disorder H359); Diabetes mellitus 250; Unspecified endocrine disorder 259.9 (Endocrine disorder, unspecified E349); Unspecified disorder of metabolism 277.9 (Metabolic disorder, unspecified E889)	
Disorder of eye, unspecified 379.90/H579 with hyphema D006988:	
Qǐjúdìhuángwán 5g zīshènmíngmùtāng 5g to ♀	Qǐjúdìhuángwán 5g xǐgānmíngmùtāng 5g zīshènmíngmùtāng 5g to ♂
Primary open angle glaucoma 365.11/H401110,H401111,H401112,H401113,H401114,H401120,H401121,H401122,H401123, H401124,H401130,H401131,H401132,H401133,H401134,H401190,H401191,H401192, H401193,H401194 with Hyphema D006988:	
Qǐjúdìhuángwán 5g xǐgānmíngmùtāng 5g zīshènmíngmùtāng 5g to ♀	Qǐjúdìhuángwán 5g xǐgānmíngmùtāng 5g zīshènmíngmùtāng 5g to ♂
Cardiovascular disease, unspecified 429.2/I2510 with hyphema D006988:	
Yùzhú 5g sìnìtāng 5g gānlùyǐn 5g to ♀	Sìnìtāng 5g gānlùyǐn 5g lóngdǎnxiègāntāng 5g to ♂

8.4. Vitreous Hemorrhage

Vitreous hemorrhage is blood in the space between the lens and retina in the eye, called the vitreous chamber, which contains mostly water and helps maintain the spherical shape of the eye. Blood in the vitreous humor can blur the vision. Diabetic retinopathy, age-related macular degeneration, intraocular tumor, and trauma can cause vitreous hemorrhage.

Table 8.4. Herbal prescriptions for vitreous hemorrhage

<table>
<tr><td colspan="2">Vitreous Hemorrhage: https://meshb.nlm.nih.gov/record/ui?ui=D014823.</td></tr>
<tr><td colspan="2">Common prescriptions:</td></tr>
<tr><td colspan="2">Qǐjúdìhuángwán 5g zīshènmíngmùtāng 5g
Qǐjúdìhuángwán 5g xǐgānmíngmùtāng 5g zīshènmíngmùtāng 5g
Qǐjúdìhuángwán 5g xǐgānmíngmùtāng 5g
Qǐjúdìhuángwán 5g xǐgānmíngmùtāng 5g zīshènmíngmùtāng 5g mùzéicǎo 1g cǎojuémíng 1g mìmēnghuā 1g
Qǐjúdìhuángwán 5g zīshènmíngmùtāng 5g mùzéicǎo 1g juémíngzǐ 1g mìmēnghuā 1g</td></tr>
<tr><td colspan="2">Alternative prescriptions:</td></tr>
<tr><td colspan="2">Qǐjúdìhuángwán 5g xǐgānmíngmùtāng 5g zīshènmíngmùtāng 5g lóngdǎnxiègāntāng 5g
Qǐjúdìhuángwán 5g zīshènmíngmùtāng 5g mùzéicǎo 1g gǔjīngcǎo 1g
Qǐjúdìhuángwán 5g xǐgānmíngmùtāng 5g zīshènmíngmùtāng 5g cǎojuémíng 1g mànjīngzǐ 1g
Xǐgānmíngmùtāng 5g qǐjúdìhuángwán 4g zīshènmíngmùtāng 4g gǒuqǐzǐ 1g júhuā 1g</td></tr>
<tr><td colspan="2">Indicated diseases:</td></tr>
<tr><td colspan="2">Unspecified retinal detachment 361.9 (Serous retinal detachment, unspecified eye H3320); Unspecified retinal disorder 362.9 (Unspecified retinal disorder H359); Disorder of eye, unspecified 379.90 (Unspecified disorder of eye and adnexa H579); Cardiovascular disease, unspecified 429.2 (Atherosclerotic heart disease of native coronary artery without angina pectoris I2510); Malignant neoplasm of retina 190.5 (Malignant neoplasm of unspecified retina C6920); Unspecified hemorrhagic conditions 287.9 (Hemorrhagic condition, unspecified D699); Malignant neoplasm of other specified sites of eye 190.8 (Malignant neoplasm of overlapping sites of unspecified eye and adnexa C6980); Hemangioma of unspecified site 228.00 (Hemangioma unspecified site D1800); Unspecified diseases of blood and blood-forming organs 289.9 (Disease of blood and blood-forming organs, unspecified D759); Diabetic retinopathy 362.0; Diabetes with peripheral circulatory disorders 250.7; Diabetes mellitus 250; Unspecified endocrine disorder 259.9 (Endocrine disorder, unspecified E349); Unspecified disorder of metabolism 277.9 (Metabolic disorder, unspecified E889)</td></tr>
<tr><td colspan="2">Unspecified retinal detachment 361.9/H3320 with vitreous hemorrhage D014823:</td></tr>
<tr><td>Qǐjúdìhuángwán 5g zīshènmíngmùtāng 5g to ♀</td><td>Qǐjúdìhuángwán 5g zīshènmíngmùtāng 5g to ♂</td></tr>
<tr><td colspan="2">Cardiovascular disease, unspecified 429.2/I2510 with vitreous hemorrhage D014823:</td></tr>
<tr><td>Yùzhú 5g sìnìtāng 5g gānlùyǐn 5g to ♀</td><td>Sìnìtāng 5g gānlùyǐn 5g lóngdǎnxiègāntāng 5g to ♂</td></tr>
</table>

Cǎojuémíng, Mìmēnghuā, Gǒuqǐzǐ, Júhuā and Mànjīngzǐ have long been appreciated for their benefits to the health of the eye. In particular, specific uses of Cǎojuémíng for glaucoma, Mìmēnghuā for inflammation of eyelids and disorders of conjunctiva, and Gǒuqǐzǐ for disorders of lacrimal system are recently documented (Wang, 2019). Specific uses of Júhuā for unspecified disorder of globe, unspecified dacryoadenitis, and acute conjunctivitis are also listed, so are Mànjīngzǐ for unspecified disorder of globe, unspecified disorder of lacrimal system, unspecified dacryoadenitis, unspecified glaucoma, and unspecified acute conjunctivitis (Wang, 2020).

8.5. Choroid Hemorrhage

Choroid hemorrhage is bleeding of the blood vessels in the choroid, a concentric layer between the sclera and retina. The choroid provides oxygen and nutrients to the retina. Intraocular surgery such as glaucoma surgery can cause choroid hemorrhage. As the choroid is loaded with blood vessels, it is the most common site of ocular metastasis originating from breast or lung cancers.

Table 8.5. Herbal prescriptions for choroid hemorrhage

Choroid Hemorrhage: https://meshb.nlm.nih.gov/record/ui?ui=D002832.	
Common prescriptions:	
Sìnìtāng 5g bànxià 1g dàhuáng 0g Sìnìtāng 5g bànxià 1g shēngjiāng 1g guìzhī 1g Guìzhītāng 5g gégēn 1g Sìnìtāng 5g bànxià 1g guìzhī 1g máhuáng 1g xìxīn 1g	
Alternative prescriptions:	
Sháoyàogāncǎotāng 5g tiānhuā 1g xuánshēn 1g mǔlì 1g màiméndōng 1g fùzǐ 0g Guìzhītāng 5g shēngjiāng 1g guìzhī 1g Sháoyàogāncǎotāng 5g xuánshēn 2g màiméndōng 2g tiānhuā 1g mǔlì 1g fùzǐ 1g Sìnìtāng 5g jiégěng 2g bànxià 1g dàhuáng 0g Sìnìtāng 5g rénshēn 1g bànxià 1g gānjiāng 1g dàhuáng 0g	
Indicated diseases:	
Unspecified disorder of choroid 363.9 (Unspecified disorder of choroid H319); Malignant neoplasm of choroid 190.6 (Malignant neoplasm of unspecified choroid C6930); Disorder of eye, unspecified 379.90 (Unspecified disorder of eye and adnexa H579); Malignant neoplasm of other specified sites of eye 190.8 (Malignant neoplasm of overlapping sites of unspecified eye and adnexa C6980); Neuroendocrine tumors 209; Malignant neoplasm of nervous system, part unspecified 192.9 (Malignant neoplasm of central nervous system, unspecified C729); Glaucoma 365; Ocular hypertension 365.04 (Ocular hypertension, unspecified eye H40059); Cardiovascular disease, unspecified 429.2 (Atherosclerotic heart disease of native coronary artery without angina pectoris I2510); Macular degeneration (senile), unspecified 362.50 (Unspecified macular degeneration H3530); Unspecified retinal disorder 362.9 (Unspecified retinal disorder H359)	
Unspecified disorder of choroid 363.9/H319 with choroid hemorrhage D002832:	
Qǐjúdìhuángwán 5g zīshènmíngmùtāng 5g to ♀	Qǐjúdìhuángwán 5g zīshènmíngmùtāng 5g to ♂
Cardiovascular disease, unspecified 429.2/I2510 withc hemorrhage D002832:	
Yùzhú 5g sìnìtāng 5g zhìgāncǎotāng 5g to ♀	Sìnìtāng 5g gānlùyǐn 5g mǔdānpí 1g zhīzǐ 1g huánglián 0g to ♂
Macular degeneration (senile), unspecified 362.50/H3530 with choroid hemorrhage D002832:	
Qǐjúdìhuángwán 5g zīshènmíngmùtāng 5g to ♀	Qǐjúdìhuángwán 5g zīshènmíngmùtāng 5g to ♂

As metastasis typically occurs in late stages of the primary cancer, Sìnìtāng is prescribed to help the frail health of the patients with metastasis.

8.6. Retinal Hemorrhage

Retinal hemorrhage is bleeding of the blood vessels in the retina, a layer in the back of the eye that is sensitive to light. Causes of retinal hemorrhage include head trauma, macular degeneration, hypertension, diabetes, anemia and leukemia.

The modern use of both Shíhú and Chōngwèizǐ is for essential hypertension (Wang, 2019). However, when used alone, Chōngwèizǐ is for disorder of lacrimal system (Wang, 2020). And when Chōngwèizǐ is paired with Gǔjīngcǎo, Júhuā or Mùzéicǎo, the herbal dyads are used for disorder of globe (Wang, 2020).

Table 8.6. Herbal prescriptions for retinal hemorrhage

<table>
<tr><td colspan="2">Retinal Hemorrhage: https://meshb.nlm.nih.gov/record/ui?ui=D012166.</td></tr>
<tr><td colspan="2">Common prescriptions:</td></tr>
<tr><td colspan="2">Qǐjúdìhuángwán 5g zīshènmíngmùtāng 5g
Jiāwèixiāoyáosǎn 5g qǐjúdìhuángwán 5g mùzéicǎo 1g shíhú 1g chōngwèizǐ 1g gǔjīngcǎo 1g
Qǐjúdìhuángwán 5g xǐgānmíngmùtāng 5g zīshènmíngmùtāng 5g
Jiāwèixiāoyáosǎn 5g qǐjúdìhuángwán 5g mùzéicǎo 1g shíhú 1g chōngwèizǐ 1g mìmēnghuā 1g
Jiāwèixiāoyáosǎn 5g qǐjúdìhuángwán 5g mùzéicǎo 1g shíhú 1g chōngwèizǐ 1g cǎojuémíng 1g</td></tr>
<tr><td colspan="2">Alternative prescriptions:</td></tr>
<tr><td colspan="2">Qǐjúdìhuángwán 5g xǐgānmíngmùtāng 5g zīshènmíngmùtāng 5g mùzéicǎo 1g cǎojuémíng 1g mìmēnghuā 1g
Qǐjúdìhuángwán 5g jiāwèixiāoyáosǎn 4g dānshēn 2g shíhú 2g yuǎnzhì 2g yùjīn 1g
Qǐjúdìhuángwán 5g zīshènmíngmùtāng 4g mùzéicǎo 1g cǎojuémíng 1g mìmēnghuā 1g gǔjīngcǎo 1g
Jiāwèixiāoyáosǎn 5g qǐjúdìhuángwán 5g suānzǎoréntāng 5g yèjiāoténg 1g fúshén 1g yuǎnzhì 1g</td></tr>
<tr><td colspan="2">Indicated diseases:</td></tr>
<tr><td colspan="2">Hypertensive heart and chronic kidney disease 404; Unspecified retinal disorder 362.9 (Unspecified retinal disorder H359); Secondary hypertension 405; Essential hypertension 401; Hypertensive chronic kidney disease 403; Hypertensive heart disease 402;
Cardiovascular disease, unspecified 429.2 (Atherosclerotic heart disease of native coronary artery without angina pectoris I2510); Disorder of eye, unspecified 379.90
(Unspecified disorder of eye and adnexa H579); Diabetic retinopathy 362.0;
Diabetes with peripheral circulatory disorders 250.7; Diabetes mellitus 250; Unspecified endocrine disorder 259.9 (Endocrine disorder, unspecified E349); Unspecified disorder of metabolism 277.9 (Metabolic disorder, unspecified E889); Multiple myeloma 203.0; Unspecified hemorrhagic conditions 287.9 (Hemorrhagic condition, unspecified D699); Unspecified diseases of blood and blood-forming organs 289.9 (Disease of blood and blood-forming organs, unspecified D759); Macroglobulinemia 273.3 (Waldenstrom macroglobulinemia C880)</td></tr>
<tr><td colspan="2">Hypertensive heart and chronic kidney disease 404 with retinal hemorrhage D012166:</td></tr>
<tr><td>Tiānmágōuténgyǐn 5g jiāwèixiāoyáosǎn 5g qǐjúdìhuángwán 5g to ♀</td><td>Tiānmágōuténgyǐn 5g qǐjúdìhuángwán 5g to ♂</td></tr>
<tr><td colspan="2">Cardiovascular disease, unspecified 429.2/I2510 with retinal hemorrhage D012166:</td></tr>
<tr><td>Yùzhú 5g sìnìtāng 5g gānlùyǐn 5g to ♀</td><td>Sìnìtāng 5g gānlùyǐn 5g lóngdǎnxiègāntāng 5g to ♂</td></tr>
</table>

References

Wang, S. C. (2019). *Clinical Herbal Prescriptions: Principles and Practices of Herbal Formulations from Deep Learning Health Insurance Herbal Prescription Big Data.* WSPC. https://doi.org/10.1142/11211.

Wang, S. C. (2020). *Veterinary Herbal Pharmacopoeia.* Nova Science Publishers. https://doi.org/10.52305/GHTR1903.

Chapter 9

Urological Manifestations

The human urinary system, also known as the urinary tract, consists of the kidneys, ureters, bladder and urethra. We ingest food and beverage as the source of material and energy for growth, maintenance, repair and movement of our body, as pointed out in Chapter 4. Solid or semisolid wastes, resulting from undigested food as well as dead gut epithelial and bacterial cells, are eliminated through the anus as feces. Excessive water and products of amino acid breakdown in the liver, known as urea, make up liquid wastes. The function of the kidneys in the urinary system is to filter the metabolic wastes from the blood, producing urine. Urine then transports through the ureters to the bladder for storage. Once the bladder is full, the brain signals the muscle in the bladder neck to release urine out of the body through the urethra. In addition to eliminating liquid wastes from the body, the urinary system also regulates blood volume, blood pressure and blood pH. To achieve these, it works closely with the circulatory system, nervous system and endocrine system. Figure 9.1 shows clinical disturbances of the urinary system.

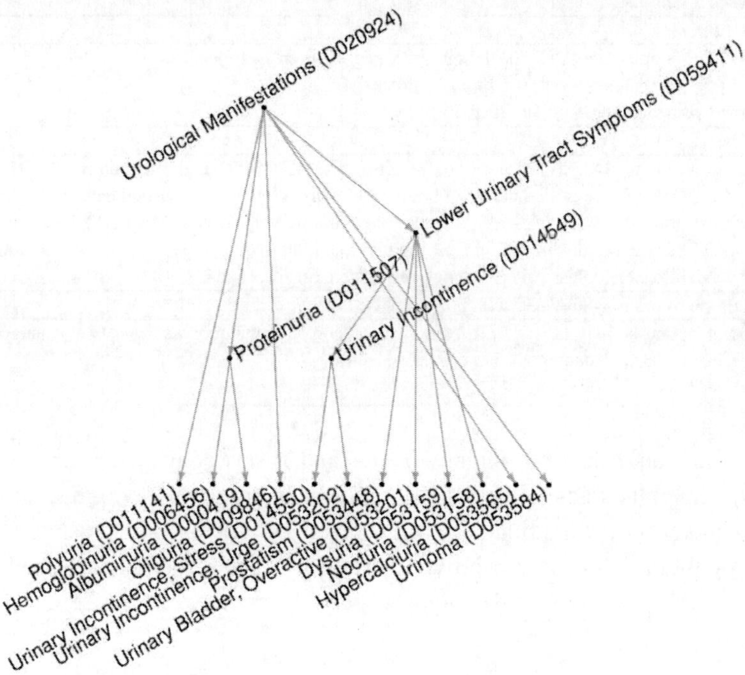

Figure 9.1. Pathological manifestations relating to urine and urination.

The formulas that are commonly prescribed for the urological manifestations in Figure 9.1 are Sāngpiāoxiāosǎn, Bāwèidìhuángwán, Bǔzhōngyìqìtāng, Sìnìtāng, Jìshēngshènqìwán, Guìzhīfúlíngwán, and Guìzhītāng. Many of them are known to benefit the Kidney. The supportive herbs that are commonly used include Yìzhìrén, Fùpénzǐ, Fùzǐ, Yánhúsuǒ, Shéchuángzǐ, Tǔfúlíng, and Dàhuáng.

The diseases that frequently cause or accompany the urological manifestations are unspecified cardiovascular disease, unspecified disorder of bladder, unspecified endocrine disorder, unspecified disorder of metabolism, unspecified condition of brain, unspecified disorders of nervous system, and proteinuria.

9.1. Polyuria

Polyuria is excessive production and passage of urine. More precisely, if an adult urinates more than 40 milliliters per kilogram of his weight per day, he urinates too much. Common causes of polyuria are excessive thirst, diabetes mellitus, kidney disease, urinary tract infection and diuretic medication.

Table 9.1. Herbal prescriptions for polyuria

Polyuria: https://meshb.nlm.nih.gov/record/ui?ui=D011141.	
Common prescriptions:	
Bāwèidìhuángwán 5g bǔzhōngyìqìtāng 5g Bāwèidìhuángwán 5g sāngpiāoxiāosǎn 5g bǔzhōngyìqìtāng 5g Bāwèidìhuángwán 5g sāngpiāoxiāosǎn 5g	
Alternative prescriptions:	
Bāwèidìhuángwán 5g sāngpiāoxiāosǎn 5g bǔzhōngyìqìtāng 5g yìzhìrén 1g fùpénzǐ 1g Bāwèidìhuángwán 5g sāngpiāoxiāosǎn 5g yìzhìrén 1g fùpénzǐ 1g Bāwèidìhuángwán 5g bǔzhōngyìqìtāng 4g fùpénzǐ 1g	
Indicated diseases:	
Unspecified condition of brain 348.9 (Disorder of brain, unspecified G939); Diabetes insipidus 253.5 (Diabetes insipidus E232); Neoplasm of unspecified nature of brain 239.6 (Neoplasm of unspecified behavior of brain D496); Unspecified disorders of nervous system 349.9 (Disorder of central nervous system, unspecified G969); Unspecified endocrine disorder 259.9 (Endocrine disorder, unspecified E349); Malignant neoplasm of nervous system, part unspecified 192.9 (Malignant neoplasm of central nervous system, unspecified C729)	
Unspecified condition of brain 348.9/G939 with polyuria D011141:	
Bǔyánghuánwǔtāng 5g dānshēn 1g shíchāngpú 1g yuǎnzhì 1g + acupuncture to ♀	Bǔyánghuánwǔtāng 5g chuānqī 1g dānshēn 1g shíchāngpú 1g yuǎnzhì 1g + acupuncture to ♂

Bāwèidìhuángwán ‘nourishes Kidney Yang’ and is nowadays used for diabetes mellitus (Wang, 2019). Sāngpiāoxiāosǎn has traditionally been used for nocturnal emission or wet dreams and is today used for urinary frequency and hypertrophy of prostate (Wang, 2019). Combination of them in the prescriptions therefore targets both diabetes and urinary tract conditions. Polyuria often occurs after brain surgery (Hannon et al., 2012).

9.2. Proteinuria

Proteinuria is excessive levels of proteins in the urine, forming foams in the urine. In a healthy individual, proteins in serum are absorbed in the kidneys. Proteinuria indicates problems with absorption or filtration of proteins by the kidneys. The most common cause of proteinuria is diabetes, which damages the kidneys.

Table 9.2. Herbal prescriptions for proteinuria

Proteinuria: https://meshb.nlm.nih.gov/record/ui?ui=D011507.	
Common prescriptions:	
Bāzhèngsǎn 5g wǔlínsǎn 5g dǐdāngtāng 5g Bāzhèngsǎn 5g wǔlínsǎn 5g táohéchéngqìtāng 5g Bāzhèngsǎn 5g wǔlínsǎn 5g dǐdāngtāng 4g Wǔlínsǎn 5g bāzhèngsǎn 4g dǐdāngtāng 4g Bāzhèngsǎn 5g wǔlínsǎn 5g	
Alternative prescriptions:	
Wǔlínsǎn 5g bāzhèngsǎn 3g púgōngyīng 1g Wǔlíngsǎn 5g dǎochìsǎn 5g niúxī 1g chēqiánzǐ 1g Bāzhèngsǎn 5g wǔlínsǎn 3g dǐdāngtāng 3g	
Indicated diseases:	
Cardiovascular disease, unspecified 429.2 (Atherosclerotic heart disease of native coronary artery without angina pectoris I2510); Diabetic retinopathy 362.0; Diabetes with peripheral circulatory disorders 250.7; Proteinuria 791.0 (Bence Jones proteinuria R803, Proteinuria, unspecified R809); Unspecified retinal disorder 362.9 (Unspecified retinal disorder H359); Disorder of eye, unspecified 379.90 (Unspecified disorder of eye and adnexa H579); Diabetes mellitus 250; Unspecified endocrine disorder 259.9 (Endocrine disorder, unspecified E349); Unspecified disorder of metabolism 277.9 (Metabolic disorder, unspecified E889); Multiple myeloma 203.0; Unspecified hemorrhagic conditions 287.9 (Hemorrhagic condition, unspecified D699); Unspecified diseases of blood and blood-forming organs 289.9 (Disease of blood and blood-forming organs, unspecified D759)	
Cardiovascular disease, unspecified 429.2/I2510 with proteinuria D011507:	
Sìnìtāng 5g gānlùyǐn 5g lóngdǎnxiègāntāng 5g to ♀	Sìnìtāng 5g gānlùyǐn 5g jìshēngshènqìwán 5g to ♂

Bāzhèngsǎn 'clears Heat, extinguishes Fire,' 'helps drainage, unblocks urination,' and has traditionally been used for problems of the kidneys and bladder. Wǔlíngsǎn 'helps drainage, soaks Dampness,' 'warms up Yang, helps vaporization,' and is today used for edema (Wang, 2019). Use of both Bāzhèngsǎn and Wǔlínsǎn in the prescriptions is believed to alleviate edema, a complication of severe proteinuria.

9.3. Hemoglobinuria

Hemoglobinuria is high concentration of free hemoglobin in the urine. Rupturing of red blood cells releases the cell contents, including hemoglobin, into blood plasma in a process called intravascular hemolysis. Extensive intravascular hemolysis leads to hemoglobinuria. Intravascular hemolysis can be triggered by autoimmune response following viral infection such as syphilis in adults. As free hemoglobin is pro-oxidant, hemoglobinuria can damage the kidneys.

Both Bāwèidàixiàfāng and Wándàitāng have traditionally been used for 'Damp Heat in the lower abdomen' and are today used for leukorrhea (Wang, 2019). As the primary symptom of genitourinary tract infection is leukorrhea in female, the prescriptions look to address the viral origin of hemoglobinuria.

Table 9.3. Herbal prescriptions for hemoglobinuria

Hemoglobinuria: https://meshb.nlm.nih.gov/record/ui?ui=D006456.	
Common prescriptions:	
Bāwèidàixiàfāng 5g lóngdǎnxiègāntāng 5g tǔfúlíng 1g shéchuángzǐ 1g Wándàitāng 5g dāngguīsháoyàosǎn 5g tǔfúlíng 1g shéchuángzǐ 1g Wándàitāng 5g lóngdǎnxiègāntāng 5g tǔfúlíng 1g shéchuángzǐ 1g Bāwèidàixiàfāng 5g lóngdǎnxiègāntāng 5g tǔfúlíng 1g shéchuángzǐ 1g huángbò 1g	
Alternative prescriptions:	
Lóngdǎnxiègāntāng 5g tǔfúlíng 0g jīnyínhuā 0g liánqiáo 0g Wándàitāng 5g bāwèidàixiàfāng 4g tǔfúlíng 1g báixiānpí 1g dìfūzǐ 1g shéchuángzǐ 1g Wándàitāng 5g tǔfúlíng 1g shéchuángzǐ 1g huángbò 1g bìxiè 1g chūngēnpí 1g Lóngdǎnxiègāntāng 5g Jiāwèixiāoyáosǎn 5g wándàitāng 5g tǔfúlíng 1g dìfūzǐ 1g shéchuángzǐ 1g púgōngyīng 1g	
Indicated diseases:	
Unspecified disorder of metabolism 277.9 (Metabolic disorder, unspecified E889); Hereditary hemolytic anemias 282; Hemoglobinuria 791.2 (Hemoglobinuria R823); Anemia, unspecified 285.9 (Anemia, unspecified D649); Unspecified diseases of blood and blood-forming organs 289.9 (Disease of blood and blood-forming organs, unspecified D759); Proteinuria 791.0 (Bence Jones proteinuria R803, Proteinuria, unspecified R809); Cardiovascular disease, unspecified 429.2 (Atherosclerotic heart disease of native coronary artery without angina pectoris I2510); Multiple myeloma 203.0; Unspecified hemorrhagic conditions 287.9 (Hemorrhagic condition, unspecified D699); Heart disease, unspecified 429.9 (Heart disease, unspecified I519); Unspecified congenital anomaly of heart 746.9 (Congenital malformation of cardiac chambers and connections, unspecified Q209, Congenital malformation of heart, unspecified Q249)	
Unspecified disorder of metabolism 277.9/E889 with hemoglobinuria D006456:	
Jiāwèixiāoyáosǎn 5g wándàitāng 5g tǔfúlíng 1g shéchuángzǐ 1g to ♀	Liùwèidìhuángwán 5g qīngxīnliánzǐyǐn 5g tǔfúlíng 1g bìxiè 1g to ♂
Cardiovascular disease, unspecified 429.2/I2510 with hemoglobinuria D006456:	
Yùzhú 5g sìnìtāng 5g mǔdānpí 1g zhīzǐ 1g huánglián 0g to ♀	Sìnìtāng 5g gānlùyǐn 5g mǔdānpí 1g zhīzǐ 1g huánglián 0g to ♂
Heart disease, unspecified 429.9/I519 with hemoglobinuria D006456:	
Sìnìtāng 5g gānlùyǐn 5g lóngdǎnxiègāntāng 5g to ♀	Sìnìtāng 5g gānlùyǐn 5g mǔdānpí 1g zhīzǐ 1g huánglián 0g to ♂

9.4. Albuminuria

Albuminuria is high amount of albumin in the urine. Albumin, an important transport protein needed by the body, is normally present in the blood. The kidneys filter blood to remove waste and extra water, not albumin, from the blood. Albuminuria therefore signals problems with the kidneys, which in turn can be damaged by high blood pressure and diabetes mellitus.

Table 9.4. Herbal prescriptions for albuminuria

Albuminuria: https://meshb.nlm.nih.gov/record/ui?ui=D000419.
Common prescriptions:
Liùwèidìhuángwán 5g Yùquánwán 5g zhībódìhuángwán 5g Bāwèidìhuángwán 5g Yùquánwán 5g jìshēngshènqìwán 5g Liùwèidìhuángwán 5g báihǔjiārénshēntāng 5g
Alternative prescriptions:
Liùwèidìhuángwán 5g yùquánwán 5g Báihǔjiārénshēntāng 5g qǐjúdìhuángwán 5g tiānhuā 1g Bāwèidìhuángwán 5g qīngxīnliánzǐyǐn 5g shānyào 1g yìzhìrén 1g Bāwèidìhuángwán 5g shānyào 1g huángqí 0g dǎngshēn 0g

Albuminuria: https://meshb.nlm.nih.gov/record/ui?ui=D000419.	
Indicated diseases:	
Cardiovascular disease, unspecified 429.2 (Atherosclerotic heart disease of native coronary artery without angina pectoris I2510); Diabetic retinopathy 362.0; Diabetes with peripheral circulatory disorders 250.7; Proteinuria 791.0 (Bence Jones proteinuria R803, Proteinuria, unspecified R809); Unspecified retinal disorder 362.9 (Unspecified retinal disorder H359); Disorder of eye, unspecified 379.90 (Unspecified disorder of eye and adnexa H579); Diabetes mellitus 250; Unspecified endocrine disorder 259.9 (Endocrine disorder, unspecified E349); Unspecified disorder of metabolism 277.9 (Metabolic disorder, unspecified E889); Hypertensive heart and chronic kidney disease 404; Secondary hypertension 405; Essential hypertension 401; Hypertensive chronic kidney disease 403; Hypertensive heart disease 402	
Cardiovascular disease, unspecified 429.2/I2510 with albuminuria D000419:	
Yùzhú 5g sìnìtāng 5g gānlùyǐn 5g to ♀	Sìnìtāng 5g gānlùyǐn 5g báihǔtāng 5g to ♂
Hypertensive heart and chronic kidney disease 404 with albuminuria D000419:	
Tiānmágōuténgyǐn 5g báihǔjiārénshēntāng 5g zhībódìhuángwán 5g to ♀	Liùwèidìhuángwán 5g to ♂

Liùwèidìhuángwán, Yùquánwán, Zhībódìhuángwán, Bāwèidìhuángwán, Báihǔjiārénshēntāng and Jìshēngshènqìwán are all nowadays used for diabetes mellitus (Wang, 2019). In addition, Jìshēngshènqìwán is also used for hypertrophy of prostate and edema (Wang, 2019).

9.5. Oliguria

Oliguria is too little urine output. Specifically, urinating less than 12 milliliters per kilogram of the body weight per day is considered oliguria in adults. Causes of oliguria include blockage in the urinary tract and dehydration due to vomiting, diarrhea, hemorrhage or burns.

Table 9.5. Herbal prescriptions for oliguria

Oliguria https://meshb.nlm.nih.gov/record/ui?ui=D009846	
Common prescriptions:	
Wǔlíngsǎn 5g fùzǐ 1g huángqín 1g Wǔlíngsǎn 5g fùzǐ 1g huángqín 1g dìdǎngtāng 0g Zhēnwǔtāng 5g fùzǐ 1g gānjiāng 1g Wǔlíngsǎn 5g fùzǐ 1g huángqín 1g tiáowèichéngqìtāng 1g Zhēnwǔtāng 5g fùzǐ 1g xìxīn 1g	
Alternative prescriptions:	
Wǔlíngsǎn 5g báisháo 1g huángqín 1g tiáowèichéngqìtāng 0g Zhēnwǔtāng 5g fùzǐ 0g Zhēnwǔtāng 5g fùzǐ 1g xiǎochéngqìtāng 0g Zhēnwǔtāng 5g fùzǐ 1g suānzǎorén 1g xiǎochéngqìtāng 1g dàhuáng 0g Língguìshùgāntāng 5g fùzǐ 1g xiǎochéngqìtāng 1g dàhuáng 0g	
Indicated diseases:	
Cardiovascular disease, unspecified 429.2 (Atherosclerotic heart disease of native coronary artery without angina pectoris I2510); Myopathy, unspecified 359.9 (Myopathy, unspecified G729); Compartment syndrome, unspecified 958.90 (Compartment syndrome, unspecified, initial encounter T79A0XA); Multiple myeloma 203.0; Unspecified hemorrhagic conditions 287.9 (Hemorrhagic condition, unspecified D699); Unspecified diseases of blood and blood-forming organs 289.9 (Disease of blood and blood-forming organs, unspecified D759); Renal failure, unspecified 586 (Unspecified kidney failure N19); Congestive heart failure, unspecified 428.0 (Right heart failure due to left heart failure I50814, Heart failure, unspecified I509); Heart disease, unspecified 429.9 (Heart disease, unspecified I519)	
Cardiovascular disease, unspecified 429.2/I2510 with oliguria D009846:	
Yùzhú 5g sìnìtāng 5g mǔdānpí 1g zhīzǐ 1g to ♀	Sìnìtāng 5g gānlùyǐn 5g mǔdānpí 1g zhīzǐ 1g huánglián 0g to ♂
Congestive heart failure, unspecified 428.0/I50814,I509 with oliguria D009846:	
Shēngmàiyǐn 5g xuèfǔzhúyūtāng 5g dānshēn 1g yùjīn 1g to ♀	Shēngmàiyǐn 5g xuèfǔzhúyūtāng 5g dānshēn 1g yùjīn 1g to ♂

Zhēnwǔtāng 'warms up Kidney Yang, helps draining and vaporizing,' and is used today for hypertension (Wang, 2019). Wǔlíngsǎn and Zhēnwǔtāng are apparently used here to relieve the complications of water retention in the body due to oliguria. Multiple myeloma manifests renal impairment which in turn presents oliguria (Jung et al., 2015).

9.6. Lower Urinary Tract Symptoms

Lower urinary tract symptoms are a group of signs and symptoms regarding filling and voiding of urine, such as urgent urination and painful urination, as shown in Figure 9.1. Irritation, by infections, or obstruction, by stones, of the lower urinary tract can cause lower urinary tract symptoms.

Table 9.6. Herbal prescriptions for lower urinary tract symptoms

Lower Urinary Tract Symptoms: https://meshb.nlm.nih.gov/record/ui?ui=D059411.	
Common prescriptions:	
Jīnsuǒgùjīngwán 5g huánshǎodān 5g bājǐtiān 1g ròucōngróng 1g yínyánghuò 1g Jīnsuǒgùjīngwán 5g huánshǎodān 5g ròucōngróng 1g yínyánghuò 1g Jīnsuǒgùjīngwán 5g huánshǎodān 5g yínyánghuò 1g shéchuángzǐ 1g Jīnsuǒgùjīngwán 5g huánshǎodān 5g bājǐtiān 1g ròucōngróng 1g yínyánghuò 1g tùsīzǐ 1g Jīnsuǒgùjīngwán 5g huánshǎodān 5g ròucōngróng 1g yínyánghuò 1g shéchuángzǐ 1g	
Alternative prescriptions:	
Jīnsuǒgùjīngwán 5g huánshǎodān 5g huánshǎodān 5g ròucōngróng 1g yínyánghuò 1g Jīnsuǒgùjīngwán 5g zhībódìhuángwán 4g bājǐtiān 1g yínyánghuò 1g tùsīzǐ 1g Jīnsuǒgùjīngwán 5g jìshēngshènqìwán 5g yínyánghuò 2g Jīnsuǒgùjīngwán 5g huánshǎodān 3g ròucōngróng 1g yínyánghuò 1g tùsīzǐ 1g fùpénzǐ 1g Jīnsuǒgùjīngwán 5g huánshǎodān 5g ròucōngróng 2g yínyánghuò 2g tùsīzǐ 2g fùpénzǐ 2g suǒyáng 2g	
Indicated diseases:	
Bladder neck obstruction 596.0 (Bladder-neck obstruction N320); Unspecified disorder of prostate 602.9 (Disorder of prostate, unspecified N429); Unspecified disorder of bladder 596.9 (Bladder disorder, unspecified N329); Unspecified disorder of male genital organs 608.9 (Disorder of male genital organs, unspecified N509, Pelvic and perineal pain R102); Dysmetabolic syndrome X 277.7 (Metabolic syndrome E8881); Unspecified disorder of metabolism 277.9 (Metabolic disorder, unspecified E889); Hypoactive sexual desire disorder 302.71 (Hypoactive sexual desire disorder F520); Cardiovascular disease, unspecified 429.2 (Atherosclerotic heart disease of native coronary artery without angina pectoris I2510)	
Bladder neck obstruction 596.0/N320 with lower urinary tract symptoms D059411:	
Bāzhèngsǎn 5g wǔlínsǎn 5g dǐdāngtāng 5g to ♀	Bāwèidìhuángwán 5g sāngpiāoxiāosǎn 5g bǔzhōngyìqìtāng 5g to ♂
Dysmetabolic syndrome X 277.7/E8881 with lower urinary tract symptoms D059411:	
Zhēnwǔtāng 5g fùzǐ 1g gānjiāng 1g dǐdāngtāng 0g to ♀	Jīnsuǒgùjīngwán 5g huánshǎodān 5g to ♂
Unspecified disorder of prostate 602.9/N429 with lower urinary tract symptoms D059411:	
Bāzhèngsǎn 5g wǔlínsǎn 5g dǐdāngtāng 5g to ♀	Bāwèidìhuángwán 5g jīnsuǒgùjīngwán 5g sāngpiāoxiāosǎn 5g to ♂
Cardiovascular disease, unspecified 429.2/I2510 with lower urinary tract symptoms D059411:	
Yùzhú 5g sìnìtāng 5g mǔdānpí 1g zhīzǐ 1g huánglián 1g to ♀	Sìnìtāng 5g gānlùyǐn 5g lóngdǎnxiègāntāng 5g to ♂

Jīnsuǒgùjīngwán has traditionally been used to prevent nocturnal emission and nocturnal enuresis. It 'nourishes the Kidney,' which in traditional Chinese medicine is responsible for sexual potency. Huánshǎodān 'nourishes Yin, benefits the Kidney,' and has traditionally been used for not only nocturnal emission and enuresis but also aging. Yínyánghuò, Ròucōngróng and Tùsīzǐ are all used for female infertility (Wang, 2020). Yínyánghuò and Tùsīzǐ are also used for impotence of organic origin (Wang, 2020). It therefore looks that herbal doctors, and their patients, are especially concerned about the sexual performance affected by lower urinary tract symptoms.

9.7. Stress Urinary Incontinence

Stress urinary incontinence is leaking out of urine from the bladder during physical activity or exertion such as coughing, sneezing, laughing, lifting weights or exercising. Weakness of or damage to the muscles that control urination can cause stress urinary incontinence.

Table 9.7. Herbal prescriptions for stress urinary incontinence

Stress Urinary Incontinence: https://meshb.nlm.nih.gov/record/ui?ui=D014550.	
Common prescriptions:	
Sāngpiāoxiāosǎn 5g jìshēngshènqìwán 5g yìzhìrén 1g fùpénzǐ 1g Bāwèidìhuángwán 5g sāngpiāoxiāosǎn 5g bǔzhōngyìqìtāng 5g Sāngpiāoxiāosǎn 5g jìshēngshènqìwán 5g Jīnsuǒgùjīngwán 5g sāngpiāoxiāosǎn 5g jìshēngshènqìwán 5g	
Alternative prescriptions:	
Sāngpiāoxiāosǎn 5g yìzhìrén 1g fùpénzǐ 1g Sāngpiāoxiāosǎn 5g jìshēngshènqìwán 5g yìzhìrén 2g fùpénzǐ 2g Sāngpiāoxiāosǎn 5g bāwèidìhuángwán 2g yìzhìrén 1g fùpénzǐ 1g Sāngpiāoxiāosǎn 5g yìzhìrén 1g	
Indicated diseases:	
Unspecified disorder of uterus 621.9 (Noninflammatory disorder of uterus, unspecified N859); Unspecified disorder of bladder 596.9 (Bladder disorder, unspecified N329); Unspecified disorder of female genital organs 629.9 (Unspecified condition associated with female genital organs and menstrual cycle N949); Unspecified disorder of intestine 569.9 (Disease of intestine, unspecified K639); Malignant neoplasm of rectum 154.1 (Malignant neoplasm of rectum C20); Diseases of the jaws 526; Bladder neck obstruction 596.0 (Bladder-neck obstruction N320)	
Unspecified disorder of uterus 621.9/N859 with urinary incontinence, stress D014550:	
Guìzhīfúlíngwán 5g dāngguīsháoyàosǎn 5g yánhúsuǒ 1g xiāngfù 1g to ♀	
Unspecified disorder of intestine 569.9/K639 with urinary incontinence, stress D014550:	
Xiāngshāliùjūnzǐtāng 5g cānlíngbáizhúsǎn 5g to ♀	Gégēnhuángqínhuángliántāng 5g huòxiāngzhèngqìsǎn 5g to ♂
Bladder neck obstruction 596.0/N320 with urinary incontinence, stress D014550:	
Bāzhèngsǎn 5g wǔlínsǎn 5g dǐdāngtāng 5g to ♀	Bāwèidìhuángwán 5g sāngpiāoxiāosǎn 5g bǔzhōngyìqìtāng 5g to ♂
Unspecified disorder of bladder 596.9/N329 with urinary incontinence, stress D014550:	
Sāngpiāoxiāosǎn 5g bǔzhōngyìqìtāng 5g jìshēngshènqìwán 5g yìzhìrén 2g fùpénzǐ 2g to ♀	Sāngpiāoxiāosǎn 5g bǔzhōngyìqìtāng 5g jìshēngshènqìwán 5g to ♂

Yìzhìrén is currently used for symptoms involving urinary system and hyperplasia of prostate while Fùpénzǐ is used for nephritis and nephropathy (Wang, 2019). The single herbs therefore further enhance effects of the formulas in the prescriptions. Note that jawbone joint disorders may lead to pelvic floor disorders (Tim and Mazur-Bialy, 2021).

9.8. Urge Urinary Incontinence

Urge urinary incontinence is urine leakage following a sudden and strong need to urinate. Problems with the bladder muscles and nerves that control the urinary system cause urge urinary incontinence. Examples are bladder inflammation and prostatic hyperplasia.

Table 9.8. Herbal prescriptions for urge urinary incontinence

Urge Urinary Incontinence: https://meshb.nlm.nih.gov/record/ui?ui=D053202.	
Common prescriptions:	
Jīnsuǒgùjīngwán 5g sāngpiāoxiāosǎn 5g jìshēngshènqìwán 5g Jīnsuǒgùjīngwán 5g sāngpiāoxiāosǎn 5g huánshǎodān 5g Jīnsuǒgùjīngwán 5g huánshǎodān 5g yínyánghuò 2g shéchuángzǐ 2g	
Alternative prescriptions:	
Bāwèidìhuángwán 5g sāngpiāoxiāosǎn 4g yìzhìrén 1g fùpénzǐ 1g Bāwèidìhuángwán 5g bǔzhōngyìqìtāng 5g huánshǎodān 5g Jìshēngshènqìwán 5g yínyánghuò 1g shéchuángzǐ 1g tùsīzǐ 1g Sāngpiāoxiāosǎn 5g bāwèidìhuángwán 3g bǔzhōngyìqìtāng 3g yìzhìrén 1g fùpénzǐ 1g Jīnsuǒgùjīngwán 5g sāngpiāoxiāosǎn 5g jìshēngshènqìwán 5g yìzhìrén 2g yínyánghuò 2g fùpénzǐ 2g	
Indicated diseases:	
Malignant neoplasm of male genital organ, site unspecified 187.9 (Malignant neoplasm of male genital organ, unspecified C639); Unspecified disorder of prostate 602.9 (Disorder of prostate, unspecified N429); Unspecified disorder of male genital organs 608.9 (Disorder of male genital organs, unspecified N509, Pelvic and perineal pain R102); Unspecified disorder of intestine 569.9 (Disease of intestine, unspecified K639); Diseases of the jaws 526; Diseases of the oral soft tissues, excluding lesions specific for gingiva and tongue 528; Unspecified disorder of uterus 621.9 (Noninflammatory disorder of uterus, unspecified N859); Unspecified disorder of female genital organs 629.9 (Unspecified condition associated with female genital organs and menstrual cycle N949); Malignant neoplasm of rectum 154.1 (Malignant neoplasm of rectum C20); Unspecified disorder of bladder 596.9 (Bladder disorder, unspecified N329)	
Malignant neoplasm of male genital organ, site unspecified 187.9/C639 with urinary incontinence, urge D053202:	
Guīlùèrxiānjiāo 5g bànzhīlián 2g báihuāshéshécǎo 2g zhìgāncǎotāng 2g xiāngshāliùjūnzǐtāng 2g zhēnrénhuómìngyǐnqùchuānshānjiǎ 2g to ♂	
Unspecified disorder of intestine 569.9/K639 with urinary incontinence, urge D053202:	
Lǐzhōngtāng 5g fùzǐ 1g to ♀	Xiāngshāliùjūnzǐtāng 5g cānlíngbáizhúsǎn 5g to ♂
Unspecified disorder of uterus 621.9/N859 with urinary incontinence, urge D053202:	
Guìzhīfúlíngwán 5g dāngguīsháoyàosǎn 5g sānléng 1g éshù 1g to ♀	
Unspecified disorder of bladder 596.9/N329 with urinary incontinence, urge D053202:	
Bāwèidìhuángwán 5g sāngpiāoxiāosǎn 5g bǔzhōngyìqìtāng 5g to ♀	Bāwèidìhuángwán 5g sāngpiāoxiāosǎn 5g bǔzhōngyìqìtāng 5g to ♂

Jīnsuǒgùjīngwán has traditionally been used to prevent nocturnal emission and enuresis. It is therefore used here to help the bladder hold urine. Bowel cancer and bladder cancer, and their treatment side-effects, can cause bladder incontinence.

9.9. Prostatism

Prostatism is a group of lower urinary tract symptoms, including difficulty initiating urination and passing only small volumes of urine. Prostatism is caused by non-cancerous enlargement of the prostate gland, which is in turn caused mainly by aging-related hormonal changes. Complications of prostatism are recurrent bladder or urethra infections.

Guìzhītāng has traditionally been used for fever from infections and is presumably used here for the lower urinary tract infections. Prostate cancer can metastasize to the central nervous system including the brain (Benjamin, 2002). Moreover, the size of prostate correlates with the risk of cardiovascular disease in men with prostatism (Sandfeldt and Hahn, 2003).

Table 9.9. Herbal prescriptions for prostatism

Prostatism: https://meshb.nlm.nih.gov/record/ui?ui=D053448.
Common prescriptions:
Bǔzhōngyìqìtāng 5g Guìzhītāng 5g huángqí 1g Sìnìtāng 5g bǔzhōngyìqìtāng 5g Guìzhītāng 5g huángqí 2g gégēn 2g
Alternative prescriptions:
Guìzhītāng 5g huángqí 2g dāngguī 0g Guìzhītāng 5g shēngjiāng 1g báisháo 1g Guìzhītāng 5g gégēn 2g Xiǎojiànzhōngtāng 5g huángqí 2g dāngguī 1g
Indicated diseases:
Unspecified cerebrovascular disease 437.9 (Cerebrovascular disease, unspecified I679); Unspecified condition of brain 348.9 (Disorder of brain, unspecified G939); Cardiovascular disease, unspecified 429.2 (Atherosclerotic heart disease of native coronary artery without angina pectoris I2510); Unspecified disorders of nervous system 349.9 (Disorder of central nervous system, unspecified G969); Neoplasm of unspecified nature of brain 239.6 (Neoplasm of unspecified behavior of brain D496); Malignant neoplasm of nervous system, part unspecified 192.9 (Malignant neoplasm of central nervous system, unspecified C729); Unspecified disorder of metabolism 277.9 (Metabolic disorder, unspecified E889)
Unspecified cerebrovascular disease 437.9/I679 with prostatism D053448:
Bǔyánghuánwǔtāng 5g chuānqī 2g dānshēn 1g shíchāngpú 1g yuǎnzhì 1g + acupuncture to ♂
Unspecified condition of brain 348.9/G939 with prostatism D053448:
Bǔyánghuánwǔtāng 5g tiānmá 1g shíchāngpú 1g yuǎnzhì 1g gōuténg 1g + acupuncture to ♂
Unspecified disorder of metabolism 277.9/E889 with prostatism D053448:
Shàngzhōngxiàtōngyòngtòngfēngwán 5g dāngguīniāntòngtāng 5g niúxī 1g huángbò 1g cangzhú 1g yìyǐrén 1g to ♂

9.10. Overactive Urinary Bladder

An overactive urinary bladder causes a sudden urge to urinate, with or without urinary incontinence. Causes of overactive urinary bladder include abdominal trauma, pelvic trauma, medications, and frequent or chronic urinary tract infections.

Table 9.10. Herbal prescriptions for overactive urinary bladder

Overactive Urinary Bladder: https://meshb.nlm.nih.gov/record/ui?ui=D053201.
Common prescriptions:
Bāwèidìhuángwán 5g sāngpiāoxiāosǎn 5g yìzhìrén 1g fùpénzǐ 1g Bāwèidìhuángwán 5g sāngpiāoxiāosǎn 5g bǔzhōngyìqìtāng 5g Bāwèidìhuángwán 5g sāngpiāoxiāosǎn 5g bǔzhōngyìqìtāng 5g fùpénzǐ 2g Bāwèidìhuángwán 5g sāngpiāoxiāosǎn 5g
Alternative prescriptions:
Sāngpiāoxiāosǎn 5g yìzhìrén 1g fùpénzǐ 1g Sāngpiāoxiāosǎn 5g jìshēngshènqìwán 5g yìzhìrén 2g fùpénzǐ 2g Jìshēngshènqìwán 5g sāngpiāoxiāosǎn 4g wūyào 1g yìzhìrén 1g Bāwèidìhuángwán 5g sāngpiāoxiāosǎn 4g yìzhìrén 1g

Table 9.10. (Continued)

Overactive Urinary Bladder: https://meshb.nlm.nih.gov/record/ui?ui=D053201.	
Indicated diseases:	
Bladder neck obstruction 596.0 (Bladder-neck obstruction N320); Unspecified disorder of prostate 602.9 (Disorder of prostate, unspecified N429); Unspecified disorder of bladder 596.9 (Bladder disorder, unspecified N329); Unspecified disorder of male genital organs 608.9 (Disorder of male genital organs, unspecified N509, Pelvic and perineal pain R102); Unspecified disorder of intestine 569.9 (Disease of intestine, unspecified K639); Diseases of the jaws 526; Hypoactive sexual desire disorder 302.71 (Hypoactive sexual desire disorder F520); Unspecified disorder of female genital organs 629.9 (Unspecified condition associated with female genital organs and menstrual cycle N949); Dysmetabolic syndrome X 277.7 (Metabolic syndrome E8881); Unspecified disorder of metabolism 277.9 (Metabolic disorder, unspecified E889)	
Bladder neck obstruction 596.0/N320 with urinary bladder, overactive D053201:	
Bāzhèngsǎn 5g wǔlínsǎn 5g dǐdāngtāng 5g to ♀	Bāwèidìhuángwán 5g sāngpiāoxiāosǎn 5g bǔzhōngyìqìtāng 5g to ♂
Unspecified disorder of intestine 569.9/K639 with urinary bladder, overactive D053201:	
Jiāwèixiāoyáosǎn 5g xiāngshāliùjūnzǐtāng 5g sāngpiāoxiāosǎn 5g bǔzhōngyìqìtāng 5g to ♀	Xiāngshāliùjūnzǐtāng 5g sāngpiāoxiāosǎn 5g bǔzhōngyìqìtāng 5g to ♂
Unspecified disorder of bladder 596.9/N329 with urinary bladder, overactive D053201:	
Sāngpiāoxiāosǎn 5g bǔzhōngyìqìtāng 5g jìshēngshènqìwán 5g to ♀	Sāngpiāoxiāosǎn 5g jìshēngshènqìwán 5g yìzhìrén 1g fùpénzǐ 1g to ♂
Dysmetabolic syndrome X 277.7/E8881 with urinary bladder, overactive D053201:	
Sāngpiāoxiāosǎn 5g jìshēngshènqìwán 5g yìzhìrén 1g fùpénzǐ 1g to ♀	Sāngpiāoxiāosǎn 5g jìshēngshènqìwán 5g yìzhìrén 1g fùpénzǐ 1g to ♂

Wūyào is mainly for disorders of function of stomach (Wang, 2019). However, one of its major uses is for urinary frequency when it is used alone or together with Fùpénzǐ (Wang, 2020).

9.11. Neurogenic Urinary Bladder

Neurogenic urinary bladder is bladder dysfunction due to damage to the brain, spinal cord and nerve that control the filling and emptying of the bladder. Causes of neurogenic urinary bladder include multiple sclerosis, stroke, spinal cord injury, pelvic surgery and diabetes.

Table 9.11. Herbal prescriptions for neurogenic urinary bladder

Neurogenic Urinary Bladder: https://meshb.nlm.nih.gov/record/ui?ui=D001750.
Common prescriptions:
Bāwèidìhuángwán 5g yìzhìrén 1g fùpénzǐ 1g Bāwèidìhuángwán 5g Bāwèidìhuángwán 5g sāngpiāoxiāosǎn 5g bǔzhōngyìqìtāng 5g Bāwèidìhuángwán 5g bǔzhōngyìqìtāng 5g Bāwèidìhuángwán 5g sāngpiāoxiāosǎn 5g
Alternative prescriptions:
Bāwèidìhuángwán 5g sāngpiāoxiāosǎn 5g yìzhìrén 2g fùpénzǐ 2g Bāwèidìhuángwán 5g yìzhìrén 0g Bāwèidìhuángwán 5g wǔlíngsǎn 5g
Indicated diseases:
Unspecified disease of spinal cord 336.9 (Disease of spinal cord, unspecified G959); Neurogenic bladder NOS 596.54 (Neuromuscular dysfunction of bladder, unspecified N319); Unspecified disorders of nervous system 349.9 (Disorder of central nervous system, unspecified G969); Unspecified disorder of bladder 596.9 (Bladder disorder, unspecified

Neurogenic Urinary Bladder: https://meshb.nlm.nih.gov/record/ui?ui=D001750.	
N329); Spina bifida 741; Herpes zoster 053; Polyneuropathy in diabetes 357.2 (Diabetes mellitus due to underlying condition with diabetic polyneuropathy E0842, Drug or chemical induced diabetes mellitus with neurological complications with diabetic polyneuropathy E0942, Type 1 diabetes mellitus with diabetic polyneuropathy E1042, Type 2 diabetes mellitus with diabetic polyneuropathy E1142, Other specified diabetes mellitus with diabetic polyneuropathy E1342); Diabetes with neurological manifestations 250.6; Myoneural disorders 358; Diabetes mellitus 250; Unspecified endocrine disorder 259.9 (Endocrine disorder, unspecified E349); Vesicoureteral reflux 593.7; Hydronephrosis 591 (Unspecified hydronephrosis N1330)	
Unspecified disease of spinal cord 336.9/G959 with urinary bladder, neurogenic D001750:	
Guīlùèrxiānjiāo 5g shūjīnghuóxuètāng 2g dāngguīniāntòngtāng 2g xiǎohuóluòdān 1g xiāngshāliùjūnzǐtāng 1g to ♀	Guīlùèrxiānjiāo 5g + acupuncture to ♂
Unspecified disorders of nervous system 349.9/G969 with urinary bladder, neurogenic D001750:	
Huángqíwǔwùtāng 5g dānshēn 1g zhúrú 1g sāngzhī 1g jiānghuáng 1g to ♀	Huángqíwǔwùtāng 5g dānshēn 1g zhúrú 1g sāngzhī 1g jiānghuáng 1g to ♂
Polyneuropathy in diabetes 357.2/E0842,E0942,E1042,E1142,E1342 with urinary bladder, neurogenic D001750:	
Bāwèidìhuángwán 5g huángqíwǔwùtāng 5g dānshēn 1g zhúrú 1g sāngzhī 1g jiānghuáng 1g to ♀	Bāwèidìhuángwán 5g báihǔjiārénshēntāng 5g dānshēn 1g tiānhuā 1g to ♂

Wǔlíngsǎn is used in Section 9.5 for oliguria. As neurogenic urinary bladder can manifest decreased urine output, we see its use here for neurogenic urinary bladder.

9.12. Dysuria

Dysuria, also known as painful urination, is a sharp, uncomfortable or burning sensation when one urinates. Bladder stones, bladder inflammation, urethra inflammation, and sexually transmitted infections can cause painful urination.

Table 9.12. Herbal prescriptions for dysuria

Dysuria: https://meshb.nlm.nih.gov/record/ui?ui=D053159.	
Common prescriptions:	
Guìzhīfúlíngwán 5g dāngguīsháoyàosǎn 5g yánhúsuǒ 1g xiāngfù 1g Guìzhīfúlíngwán 5g dāngguīsháoyàosǎn 5g Guìzhīfúlíngwán 5g dāngguīsháoyàosǎn 5g yánhúsuǒ 1g xiāngfù 1g yìmǔcǎo 1g Guìzhīfúlíngwán 5g dāngguīsháoyàosǎn 5g yánhúsuǒ 1g xiāngfù 1g yìmǔcǎo 1g zélán 1g Guìzhīfúlíngwán 5g dāngguīsháoyàosǎn 5g yánhúsuǒ 1g xiāngfù 1g yìmǔcǎo 1g + acupuncture	
Alternative prescriptions:	
Guìzhīfúlíngwán 5g dāngguīsháoyàosǎn 5g sānléng 1g éshù 1g Shǎofùzhúyūtāng 5g guìzhīfúlíngwán 5g chuānliànzǐ 1g yánhúsuǒ 1g Táohóngsìwùtāng 5g wángbùliúxíng 1g wángbùliúxíng 1g gāncǎo 0g Guìzhīfúlíngwán 5g dāngguīsháoyàosǎn 5g niúxī 1g xiāngfù 1g yìmǔcǎo 1g Guìzhīfúlíngwán 5g yánhúsuǒ 1g xiāngfù 1g + acupuncture	
Indicated diseases:	
Chronic interstitial cystitis 595.1 (Interstitial cystitis (chronic) without hematuria N3010, Interstitial cystitis (chronic) with hematuria N3011); Cystitis 595; Unspecified disorder of bladder 596.9 (Bladder disorder, unspecified N329); Unspecified disorder of intestine 569.9 (Disease of intestine, unspecified K639); Malignant neoplasm of rectum 154.1 (Malignant neoplasm of rectum C20); Diseases of the jaws 526; Exstrophy of urinary bladder 753.5 (Exstrophy of urinary bladder, unspecified Q6410, Other exstrophy of urinary bladder Q6419)	
Chronic interstitial cystitis 595.1/N3010,N3011 with dysuria D053159:	
Bāzhèngsǎn 5g wǔlínsǎn 5g to ♀	Bāzhèngsǎn 5g wǔlínsǎn 5g to ♂

Table 9.12. (Continued)

Dysuria: https://meshb.nlm.nih.gov/record/ui?ui=D053159.	
Cystitis 595 with dysuria D053159:	
Bāzhèngsǎn 5g wǔlínsǎn 5g dǐdāngtāng 5g to ♀	Bāzhèngsǎn 5g wǔlínsǎn 5g dǐdāngtāng 5g to ♂
Unspecified disorder of intestine 569.9/K639 with dysuria D053159:	
Lǐzhōngtāng 5g báisháo 1g guìzhī 1g to ♀	Lǐzhōngtāng 5g fúlíng 2g bànxià 1g shārén 1g to ♂
Unspecified disorder of bladder 596.9/N329 with dysuria D053159:	
Bāwèidìhuángwán 5g sāngpiāoxiāosǎn 5g bǔzhōngyìqìtāng 5g to ♀	Bāwèidìhuángwán 5g sāngpiāoxiāosǎn 5g bǔzhōngyìqìtāng 5g to ♂

Guìzhīfúlíngwán has traditionally been used to 'eliminate accumulation and disperse obstruction.' Dāngguīsháoyàosǎn is today used for dysmenorrhea (Wang, 2019). Their use in the prescriptions is believed to focus on pain relieving in dysuria.

9.13. Nocturia

Nocturia is a need to wake up more than once in the night to urinate. Age-related deficiency in the production, in the brain, of antidiuretic hormone that controls urine production in the kidneys can cause nocturia, so can administration of diuretic medications.

Table 9.13. Herbal prescriptions for nocturia

Nocturia: https://meshb.nlm.nih.gov/record/ui?ui=D053158.	
Common prescriptions:	
Sìnìtāng 5g ròuguì 1g wúzhūyú 1g Sìnìtāng 5g rénshēn 1g wúzhūyú 1g Sìnìtāng 5g ròuguì 1g wúzhūyú 1g yánhúsuǒ 1g Sìnìtāng 5g rénshēn 1g Sìnìtāng 5g ròuguì 1g yánhúsuǒ 1g	
Alternative prescriptions:	
Sìnìtāng 5g guìzhī 2g máhuáng 2g xìxīn 1g Sìnìtāng 5g ròuguì 1g wúzhūyú 1g gānjiāng 1g zhìgāncǎotāng 1g Sìnìtāng 5g dāngguīsìnìtāng 5g wúzhūyú 1g gānjiāng 1g Sìnìtāng 5g rénshēn 1g yìzhìrén 1g fùpénzǐ 1g dàhuáng 0g	
Indicated diseases:	
Hypertensive heart and chronic kidney disease 404; Secondary hypertension 405; Essential hypertension 401; Hypertensive chronic kidney disease 403; Hypertensive heart disease 402; Cardiovascular disease, unspecified 429.2 (Atherosclerotic heart disease of native coronary artery without angina pectoris I2510); Dysmetabolic syndrome X 277.7 (Metabolic syndrome E8881); Unspecified disorder of metabolism 277.9 (Metabolic disorder, unspecified E889); Diabetes mellitus 250; Unspecified endocrine disorder 259.9 (Endocrine disorder, unspecified E349); Unspecified disorder of prostate 602.9 (Disorder of prostate, unspecified N429); Unspecified disorder of male genital organs 608.9 (Disorder of male genital organs, unspecified N509, Pelvic and perineal pain R102)	
Hypertensive heart and chronic kidney disease 404 with nocturia D053158:	
Tiānmágōuténgyǐn 5g bǔyánghuánwǔtāng 5g to ♀	Tiānmágōuténgyǐn 5g bǔyánghuánwǔtāng 5g to ♂
Dysmetabolic syndrome X 277.7/E8881 with nocturia D053158:	
Zhēnwǔtāng 5g fùzǐ 1g gānjiāng 1g dǐdāngtāng 0g to ♀	Zhēnwǔtāng 5g fùzǐ 1g gānjiāng 1g dǐdāngtāng 0g to ♂

Nocturia: https://meshb.nlm.nih.gov/record/ui?ui=D053158.	
Diabetes mellitus 250 with nocturia D053158:	
Bāwèidìhuángwán 5g báihǔjiārénshēntāng 5g to ♀	Bāwèidìhuángwán 5g yùquánwán 5g to ♂
Cardiovascular disease, unspecified 429.2/I2510 with nocturia D053158:	
Sìnìtāng 5g gānlùyǐn 5g mǔdānpí 1g zhīzǐ 1g huánglián 0g to ♀	Sìnìtāng 5g gānlùyǐn 5g mǔdānpí 1g zhīzǐ 1g huánglián 1g to ♂

Sìnìtāng 'recovers Yang and overcomes adversity.' Ròuguì 'augments Fire and helps Yang.' Wúzhūyú 'helps Yang and stops draining.' As body fluids, including urine, belong to Yin, nocturia is considered to be a state of excessive Yin or deficient Yang. The strategy of herbal doctors for nocturia is to supplement Yang in an effort to restore Yin-Yang balance. Nocturia is associated with coronary heart disease mortality (Lightner et al., 2012).

9.14. Hypercalciuria

Hypercalciuria is excessive calcium in the urine. Calcium is needed not only as material for bones and teeth but also as a charge carrier for synaptic transmission. Symptoms of hypercalciuria depend on which parts of the body are affected and include osteoporosis and kidney stones. The commonest cause of hypercalciuria is overproduction of parathyroid hormone which stimulates release of calcium from the bones into blood.

Table 9.14. Herbal prescriptions for hypercalciuria

Hypercalciuria: https://meshb.nlm.nih.gov/record/ui?ui=D053565.	
Common prescriptions:	
Guìzhītāng 5g jiégěng 1g dàhuáng 0g Máhuángfùzǐxìxīntāng 5g shēngjiāng 2g guìzhī 2g zhìgāncǎo 1g Máhuángfùzǐxìxīntāng 5g shēngjiāng 2g zhìgāncǎo 2g guìzhī 2g Máhuángfùzǐxìxīntāng 5g shēngjiāng 2g zhìgāncǎo 2g guìzhī 2g dàzǎo 1g	
Alternative prescriptions:	
Guìzhītāng 5g gégēn 2g bànxià 1g dàhuáng 0g Sìnìtāng 5g bànxià 1g guìzhī 1g xìxīn 1g dàhuáng 0g Língguìshùgāntāng 5g bànxià 1g shārén 1g fùzǐ 1g dàhuáng 0g Guìzhītāng 5g gégēn 2g jiégěng 1g dàhuáng 0g Guìzhītāng 5g jiégěng 1g gégēn 1g	
Indicated diseases:	
Osteoporosis 733.0; Hyperparathyroidism 252.0; Unspecified disorder of parathyroid gland 252.9 (Disorder of parathyroid gland, unspecified E215); Unspecified endocrine disorder 259.9 (Endocrine disorder, unspecified E349); Unspecified disorder of metabolism 277.9 (Metabolic disorder, unspecified E889); Malignant neoplasm of parathyroid gland 194.1 (Malignant neoplasm of parathyroid gland C750); Malignant neoplasm of endocrine gland, site unspecified 194.9 (Malignant neoplasm of endocrine gland, unspecified C759); End stage renal disease 585.6 (End stage renal disease N186); Renal failure, unspecified 586 (Unspecified kidney failure N19)	
Osteoporosis 733.0 with hypercalciuria D053565:	
Guīlùèrxiānjiāo 5g to ♀	Guīlùèrxiānjiāo 5g to ♂
Unspecified disorder of parathyroid gland 252.9/E215 with hypercalciuria D053565:	
Jiāwèixiāoyáosǎn 5g zhìgāncǎotāng 5g dānshēn 1g xuánshēn 1g mǔlì 1g bèimǔ 1g xiàkūcǎo 1g to ♀	Jiāwèixiāoyáosǎn 5g zhībódìhuángwán 5g dānshēn 1g xuánshēn 1g mǔlì 1g bèimǔ 1g xiàkūcǎo 1g to ♂
Hyperparathyroidism 252.0 with hypercalciuria D053565:	
Jiāwèixiāoyáosǎn 5g zhìgāncǎotāng 5g dānshēn 1g xuánshēn 1g mǔlì 1g bèimǔ 1g xiàkūcǎo 1g to ♀	Jiāwèixiāoyáosǎn 5g zhìgāncǎotāng 5g dānshēn 1g xuánshēn 1g mǔlì 1g bèimǔ 1g xiàkūcǎo 1g to ♂

Guìzhītāng and Máhuángfùzǐxìxīntāng have traditionally been used for respiratory tract infections such as the common cold. Jiégěng is for symptoms involving respiratory system and other chest symptoms (Wang, 2019). As urinary calcium is correlated to the clinical status of sarcoidosis (Cameli et al., 2020), which mainly affects the lung with such inflammatory symptoms as dry cough, shortness of breath, and chest pain, we see that the herbal doctors may treat hypercalciuria as secondary to a disease such as sarcoidosis.

9.15. Urinoma

Urinoma is an encapsulated mass of urine outside the urinary tract as a result of disruption to the urine collection and excretion. Urinomas commonly form in the retroperitoneal space so the major symptom is abdominal pain. Causes of urinoma are traumatic injuries to the abdomen and pelvis, obstruction of the ureter or urethra, bladder stones and bladder cancer.

Table 9.15. Herbal prescriptions for urinoma

Urinoma: https://meshb.nlm.nih.gov/record/ui?ui=D053584.	
Common prescriptions:	
Sháoyàogāncǎotāng 5g shūjīnghuóxuètāng 5g dāngguīniāntòngtāng 5g + acupuncture Sháoyàogāncǎotāng 5g shūjīnghuóxuètāng 5g + acupuncture	
Alternative prescriptions:	
Liùwèidìhuángwán 5g shūjīnghuóxuètāng 5g niúxī 1g mòyào 1g rǔxiāng 1g yánhúsuǒ 1g fùzǐ 1g guìzhī 1g jīxuèténg 1g + acupuncture Bǔzhōngyìqìtāng 5g + acupuncture Xiǎocháihútāng 5g sháoyàogāncǎotāng 5g shūjīnghuóxuètāng 5g Zhènggǔzǐjīndān 5g dāngguīniāntòngtāng 2g sānqī 1g dàdīnghuáng 1g gāncǎo 1g dǎodìwúgōng 1g dǎodìwúgōng 1g sūmù 1g xùduàn 1g + acupuncture Sháoyàogāncǎotāng 5g yánhúsuǒ 1g mòyào 1g rǔxiāng 1g + acupuncture	
Indicated diseases:	
Cardiovascular disease, unspecified 429.2 (Atherosclerotic heart disease of native coronary artery without angina pectoris I2510); Multiple myeloma 203.0; Unspecified hemorrhagic conditions 287.9 (Hemorrhagic condition, unspecified D699); Unspecified diseases of blood and blood-forming organs 289.9 (Disease of blood and blood-forming organs, unspecified D759); Unspecified disorder of metabolism 277.9 (Metabolic disorder, unspecified E889)	
Cardiovascular disease, unspecified 429.2/I2510 with urinoma D053584:	
Sìnìtāng 5g gānlùyǐn 5g mǔdānpí 1g zhīzǐ 1g huánglián 0g to ♀	Xuèfǔzhúyūtāng 5g zhìgāncǎotāng 5g to ♂
Unspecified disorder of metabolism 277.9/E889 with urinoma D053584:	
Rénshēnbàidúsǎn 5g xiǎocháihútāngqùrénshēn 5g yīnchénhāotāng 2g mùxiāng 1g yùjīn 1g to ♀	Dānshēn 5g tiānmágōuténgyǐn 5g sǎnzhǒngkuìjiāntāng 5g bǔyánghuánwǔtāng 5g to ♂

Sháoyàogāncǎotāng, Shūjīnghuóxuètāng or Dāngguīniāntòngtāng are used for pains in the first chapter of the book. Yánhúsuǒ, Mòyào and Rǔxiāng are also well-known pain relievers (Wang, 2020), so is acupuncture. The prescriptions therefore cope with pain associated with urinoma. A case of fetal urinoma due to vascular disorder was reported (Kozlova et al., 2021).

References

Benjamin, R. (2002). Neurologic complications of prostate cancer. *American Family Physician, 65*(9), 1834–1840.

Cameli, P., Gonnelli, S., Bargagli, E., d'Alessandro, M., Bergantini, L., Favetta, V., Tomai Pitinca, M., Lisi, E., Refini, R., Pieroni, M., Sestini, P., & Caffarelli, C. (2020). The Role of Urinary Calcium and Chitotriosidase in a Cohort of Chronic Sarcoidosis Patients. *Respiration*, *99*(3), 207–212. https://doi.org/10.1159/000505653.

Hannon, M. J., Finucane, F. M., Sherlock, M., Agha, A., & Thompson, C. J. (2012). Disorders of Water Homeostasis in Neurosurgical Patients. *The Journal of Clinical Endocrinology & Metabolism*, *97*(5), 1423–1433. https://doi.org/10.1210/jc.2011-3201.

Jung, S.-H., Ahn, J.-S., Yang, D.-H., Cho, M.-S., Kim, J.-Y., Ahn, S.-Y., Kim, Y.-K., Kim, H.-J., & Lee, J.-J. (2015). Oliguria as an early indicator of mortality risk in patients with multiple myeloma and renal impairment. *Blood Research*, *50*(3), 167–172. https://doi.org/10.5045/br.2015.50.3.167.

Kozlova, D., Gilboa, Y., Sade-Zalts, C., Gielchinsky, Y., Shteingart, S., & Kidron, D. (2021). Fetal Urinoma Due to Circulatory Disorders in an Umbilical Artery: Case Report. *Pediatric and Developmental Pathology*, *24*(4), 383–387. https://doi.org/10.1177/10935266211002730.

Lightner, D. J., Krambeck, A. E., Jacobson, D. J., McGree, M. E., Jacobsen, S. J., Lieber, M. M., Roger, V. L., Girman, C. J., & St. Sauver, J. L. (2012). Nocturia is associated with an increased risk of coronary heart disease and death. *BJU International*, *110*(6), 848–853. https://doi.org/10.1111/j.1464-410x.2011.10806.x.

Sandfeldt, L., & Hahn, R. G. (2003). Cardiovascular risk factors correlate with prostate size in men with bladder outlet obstruction. *BJU International*, *92*(1), 64–68. https://doi.org/10.1046/j.1464-410x.2003.04277.x.

Tim, S., & Mazur-Bialy, A. I. (2021). The Most Common Functional Disorders and Factors Affecting Female Pelvic Floor. *Life*, *11*(12), 1397. https://doi.org/10.3390/life11121397.

Wang, S. C. (2019). *Clinical Herbal Prescriptions: Principles and Practices of Herbal Formulations from Deep Learning Health Insurance Herbal Prescription Big Data*. WSPC. https://doi.org/10.1142/11211.

Wang, S. C. (2020). *Veterinary Herbal Pharmacopoeia*. Nova Science Publishers. https://doi.org/10.52305/GHTR1903.

Chapter 10

Paralysis and Paresis

Chapter 5 discusses abnormal involuntary movements of the body part(s). In contrast, this chapter focuses on paralysis, which refers to severe or complete loss of movement of the body part(s). As a manifestation of nervous system dysfunction or injury, paralysis can affect different parts of the body, giving rise to varying signs and symptoms. Examples include vocal cord paralysis and paralysis of the body below the neck, as illustrated in Figure 10.1.

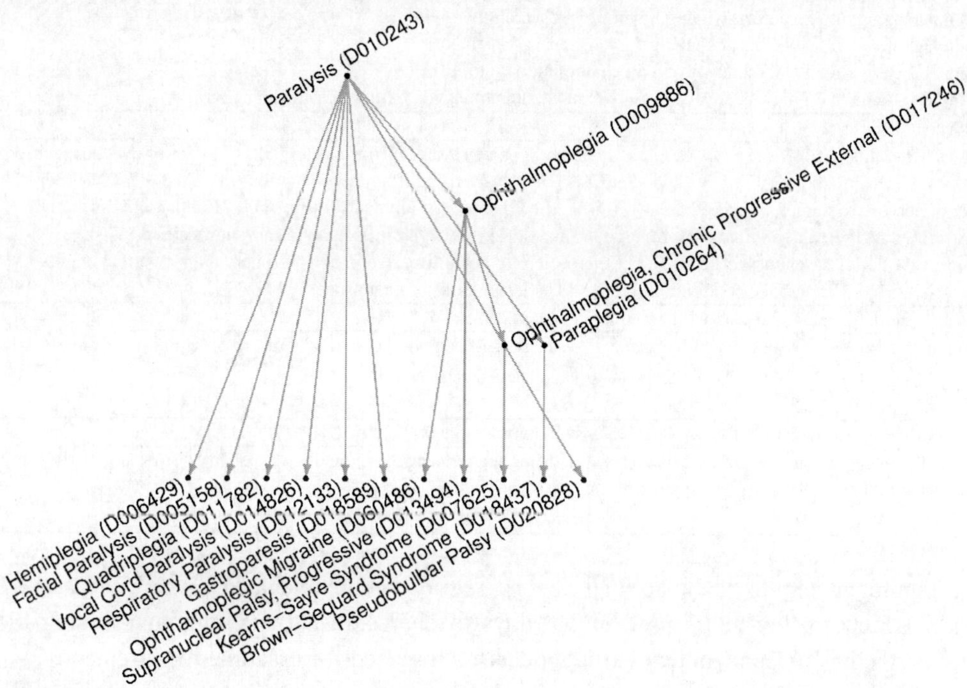

Figure 10.1. Paralysis that affects different anatomical part or physiological system of the body.

The formulas and herbs that are frequently prescribed for paralysis are Jiégěngtāng, Xuèfǔzhúyūtāng, Gégēnhuángqínhuángliántāng, Rénshēnbàidúsǎn, Bāwèidìhuángwán, Jiāwèixiāoyáosǎn, Shūjīnghuóxuètāng, Bǔzhōngyìqìtāng, Bǔyánghuánwǔtāng, Dàhuáng, Dānshēn, Mǔlì, Bèimǔ, Zhīzǐ, Liánqiáo, Xuánshēn, Bànxià, and Shēngjiāng. They tend to attend to the brain or the part of the body with paralyzed muscles. Note that acupuncture is frequently recommended as a complementary therapy to herbal medicine for the treatment of paralysis and paresis.

The diseases that commonly present or co-occur with paralysis are unspecified disorders of nervous system, unspecified disorder of cranial nerves, unspecified cardiovascular disease, unspecified condition of brain, unspecified disorder of metabolism, and unspecified disorder of eye.

10.1. Hemiplegia

Hemiplegia is paralysis of the muscles of the lower face, arm and leg on one side of the body. Hemiplegia is commonly caused by brain damage such as ischemic stroke and cerebral hemorrhage. Traumatic injury to the spinal cord can also cause hemiplegia.

Table 10.1. Herbal prescriptions for hemiplegia

<table>
<tr><td colspan="2">Hemiplegia: https://meshb.nlm.nih.gov/record/ui?ui=D006429.</td></tr>
<tr><td colspan="2">Common prescriptions:</td></tr>
<tr><td colspan="2">Tiānmágōuténgyǐn 5g jiāwèixiāoyáosǎn 5g zhībódìhuángwán 5g
Tiānmágōuténgyǐn 5g jiāwèixiāoyáosǎn 5g qǐjúdìhuángwán 5g</td></tr>
<tr><td colspan="2">Alternative prescriptions:</td></tr>
<tr><td colspan="2">Tiānmágōuténgyǐn 5g xuèfǔzhúyūtāng 5g zhībódìhuángwán 5g sānqī 1g dānshēn 1g
Tiānmágōuténgyǐn 5g xuèfǔzhúyūtāng 4g niúxī 1g chēqiánzǐ 1g
Tiānmágōuténgyǐn 5g cháihúshūgāntāng 5g dānshēn 1g xiàkūcǎo 1g
Tiānmágōuténgyǐn 5g zhībódìhuángwán 5g cháihújiālónggǔmǔlìtāng 3g
Tiānmágōuténgyǐn 5g jiāwèixiāoyáosǎn 5g bànxiàbáizhútiānmátāng 5g língguìshùgāntāng 5g</td></tr>
<tr><td colspan="2">Indicated diseases:</td></tr>
<tr><td colspan="2">Infantile hemiplegia 343.4 (Spastic hemiplegic cerebral palsy G802); Herpes zoster 053; Disorder of eye, unspecified 379.90 (Unspecified disorder of eye and adnexa H579); Unspecified disorders of nervous system 349.9 (Disorder of central nervous system, unspecified G969); Unspecified disorder of joint, site unspecified 719.90 (Joint disorder, unspecified M259); Unspecified cerebrovascular disease 437.9 (Cerebrovascular disease, unspecified I679); Cardiovascular disease, unspecified 429.2 (Atherosclerotic heart disease of native coronary artery without angina pectoris I2510); Unspecified condition of brain 348.9 (Disorder of brain, unspecified G939)</td></tr>
<tr><td colspan="2">Infantile hemiplegia 343.4/G802 with hemiplegia D006429:</td></tr>
<tr><td>Tiānmágōuténgyǐn 5g bànxiàbáizhútiānmátāng 5g qǐjúdìhuángwán 5g xuèfǔzhúyūtāng 4g sānqī 1g to ♀</td><td>Tiānmágōuténgyǐn 5g xuèfǔzhúyūtāng 5g qǐjúdìhuángwán 5g sānqī 1g dānshēn 1g to ♂</td></tr>
<tr><td colspan="2">Unspecified cerebrovascular disease 437.9/I679 with hemiplegia D006429:</td></tr>
<tr><td>Bǔyánghuánwǔtāng 5g chuānqī 2g dānshēn 1g shíchāngpú 1g yuǎnzhì 1g + acupuncture to ♀</td><td>Bǔyánghuánwǔtāng 5g chuānqī 2g dānshēn 1g shíchāngpú 1g yuǎnzhì 1g + acupuncture to ♂</td></tr>
</table>

Tiānmágōuténgyǐn has historically been used to 'quench elevated Liver Yang and Liver Wind,' which are the terms used in old days to characterize the symptoms of high blood pressure. Today, Tiānmágōuténgyǐn is indeed mainly used for essential hypertension (Wang, 2019). Transient blindness of one eye can also happen to patients with hemiplegia (Fisher, 1952).

10.2. Facial Paralysis

Facial paralysis is the inability to move one or many muscles on one or both sides of the face. Damage, such as swelling or inflammation, to the nerves that control the muscles of the face can cause facial paralysis.

Chuānxiōngchádiàosǎn 'disperses Wind, clears Heat, stops pain,' and has traditionally been used for headache due to infections. It is thought to be used here to relieve the inflamed nerves that paralyze the face.

Table 10.2. Herbal prescriptions for facial paralysis

Facial Paralysis: https://meshb.nlm.nih.gov/record/ui?ui=D005158.	
Common prescriptions:	
Chuānxiōngchádiàosǎn 5g gégēntāng 5g Chuānxiōngchádiàosǎn 5g jiāwèixiāoyáosǎn 5g cháigéjiějītāng 5g	
Alternative prescriptions:	
Chuānxiōngchádiàosǎn 5g cháigéjiějītāng 5g yínqiàosǎn 5g huángqín 1g bòhé 1g + acupuncture Xiǎocháihútāng 5g chuānxiōngchádiàosǎn 5g Chuānxiōngchádiàosǎn 5g jiāwèixiāoyáosǎn 5g báizhǐ 1g hángjú 1g xiāngfù 1g huángqín 1g mànjīngzǐ 1g Chuānxiōngchádiàosǎn 5g Chuānxiōngchádiàosǎn 5g gégēntāng 5g + acupuncture	
Indicated diseases:	
Other dermatoses 702; Cholesteatoma of middle ear 385.32 (Cholesteatoma of tympanum, bilateral H7113, Polyp of middle ear, unspecified ear H7440); Cholesteatoma, unspecified 385.30 (Unspecified cholesteatoma, bilateral H7193); Unspecified disorder of ear 388.9 (Unspecified disorder of ear, bilateral H9393); Unspecified disorders of nervous system 349.9 (Disorder of central nervous system, unspecified G969); Geniculate ganglionitis 351.1 (Geniculate ganglionitis G511); Malignant neoplasm of cranial nerves 192.0 (Malignant neoplasm of unspecified cranial nerve C7250); Facial nerve disorders 351; Unspecified disorder of cranial nerves 352.9 (Cranial nerve disorder, unspecified G529); Neuroendocrine tumors 209; Malignant neoplasm of nervous system, part unspecified 192.9 (Malignant neoplasm of central nervous system, unspecified C729); Cardiovascular disease, unspecified 429.2 (Atherosclerotic heart disease of native coronary artery without angina pectoris I2510); Multiple myeloma 203.0; Unspecified hemorrhagic conditions 287.9 (Hemorrhagic condition, unspecified D699);	
Unspecified diseases of blood and blood-forming organs 289.9	
(Disease of blood and blood-forming organs, unspecified D759); Malignant neoplasm of parotid gland 142.0 (Malignant neoplasm of parotid gland C07)	
Other dermatoses 702 with facial paralysis D005158:	
Qīngshàngfángfēngtāng 5g jīnyínhuā 1g liánqiáo 1g to ♀	Qīngshàngfángfēngtāng 5g jīnyínhuā 1g liánqiáo 1g to ♂
Geniculate ganglionitis 351.1/G511 with facial paralysis D005158:	
Wūyàoshùnqìsǎn 5g gégēntāng 5g + acupuncture to ♀	Xiǎoxùmìngtāng 5g wūyàoshùnqìsǎn 5g báijiāngcán 1g dìlóng 1g + acupuncture to ♂
Cardiovascular disease, unspecified 429.2/I2510 with facial paralysis D005158:	
Yùzhú 5g sìnìtāng 5g mǔdānpí 1g zhīzǐ 1g huánglián 1g to ♀	Sìnìtāng 5g gānlùyǐn 5g lóngdǎnxiègāntāng 5g to ♂
Unspecified disorders of nervous system 349.9/G969 with facial paralysis D005158:	
Huángqíwǔwùtāng 5g chuānxiōng 1g dānshēn 1g zhúrú 1g sāngzhī 1g dāngguī 1g jiānghuáng 1g to ♀	Huángqíwǔwùtāng 5g chuānxiōng 1g dānshēn 1g zhúrú 1g sāngzhī 1g dāngguī 1g jiānghuáng 1g to ♂

10.3. Quadriplegia

Quadriplegia is paralysis of the body from the neck down, including the hands, torso and legs. Common causes of quadriplegia are traumatic spinal cord injuries at the base of the skull or neck.

Bāwèidìhuángwán helps the kidneys; Sāngpiāoxiāosǎn the lower urinary tract; and Bǔzhōngyìqìtāng the respiratory and digestive systems. We see that the prescriptions attend to many of the affected systems at the same time. Cardiovascular dysfunctions are common complications of spinal cord injuries (Grigorean et al., 2009).

Table 10.3. Herbal prescriptions for quadriplegia

Quadriplegia: https://meshb.nlm.nih.gov/record/ui?ui=D011782.	
Common prescriptions:	
Bāwèidìhuángwán 5g sāngpiāoxiāosǎn 5g yìzhìrén 1g fùpénzǐ 1g Bāwèidìhuángwán 5g sāngpiāoxiāosǎn 5g bǔzhōngyìqìtāng 5g Bāwèidìhuángwán 5g sāngpiāoxiāosǎn 5g Bāwèidìhuángwán 5g sāngpiāoxiāosǎn 5g bǔzhōngyìqìtāng 5g fùpénzǐ 2g	
Alternative prescriptions:	
Bāwèidìhuángwán 5g yìzhìrén 0g fùpénzǐ 0g Bāwèidìhuángwán 5g sāngpiāoxiāo 1g yìzhìrén 1g fùpénzǐ 1g Bāwèidìhuángwán 5g sāngpiāoxiāosǎn 5g bǔzhōngyìqìtāng 5g yìzhìrén 1g fùpénzǐ 1g Bāwèidìhuángwán 5g sāngpiāoxiāosǎn 5g wǔwèizǐ 1g wūyào 1g yìzhìrén 1g fùpénzǐ 1g Jìshēngshènqìwán 5g sāngpiāoxiāosǎn 4g yìzhìrén 1g fùpénzǐ 1g	
Indicated diseases:	
Heart disease, unspecified 429.9 (Heart disease, unspecified I519); Quadriplegia, unspecified 344.00 (Quadriplegia, unspecified G8250); Cardiovascular disease, unspecified 429.2 (Atherosclerotic heart disease of native coronary artery without angina pectoris I2510); Unspecified disorders of nervous system 349.9 (Disorder of central nervous system, unspecified G969); Unspecified disorder of joint, site unspecified 719.90 (Joint disorder, unspecified M259); Unspecified disease of spinal cord 336.9 (Disease of spinal cord, unspecified G959); Malignant neoplasm of spinal cord 192.2 (Malignant neoplasm of spinal cord C720, Malignant neoplasm of cauda equina C721); Unspecified disorder of metabolism 277.9 (Metabolic disorder, unspecified E889); Malignant neoplasm of nervous system, part unspecified 192.9 (Malignant neoplasm of central nervous system, unspecified C729)	
Heart disease, unspecified 429.9/I519 with quadriplegia D011782:	
Sìnìtāng 5g gānlùyǐn 5g mǔdānpí 1g zhīzǐ 1g huánglián 0g to ♀	Sìnìtāng 5g gānlùyǐn 5g mǔdānpí 1g zhīzǐ 1g huánglián 0g to ♂
Quadriplegia, unspecified 344.00/G8250 with quadriplegia D011782:	
Huángqíwǔwùtāng 5g dāngguīsìnìtāng 5g to ♀	Bǔyánghuánwǔtāng 5g dúhuójìshēngtāng 5g to ♂
Unspecified disease of spinal cord 336.9/G959 with quadriplegia D011782:	
Shūjīnghuóxuètāng 5g dúhuójìshēngtāng 5g niúxī 1g dùzhòng 1g xùduàn 1g to ♀	Bǔyánghuánwǔtāng 5g dúhuójìshēngtāng 5g niúxī 1g dùzhòng 1g xùduàn 1g to ♂

10.4. Vocal Cord Paralysis

Vocal cord paralysis is inability to move one or both of the vocal cords. Vocal cord paralysis affects not only voicing, but also swallowing and breathing. Damage of the nerves to the larynx due to tumor, infection or surgery can cause vocal cord paralysis.

Table 10.4. Herbal prescriptions for vocal cord paralysis

Vocal Cord Paralysis: https://meshb.nlm.nih.gov/record/ui?ui=D014826.
Common prescriptions:
Jiégěngtāng 5g xuánshēn 2g mǔlì 2g bèimǔ 2g liánqiáo 2g zhīzǐ 1g dàhuáng 0g Jiégěngtāng 5g xuánshēn 2g mǔlì 2g bèimǔ 2g dàzǎo 2g shēngjiāng 2g zhīzǐ 1g liánqiáo 1g dàhuáng 0g Jiégěngtāng 5g xuánshēn 2g mǔlì 2g bèimǔ 2g liánqiáo 2g zhīzǐ 1g Jiégěngtāng 5g xuánshēn 2g mǔlì 2g bèimǔ 2g dàzǎo 2g shēngjiāng 2g zhīzǐ 1g liánqiáo 1g Jiégěngtāng 5g xuánshēn 2g mǔlì 2g bèimǔ 2g liánqiáo 2g dàzǎo 1g shēngjiāng 1g zhīzǐ 1g
Alternative prescriptions:
Guìzhītāng 5g jiégěng 1g dàhuáng 0g Jiégěngtāng 5g xuánshēn 2g mǔlì 2g bèimǔ 2g liánqiáo 2g huángqín 2g zhīzǐ 1g dàhuáng 0g Guìzhītāng 5g xìngrén 1g hòupò 1g dàhuáng 0g Yínqiàosǎn 5g jiégěng 3g cāngěrsǎn 3g gānlùyǐn 2g qīngzàojiùfèitāng 2g yúxīngcǎo 1g ǒujiē 1g Jiégěngtāng 5g xuánshēn 2g mǔlì 2g bèimǔ 2g dàzǎo 2g shēngjiāng 2g liánqiáo 2g zhīzǐ 1g

Vocal Cord Paralysis: https://meshb.nlm.nih.gov/record/ui?ui=D014826.	
Indicated diseases:	
Unspecified disease of larynx 478.70 (Other diseases of larynx J387); Disorders of pneumogastric [10th] nerve 352.3 (Disorders of vagus nerve G522); Unspecified disorder of thyroid 246.9 (Disorder of thyroid, unspecified E079); Malignant neoplasm of endocrine gland, site unspecified 194.9 (Malignant neoplasm of endocrine gland, unspecified C759); Unspecified disorder of cranial nerves 352.9 (Cranial nerve disorder, unspecified G529); Unspecified disorders of nervous system 349.9 (Disorder of central nervous system, unspecified G969); Unspecified endocrine disorder 259.9 (Endocrine disorder, unspecified E349); Hypoparathyroidism 252.1 (Hypoparathyroidism, unspecified E209); Unspecified disorder of parathyroid gland 252.9 (Disorder of parathyroid gland, unspecified E215); Heart disease, unspecified 429.9 (Heart disease, unspecified I519); Cardiovascular disease, unspecified 429.2 (Atherosclerotic heart disease of native coronary artery without angina pectoris I2510)	
Unspecified disease of larynx 478.70/J387 with vocal cord paralysis D014826:	
Jiégěngtāng 5g xuánshēn 2g mǔlì 2g bèimǔ 2g dàzǎo 2g shēngjiāng 2g zhīzǐ 1g liánqiáo 1g dàhuáng 0g to ♀	Yínqiàosǎn 5g jiégěng 2g cāngěrsǎn 2g gānlùyǐn 1g qīngzàojiùfèitāng 1g shíhúsuī 1g yúxīngcǎo 1g to ♂
Heart disease, unspecified 429.9/I519 with vocal cord paralysis D014826:	
Sìnìtāng 5g gānlùyǐn 5g mǔdānpí 1g zhīzǐ 1g huánglián 0g to ♀	Sìnìtāng 5g gānlùyǐn 5g mǔdānpí 1g zhīzǐ 1g huánglián 0g to ♂

Jiégěngtāng has traditionally been used to remove phlegm and exudate from the respiratory tract. It is not surprising to see its use here for vocal cord paralysis. Note that not only neck surgery but also open-heart surgery can cause vocal cord paralysis (Hamdan et al., 2002).

10.5. Respiratory Paralysis

Respiratory paralysis is paralysis of the muscles of respiration. Patients with respiratory paralysis will depend on mechanical ventilation. Damage to the spinal cord or phrenic nerve can cause respiratory paralysis.

Table 10.5. Herbal prescriptions for respiratory paralysis

Respiratory Paralysis: https://meshb.nlm.nih.gov/record/ui?ui=D012133.
Common prescriptions:
Èrshùtāng 5g sháoyàogāncǎotāng 5g shūjīnghuóxuètāng 5g + acupuncture Èrshùtāng 5g sháoyàogāncǎotāng 5g shūjīnghuóxuètāng 5g Èrshùtāng 5g shūjīnghuóxuètāng 5g + acupuncture
Alternative prescriptions:
Gégēntāng 5g + acupuncture Èrshùtāng 5g gégēntāng 5g yánhúsuǒ 1g + acupuncture Èrshùtāng 5g jiāwèixiāoyáosǎn 5g cháihúshūgāntāng 5g xùduàn 1g Guìzhītāng 5g gégēn 2g yánhúsuǒ 1g Èrshùtāng 5g sháoyàogāncǎotāng 4g shūjīnghuóxuètāng 4g sāngzhī 1g
Indicated diseases:
Heart disease, unspecified 429.9 (Heart disease, unspecified I519); Unspecified disorders of nervous system 349.9 (Disorder of central nervous system, unspecified G969); Unspecified congenital anomaly of heart 746.9 (Congenital malformation of cardiac chambers and connections, unspecified Q209, Congenital malformation of heart, unspecified Q249); Cardiovascular disease, unspecified 429.2 (Atherosclerotic heart disease of native coronary artery without angina pectoris I2510); Unspecified disease of spinal cord 336.9 (Disease of spinal cord, unspecified G959); Acute poliomyelitis 045; Myoneural disorders 358; Acute paralytic poliomyelitis specified as bulbar 045.0; Diseases of the jaws 526; Diseases of the oral soft tissues, excluding lesions specific for gingiva and tongue 528

Table 10.5. (Continued)

Respiratory Paralysis: https://meshb.nlm.nih.gov/record/ui?ui=D012133.	
Heart disease, unspecified 429.9/I519 with respiratory paralysis D012133:	
Sìnìtāng 5g gānlùyǐn 5g mǔdānpí 1g zhīzǐ 1g huánglián 0g to ♀	Sìnìtāng 5g gānlùyǐn 5g mǔdānpí 1g zhīzǐ 1g huánglián 0g to ♂
Unspecified disease of spinal cord 336.9/G959 with respiratory paralysis D012133:	
Guīlùèrxiānjiāo 5g shūjīnghuóxuètāng 2g dúhuójìshēngtāng 2g xiǎohuóluòdān 1g xiāngshāliùjūnzǐtāng 1g to ♀	Guīlùèrxiānjiāo 5g + acupuncture to ♂
Diseases of the jaws 526 with respiratory paralysis D012133:	
Guìzhītāng 5g báisháo 1g dàhuáng 0g to ♀	Gégēnhuángqínhuángliántāng 5g bànxià 1g dàhuáng 0g to ♂

Èrshùtāng 'dries Dampness, dissolves Phlegm,' and has traditionally been used for syndromes due to Damp-Heat accumulated in the upper body above the diaphragm. Sháoyàogāncǎotāng and Shūjīnghuóxuètāng are used for a plethora of neuromuscular signs and symptoms over the body in previous chapters. Combining them all here is thought to relieve respiratory paralysis. Respiratory muscle strength was found to be correlated with the prognosis of congested heart failure (Meyer et al., 2001). Mandibular movement and diaphragmatic effort during sleep are associated (Martinot et al., 2019).

10.6. Gastroparesis

Gastroparesis is delayed gastric emptying due to weakening of the movements of the muscles in the stomach. A known common cause of gastroparesis is damage to the vagus nerve which innervates and contracts the stomach muscles. Symptoms of gastroparesis include fullness soon after starting a meal, fullness long after finishing a meal, nausea, acid reflux and heartburn. Complications of gastroparesis include weight loss, malnutrition, and overgrowth of intestinal bacteria. Gastroparesis can be caused by chemotherapy, diabetes and abdominal surgery.

Table 10.6. Herbal prescriptions for gastroparesis

Gastroparesis: https://meshb.nlm.nih.gov/record/ui?ui=D018589.
Common prescriptions:
Gégēnhuángqínhuángliántāng 5g bànxià 1g dàhuáng 0g Gégēnhuángqínhuángliántāng 5g mùxiāng 1g bànxià 1g dàhuáng 0g Gégēnhuángqínhuángliántāng 5g bànxià 1g fúlíng 1g dàhuáng 0g Gégēnhuángqínhuángliántāng 5g mùxiāng 1g bànxià 1g fúlíng 1g dàhuáng 0g Gégēnhuángqínhuángliántāng 5g mùxiāng 1g bànxià 1g fúlíng 1g
Alternative prescriptions:
Gégēnhuángqínhuángliántāng 5g bànxià 2g fúlíng 2g dàhuáng 0g Gégēnhuángqínhuángliántāng 5g bànxià 1g fúlíng 1g Gégēnhuángqínhuángliántāng 5g mùxiāng 1g bànxià 1g
Indicated diseases:
Gastroparesis 536.3 (Gastroparesis K3184); Diabetes mellitus 250; Diseases of the jaws 526; Unspecified disorder of metabolism 277.9 (Metabolic disorder, unspecified E889); Polyneuropathy in diabetes 357.2 (Diabetes mellitus due to underlying condition with diabetic polyneuropathy E0842, Drug or chemical induced diabetes mellitus with neurological complications with diabetic polyneuropathy E0942, Type 1 diabetes mellitus with diabetic polyneuropathy E1042, Type 2 diabetes mellitus with diabetic polyneuropathy E1142, Other specified diabetes mellitus

Gastroparesis: https://meshb.nlm.nih.gov/record/ui?ui=D018589.	
with diabetic polyneuropathy E1342); Diabetes with neurological manifestations 250.6; Unspecified disorders of nervous system 349.9 (Disorder of central nervous system, unspecified G969); Unspecified endocrine disorder 259.9 (Endocrine disorder, unspecified E349); Malignant neoplasm of endocrine gland, site unspecified 194.9 (Malignant neoplasm of endocrine gland, unspecified C759)	
Gastroparesis 536.3/K3184 with gastroparesis D018589:	
Píngwèisǎn 5g ānzhōngsǎn 5g xiāngshāliùjūnzǐtāng 5g to ♀	Píngwèisǎn 5g cānlíngbáizhúsǎn 5g huòxiāngzhèngqìsǎn 5g to ♂

Gégēnhuángqínhuángliántāng has traditionally been used for fever and diarrhea, and is used in Chapter 4 for dyspepsia and heartburn. Píngwèisǎn literally translates to 'powder that normalizes the Stomach.' The prescriptions therefore attend to the complications or symptoms of gastroparesis.

10.7. Ophthalmoplegia

Ophthalmoplegia is paralysis of the muscles that control eye movements. Ophthalmoplegia can be caused by viral infection, multiple sclerosis, brain tumor, migraine, diabetes and trauma.

Table 10.7. Herbal prescriptions for ophthalmoplegia

Ophthalmoplegia: https://meshb.nlm.nih.gov/record/ui?ui=D009886.	
Common prescriptions:	
Jīngfángbàidúsǎn 5g niúbàngzǐ 1g xuánshēn 1g bǎnlángēn 1g Jīngfángbàidúsǎn 5g niúbàngzǐ 1g xuánshēn 1g liánqiáo 1g Jīngfángbàidúsǎn 5g niúbàngzǐ 1g xuánshēn 1g huángqín 1g Jīngfángbàidúsǎn 5g niúbàngzǐ 1g xuánshēn 1g Jīngfángbàidúsǎn 5g niúbàngzǐ 1g xuánshēn 1g xiàkūcǎo 1g	
Alternative prescriptions:	
Rénshēnbàidúsǎn 5g sǎnzhǒngkuìjiāntāng 5g pǔjìxiāodúyǐn 5g dānshēn 4g máxìnggānshítāng 4g tiānwángbǔxīndān 2g xiāozhìwán 2g Rénshēnbàidúsǎn 5g sǎnzhǒngkuìjiāntāng 5g pǔjìxiāodúyǐn 5g dānshēn 3g máxìnggānshítāng 3g tiānwángbǔxīndān 2g xiāozhìwán 2g Rénshēnbàidúsǎn 5g xiāozhìwán 3g Fángfēngtōngshèngsǎn 5g jīngfángbàidúsǎn 2g liánggésǎn 2g shígāo 1g lóngdǎnxiègāntāng 1g	
Indicated diseases:	
Exophthalmos, unspecified 376.30 (Unspecified exophthalmos H0520); Goiter, unspecified 240.9 (Iodine-deficiency related (endemic) goiter, unspecified E012, Nontoxic goiter, unspecified E049); Unspecified disorder of orbit 376.9 (Unspecified disorder of orbit H059); Total ophthalmoplegia 378.56 (Total (external) ophthalmoplegia, unspecified eye H4930); Brown's (tendon) sheath syndrome 378.61 (Brown's sheath syndrome, right eye H50611, Brown's sheath syndrome, left eye H50612); Internuclear ophthalmoplegia 378.86 (Internuclear ophthalmoplegia, unspecified eye H5120); Unspecified disorder of eye movements 378.9 (Unspecified disorder of binocular movement H519); Unspecified disorder of cranial nerves 352.9 (Cranial nerve disorder, unspecified G529); Disorder of eye, unspecified 379.90 (Unspecified disorder of eye and adnexa H579); Unspecified disorders of nervous system 349.9 (Disorder of central nervous system, unspecified G969); Unspecified disorder of thyroid 246.9 (Disorder of thyroid, unspecified E079); Unspecified endocrine disorder 259.9 (Endocrine disorder, unspecified E349); Unspecified disorder of metabolism 277.9 (Metabolic disorder, unspecified E889); Malignant neoplasm of endocrine gland, site unspecified 194.9 (Malignant neoplasm of endocrine gland, unspecified C759); Unspecified condition of brain 348.9 (Disorder of brain, unspecified G939); Neoplasm of unspecified nature of brain 239.6 (Neoplasm of unspecified behavior of brain D496); Malignant neoplasm of nervous system, part unspecified 192.9 (Malignant neoplasm of central nervous system, unspecified C729)	
Exophthalmos, unspecified 376.30/H0520 with ophthalmoplegia D009886:	
Jiāwèixiāoyáosǎn 5g qǐjúdìhuángwán 5g mùzéicǎo 1g shíhú 1g chōngwèizǐ 1g gǔjīngcǎo 1g to ♀	Xǐgānmíngmùtāng 5g jīngfángbàidúsǎn 5g to ♂

Jīngfángbàidúsǎn has traditionally been used for early stages of Wind-Chilliness-Dampness infections manifesting fever and headache. The prescriptions therefore look to remedy ophthalmoplegia due to infections.

10.8. Ophthalmoplegic Migraine

Ophthalmoplegic migraine is characterized by recurrent bouts of unilateral headache with ophthalmoplegia on the same side. The exact cause of ophthalmoplegic migraine is unknown, however damage to the third cranial nerve is involved.

Table 10.8. Herbal prescriptions for ophthalmoplegic migraine

Ophthalmoplegic Migraine: https://meshb.nlm.nih.gov/record/ui?ui=D060486.	
Common prescriptions:	
Sháoyàogāncǎotāng 5g shūjīnghuóxuètāng 5g dāngguīniāntòngtāng 5g + acupuncture Sháoyàogāncǎotāng 5g shūjīnghuóxuètāng 5g + acupuncture	
Alternative prescriptions:	
Jiāwèixiāoyáosǎn 5g cháihúshūgāntāng 5g héhuānpí 3g dānshēn 1g shíchāngpú 1g yuǎnzhì 1g Jiāwèixiāoyáosǎn 5g xiāngshāliùjūnzǐtāng 5g gégēntāng 2g héhuānpí 1g yánhúsuǒ 1g Sháoyàogāncǎotāng 5g shūjīnghuóxuètāng 5g yánhúsuǒ 1g xiāngfù 1g + acupuncture Shūjīnghuóxuètāng 5g sháoyàogāncǎotāng 4g yánhúsuǒ 1g + acupuncture Jiāwèixiāoyáosǎn 5g gāncǎoxiǎomàidàzǎotāng 5g cháihúshūgāntāng 5g héhuānpí 1g yèjiāoténg 1g fúshén 1g	
Indicated diseases:	
Unspecified condition of brain 348.9 (Disorder of brain, unspecified G939); Unspecified disorders of nervous system 349.9 (Disorder of central nervous system, unspecified G969); Unspecified disorder of metabolism 277.9 (Metabolic disorder, unspecified E889)	
Unspecified condition of brain 348.9/G939 with ophthalmoplegic migraine D060486:	
Bǔyánghuánwǔtāng 5g + acupuncture to ♀	Bǔyánghuánwǔtāng 5g shíchāngpú 1g yuǎnzhì 1g + acupuncture to ♂
Unspecified disorder of metabolism 277.9/E889 with ophthalmoplegic migraine D060486:	
Rénshēnbàidúsǎn 5g xiǎocháihútāngqùrénshēn 5g yīnchénhāotāng 2g mùxiāng 1g yùjīn 1g to ♀	Dānshēn 5g tiānmágōuténgyǐn 5g sānzhǒngkuìjiāntāng 5g bǔyánghuánwǔtāng 5g to ♂

We have learned to combine Sháoyàogāncǎotāng, Shūjīnghuóxuètāng and Dāngguīniāntòngtāng for neuralgia and we do so here for ophthalmoplegic migraine, which is a painful, cranial neuropathy. Note that acupuncture is also co-prescribed for ophthalmoplegic migraine.

10.9. Progressive Supranuclear Palsy

Progressive supranuclear palsy is caused by deterioration and death of the neurons in specific brain regions including the cerebral cortex, basal ganglia and brain stem. One of the characteristic symptoms of progressive supranuclear palsy is ophthalmoparesis.

Rénshēnbàidúsǎn literally reads 'ginseng and detoxification powder.' It 'disperses Wind, removes Dampness,' and 'nourishes Qi, upholds uprightness.' The hallmark of progressive supranuclear palsy is aggregation of tau proteins in the affected brain regions. Tau protein aggregates are toxic and Rénshēnbàidúsǎn is thought to be used here to detoxify the tauopathy.

Table 10.9. Herbal prescriptions for progressive supranuclear palsy

<table>
<tr><td colspan="2">Progressive Supranuclear Palsy: https://meshb.nlm.nih.gov/record/ui?ui=D013494</td></tr>
<tr><td colspan="2">Common prescriptions:</td></tr>
<tr><td colspan="2">Rénshēnbàidúsǎn 5g sǎnzhǒngkuìjiāntāng 5g pǔjìxiāodúyǐn 5g dānshēn 4g máxìnggānshítāng 4g tiānwángbǔxīndān 2g xiāozhìwán 2g
Rénshēnbàidúsǎn 5g sǎnzhǒngkuìjiāntāng 5g pǔjìxiāodúyǐn 5g dānshēn 3g máxìnggānshítāng 3g tiānwángbǔxīndān 2g xiāozhìwán 2g
Rénshēnbàidúsǎn 5g xiǎocháihútāngqùrénshēn 5g yīnchénhāotāng 2g mùxiāng 1g yùjīn 1g
Rénshēnbàidúsǎn 5g sǎnzhǒngkuìjiāntāng 5g pǔjìxiāodúyǐn 5g báihǔtāng 4g liánggésǎn 4g xièbáisǎn 4g</td></tr>
<tr><td colspan="2">Alternative prescriptions:</td></tr>
<tr><td colspan="2">Rénshēnbàidúsǎn 5g xiǎocháihútāngqùrénshēn 5g yīnchénhāotāng 2g mùxiāng 0g yùjīn 0g
Rénshēnbàidúsǎn 5g sǎnzhǒngkuìjiāntāng 3g dānshēn 2g máxìnggānshítāng 2g
Rénshēnbàidúsǎn 5g sǎnzhǒngkuìjiāntāng 5g pǔjìxiāodúyǐn 5g dānshēn 4g máxìnggānshítāng 4g xiāozhìwán 2g
Rénshēnbàidúsǎn 5g sǎnzhǒngkuìjiāntāng 4g dānshēn 2g máxìnggānshítāng 2g</td></tr>
<tr><td colspan="2">Indicated diseases:</td></tr>
<tr><td colspan="2">Unspecified cerebrovascular disease 437.9 (Cerebrovascular disease, unspecified I679); Total ophthalmoplegia 378.56 (Total (external) ophthalmoplegia, unspecified eye H4930); Cardiovascular disease, unspecified 429.2 (Atherosclerotic heart disease of native coronary artery without angina pectoris I2510); Brown's (tendon) sheath syndrome 378.61 (Brown's sheath syndrome, right eye H50611, Brown's sheath syndrome, left eye H50612); Internuclear ophthalmoplegia 378.86 (Internuclear ophthalmoplegia, unspecified eye H5120); Unspecified disorder of eye movements 378.9 (Unspecified disorder of binocular movement H519); Unspecified disorder of cranial nerves 352.9 (Cranial nerve disorder, unspecified G529); Disorder of eye, unspecified 379.90 (Unspecified disorder of eye and adnexa H579); Unspecified condition of brain 348.9 (Disorder of brain, unspecified G939); Unspecified disorders of nervous system 349.9 (Disorder of central nervous system, unspecified G969); Dementia with Lewy bodies 331.82 (Dementia with Lewy bodies G3183); Unspecified disorder of metabolism 277.9 (Metabolic disorder, unspecified E889)</td></tr>
<tr><td colspan="2">Unspecified cerebrovascular disease 437.9/I679 with supranuclear palsy, progressive D013494:</td></tr>
<tr><td>Xiǎoxùmìngtāng 5g wūyàoshùnqìsǎn 5g bǔyánghuánwǔtāng 5g to ♀</td><td>Xiǎoxùmìngtāng 5g bǔyánghuánwǔtāng 5g + acupuncture to ♂</td></tr>
<tr><td colspan="2">Dementia with Lewy bodies 331.82/G3183 with supranuclear palsy, progressive D013494:</td></tr>
<tr><td>Bǔyánghuánwǔtāng 5g tiānmá 1g shíchāngpú 1g yuǎnzhì 1g to ♀</td><td>Bǔyánghuánwǔtāng 5g tiānmá 1g shíchāngpú 1g yuǎnzhì 1g to ♂</td></tr>
<tr><td colspan="2">Total ophthalmoplegia 378.56/H4930 with supranuclear palsy, progressive D013494:</td></tr>
<tr><td>Rénshēnbàidúsǎn 5g liánggésǎn 5g xièbáisǎn 5g to ♀</td><td>Rénshēnbàidúsǎn 5g liùjūnzǐtāng 5g gānlùyǐn 5g sāngjúyǐn 5g gégēntāng 5g yínqiàosǎn 5g lóngdǎnxiègāntāng 5g to ♂</td></tr>
</table>

10.10. Chronic Progressive External Ophthalmoplegia

Chronic progressive external ophthalmoplegia is inability of eye and eyelid movements that develops slowly and progressively. The commonest cause of chronic progressive external ophthalmoplegia is mitochondrial myopathy, which can also affect the skeletal muscles.

The combination of Sháoyàogāncǎotāng, Shūjīnghuóxuètāng, Dāngguīniāntòngtāng and acupuncture is prescribed presumably as pain of neuropathic nature is common in mitochondrial diseases (van den Ameele et al., 2020).

Table 10.10. Herbal prescriptions for chronic progressive external ophthalmoplegia

Chronic Progressive External Ophthalmoplegia: https://meshb.nlm.nih.gov/record/ui?ui=D017246.	
Common prescriptions:	
Sháoyàogāncǎotāng 5g shūjīnghuóxuètāng 5g dāngguīniāntòngtāng 5g + acupuncture Sháoyàogāncǎotāng 5g shūjīnghuóxuètāng 5g dāngguīniāntòngtāng 5g	
Alternative prescriptions:	
Dāngguīniāntòngtāng 5g sháoyàogāncǎotāng 4g shūjīnghuóxuètāng 4g Dāngguīsìnìtāng 5g dāngguīniāntòngtāng 5g mùguā 1g niúxī 1g huángbò 1g cāngzhú 1g yìyǐrén 1g Shūjīnghuóxuètāng 5g dāngguīniāntòngtāng 5g niúxī 1g jīxuèténg 1g + acupuncture Guìzhītāng 5g yánhúsuǒ 1g Shūjīnghuóxuètāng 5g gégēntāng 5g dúhuójìshēngtāng 5g	
Indicated diseases:	
Progressive external ophthalmoplegia 378.72 (Other specified strabismus H5089); Unspecified disorder of metabolism 277.9 (Metabolic disorder, unspecified E889); Total ophthalmoplegia 378.56 (Total (external) ophthalmoplegia, unspecified eye H4930); Brown's (tendon) sheath syndrome 378.61 (Brown's sheath syndrome, right eye H50611, Brown's sheath syndrome, left eye H50612); Internuclear ophthalmoplegia 378.86 (Internuclear ophthalmoplegia, unspecified eye H5120); Unspecified disorder of eye movements 378.9 (Unspecified disorder of binocular movement H519); Myopathy, unspecified 359.9 (Myopathy, unspecified G729); Unspecified disorder of cranial nerves 352.9 (Cranial nerve disorder, unspecified G529); Myoneural disorders 358; Disorder of eye, unspecified 379.90 (Unspecified disorder of eye and adnexa H579); Unspecified disorders of nervous system 349.9 (Disorder of central nervous system, unspecified G969); Optic atrophy 377.1; Foster-Kennedy syndrome 377.04 (Foster-Kennedy syndrome, unspecified eye H47149); Ptosis of eyelid 374.3; Unspecified disorder of eyelid 374.9 (Unspecified disorder of eyelid H029); Unspecified condition of brain 348.9 (Disorder of brain, unspecified G939)	
Progressive external ophthalmoplegia 378.72/H5089 with ophthalmoplegia, chronic progressive external D017246:	
Rénshēnbàidúsǎn 5g sǎnzhǒngkuìjiāntāng 5g pǔjìxiāodúyǐn 5g dānshēn 4g máxìnggānshítāng 4g tiānwángbǔxīndān 2g xiāozhìwán 2g to ♀	Sǎnzhǒngkuìjiāntāng 5g pǔjìxiāodúyǐn 5g dānshēn 2g gégēntāng 2g to ♂

10.11. Paraplegia

Paraplegia is paralysis of the lower part of the body. Paraplegia is most often caused by spinal cord injury.

Table 10.11. Herbal prescriptions for paraplegia

Paraplegia: https://meshb.nlm.nih.gov/record/ui?ui=D010264.
Common prescriptions:
Shūjīnghuóxuètāng 5g dāngguīniāntòngtāng 5g dúhuójìshēngtāng 5g sháoyàogāncǎotāng 3g gégēntāng 3g guīlùèrxiānjiāo 3g niúxī 2g yánhúsuǒ 2g Shūjīnghuóxuètāng 5g dāngguīniāntòngtāng 5g dúhuójìshēngtāng 5g sháoyàogāncǎotāng 3g gégēntāng 3g guīlùèrxiānjiāo 3g niúxī 2g gǔsuìbǔ 2g Shūjīnghuóxuètāng 5g dāngguīniāntòngtāng 5g dúhuójìshēngtāng 5g sháoyàogāncǎotāng 3g gégēntāng 3g guīlùèrxiānjiāo 3g niúxī 2g yánhúsuǒ 2g guìzhīsháoyàozhīmǔtāng 2g Shūjīnghuóxuètāng 5g dāngguīniāntòngtāng 5g dúhuójìshēngtāng 5g sháoyàogāncǎotāng 3g gégēntāng 3g guīlùèrxiānjiāo 3g niúxī 2g Shūjīnghuóxuètāng 5g dāngguīniāntòngtāng 5g dúhuójìshēngtāng 5g sháoyàogāncǎotāng 3g gégēntāng 3g guīlùèrxiānjiāo 3g niúxī 2g guìzhīsháoyàozhīmǔtāng 2g
Alternative prescriptions:
Dāngguīniāntòngtāng 5g dúhuójìshēngtāng 5g sháoyàogāncǎotāng 3g shūjīnghuóxuètāng 3g gégēntāng 3g guīlùèrxiānjiāo 3g niúxī 2g qiānghuóshèngshītāng 2g Shūjīnghuóxuètāng 5g niúxī 1g dùzhòng 1g xùduàn 1g + acupuncture Dúhuójìshēngtāng 5g sháoyàogāncǎotāng 2g yánhúsuǒ 1g xùduàn 1g + acupuncture Shūjīnghuóxuètāng 5g dúhuójìshēngtāng 5g sháoyàogāncǎotāng 2g + acupuncture

Paraplegia: https://meshb.nlm.nih.gov/record/ui?ui=D010264.	
Indicated diseases:	
Cardiovascular disease, unspecified 429.2 (Atherosclerotic heart disease of native coronary artery without angina pectoris I2510); Paraplegia 344.1 (Paraplegia, unspecified G8220); Hemangioma of unspecified site 228.00 (Hemangioma unspecified site D1800); Unspecified hemorrhagic conditions 287.9 (Hemorrhagic condition, unspecified D699); Unspecified disorders of nervous system 349.9 (Disorder of central nervous system, unspecified G969); Unspecified diseases of blood and blood-forming organs 289.9 (Disease of blood and blood-forming organs, unspecified D759); Malignant neoplasm of spinal cord 192.2 (Malignant neoplasm of spinal cord C720, Malignant neoplasm of cauda equina C721); Unspecified disease of spinal cord 336.9 (Disease of spinal cord, unspecified G959); Multiple myeloma 203.0; Malignant neoplasm of nervous system, part unspecified 192.9 (Malignant neoplasm of central nervous system, unspecified C729)	
Cardiovascular disease, unspecified 429.2/I2510 with paraplegia D010264:	
Yùzhú 5g sìnìtāng 5g mǔdānpí 1g zhīzǐ 1g huánglián 0g to ♀	Yùzhú 5g sìnìtāng 5g mǔdānpí 1g zhīzǐ 1g to ♂
Paraplegia 344.1/G8220 with paraplegia D010264:	
Shūjīnghuóxuètāng 5g dúhuójìshēngtāng 5g niúxī 1g mòyào 1g rǔxiāng 1g yánhúsuǒ 1g fùzǐ 1g guìzhī 1g jīxuèténg 1g to ♀	Shūjīnghuóxuètāng 5g dúhuójìshēngtāng 5g niúxī 1g mòyào 1g rǔxiāng 1g yánhúsuǒ 1g fùzǐ 1g guìzhī 1g jīxuèténg 1g to ♂

Dúhuójìshēngtāng is literally translated to ‘decoction for living independently and parasitically.’ It ‘eliminates Wind-Chilliness-Dampness accumulated in the lower body.’ Its incorporation into the prescriptions is thought to improve the abdomen and enhance the lower extremities. Patients with paraplegia are at a high risk for cardiovascular disease risk factors such as hypertension (Wahman et al., 2010). Spinal hemangiomas can present acute paraplegia (Eguchi et al., 2022).

10.12. Brown-Sequard Syndrome

Brown-Sequard syndrome is caused by an injury to a side of the spine, leading to paralysis on the side of the spinal cord injury and loss of pain and temperature sensation on the side of the body opposite to the injury, below the level of the spinal cord injury.

Bǔzhōngyìqìtāng, which helps the bowels, and Jìshēngshènqìwán, which benefits the Kidney, are prescribed here as control of the bowels and bladder is most likely affected by the spinal cord injury.

Table 10.12. Herbal prescriptions for Brown-Sequard syndrome

Brown-Sequard Syndrome: https://meshb.nlm.nih.gov/record/ui?ui=D018437.
Common prescriptions:
Bǔzhōngyìqìtāng 5g Bǔzhōngyìqìtāng 5g dúhuójìshēngtāng 5g Bǔzhōngyìqìtāng 5g bǔyánghuánwǔtāng 5g Bǔzhōngyìqìtāng 5g jìshēngshènqìwán 5g
Alternative prescriptions:
Wūyàoshùnqìsǎn 5g bǔzhōngyìqìtāng 5g bǔyánghuánwǔtāng 5g Bǔzhōngyìqìtāng 5g bāwèidìhuángwán 3g Sìnìtāng 5g bǔyánghuánwǔtāng 5g + acupuncture Bǔyánghuánwǔtāng 5g Máhuángfùzǐxìxīntāng 5g báizhú 2g guìzhī 2g gānjiāng 2g gāncǎo 1g

Table 10.12. (Continued)

Brown-Sequard Syndrome: https://meshb.nlm.nih.gov/record/ui?ui=D018437.	
Indicated diseases:	
Cardiovascular disease, unspecified 429.2 (Atherosclerotic heart disease of native coronary artery without angina pectoris I2510); Paraplegia 344.1 (Paraplegia, unspecified G8220); Hemangioma of unspecified site 228.00 (Hemangioma unspecified site D1800); Unspecified hemorrhagic conditions 287.9 (Hemorrhagic condition, unspecified D699); Unspecified disorders of nervous system 349.9 (Disorder of central nervous system, unspecified G969); Unspecified diseases of blood and blood-forming organs 289.9 (Disease of blood and blood-forming organs, unspecified D759); Malignant neoplasm of spinal cord 192.2 (Malignant neoplasm of spinal cord C720, Malignant neoplasm of cauda equina C721); Unspecified disease of spinal cord 336.9 (Disease of spinal cord, unspecified G959); Unspecified cerebrovascular disease 437.9 (Cerebrovascular disease, unspecified I679); Unspecified condition of brain 348.9 (Disorder of brain, unspecified G939); Malignant neoplasm of nervous system, part unspecified 192.9 (Malignant neoplasm of central nervous system, unspecified C729)	
Cardiovascular disease, unspecified 429.2/I2510 with Brown-Sequard syndrome D018437:	
Yùzhú 5g sìnìtāng 5g mǔdānpí 1g zhīzǐ 1g huánglián 1g to ♀	Sìnìtāng 5g gānlùyǐn 5g mǔdānpí 1g zhīzǐ 1g huánglián 1g to ♂
Paraplegia 344.1/G8220 with Brown-Sequard syndrome D018437:	
Shūjīnghuóxuètāng 5g dāngguīniāntòngtāng 5g niúxī 1g mòyào 1g rǔxiāng 1g yánhúsuǒ 1g fùzǐ 1g guìzhī 1g jīxuèténg 1g + acupuncture to ♀	Shūjīnghuóxuètāng 5g dāngguīniāntòngtāng 5g niúxī 1g mòyào 1g rǔxiāng 1g yánhúsuǒ 1g fùzǐ 1g guìzhī 1g jīxuèténg 1g + acupuncture to ♂
Unspecified cerebrovascular disease 437.9/I679 with Brown-Sequard syndrome D018437:	
Bǔyánghuánwǔtāng 5g dānshēn 1g shíchāngpú 1g yuǎnzhì 1g + acupuncture to ♀	Bǔyánghuánwǔtāng 5g dānshēn 1g shíchāngpú 1g yuǎnzhì 1g + acupuncture to ♂
Unspecified disease of spinal cord 336.9/G959 with Brown-Sequard syndrome D018437:	
Shūjīnghuóxuètāng 5g dāngguīniāntòngtāng 5g dúhuójìshēngtāng 5g to ♀	Guīlùèrxiānjiāo 5g to ♂

10.13. Pseudobulbar Palsy

Pseudobulbar palsy is characterized by difficulty in chewing, speaking and swallowing. It is caused by impairment or degeneration of the corticobulbar tracts, which are located in a region of the brainstem.

Table 10.13. Herbal prescriptions for pseudobulbar palsy

Pseudobulbar Palsy: https://meshb.nlm.nih.gov/record/ui?ui=D020828.
Common prescriptions:
Jiégěngtāng 5g xuánshēn 2g mǔlì 2g bèimǔ 2g liánqiáo 2g zhīzǐ 1g dàhuáng 0g
Jiégěngtāng 5g xuánshēn 2g mǔlì 2g bèimǔ 2g liánqiáo 2g zhīzǐ 1g
Jiégěngtāng 5g xuánshēn 2g mǔlì 2g bèimǔ 2g dàzǎo 2g shēngjiāng 2g zhīzǐ 1g liánqiáo 1g dàhuáng 0g
Jiégěngtāng 5g xuánshēn 2g mǔlì 2g bèimǔ 2g liánqiáo 2g dàzǎo 1g shēngjiāng 1g zhīzǐ 1g
Jiégěngtāng 5g xuánshēn 2g mǔlì 2g bèimǔ 2g dàzǎo 2g shēngjiāng 2g zhīzǐ 1g liánqiáo 1g
Alternative prescriptions:
Guìzhītāng 5g jiégěng 1g dàhuáng 0g
Jiégěngtāng 5g xuánshēn 2g mǔlì 2g bèimǔ 2g liánqiáo 2g dàzǎo 1g shēngjiāng 1g zhīzǐ 1g dàhuáng 0g
Guìzhītāng 5g bànxià 1g xìngrén 1g hòupò 1g dàhuáng 0g
Guìzhītāng 5g shēngjiāng 1g guìzhī 1g dàhuáng 0g + acupuncture
Guìzhītāng 5g bànxià 1g shēngjiāng 1g guìzhī 1g dàhuáng 0g

Pseudobulbar Palsy: https://meshb.nlm.nih.gov/record/ui?ui=D020828.	
Indicated diseases:	
Pseudobulbar palsy 335.23 (Other spinal muscular atrophies and related syndromes G128); Unspecified disorder of metabolism 277.9 (Metabolic disorder, unspecified E889); Primary lateral sclerosis 335.24 (Primary lateral sclerosis G1223); Motor neuron disease 335.2; Anterior horn cell disease 335; Unspecified disease of spinal cord 336.9 (Disease of spinal cord, unspecified G959); Myoneural disorders 358; Unspecified disorders of nervous system 349.9 (Disorder of central nervous system, unspecified G969); Unspecified condition of brain 348.9 (Disorder of brain, unspecified G939); Epilepsy, unspecified 345.9; Unspecified disease of pharynx 478.20 (Other diseases of pharynx J392); Unspecified disorder of esophagus 530.9 (Disease of esophagus, unspecified K229)	
Pseudobulbar palsy 335.23/G128 with pseudobulbar palsy D020828:	
Huángqíwǔwùtāng 5g bǔyánghuánwǔtāng 5g dānshēn 1g sāngzhī 1g jīxuèténg 1g to ♀	Cháihújiālónggǔmǔlìtāng 5g bǔyánghuánwǔtāng 5g shíchāngpú 1g yuǎnzhì 1g + acupuncture to ♂
Unspecified disease of pharynx 478.20/J392 with pseudobulbar palsy D020828:	
Bànxiàhòupòtāng 5g màiméndōngtāng 5g xuánshēn 1g jiégěng 1g to ♀	Bànxiàhòupòtāng 5g màiméndōngtāng 5g jiégěng 1g to ♂

Jiégěngtāng is used in Section 10.4 for vocal cord paralysis. It is used here to relieve difficulty swallowing and speaking. When the underlying disease of pseudobulbar palsy is pseudobulbar palsy itself, Bǔyánghuánwǔtāng, which benefits the brain, is prescribed as the cause of pseudobulbar palsy involves brain lesions.

10.14. Paresis

Paresis, i.e., mild or partial paralysis, is weakening of a muscle or a group of muscles, through damage to the nerve that serves the affected muscle. Stroke and spinal cord injury commonly cause paresis.

Modern uses of Niúxī and Gǔsuìbǔ include other and unspecified disorders of back, and other and unspecified disorder of joint (Wang, 2019).

Table 10.14. Herbal prescriptions for paresis

Paresis: https://meshb.nlm.nih.gov/record/ui?ui=D010291.
Common prescriptions:
Dāngguīniāntòngtāng 5g dúhuójìshēngtāng 5g sháoyàogāncǎotāng 3g shūjīnghuóxuètāng 3g gégēntāng 3g guīlùèrxiānjiāo 3g niúxī 2g yánhúsuǒ 2g Dāngguīniāntòngtāng 5g dúhuójìshēngtāng 5g sháoyàogāncǎotāng 3g shūjīnghuóxuètāng 3g gégēntāng 3g guīlùèrxiānjiāo 3g niúxī 2g gǔsuìbǔ 2g Dāngguīniāntòngtāng 5g dúhuójìshēngtāng 5g sháoyàogāncǎotāng 3g shūjīnghuóxuètāng 3g gégēntāng 3g guīlùèrxiānjiāo 3g niúxī 2g guìzhīsháoyàozhīmǔtāng 2g Dāngguīniāntòngtāng 5g dúhuójìshēngtāng 5g sháoyàogāncǎotāng 4g shūjīnghuóxuètāng 4g gégēntāng 4g niúxī 1g yánhúsuǒ 1g Dāngguīniāntòngtāng 5g dúhuójìshēngtāng 5g sháoyàogāncǎotāng 3g shūjīnghuóxuètāng 3g gégēntāng 3g guīlùèrxiānjiāo 3g niúxī 2g
Alternative prescriptions:
Dāngguīniāntòngtāng 5g dúhuójìshēngtāng 4g sháoyàogāncǎotāng 2g shūjīnghuóxuètāng 2g gégēntāng 2g guīlùèrxiānjiāo 2g niúxī 1g yánhúsuǒ 1g Dāngguīniāntòngtāng 5g dúhuójìshēngtāng 4g sháoyàogāncǎotāng 2g shūjīnghuóxuètāng 2g gégēntāng 2g guīlùèrxiānjiāo 2g niúxī 1g Dāngguīniāntòngtāng 5g dúhuójìshēngtāng 5g sháoyàogāncǎotāng 2g shūjīnghuóxuètāng 2g gégēntāng 2g niúxī 1g guīlùèrxiānjiāo 1g Dāngguīniāntòngtāng 5g dúhuójìshēngtāng 5g sháoyàogāncǎotāng 4g shūjīnghuóxuètāng 4g gégēntāng 4g niúxī 1g Dúhuójìshēngtāng 5g shūjīnghuóxuètāng 2g niúxī 1g dùzhòng 1g xùduàn 1g + acupuncture

Table 10.14. (Continued)

Paresis: https://meshb.nlm.nih.gov/record/ui?ui=D010291.	
Indicated diseases:	
Cardiovascular disease, unspecified 429.2 (Atherosclerotic heart disease of native coronary artery without angina pectoris I2510); Unspecified condition of brain 348.9 (Disorder of brain, unspecified G939); Hemangioma of unspecified site 228.00 (Hemangioma unspecified site D1800); Unspecified hemorrhagic conditions 287.9 (Hemorrhagic condition, unspecified D699); Unspecified disorders of nervous system 349.9 (Disorder of central nervous system, unspecified G969); Neoplasm of unspecified nature of brain 239.6 (Neoplasm of unspecified behavior of brain D496); Unspecified diseases of blood and blood-forming organs 289.9 (Disease of blood and blood-forming organs, unspecified D759); Unspecified cerebrovascular disease 437.9 (Cerebrovascular disease, unspecified I679); Conversion disorder 300.11 (Conversion disorder with motor symptom or deficit F444, Conversion disorder with sensory symptom or deficit F446); Somatization disorder 300.81 (Somatization disorder F450)	
Cardiovascular disease, unspecified 429.2/I2510 with paresis D010291:	
Yùzhú 5g sìnìtāng 5g mǔdānpí 1g zhīzǐ 1g huánglián 0g to ♀	Yùzhú 5g sìnìtāng 5g zhìgāncǎotāng 5g to ♂
Unspecified cerebrovascular disease 437.9/I679 with paresis D010291:	
Bǔyánghuánwǔtāng 5g chuānqī 2g dānshēn 1g shíchāngpú 1g yuǎnzhì 1g + acupuncture to ♀	Bǔyánghuánwǔtāng 5g chuānqī 2g dānshēn 1g shíchāngpú 1g yuǎnzhì 1g + acupuncture to ♂
Unspecified disorders of nervous system 349.9/G969 with paresis D010291:	
Huángqíwǔwùtāng 5g chuānxiōng 1g dānshēn 1g zhúrú 1g sāngzhī 1g dāngguī 1g jiānghuáng 1g to ♀	Huángqíwǔwùtāng 5g chuānxiōng 1g dānshēn 1g zhúrú 1g sāngzhī 1g dāngguī 1g jiānghuáng 1g to ♂

10.15. Paraparesis

Paraparesis is partial loss of the motor function of the lower body including the legs. Spinal tuberculosis, acute transverse myelitis, spinal cord tumor, and spinal cord injury can cause paraparesis.

Table 10.15. Herbal prescriptions for paraparesis

Paraparesis https://meshb.nlm.nih.gov/record/ui?ui=D020335
Common prescriptions:
Sānbìtāng 5g shūjīnghuóxuètāng 5g dāngguīniāntòngtāng 5g + acupuncture Sānbìtāng 5g shūjīnghuóxuètāng 5g dúhuójìshēngtāng 5g Sānbìtāng 5g shūjīnghuóxuètāng 5g + acupuncture
Alternative prescriptions:
Sānbìtāng 5g Sānbìtāng 5g shàngzhōngxiàtōngyòngtòngfēngwán 4g huǒmárén 1g yánhúsuǒ 1g Sānbìtāng 5g wǔjīsǎn 2g Dúhuójìshēngtāng 5g dùzhòng 1g xùduàn 1g Dúhuójìshēngtāng 5g sháoyàogāncǎotāng 2g + acupuncture
Indicated diseases:
Unspecified disease of spinal cord 336.9 (Disease of spinal cord, unspecified G959); Malignant neoplasm of spinal cord 192.2 (Malignant neoplasm of spinal cord C720, Malignant neoplasm of cauda equina C721); Unspecified disorders of nervous system 349.9 (Disorder of central nervous system, unspecified G969); Malignant neoplasm of nervous system, part unspecified 192.9 (Malignant neoplasm of central nervous system, unspecified C729); Cardiovascular disease, unspecified 429.2 (Atherosclerotic heart disease of native coronary artery without angina pectoris I2510); Multiple myeloma 203.0; Unspecified hemorrhagic conditions 287.9 (Hemorrhagic condition, unspecified D699); Unspecified diseases of blood and blood-forming organs 289.9 (Disease of blood and blood-forming organs, unspecified D759); Hemangioma of unspecified site 228.00 (Hemangioma unspecified site D1800)

Paraparesis https://meshb.nlm.nih.gov/record/ui?ui=D020335	
Unspecified disease of spinal cord 336.9/G959 with paraparesis D020335:	
Shūjīnghuóxuètāng 5g dāngguīniāntòngtāng 5g dúhuójìshēngtāng 5g guīlùèrxiānjiāo 5g to ♀	Shūjīnghuóxuètāng 5g dāngguīniāntòngtāng 5g dúhuójìshēngtāng 5g guīlùèrxiānjiāo 5g to ♂
Cardiovascular disease, unspecified 429.2/I2510 with paraparesis D020335:	
Yùzhú 5g sìnìtāng 5g mǔdānpí 1g zhīzǐ 1g huánglián 0g to ♀	Yùzhú 5g sìnìtāng 5g mǔdānpí 1g zhīzǐ 1g to ♂

Sānbìtāng has traditionally been used for paralysis due to Wind, Dampness and chills and is today used for lumbago (Wang, 2019). Shàngzhōngxiàtōngyòngtòngfēngwán 'expels Wind, eliminates Dampness,' 'activates Blood, clears Heat,' and is today used for unspecified gout (Wang, 2019).

References

Eguchi, K., Malhotra, A. R., Malhotra, A. K., Harrington, E. M., Munoz, D. G., Nishimura, Y., Wilson, J. R., & Witiw, C. D. (2022). Pure extraosseous spinal epidural cavernous hemangioma presenting with acute paraplegia: a case report. *Spinal Cord Series and Cases*, *8*, 63. https://doi.org/10.1038/s41394-022-00531-9.

Fisher, M. (1952). Transient Monocular Blindness Associated with Hemiplegia. *Archives of Ophthalmology*, *47*(2), 167–203. https://doi.org/10.1001/archopht.1952.01700030174005.

Grigorean, V. T., Sandu, A. M., Popescu, M., Iacobini, M. A., Stoian, R., Neascu, C. & Popa, F. (2009). Cardiac dysfunctions following spinal cord injury. *Journal of Medicine and Life, 2*(2), 133–145.

Hamdan, A. L., Moukarbel, R. V., Farhat, F., & Obeid, M. (2002). Vocal cord paralysis after open-heart surgery. *European Journal of Cardio-Thoracic Surgery*, *21*(4), 671–674. https://doi.org/10.1016/s1010-7940(02)00019-2.

Martinot, J.-B., Le-Dong, N.-N., Cuthbert, V., Denison, S., Borel, J. C., Gozal, D., & Pépin, J. L. (2019). Respiratory Mandibular Movement Signals Reliably Identify Obstructive Hypopnea Events During Sleep. *Frontiers in Neurology*, *10*, 828. https://doi.org/10.3389/fneur.2019.00828.

Meyer, F. J., Borst, M. M., Zugck, C., Kirschke, A., Schellberg, D., KüblerW., & Haass, M. (2001). Respiratory Muscle Dysfunction in Congestive Heart Failure. *Circulation*, *103*(17), 2153–2158. https://doi.org/10.1161/01.cir.103.17.2153.

van den Ameele, J., Fuge, J., Pitceathly, R. D. S., Berry, S., McIntyre, Z., Hanna, M. G., Lee, M., & Chinnery, P. F. (2020). Chronic pain is common in mitochondrial disease. *Neuromuscular Disorders*, *30*(5), 413–419. https://doi.org/10.1016/j.nmd.2020.02.017.

Wahman, K., Nash, M., Westgren, N., Lewis, J., Seiger, Å., & Levi, R. (2010). Cardiovascular disease risk factors in persons with paraplegia: The Stockholm spinal cord injury study. *Journal of Rehabilitation Medicine*, *42*(3), 272–278. https://doi.org/10.2340/16501977-0510.

Wang, S. C. (2019). *Clinical Herbal Prescriptions: Principles and Practices of Herbal Formulations from Deep Learning Health Insurance Herbal Prescription Big Data*. WSPC. https://doi.org/10.1142/11211.

Chapter 11

Body Weight

Body weight is the quantity of heaviness of an individual expressed in kilograms or pounds. A very simple formula to calculate one's ideal body weight is the so-called Devine formula: 50 kilograms + 0.9 kilograms per centimeter over 152 centimeters for adult men. For women, we subtract 4.5 kilograms from the above result. The Devine formulas was first proposed by Ben J. Devine in 1974 to estimate the maximum drug dosage based on one's renal creatinine clearance whose estimation requires one's lean body weight, instead of total body weight. The formula therefore actually estimates one's lean body weight given his or her height. Since adipose tissue is needed as a cushion underneath the skin for both men and women and as an endocrine organ for female reproduction, the formula gives a value too low, especially for women. The other way is to calculate one's body mass index using the ratio of weight in kilograms to height in meters squared. A body mass index of 22 is considered ideal. Daily fluctuations in one's body weight are normal as one varies in his food and water consumption and elimination. However, excessive gain or loss of body weight, as shown in Figure 11.1, can indicate underlying diseases.

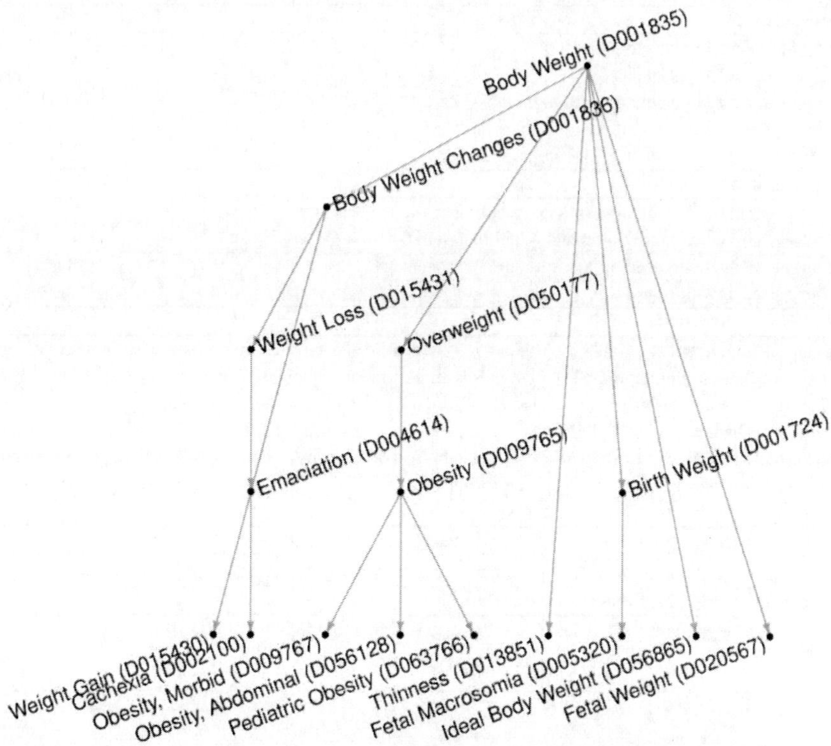

Figure 11.1. Signs and symptoms related to deviations from a healthy body weight.

The formulas and herbs commonly prescribed for the body weight signs and symptoms of Figure 11.1 include Fángfēngtōngshèngsǎn, Guìzhītāng, Sìnìtāng, Huòxiāngzhèngqìsǎn, Fángjǐhuángqítāng, Shānzhā, Dàhuáng, Shēngjiāng, Cǎojuémíng, and Wúzhūyú. Many of them are known for their effects on digestion.

The diseases that are commonly indicated or associated in this chapter are unspecified disorder of metabolism, unspecified cardiovascular disease, dysmetabolic syndrome X, unspecified endocrine disorder, and unspecified obesity.

11.1. Weight Gain

Weight gain is an increase in body weight, including muscle masses, fat deposits and water retention in the body. When the number of calories consumed through food exceeds the number of calories burned through daily activities such as work, commuting, grocery shopping, housekeeping and exercise, a person will gain weight.

Wǔlíngsǎn, Huòxiāngzhèngqìsǎn and Wèilíngtāng all 'help drain off Dampness' in addition to their modern uses for digestive conditions (Wang, 2019). Eye problems can be caused by retinopathy of diabetes which is associated with obesity.

Table 11.1. Herbal prescriptions for weight gain

Weight Gain: https://meshb.nlm.nih.gov/record/ui?ui=D015430.	
Common prescriptions:	
Wǔlíngsǎn 5g huòxiāngzhèngqìsǎn 5g Wèilíngtāng 5g huòxiāngzhèngqìsǎn 5g Huòxiāngzhèngqìsǎn 5g gégēnhuángqínhuángliántāng 2g Gégēnhuángqínhuángliántāng 5g huòxiāngzhèngqìsǎn 5g Huòxiāngzhèngqìsǎn 5g gégēnhuángqínhuángliántāng 3g	
Alternative prescriptions:	
Wèilíngtāng 5g gégēnhuángqínhuángliántāng 5g huòxiāngzhèngqìsǎn 5g Huòxiāngzhèngqìsǎn 5g huángqín 0g huángbò 0g huánglián 0g Wǔlíngsǎn 5g huòxiāngzhèngqìsǎn 5g xiāngfù 1g Huòxiāngzhèngqìsǎn 5g wǔlíngsǎn 2g	
Indicated and associated diseases:	
Cardiovascular disease, unspecified 429.2 (Atherosclerotic heart disease of native coronary artery without angina pectoris I2510); Diabetic retinopathy 362.0; Diabetes with peripheral circulatory disorders 250.7; Unspecified retinal disorder 362.9 (Unspecified retinal disorder H359); Disorder of eye, unspecified 379.90 (Unspecified disorder of eye and adnexa H579); Diabetes mellitus 250; Unspecified endocrine disorder 259.9 (Endocrine disorder, unspecified E349); Unspecified disorder of metabolism 277.9 (Metabolic disorder, unspecified E889); Dysmetabolic syndrome X 277.7 (Metabolic syndrome E8881); Schizophreniform disorder 295.4; Schizoaffective disorder 295.7; Schizophrenic disorders 295	
Cardiovascular disease, unspecified 429.2/I2510 with weight gain D015430:	
Yùzhú 5g sìnìtāng 5g gānlùyǐn 5g to ♀	Sìnìtāng 5g gānlùyǐn 5g mǔdānpí 1g zhīzǐ 1g huánglián 1g to ♂
Dysmetabolic syndrome X 277.7/E8881 with weight gain D015430:	
Zhēnwǔtāng 5g fùzǐ 1g gānjiāng 1g dìdāngtāng 0g to ♀	Gānlùyǐn 5g sìnìtāng 2g mǔdānpí 1g shānzhīzǐ 1g guālóurén 1g xièbái 1g to ♂

11.2. Weight Loss

Weight loss is a decrease in total body weight including body fluids, fats and other lean mass such as muscles, bones and connective tissues. Unintentional weight loss can be caused by malnutrition, medications, or diseases such as diabetes and cancer.

Guìzhītāng helps not only defense (against infection) but also digestion as we have learned in previous chapters. Weight loss improves cardiovascular disease risk factors (Brown et al., 2016) and also dermatological conditions (Rout and Das, 2022).

Table 11.2. Herbal prescriptions for weight loss

Weight Loss: https://meshb.nlm.nih.gov/record/ui?ui=D015431.	
Common prescriptions:	
Guìzhītāng 5g bànxià 1g dàhuáng 0g Guìzhītāng 5g báisháo 1g dàhuáng 0g Guìzhītāng 5g dàhuáng 0g Guìzhītāng 5g bànxià 1g shēngjiāng 1g guìzhī 1g Guìzhītāng 5g bànxià 1g shēngjiāng 1g guìzhī 1g dàhuáng 0g	
Alternative prescriptions:	
Guìzhītāng 5g bànxià 1g huángqín 1g dàhuáng 0g Guìzhītāng 5g bànxià 1g Guìzhītāng 5g gégēn 2g bànxià 1g dàhuáng 0g Guìzhītāng 5g yánhúsuǒ 1g dàhuáng 0g	
Indicated diseases:	
Cardiovascular disease, unspecified 429.2 (Atherosclerotic heart disease of native coronary artery without angina pectoris I2510); Diabetic retinopathy 362.0; Diabetes with peripheral circulatory disorders 250.7; Unspecified retinal disorder 362.9 (Unspecified retinal disorder H359); Disorder of eye, unspecified 379.90 (Unspecified disorder of eye and adnexa H579); Diabetes mellitus 250; Unspecified endocrine disorder 259.9 (Endocrine disorder, unspecified E349); Unspecified disorder of metabolism 277.9 (Metabolic disorder, unspecified E889); Other dermatoses 702; Polyneuropathy in diabetes 357.2 (Diabetes mellitus due to underlying condition with diabetic polyneuropathy E0842, Drug or chemical induced diabetes mellitus with neurological complications with diabetic polyneuropathy E0942, Type 1 diabetes mellitus with diabetic polyneuropathy E1042, Type 2 diabetes mellitus with diabetic polyneuropathy E1142, Other specified diabetes mellitus with diabetic polyneuropathy E1342); Diabetes with neurological manifestations 250.6; Dysmetabolic syndrome X 277.7 (Metabolic syndrome E8881)	
Cardiovascular disease, unspecified 429.2/I2510 with weight loss D015431:	
Yùzhú 5g sìnìtāng 5g mǔdānpí 1g zhīzǐ 1g huánglián 0g to ♀	Sìnìtāng 5g gānlùyǐn 5g mǔdānpí 1g zhīzǐ 1g huánglián 0g to ♂

11.3. Emaciation

Emaciation is extreme thinness and weakness of the body. Causes of emaciation include undernutrition, bacterial infections such as malaria and tuberculosis, and parasitic infections. Emaciation can lead to death if not treated.

Guìzhītāng is used in Section 4.2 for anorexia which is associated with emaciation. It is presumably used here to boost patient's immunity and digestion. Shēngjiāng and Hòupò are today used for functional digestive disorders (Wang, 2019). Hòupò is in addition for disorders of function of stomach (Wang, 2019). Sunken eyes and dry skin are among the physical characteristics of emaciation.

Table 11.3. Herbal prescriptions for emaciation

Emaciation: https://meshb.nlm.nih.gov/record/ui?ui=D004614.	
Common prescriptions:	
Guìzhītāng 5g báisháo 1g dàhuáng 0g Guìzhītāng 5g shēngjiāng 1g báisháo 1g dàhuáng 0g Guìzhītāng 5g shēngjiāng 1g guìzhī 1g Guìzhītāng 5g shēngjiāng 1g báisháo 1g	
Alternative prescriptions:	
Guìzhītāng 5g hòupò 1g zhǐshí 1g dàhuáng 0g Guìzhītāng 5g shēngjiāng 1g guìzhī 1g dàhuáng 0g Guìzhītāng 5g shēngjiāng 0g guìzhī 0g Guìzhītāng 5g wúzhūyútāng 3g fùzǐ 1g gānjiāng 1g	
Indicated diseases:	
Cardiovascular disease, unspecified 429.2 (Atherosclerotic heart disease of native coronary artery without angina pectoris I2510); Vascular disorders of skin 709.1 (Vasculitis limited to the skin, unspecified L959); Panuveitis 360.12 (Panuveitis, unspecified eye H44119); Behcet's syndrome 136.1 (Behcet's disease M352); Other dermatoses 702; Disorder of eye, unspecified 379.90 (Unspecified disorder of eye and adnexa H579); Unspecified condition of brain 348.9 (Disorder of brain, unspecified G939); Neoplasm of unspecified nature of brain 239.6 (Neoplasm of unspecified behavior of brain D496); Unspecified disorders of nervous system 349.9 (Disorder of central nervous system, unspecified G969); Malignant neoplasm of nervous system, part unspecified 192.9 (Malignant neoplasm of central nervous system, unspecified C729); Unspecified disorder of liver 573.9 (Liver disease, unspecified K769); Malignant neoplasm of liver, not specified as primary or secondary 155.2 (Malignant neoplasm of liver, not specified as primary or secondary C229); Diseases of the jaws 526	
Cardiovascular disease, unspecified 429.2/I2510 with emaciation D004614:	
Yùzhú 5g sìnìtāng 5g mǔdānpí 1g zhīzǐ 1g huánglián 1g to ♀	Yùzhú 5g sìnìtāng 5g zhìgāncǎotāng 2g to ♂
Unspecified condition of brain 348.9/G939 with emaciation D004614:	
Bǔyánghuánwǔtāng 5g dānshēn 1g tiānmá 1g shíchāngpú 1g yuǎnzhì 1g gōuténg 1g + acupuncture to ♀	Bǔyánghuánwǔtāng 5g + acupuncture to ♂
Unspecified disorder of liver 573.9/K769 with emaciation D004614:	
Xuèfǔzhúyūtāng 5g cháihúshūgāntāng 5g to ♀	Xuèfǔzhúyūtāng 5g cháihúshūgāntāng 5g to ♂

11.4. Cachexia

Cachexia, or wasting syndrome, is characterized by muscle mass loss, with or without fat mass loss, that is related to an underlying disease such as cancer, congestive heart failure, chronic obstructive pulmonary disease, and chronic kidney disease. The exact cause of cachexia is unknown but involves cytokine excess.

Table 11.4. Herbal prescriptions for cachexia

Cachexia: https://meshb.nlm.nih.gov/record/ui?ui=D002100.
Common prescriptions:
Guìzhītāng 5g bànxià 1g dàhuáng 0g Guìzhītāng 5g shēngjiāng 1g báisháo 1g dàhuáng 0g Guìzhītāng 5g shēngjiāng 1g guìzhī 1g Guìzhītāng 5g shēngjiāng 1g báisháo 1g
Alternative prescriptions:
Guìzhītāng 5g xìngrén 1g hòupò 1g dàhuáng 0g Guìzhītāng 5g báizhú 2g fùzǐ 2g báisháo 2g fúlíng 2g dǎngshēn 1g shēngjiāng 1g Guìzhītāng 5g xìngrén 1g hòupò 1g bànxià 1g dàhuáng 0g Guìzhītāng 5g báizhú 1g fùzǐ 1g Guìzhītāng 5g báisháo 1g dàhuáng 0g

Cachexia: https://meshb.nlm.nih.gov/record/ui?ui=D002100.	
Indicated diseases:	
Unspecified endocrine disorder 259.9 (Endocrine disorder, unspecified E349); Malignant neoplasm of ovary 183.0 (Malignant neoplasm of unspecified ovary C569); Unspecified disorder of female genital organs 629.9 (Unspecified condition associated with female genital organs and menstrual cycle N949); Malignant neoplasm of other and unspecified female genital organs 184; Malignant neoplasm of endocrine gland, site unspecified 194.9 (Malignant neoplasm of endocrine gland, unspecified C759); Malignant neoplasm of male genital organ, site unspecified 187.9 (Malignant neoplasm of male genital organ, unspecified C639); Unspecified disorder of male genital organs 608.9 (Disorder of male genital organs, unspecified N509, Pelvic and perineal pain R102); Malignant neoplasm of testis 186; Cardiovascular disease, unspecified 429.2 (Atherosclerotic heart disease of native coronary artery without angina pectoris I2510); Multiple myeloma 203.0; Unspecified hemorrhagic conditions 287.9 (Hemorrhagic condition, unspecified D699); Unspecified diseases of blood and blood-forming organs 289.9 (Disease of blood and blood-forming organs, unspecified D759); Diseases of the jaws 526; Unspecified disorder of intestine 569.9 (Disease of intestine, unspecified K639); Unspecified disorder of metabolism 277.9 (Metabolic disorder, unspecified E889); Whipple's disease 040.2 (Whipple's disease K9081)	
Unspecified endocrine disorder 259.9/E349 with cachexia D002100:	
Jiāwèixiāoyáosǎn 5g zuǒguīwán 5g nǚzhēnzǐ 1g hànliáncǎo 1g to ♀	Yòuguīwán 5g huánshǎodān 5g bājǐtiān 1g ròucōngróng 1g yínyánghuò 1g to ♂
Cardiovascular disease, unspecified 429.2/I2510 with cachexia D002100:	
Sìnìtāng 5g gānlùyǐn 5g mǔdānpí 1g zhīzǐ 1g huánglián 0g to ♀	Sìnìtāng 5g gānlùyǐn 5g mǔdānpí 1g zhīzǐ 1g huánglián 0g to ♂
Diseases of the jaws 526 with cachexia D002100:	
Guìzhītāng 5g dàhuáng 0g to ♀	Lǐzhōngtāng 5g bànxià 1g shārén 1g fúlíng 1g to ♂
Unspecified disorder of intestine 569.9/K639 with cachexia D002100:	
Lǐzhōngtāng 5g báisháo 1g guìzhī 1g to ♀	Lǐzhōngtāng 5g báisháo 1g guìzhī 1g to ♂

Xìngrén is today used for symptoms involving respiratory system and other chest symptoms, and allergic rhinitis (Wang, 2019), while Báizhú for allergic rhinitis, and functional digestive disorders (Wang, 2019).

11.5. Overweight

A person is overweight if his or her body mass index is in the range between 25 and 29.9 in kg/m/m. Causes of overweight include stress, insufficient or poor sleep, sedentary lifestyles, overeating, and hormone imbalance.

Table 11.5. Herbal prescriptions for overweight

Overweight: https://meshb.nlm.nih.gov/record/ui?ui=D050177.
Common prescriptions:
Shūjīnghuóxuètāng 5g dāngguīniāntòngtāng 5g niúxī 1g mòyào 1g rǔxiāng 1g yánhúsuǒ 1g fùzǐ 1g guìzhī 1g jīxuèténg 1g Shūjīnghuóxuètāng 5g dāngguīniāntòngtāng 5g niúxī 1g mòyào 1g rǔxiāng 1g yánhúsuǒ 1g fùzǐ 1g guìzhī 1g jīxuèténg 1g + acupuncture Shūjīnghuóxuètāng 5g dāngguīniāntòngtāng 5g niúxī 1g mòyào 1g rǔxiāng 1g yánhúsuǒ 1g fùzǐ 1g jīxuèténg 1g + acupuncture Shūjīnghuóxuètāng 5g dāngguīniāntòngtāng 5g niúxī 1g mòyào 1g rǔxiāng 1g yánhúsuǒ 1g fùzǐ 1g jīxuèténg 1g
Alternative prescriptions:
Shūjīnghuóxuètāng 5g dāngguīniāntòngtāng 5g niúxī 1g yánhúsuǒ 1g huángbò 1g cāngzhú 1g Shūjīnghuóxuètāng 5g dāngguīniāntòngtāng 2g chuānqī 1g dānshēn 1g wēilíngxiān 1g jīxuèténg 1g + acupuncture Shūjīnghuóxuètāng 5g dāngguīniāntòngtāng 2g chuānqī 1g mùguā 1g xùduàn 1g + acupuncture Shūjīnghuóxuètāng 5g dāngguīniāntòngtāng 5g sháoyàogāncǎotāng 3g + acupuncture

Table 11.5. (Continued)

Overweight: https://meshb.nlm.nih.gov/record/ui?ui=D050177.	
Indicated and associated diseases:	
Cardiovascular disease, unspecified 429.2 (Atherosclerotic heart disease of native coronary artery without angina pectoris I2510); Diabetic retinopathy 362.0; Diabetes with peripheral circulatory disorders 250.7; Unspecified retinal disorder 362.9 (Unspecified retinal disorder H359); Disorder of eye, unspecified 379.90 (Unspecified disorder of eye and adnexa H579); Diabetes mellitus 250; Unspecified endocrine disorder 259.9 (Endocrine disorder, unspecified E349); Unspecified disorder of metabolism 277.9 (Metabolic disorder, unspecified E889); Heart disease, unspecified 429.9 (Heart disease, unspecified I519); Dysmetabolic syndrome X 277.7 (Metabolic syndrome E8881)	
Cardiovascular disease, unspecified 429.2/I2510 with overweight D050177:	
Yùzhú 5g sìnìtāng 5g mǔdānpí 1g zhīzǐ 1g huánglián 0g to ♀	Yùzhú 5g sìnìtāng 5g zhìgāncǎotāng 2g to ♂
Heart disease, unspecified 429.9/I519 with overweight D050177:	
Sìnìtāng 5g gānlùyǐn 5g mǔdānpí 1g zhīzǐ 1g huánglián 0g to ♀	Sìnìtāng 5g gānlùyǐn 5g mǔdānpí 1g zhīzǐ 1g huánglián 0g to ♂

Shūjīnghuóxuètāng 'dredges meridians and cheers up Blood.' Dāngguīniāntòngtāng 'stops pain.' Their use here is supposed to promote physical activity of overweight patients.

11.6. Obesity

A body mass index equal to or greater than 30 kg/m/m is obesity. Normal body mass indexes fall in the range from 18.5 to 24.9 kg/m/m. Overweight and obesity incur too much body fat and can impair health.

Table 11.6. Herbal prescriptions for obesity

Obesity: https://meshb.nlm.nih.gov/record/ui?ui=D009765.	
Common prescriptions:	
Píngwèisǎn 5g ānzhōngsǎn 5g Píngwèisǎn 5g ānzhōngsǎn 5g xiāngshāliùjūnzǐtāng 5g Bànxiàxièxīntāng 5g píngwèisǎn 5g ānzhōngsǎn 5g	
Alternative prescriptions:	
Xiāngshāliùjūnzǐtāng 5g huòxiāngzhèngqìsǎn 5g sānqī 1g yánhúsuǒ 1g shārén 1g zhǐshí 1g Ānzhōngsǎn 5g xiāngshāliùjūnzǐtāng 5g Bànxiàxièxīntāng 5g jiāwèixiāoyáosǎn 4g chuānliànzǐ 1g bèimǔ 1g yánhúsuǒ 1g hǎipiāoxiāo 1g Xiāngshāliùjūnzǐtāng 5g jiāwèixiāoyáosǎn 4g bànxiàxièxīntāng 2g héhuānpí 1g yánhúsuǒ 1g	
Indicated diseases:	
Cardiovascular disease, unspecified 429.2 (Atherosclerotic heart disease of native coronary artery without angina pectoris I2510); Diabetic retinopathy 362.0; Diabetes with peripheral circulatory disorders 250.7; Unspecified retinal disorder 362.9 (Unspecified retinal disorder H359); Disorder of eye, unspecified 379.90 (Unspecified disorder of eye and adnexa H579); Diabetes mellitus 250; Obesity, unspecified 278.00 (Obesity, unspecified E669); Unspecified endocrine disorder 259.9 (Endocrine disorder, unspecified E349); Unspecified disorder of metabolism 277.9 (Metabolic disorder, unspecified E889); Hypertensive heart and chronic kidney disease 404; Secondary hypertension 405; Essential hypertension 401; Hypertensive chronic kidney disease 403; Hypertensive heart disease 402	
Cardiovascular disease, unspecified 429.2/I2510 with obesity D009765:	
Sìnìtāng 5g gānlùyǐn 5g mǔdānpí 1g zhīzǐ 1g huánglián 0g to ♀	Sìnìtāng 5g gānlùyǐn 5g mǔdānpí 1g zhīzǐ 1g huánglián 0g to ♂
Hypertensive heart and chronic kidney disease 404 with obesity D009765:	
Tiānmágōuténgyǐn 5g xuèfǔzhúyūtāng 5g to ♀	Tiānmágōuténgyǐn 5g xuèfǔzhúyūtāng 5g to ♂

Any of Píngwèisǎn, Ānzhōngsǎn, and Bànxiàxièxīntāng 'eases the Stomach.' The standard weight loss surgeries in conventional medicine–gastric sleeve, gastric bypass and adjustable gastric band–all involve stomach remodelling. We see in the table that the herbal prescriptions also focus on the stomach to reign in obesity.

11.7. Morbid Obesity

Morbid obesity is a body mass index of 40 or greater. Morbid obesity can interfere with one's basic physical functions so that the affected individuals become bedridden. The immobility burns off less calories, worsening the obesity. Multiple factors cause morbid obesity including genes, metabolism and behaviors.

Fángjǐhuángqítāng 'benefits Qi, strengthens the Spleen' and 'fends off Wind, drains off fluids.' Fángfēngtōngshèngsǎn 'releases exterior, targets interior' and 'guides Wind, clears Heat.' Modern uses of the former are for essential hypertension, and edema; and those of the latter are for constipation, and contact dermatitis and other eczema (Wang, 2019). They are believed to relieve the complications of morbid obesity. Jaw-wiring was found to be a safe but ineffective means of weight controlling for unmotivated patients (Castelnuovo-Tedesco et al., 1980).

Table 11.7. Herbal prescriptions for morbid obesity

<table>
<tr><td colspan="2">Morbid Obesity: https://meshb.nlm.nih.gov/record/ui?ui=D009767.</td></tr>
<tr><td colspan="2">Common prescriptions:</td></tr>
<tr><td colspan="2">Fángjǐhuángqítāng 5g fángfēngtōngshèngsǎn 5g shānzhā 1g cǎojuémíng 1g héyè 1g
Fángjǐhuángqítāng 5g fángfēngtōngshèngsǎn 5g shānzhā 1g cǎojuémíng 1g héyè 1g zéxiè 1g
Fángjǐhuángqítāng 5g fángfēngtōngshèngsǎn 5g shānzhā 1g cǎojuémíng 1g héyè 1g chénpí 1g
Fángjǐhuángqítāng 5g fángfēngtōngshèngsǎn 5g
Fángjǐhuángqítāng 5g fángfēngtōngshèngsǎn 5g shānzhā 1g cǎojuémíng 1g</td></tr>
<tr><td colspan="2">Alternative prescriptions:</td></tr>
<tr><td colspan="2">Fángfēngtōngshèngsǎn 5g liánggésǎn 2g shígāo 1g lóngdǎnxiègāntāng 1g zhīmǔ 0g huángbò 0g
Fángjǐhuángqítāng 5g fángfēngtōngshèngsǎn 2g máhuáng 2g gāncǎo 1g fùzǐ 1g fúlíng 1g gānjiāng 1g dǎngshēn 1g
Fángfēngtōngshèngsǎn 5g dàhuáng 2g gāncǎo 1g báizhú 1g fùzǐ 1g fúlíng 1g gānjiāng 1g máhuáng 1g dǎngshēn 1g
Fángfēngtōngshèngsǎn 5g liánggésǎn 3g shígāo 1g lóngdǎnxiègāntāng 1g dàhuáng 1g
Fángjǐhuángqítāng 5g fángfēngtōngshèngsǎn 5g dàhuáng 2g gāncǎo 1g fùzǐ 1g fúlíng 1g gānjiāng 1g dǎngshēn 1g</td></tr>
<tr><td colspan="2">Indicated and associated diseases:</td></tr>
<tr><td colspan="2">Unspecified disorder of intestine 569.9 (Disease of intestine, unspecified K639); Morbid obesity 278.01 (Morbid (severe) obesity due to excess calories E6601); Diseases of the jaws 526; Neoplasm of unspecified nature of digestive system 239.0 (Neoplasm of unspecified behavior of digestive system D490); Heart disease, unspecified 429.9 (Heart disease, unspecified I519); Cardiovascular disease, unspecified 429.2 (Atherosclerotic heart disease of native coronary artery without angina pectoris I2510); Obesity, unspecified 278.00 (Obesity, unspecified E669); Phobia, unspecified 300.20 (Phobic anxiety disorder, unspecified F409); Malignant neoplasm of colon 153</td></tr>
<tr><td colspan="2">Unspecified disorder of intestine 569.9/K639 with obesity, morbid D009767:</td></tr>
<tr><td>Fángfēngtōngshèngsǎn 5g mázǐrénwán 5g to ♀</td><td>Dàhuáng 5g mùxiāng 5g hòupò 5g huánglián 5g ānzhōngsǎn 5g xiāngshāliùjūnzǐtāng 5g to ♂</td></tr>
<tr><td colspan="2">Diseases of the jaws 526 with obesity, morbid D009767:</td></tr>
<tr><td>Tiáowèichéngqìtāng 5g dàhuáng 1g to ♀</td><td>Fángfēngtōngshèngsǎn 5g liánggésǎn 2g shígāo 1g lóngdǎnxiègāntāng 1g dàhuáng 1g zhīmǔ 0g huángbò 0g to ♂</td></tr>
<tr><td colspan="2">Heart disease, unspecified 429.9/I519 with obesity, morbid D009767:</td></tr>
<tr><td>Xuèfǔzhúyūtāng 5g bǔzhōngyìqìtāng 5g chuānqī 1g guìzhī 1g guālóurén 1g xièbái 1g to ♀</td><td>Shēngmàiyǐn 5g xuèfǔzhúyūtāng 5g dānshēn 2g chuānqī 1g guìzhī 1g guālóurén 1g xièbái 1g to ♂</td></tr>
</table>

Table 11.7. (Continued)

Morbid Obesity: https://meshb.nlm.nih.gov/record/ui?ui=D009767.	
Morbid obesity 278.01/E6601 with obesity, morbid D009767:	
Fángjǐhuángqítāng 5g fángfēngtōngshèngsǎn 5g shānzhā 1g cǎojuémíng 1g héyè 1g to ♀	Fángfēngtōngshèngsǎn 5g shānzhā 1g dānshēn 1g cǎojuémíng 1g héyè 1g zéxiè 1g to ♂

11.8. Abdominal Obesity

Abdominal obesity is excessive deposition of fat around the abdomen. In addition to the common causes for obesity, alcohol consumption correlates with the waist circumference in abdominally obese men. Abdominal obesity is significantly associated with cardiovascular disease and diabetes.

Xuèfǔzhúyūtāng's modern uses are for chest pain, hypercholesterolemia, and hyperglyceridemia (Wang, 2019), which are well-known risk factors for cardiovascular diseases.

Table 11.8. Herbal prescriptions for abdominal obesity

Abdominal Obesity: https://meshb.nlm.nih.gov/record/ui?ui=D056128.	
Common prescriptions:	
Fángfēngtōngshèngsǎn 5g shānzhā 1g cǎojuémíng 1g chénpí 1g Xuèfǔzhúyūtāng 5g shānzhā 1g dānshēn 1g héshǒuwū 1g cǎojuémíng 1g zéxiè 1g Xuèfǔzhúyūtāng 5g shānzhā 1g dānshēn 1g héshǒuwū 1g juémíngzǐ 1g zéxiè 1g Xuèfǔzhúyūtāng 5g shānzhā 1g dānshēn 1g héshǒuwū 1g cǎojuémíng 1g héyè 1g zéxiè 1g	
Alternative prescriptions:	
Fángfēngtōngshèngsǎn 5g shānzhā 0g juémíngzǐ 0g chénpí 0g Fángfēngtōngshèngsǎn 5g dàhuáng 1g shānzhā 1g shénqū 1g màiyá 1g Fángfēngtōngshèngsǎn 5g shānzhā 1g shénqū 1g láifúzǐ 1g Xuèfǔzhúyūtāng 5g wēndǎntāng 5g shānzhā 1g dānshēn 1g héshǒuwū 1g cǎojuémíng 1g zéxiè 1g	
Indicated diseases:	
Atherosclerosis 440; Obesity, unspecified 278.00 (Obesity, unspecified E669); Peripheral angiopathy in diseases classified elsewhere 443.81 (Other disorders of arteries, arterioles and capillaries in diseases classified elsewhere I798); Cardiovascular disease, unspecified 429.2 (Atherosclerotic heart disease of native coronary artery without angina pectoris I2510); Unspecified disorder of metabolism 277.9 (Metabolic disorder, unspecified E889); Heart disease, unspecified 429.9 (Heart disease, unspecified I519); Dysmetabolic syndrome X 277.7 (Metabolic syndrome E8881)	
Atherosclerosis 440 with obesity, abdominal D056128:	
Xuèfǔzhúyūtāng 5g to ♀	Xuèfǔzhúyūtāng 5g shānzhā 1g dānshēn 1g to ♂
Heart disease, unspecified 429.9/I519 with obesity, abdominal D056128:	
Sìnìtāng 5g gānlùyǐn 5g zhìgāncǎotāng 5g to ♀	Xuèfǔzhúyūtāng 5g dānshēn 2g chuānqī 1g guìzhī 1g guālóurén 1g xièbái 1g to ♂
Cardiovascular disease, unspecified 429.2/I2510 with obesity, abdominal D056128:	
Yùzhú 5g sìnìtāng 5g gānlùyǐn 5g to ♀	Sìnìtāng 5g gānlùyǐn 5g lóngdǎnxiègāntāng 5g to ♂

11.9. Pediatric Obesity

Pediatric obesity, or childhood obesity, is body mass index of children (ages 2-12) and adolescents (ages 13-18) above the recommended age- and sex-specific cut-off value. Family eating habits, sugary beverages and snack foods add to the causes of childhood obesity.

Table 11.9. Herbal prescriptions for pediatric obesity

Pediatric Obesity: https://meshb.nlm.nih.gov/record/ui?ui=D063766.	
Common prescriptions:	
Fángfēngtōngshèngsǎn 5g shānzhā 1g shénqū 1g màiyá 1g dàhuáng 0g Fángfēngtōngshèngsǎn 5g shānzhā 1g shénqū 1g màiyá 1g Fángfēngtōngshèngsǎn 5g shānzhā 1g dānshēn 1g héshǒuwū 1g cǎojuémíng 1g chénpí 1g zéxiè 1g	
Alternative prescriptions:	
Fángfēngtōngshèngsǎn 5g shānzhā 1g dānshēn 1g cǎojuémíng 1g zéxiè 1g Fángjǐhuángqítāng 5g fángfēngtōngshèngsǎn 5g shānzhā 1g héshǒuwū 1g cǎojuémíng 1g héyè 1g Fángfēngtōngshèngsǎn 5g shānzhā 1g shénqū 1g héyè 1g Fángfēngtōngshèngsǎn 5g fángjǐhuángqítāng 2g bǎihégùjīntāng 1g chénpí 1g Xuèfǔzhúyūtāng 5g fángfēngtōngshèngsǎn 5g shānzhā 1g dānshēn 1g chìsháo 1g	
Indicated diseases:	
Cardiovascular disease, unspecified 429.2 (Atherosclerotic heart disease of native coronary artery without angina pectoris I2510); Dysmetabolic syndrome X 277.7 (Metabolic syndrome E8881); Obesity, unspecified 278.00 (Obesity, unspecified E669); Unspecified disorder of metabolism 277.9 (Metabolic disorder, unspecified E889)	
Cardiovascular disease, unspecified 429.2/I2510 with pediatric obesity D063766:	
Yùzhú 5g sìnìtāng 5g mǔdānpí 1g zhīzǐ 1g huánglián 1g to ♀	Yùzhú 5g sìnìtāng 5g zhìgāncǎotāng 5g to ♂
Dysmetabolic syndrome X 277.7/E8881 with pediatric obesity D063766:	
Shūjīnghuóxuètāng 5g dāngguīniāntòngtāng 5g to ♀	Xuèfǔzhúyūtāng 5g wēndǎntāng 5g shānzhā 1g dānshēn 1g cǎojuémíng 1g héyè 1g zéxiè 1g to ♂

The modern uses of Shānzhā, Héshǒuwū and Héyè include disorders of lipoid metabolism (Wang, 2019). Today, Shénqū and Cǎojuémíng are used for gastritis and duodenitis, whereas Màiyá is used for disorders of function of stomach (Wang, 2019). Zéxiè is commonly used today for unspecified functional disorder of intestine (Wang, 2020), and Chénpí is used for dyspepsia and other specified disorders of function of stomach (Wang, 2020). They are believed to support the formulas in the prescriptions to normalize the patient's digestive system.

11.10. Thinness

Thinness, or underweight, is body mass index less than 18.5 kg/m/m. An underweight person has a body weight that is considered too low to be healthy. Causes of underweight include malnutrition, hyperthyroidism, cancer, tuberculosis, diabetes, gastrointestinal and liver diseases.

Table 11.10. Herbal prescriptions for thinness

Thinness: https://meshb.nlm.nih.gov/record/ui?ui=D013851.
Common prescriptions:
Guìzhītāng 5g shēngjiāng 1g báisháo 1g dàhuáng 0g Sìnìtāng 5g bànxià 1g dàhuáng 0g Guìzhītāng 5g shēngjiāng 1g guìzhī 1g Guìzhītāng 5g bànxià 1g dàhuáng 0g Guìzhītāng 5g shēngjiāng 1g báisháo 1g

Table 11.10. (Continued)

Thinness: https://meshb.nlm.nih.gov/record/ui?ui=D013851.	
Alternative prescriptions:	
Guìzhītāng 5g báisháo 1g dàhuáng 0g Sìnìtāng 5g rénshēn 1g bànxià 1g dàhuáng 0g	
Indicated diseases:	
Dysmetabolic syndrome X 277.7 (Metabolic syndrome E8881); Unspecified disorder of metabolism 277.9 (Metabolic disorder, unspecified E889); Heart disease, unspecified 429.9 (Heart disease, unspecified I519); Unspecified congenital anomaly of heart 746.9 (Congenital malformation of cardiac chambers and connections, unspecified Q209, Congenital malformation of heart, unspecified Q249); Cardiovascular disease, unspecified 429.2 (Atherosclerotic heart disease of native coronary artery without angina pectoris I2510); Human immunodeficiency virus [HIV] disease 042 (Human immunodeficiency virus [HIV] disease B20); Unspecified disorder of intestine 569.9 (Disease of intestine, unspecified K639); Diseases of the jaws 526	
Dysmetabolic syndrome X 277.7/E8881 with thinness D013851:	
Zhēnwǔtāng 5g fùzǐ 1g gānjiāng 1g dǐdāngtāng 0g to ♀	Zhēnwǔtāng 5g fùzǐ 1g gānjiāng 1g to ♂
Heart disease, unspecified 429.9/I519 with thinness D013851:	
Sìnìtāng 5g gānlùyǐn 5g mǔdānpí 1g zhīzǐ 1g huánglián 0g to ♀	Sìnìtāng 5g gānlùyǐn 5g mǔdānpí 1g zhīzǐ 1g huánglián 0g to ♂
Unspecified disorder of metabolism 277.9/E889 with thinness D013851:	
Huángqíwǔwùtāng 5g dàcháihútāng 2g xiāozhìwán 2g to ♀	Liùwèidìhuángwán 5g bǔzhōngyìqìtāng 5g dānshēn 1g to ♂
Unspecified disorder of intestine 569.9/K639 with thinness D013851:	
Lǐzhōngtāng 5g báisháo 1g guìzhī 1g to ♀	Lǐzhōngtāng 5g bànxià 1g shārén 1g fúlíng 1g to ♂
Cardiovascular disease, unspecified 429.2/I2510 with thinness D013851:	
Sìnìtāng 5g gānlùyǐn 5g mǔdānpí 1g zhīzǐ 1g huánglián 0g to ♀	Sìnìtāng 5g gānlùyǐn 5g mǔdānpí 1g zhīzǐ 1g huánglián 0g to ♂

Guìzhītāng is used for extreme thinness in Section 11.3. Its use for thinness here is imaginable. Note that underweight is a risk factor for cardiovascular disease (Park et al., 2017).

11.11. Fetal Macrosomia

Fetal macrosomia is weight of the newborn greater than 4 kilograms. Fetal macrosomia is determined retrospectively, i.e., after delivery of the baby. Fetal macrosomia incurs complications such as prolonged labor to the mother and shoulder dystocia to the fetus during birth. Common causes of fetal macrosomia are maternal diabetes and obesity.

Table 11.11. Herbal prescriptions for fetal macrosomia

Fetal Macrosomia: https://meshb.nlm.nih.gov/record/ui?ui=D005320.
Common prescriptions:
Yùquánwán 5g zhúyèshígāotāng 5g Báihǔjiārénshēntāng 5g zhībódìhuángwán 5g tiānhuā 1g xuánshēn 1g dìhuáng 1g màiméndōng 1g Báihǔjiārénshēntāng 5g zhībódìhuángwán 5g tiānhuā 1g xuánshēn 1g Báihǔjiārénshēntāng 5g zhībódìhuángwán 5g tiānhuā 1g xuánshēn 1g shíhú 1g Báihǔjiārénshēntāng 5g zhībódìhuángwán 5g tiānhuā 1g xuánshēn 1g shíhú 1g màiméndōng 1g
Alternative prescriptions:
Báihǔjiārénshēntāng 5g zhībódìhuángwán 4g tiānhuā 1g gégēn 1g Báihǔjiārénshēntāng 5g liùwèidìhuángwán 4g tiānhuā 1g Yùquánwán 5g tiānhuā 1g gégēn 1g Yùquánwán 5g zhúyèshígāotāng 5g qīngwèisǎn 5g Báihǔjiārénshēntāng 5g gānlùyǐn 2g

Fetal Macrosomia: https://meshb.nlm.nih.gov/record/ui?ui=D005320.
Indicated diseases:
Heart disease, unspecified 429.9 (Heart disease, unspecified I519); Diabetes mellitus 250; Unspecified congenital anomaly of heart 746.9 (Congenital malformation of cardiac chambers and connections, unspecified Q209, Congenital malformation of heart, unspecified Q249); Cardiovascular disease, unspecified 429.2 (Atherosclerotic heart disease of native coronary artery without angina pectoris I2510); Unspecified endocrine disorder 259.9 (Endocrine disorder, unspecified E349); Unspecified disorder of metabolism 277.9 (Metabolic disorder, unspecified E889)
Heart disease, unspecified 429.9/I519 with fetal macrosomia D005320:
Sìnìtāng 5g gānlùyǐn 5g mǔdānpí 1g zhīzǐ 1g huánglián 0g to ♀
Diabetes mellitus 250 with fetal macrosomia D005320:
Yùquánwán 5g báihǔjiārénshēntāng 5g to ♀
Cardiovascular disease, unspecified 429.2/I2510 with fetal macrosomia D005320:
Yùzhú 5g sìnìtāng 5g gānlùyǐn 5g to ♀

Yùquánwán, Zhúyèshígāotāng, Báihǔjiārénshēntāng and Zhībódìhuángwán are all used for diabetes in these days (Wang, 2019).

References

Brown, J. D., Buscemi, J., Milsom, V., Malcolm, R., & O'Neil, P. M. (2016). Effects on cardiovascular risk factors of weight losses limited to 5–10%. *Translational Behavioral Medicine*, *6*(3), 339–346. https://doi.org/10.1007/s13142-015-0353-9.

Castelnuovo-Tedesco, P., Buchanan, D. C., & Hall, H. D. (1980). Jaw-wiring for obesity. *General Hospital Psychiatry*, *2*(2), 156–159. https://doi.org/10.1016/0163-8343(80)90030-4.

Park, D., Lee, J.-H., & Han, S. (2017). Underweight: another risk factor for cardiovascular disease? *Medicine*, *96*(48), e8769. https://doi.org/10.1097/MD.0000000000008769.

Rout, A., & Das, A. (2022). Does weight loss lead to improvement of dermatological conditions: what is the evidence? *Clinical and Experimental Dermatology*, *47*(8), 1446–1453. https://doi.org/10.1111/ced.15208.

Wang, S. C. (2019). *Clinical Herbal Prescriptions: Principles and Practices of Herbal Formulations from Deep Learning Health Insurance Herbal Prescription Big Data*. WSPC. https://doi.org/10.1142/11211.

Wang, S. C. (2020). *Veterinary Herbal Pharmacopoeia*. Nova Science Publishers. https://doi.org/10.52305/GHTR1903.

Chapter 12

Delirium, Dementia, Amnestic, Cognitive Disorders

Humans adapt to changing environments not only to survive but also to thrive, and it is our high level of cognitive ability that sets us apart from other species on Earth. This distinctive cognition has been integral to the development and progression of human civilizations. Cognitive functions refer to the capabilities of attention, perception, memory, learning, problem-solving, decision-making, reasoning and language. As one ages, his or her cognitive functions decline as a result of neurodegeneration in the brain, in addition to any possible deterioration in the body. If cognitive decay affects one's independent living in the society, he or she needs medical treatment. Figure 12.1 shows the signs and symptoms of acquired cognitive disorders.

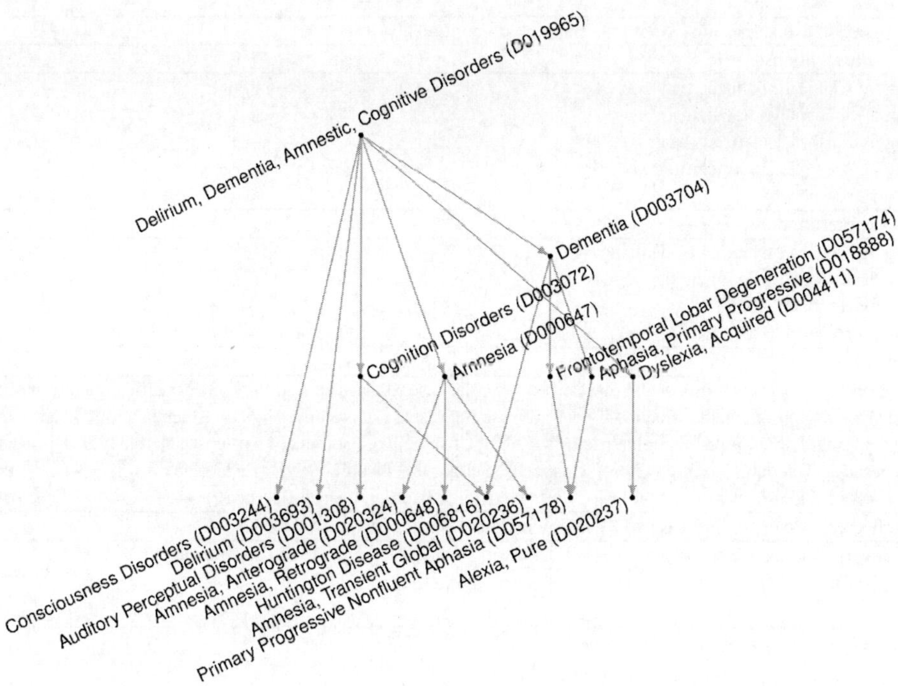

Figure 12.1. Signs and symptoms of acquired cognitive disorders.

The formulas commonly prescribed for the cognitive signs and symptoms are Sìnìtāng, Dāngguīniāntòngtāng, Sháoyàogāncǎotāng, and Dàzhēnjiāotāng. The herbs commonly supplemented in the prescriptions are Dàhuáng, Rénshēn, Bànxià, Guìzhī, Shēngjiāng, and Wúzhūyú. Note that acupuncture is also commonly prescribed along with the herbal prescriptions in this chapter.

The diseases that manifest or accompany the signs and symptoms of Figure 12.1 are unspecified disorders of nervous system, unspecified condition of brain, unspecified cardiovascular disease, unspecified cerebrovascular disease, amnestic disorder in conditions classified elsewhere, and dissociative amnesia.

12.1. Consciousness Disorders

Consciousness disorders are impairments in the ability to maintain awareness of oneself and the environment, as well as a diminished ability to respond to external stimuli. Consciousness disorders vary in their severity from intermittent minimal conscious state, persistent vegetative state, chronic coma to brain death. Consciousness disorders can be caused by traumatic brain injury or ischemic cerebrovascular disease.

Sìnìtāng 'revives Yang, rescues adversity,' and is prescribed to patients requiring critical care in previous chapters. Shēngjiāng and Rénshēn are today used for functional digestive disorders and Ròuguì for nonpsychotic mental disorders (Wang, 2019).

Table 12.1. Herbal prescriptions for consciousness disorders

<table>
<tr><td colspan="2">Consciousness Disorders: https://meshb.nlm.nih.gov/record/ui?ui=D003244.</td></tr>
<tr><td colspan="2">Common prescriptions:</td></tr>
<tr><td colspan="2">Sìnìtāng 5g bànxià 1g dàhuáng 0g
Sìnìtāng 5g shēngjiāng 1g guìzhī 1g
Sìnìtāng 5g rénshēn 1g wúzhūyú 1g
Sìnìtāng 5g shēngjiāng 1g guìzhī 1g xìxīn 1g
Sìnìtāng 5g rénshēn 1g</td></tr>
<tr><td colspan="2">Alternative prescriptions:</td></tr>
<tr><td colspan="2">Sìnìtāng 5g rénshēn 1g bànxià 1g dàhuáng 0g
Sìnìtāng 5g shēngjiāng 0g guìzhī 0g
Sìnìtāng 5g rénshēn 1g bànxià 1g
Sìnìtāng 5g ròuguì 1g wúzhūyú 1g zhìgāncǎotāng 1g</td></tr>
<tr><td colspan="2">Indicated diseases:</td></tr>
<tr><td colspan="2">Unspecified cerebrovascular disease 437.9 (Cerebrovascular disease, unspecified I679); Unspecified condition of brain 348.9 (Disorder of brain, unspecified G939); Cardiovascular disease, unspecified 429.2 (Atherosclerotic heart disease of native coronary artery without angina pectoris I2510); Unspecified disorders of nervous system 349.9 (Disorder of central nervous system, unspecified G969); Unspecified endocrine disorder 259.9 (Endocrine disorder, unspecified E349); Unspecified disorder of metabolism 277.9 (Metabolic disorder, unspecified E889)</td></tr>
<tr><td colspan="2">Unspecified cerebrovascular disease 437.9/I679 with consciousness disorders D003244:</td></tr>
<tr><td>Bǔyánghuánwǔtāng 5g dānshēn 1g shíchāngpú 1g yuǎnzhì 1g + acupuncture to ♀</td><td>Bǔyánghuánwǔtāng 5g dānshēn 1g shíchāngpú 1g yuǎnzhì 1g + acupuncture to ♂</td></tr>
</table>

12.2. Delirium

Delirium is an acute disturbance in one's attention, orientation, perception and psychomotor activities. Delirium is caused by an acute change in the function, structure or chemistry of the brain due to a disease process taking place outside of the brain. Examples of such processes are infection, medication side-effects, drug withdrawal, alcohol overconsumption, dehydration and malnutrition.

Table 12.2. Herbal prescriptions for delirium

<table>
<tr><td colspan="2">Delirium: https://meshb.nlm.nih.gov/record/ui?ui=D003693.</td></tr>
<tr><td colspan="2">Common prescriptions:</td></tr>
<tr><td colspan="2">Sìnìtāng 5g bànxià 1g dàhuáng 0g
Sìnìtāng 5g rénshēn 1g bànxià 1g dàhuáng 0g
Sìnìtāng 5g rénshēn 1g wúzhūyú 1g
Sìnìtāng 5g rénshēn 1g
Sìnìtāng 5g rénshēn 1g bànxià 1g</td></tr>
<tr><td colspan="2">Alternative prescriptions:</td></tr>
<tr><td colspan="2">Sìnìtāng 5g bànxià 1g hòupò 1g dàhuáng 0g
Sìnìtāng 5g báizhú 1g guìzhī 1g fúlíng 1g
Sìnìtāng 5g dàhuáng 0g
Máhuángfùzǐxìxīntāng 5g wúzhūyú 3g fùzǐ 3g guìzhī 2g wūméi 2g gānjiāng 2g zhìgāncǎotāng 2g</td></tr>
<tr><td colspan="2">Indicated diseases:</td></tr>
<tr><td colspan="2">Epilepsy, unspecified 345.9; Subacute delirium 293.1 (Delirium due to known physiological condition F05); Unspecified condition of brain 348.9 (Disorder of brain, unspecified G939); Unspecified disorders of nervous system 349.9 (Disorder of central nervous system, unspecified G969); Unspecified cerebrovascular disease 437.9 (Cerebrovascular disease, unspecified I679); Cardiovascular disease, unspecified 429.2 (Atherosclerotic heart disease of native coronary artery without angina pectoris I2510); Schizophreniform disorder 295.4; Schizoaffective disorder 295.7</td></tr>
<tr><td colspan="2">Epilepsy, unspecified 345.9 with delirium D003693:</td></tr>
<tr><td>Tiānmágōuténgyǐn 5g cháihújiālónggǔmǔlìtāng 4g hǎipiāoxiāo 1g nǚzhēnzǐ 1g tiānméndōng 1g dìhuáng 1g huángbò 1g to ♀</td><td>Tiānmágōuténgyǐn 5g jiāwèixiāoyáosǎn 5g cháihújiālónggǔmǔlìtāng 5g bǔyánghuánwǔtāng 5g dúhuójìshēngtāng 5g to ♂</td></tr>
<tr><td colspan="2">Unspecified cerebrovascular disease 437.9/I679 with delirium D003693:</td></tr>
<tr><td>Bǔyánghuánwǔtāng 5g chuānqī 1g dānshēn 1g shíchāngpú 1g yuǎnzhì 1g + acupuncture to ♀</td><td>Bǔyánghuánwǔtāng 5g chuānqī 1g dānshēn 1g shíchāngpú 1g yuǎnzhì 1g + acupuncture to ♂</td></tr>
</table>

Delirium is very common among hospitalized older patients. Hospitalization wears out one's Yang Qi. Sìnìtāng is therefore prescribed to replenish the Yang of delirious patients.

12.3. Auditory Perceptual Disorders

Auditory perceptual disorders, or central auditory processing disorders, are problems with how the brain understands sounds and speech, despite integrity of the outer, middle and inner ear structures and functions. It is caused by changes in an area of the brain called the auditory cortex that processes auditory information.

Table 12.3. Herbal prescriptions for auditory perceptual disorders

Auditory Perceptual Disorders: https://meshb.nlm.nih.gov/record/ui?ui=D001308.
Common prescriptions:
Xiǎocháihútāng 5g língguìshùgāntāng 5g niúxī 1g chēqiánzǐ 1g Xiǎocháihútāng 5g língguìshùgāntāng 5g shíchāngpú 1g yuǎnzhì 1g Xiǎocháihútāng 5g língguìshùgāntāng 5g niúxī 1g chēqiánzǐ 1g yuǎnzhì 1g Xiǎocháihútāng 5g língguìshùgāntāng 5g niúxī 1g chēqiánzǐ 1g yuǎnzhì 1g gōuténg 1g
Alternative prescriptions:
Sìnìtāng 5g bànxià 1g dàhuáng 0g Sìnìtāng 5g rénshēn 1g bànxià 1g yánhúsuǒ 1g dàhuáng 0g Guìzhītāng 5g bànxià 1g báisháo 1g dàhuáng 0g Xiǎocháihútāng 5g xiāngfù 2g màiyá 2g Língguìshùgāntāng 5g fùzǐ 1g xìxīn 1g xiǎochéngqìtāng 1g dàhuáng 0g

Table 12.3. (Continued)

Auditory Perceptual Disorders: https://meshb.nlm.nih.gov/record/ui?ui=D001308.	
Indicated and associated diseases:	
Unspecified disorder of ear 388.9 (Unspecified disorder of ear, bilateral H9393); Autistic disorder 299.0; Unspecified condition of brain 348.9 (Disorder of brain, unspecified G939); Unspecified disorders of nervous system 349.9 (Disorder of central nervous system, unspecified G969); Schizoaffective disorder 295.7; Schizophreniform disorder 295.4; Schizophrenic disorders 295; Unspecified cerebrovascular disease 437.9 (Cerebrovascular disease, unspecified I679); Cardiovascular disease, unspecified 429.2 (Atherosclerotic heart disease of native coronary artery without angina pectoris I2510); Schizotypal personality disorder 301.22 (Schizotypal disorder F21); Narcissistic personality disorder 301.81 (Narcissistic personality disorder F6081); Avoidant personality disorder 301.82 (Avoidant personality disorder F606)	
Unspecified disorder of ear 388.9/H9393 with auditory perceptual disorders D001308:	
Xiǎocháihútāng 5g língguìshùgāntāng 5g shíchāngpú 1g yuǎnzhì 1g to ♀	Xiǎocháihútāng 5g yìqìcōngmíngtāng 5g shíchāngpú 1g yuǎnzhì 1g to ♂
Unspecified cerebrovascular disease 437.9/I679 with auditory perceptual disorders D001308:	
Bǔyánghuánwǔtāng 5g dānshēn 1g shíchāngpú 1g yuǎnzhì 1g + acupuncture to ♀	Bǔyánghuánwǔtāng 5g chuānqī 1g dānshēn 1g shíchāngpú 1g yuǎnzhì 1g + acupuncture to ♂

Xiǎocháihútāng, Língguìshùgāntāng, Sìnìtāng and Guìzhītāng are used in Chapter 2 for an array of hearing signs and symptoms. They are used here again for auditory perceptual disorders.

12.4. Anterograde Amnesia

Anterograde amnesia is inability to form new memories, following the injury or disease that cause the amnesia. Examples of anterograde amnesia are forgetting a recent event such as meeting, meal, or phone call. Causes of anterograde amnesia are physical or organic damage to the area of the brain called the hippocampus in the temporal lobe which consolidates memory.

Table 12.4. Herbal prescriptions for anterograde amnesia

Anterograde Amnesia: https://meshb.nlm.nih.gov/record/ui?ui=D020324.
Common prescriptions:
Sìnìtāng 5g rénshēn 1g bànxià 1g dàhuáng 0g Sìnìtāng 5g rénshēn 1g wúzhūyú 1g Sìnìtāng 5g rénshēn 2g bànxià 2g dàhuáng 0g Sìnìtāng 5g rénshēn 1g Sìnìtāng 5g rénshēn 1g bànxià 1g
Alternative prescriptions:
Sìnìtāng 5g bànxià 1g yánhúsuǒ 1g dàhuáng 0g Sìnìtāng 5g rénshēn 1g wúzhūyú 0g Sìnìtāng 5g bànxià 1g Guìzhītāng 5g fùzǐ 1g dàhuáng 0g
Indicated diseases:
Unspecified cerebrovascular disease 437.9 (Cerebrovascular disease, unspecified I679); Unspecified condition of brain 348.9 (Disorder of brain, unspecified G939); Dissociative amnesia 300.12 (Dissociative amnesia F440); Cardiovascular disease, unspecified 429.2 (Atherosclerotic heart disease of native coronary artery without angina pectoris I2510); Unspecified disorders of nervous system 349.9 (Disorder of central nervous system, unspecified G969); Amnestic disorder in conditions classified elsewhere 294.0 (Amnestic disorder due to known physiological condition F04); Epilepsy, unspecified 345.9

Anterograde Amnesia: https://meshb.nlm.nih.gov/record/ui?ui=D020324.	
Unspecified cerebrovascular disease 437.9/I679 with amnesia, anterograde D020324:	
Bǔyánghuánwǔtāng 5g dānshēn 1g shíchāngpú 1g yuǎnzhì 1g + acupuncture to ♀	Bǔyánghuánwǔtāng 5g dānshēn 1g shíchāngpú 1g yuǎnzhì 1g + acupuncture to ♂
Epilepsy, unspecified 345.9 with amnesia, anterograde D020324:	
Cháihújiālónggǔmǔlìtāng 5g wēndǎntāng 5g shíchāngpú 1g yuǎnzhì 1g gōuténg 1g to ♀	Cháihújiālónggǔmǔlìtāng 5g wēndǎntāng 5g shíchāngpú 1g yuǎnzhì 1g to ♂

A modern use of Rénshēn is for unspecified vertiginous syndromes and labyrinthine disorders (Wang, 2020), which frequently co-occurs with memory loss in patients with vascular dementia.

12.5. Retrograde Amnesia

Retrograde amnesia is inability to recall memories that were formed before the event that caused the amnesia. Examples of retrograde amnesia are forgetting the name of a close childhood friend but remember that of a newly introduced friend. Causes of retrograde amnesia are damage or degeneration, such as stroke or Alzheimer's disease, to the various regions of the brain where long-term memories are stored.

Wēndǎntāng is nowadays used for insomnia and sleep disturbance (Wang, 2019).

Table 12.5. Herbal prescriptions for retrograde amnesia

Retrograde Amnesia: https://meshb.nlm.nih.gov/record/ui?ui=D000648	
Common prescriptions:	
Sìnìtāng 5g shēngjiāng 1g guìzhī 1g Sìnìtāng 5g shēngjiāng 1g guìzhī 1g dàhuáng 0g Sìnìtāng 5g rénshēn 1g wúzhūyú 1g Sìnìtāng 5g rénshēn 1g Sìnìtāng 5g shēngjiāng 1g guìzhī 1g xìxīn 1g	
Alternative prescriptions:	
Sìnìtāng 5g bànxià 1g dàhuáng 0g Sìnìtāng 5g rénshēn 1g dàhuáng 0g Sìnìtāng 5g rénshēn 1g bànxià 1g dàhuáng 0g Sìnìtāng 5g rénshēn 2g dàhuáng 0g Sìnìtāng 5g rénshēn 1g wúzhūyú 1g dàhuáng 0g	
Indicated diseases:	
Unspecified cerebrovascular disease 437.9 (Cerebrovascular disease, unspecified I679); Unspecified condition of brain 348.9 (Disorder of brain, unspecified G939); Dissociative amnesia 300.12 (Dissociative amnesia F440); Cardiovascular disease, unspecified 429.2 (Atherosclerotic heart disease of native coronary artery without angina pectoris I2510); Unspecified disorders of nervous system 349.9 (Disorder of central nervous system, unspecified G969); Amnestic disorder in conditions classified elsewhere 294.0 (Amnestic disorder due to known physiological condition F04); Neoplasm of unspecified nature of brain 239.6 (Neoplasm of unspecified behavior of brain D496); Malignant neoplasm of nervous system, part unspecified 192.9 (Malignant neoplasm of central nervous system, unspecified C729); Epilepsy, unspecified 345.9	
Unspecified cerebrovascular disease 437.9/I679 with amnesia, retrograde D000648:	
Bǔyánghuánwǔtāng 5g dānshēn 1g shíchāngpú 1g yuǎnzhì 1g + acupuncture to ♀	Bǔyánghuánwǔtāng 5g dānshēn 1g shíchāngpú 1g yuǎnzhì 1g + acupuncture to ♂
Unspecified condition of brain 348.9/G939 with amnesia, retrograde D000648:	
Bǔyánghuánwǔtāng 5g chuānqī 1g dānshēn 1g shíchāngpú 1g yuǎnzhì 1g + acupuncture to ♀	Bǔyánghuánwǔtāng 5g + acupuncture to ♂
Epilepsy, unspecified 345.9 with amnesia, retrograde D000648:	
Cháihújiālónggǔmǔlìtāng 5g báizhú 1g hǎipiāoxiāo 1g dǎngshēn 1g nǚzhēnzǐ 1g tiānméndōng 1g dìhuáng 0g to ♀	Wēndǎntāng 5g cháihújiālónggǔmǔlìtāng 4g shíchāngpú 1g yuǎnzhì 1g to ♂

12.6. Transient Global Amnesia

Transient global amnesia is temporal loss of short- and long-term memories except a few deeply rooted facts about one's childhood and family. Patients with transient global amnesia return to normal within 24 hours except forgetting about what happened during the episode. Causes of transient global amnesia are unknown but its occurrence is associated with migraine, epilepsy, emotional stress, and strenuous physical activity including sexual intercourse.

One of the modern uses of Shēngjiāng and Guìzhī is for headache (Wang, 2020). They are presumably prescribed here to alleviate migraine which can precipitate transient global amnesia.

Table 12.6. Herbal prescriptions for transient global amnesia

Transient Global Amnesia: https://meshb.nlm.nih.gov/record/ui?ui=D020236.	
Common prescriptions:	
Sìnìtāng 5g shēngjiāng 1g guìzhī 1g Sìnìtāng 5g shēngjiāng 1g guìzhī 1g dàhuáng 0g Sìnìtāng 5g shēngjiāng 1g guìzhī 1g máhuáng 1g Sìnìtāng 5g shēngjiāng 1g guìzhī 1g xìxīn 1g	
Alternative prescriptions:	
Sìnìtāng 5g shēngjiāng 1g guìzhī 1g bànxià 1g Sìnìtāng 5g dāngguīsìnìtāng 5g wúzhūyú 1g fùzǐ 1g gānjiāng 1g Sìnìtāng 5g xuèfǔzhúyūtāng 5g dānshēn 1g yánhúsuǒ 1g xiāngfù 1g yùjīn 1g Sìnìtāng 5g shēngjiāng 1g Sìnìtāng 5g dāngguīsìnìtāng 5g shēngjiāng 1g wúzhūyú 1g fùzǐ 1g	
Indicated diseases:	
Transient global amnesia 437.7 (Transient global amnesia G454); Migraine 346; Dissociative amnesia 300.12 (Dissociative amnesia F440); Unspecified condition of brain 348.9 (Disorder of brain, unspecified G939); Unspecified disorders of nervous system 349.9 (Disorder of central nervous system, unspecified G969); Amnestic disorder in conditions classified elsewhere 294.0 (Amnestic disorder due to known physiological condition F04); Epilepsy, unspecified 345.9; Unspecified cerebrovascular disease 437.9 (Cerebrovascular disease, unspecified I679); Cardiovascular disease, unspecified 429.2 (Atherosclerotic heart disease of native coronary artery without angina pectoris I2510)	
Transient global amnesia 437.7/G454 with amnesia, transient global D020236:	
Xuèfǔzhúyūtāng 5g bǔyánghuánwǔtāng 5g dānshēn 1g niúxī 1g to ♀	Xuèfǔzhúyūtāng 5g bǔyánghuánwǔtāng 5g sānqī 1g dānshēn 1g to ♂

12.7. Primary Progressive Aphasia

Aphasia is inability to auditorily comprehend, speak, read or write due to damage to the frontotemporal lobe on the left side of the brain that controls speech and language, not to the neurons and muscles responsible for the mechanics of hearing, voicing, reading and writing. Primary progressive aphasia is when the damage takes place slowly and progressively, caused by neurodegeneration such as frontotemporal dementia or Alzheimer's disease.

The difference between Sìnìtāng and Máhuángfùzǐxìxīntāng is that Gāncǎo and Gānjiāng in Sìnìtāng are replaced by Máhuáng and Xìxīn, both of which are used for allergic rhinitis (Wang, 2019). As aphasia could also be caused by brain inflammation (Marienfeld et al., 2010), Máhuángfùzǐxìxīntāng is prescribed.

Table 12.7. Herbal prescriptions for primary progressive aphasia

Primary Progressive Aphasia: https://meshb.nlm.nih.gov/record/ui?ui=D018888.	
Common prescriptions:	
Sìnìtāng 5g shēngjiāng 1g guìzhī 1g Máhuángfùzǐxìxīntāng 5g shēngjiāng 1g guìzhī 1g Máhuángfùzǐxìxīntāng 5g shēngjiāng 2g guìzhī 2g zhìgāncǎo 1g Máhuángfùzǐxìxīntāng 5g shēngjiāng 1g guìzhī 1g zhìgāncǎo 1g Máhuángfùzǐxìxīntāng 5g shēngjiāng 2g zhìgāncǎo 2g guìzhī 2g	
Alternative prescriptions:	
Sìnìtāng 5g shēngjiāng 1g guìzhī 1g dàhuáng 0g Máhuángfùzǐxìxīntāng 5g fùzǐ 3g guìzhī 3g gānjiāng 3g dàzǎo 2g zhìgāncǎotāng 2g Sìnìtāng 5g rénshēn 2g bànxià 2g dàhuáng 0g Sìnìtāng 5g bànxià 1g yánhúsuǒ 1g dàhuáng 0g	
Indicated diseases:	
Unspecified condition of brain 348.9 (Disorder of brain, unspecified G939); Unspecified disorder of metabolism 277.9 (Metabolic disorder, unspecified E889); Unspecified disorders of nervous system 349.9 (Disorder of central nervous system, unspecified G969); Unspecified cerebrovascular disease 437.9 (Cerebrovascular disease, unspecified I679); Cardiovascular disease, unspecified 429.2 (Atherosclerotic heart disease of native coronary artery without angina pectoris I2510); Pick's disease 331.11 (Pick's disease G3101)	
Unspecified condition of brain 348.9/G939 with aphasia, primary progressive D018888:	
Bǔyánghuánwǔtāng 5g chuānqī 1g dānshēn 1g shíchāngpú 1g yuǎnzhì 1g + acupuncture to ♀	Bǔyánghuánwǔtāng 5g chuānqī 1g dānshēn 1g shíchāngpú 1g yuǎnzhì 1g + acupuncture to ♂
Unspecified cerebrovascular disease 437.9/I679 with aphasia, primary progressive D018888:	
Bǔyánghuánwǔtāng 5g chuānqī 2g dānshēn 1g shíchāngpú 1g yuǎnzhì 1g + acupuncture to ♀	Bǔyánghuánwǔtāng 5g chuānqī 2g dānshēn 1g shíchāngpú 1g yuǎnzhì 1g + acupuncture to ♂
Pick's disease 331.11/G3101 with aphasia, primary progressive D018888:	
Bǔyánghuánwǔtāng 5g dānshēn 1g shíchāngpú 1g yuǎnzhì 1g + acupuncture to ♀	Bǔyánghuánwǔtāng 5g dānshēn 1g shíchāngpú 1g yuǎnzhì 1g + acupuncture to ♂

12.8. Anomia

People with anomia cannot retrieve the names of people or objects in speech or in writing, although other language capabilities are intact, due to damage to the temporal lobe of the brain. Stroke, brain tumor and Alzheimer's disease can cause anomia.

As anomia is a sine qua non of aphasia, we see aphasic prescriptions for anomia here.

Table 12.8. Herbal prescriptions for anomia

Anomia: https://meshb.nlm.nih.gov/record/ui?ui=D000849.
Common prescriptions:
Sìnìtāng 5g shēngjiāng 1g guìzhī 1g Máhuángfùzǐxìxīntāng 5g shēngjiāng 1g guìzhī 1g zhìgāncǎo 1g Máhuángfùzǐxìxīntāng 5g shēngjiāng 1g guìzhī 1g Bǔzhōngyìqìtāng 5g Máhuángfùzǐxìxīntāng 5g shēngjiāng 1g guìzhī 1g gāncǎo 1g
Alternative prescriptions:
Máhuángfùzǐxìxīntāng 5g fùzǐ 3g guìzhī 3g gānjiāng 3g dàzǎo 2g zhìgāncǎo 2g Sìnìtāng 5g shēngjiāng 0g guìzhī 0g Sìnìtāng 5g shēngjiāng 1g guìzhī 1g máhuáng 1g dàhuáng 0g Sìnìtāng 5g rénshēn 2g bànxià 2g

Table 12.8. (Continued)

Anomia: https://meshb.nlm.nih.gov/record/ui?ui=D000849.	
Indicated diseases:	
Unspecified cerebrovascular disease 437.9 (Cerebrovascular disease, unspecified I679); Unspecified condition of brain 348.9 (Disorder of brain, unspecified G939); Cardiovascular disease, unspecified 429.2 (Atherosclerotic heart disease of native coronary artery without angina pectoris I2510); Unspecified disorders of nervous system 349.9 (Disorder of central nervous system, unspecified G969); Neoplasm of unspecified nature of brain 239.6 (Neoplasm of unspecified behavior of brain D496); Malignant neoplasm of nervous system, part unspecified 192.9 (Malignant neoplasm of central nervous system, unspecified C729); Unspecified disorder of metabolism 277.9 (Metabolic disorder, unspecified E889)	
Unspecified cerebrovascular disease 437.9/I679 with anomia D000849:	
Bǔyánghuánwǔtāng 5g chuānqī 2g dānshēn 1g shíchāngpú 1g yuǎnzhì 1g + acupuncture to ♀	Bǔyánghuánwǔtāng 5g chuānqī 2g dānshēn 1g shíchāngpú 1g yuǎnzhì 1g + acupuncture to ♂
Unspecified condition of brain 348.9/G939 with anomia D000849:	
Bǔyánghuánwǔtāng 5g chuānqī 1g dānshēn 1g shíchāngpú 1g yuǎnzhì 1g + acupuncture to ♀	Bǔyánghuánwǔtāng 5g chuānqī 1g dānshēn 1g shíchāngpú 1g yuǎnzhì 1g + acupuncture to ♂

12.9. Acquired Dyslexia

Acquired dyslexia is loss of the ability to comprehend written words in previously literate individuals, despite intact vision. Traumatic brain injury, brain tumor, stroke and dementia can cause acquired dyslexia.

As memory impairment and dyslexia are associated (Lum et al., 2013), Sìnìtāng is prescribed to amnesia as it is prescribed to dyslexia here.

Table 12.9. Herbal prescriptions for acquired dyslexia

Acquired Dyslexia: https://meshb.nlm.nih.gov/record/ui?ui=D004411.	
Common prescriptions:	
Sìnìtāng 5g bànxià 1g dàhuáng 0g Sìnìtāng 5g bànxià 1g fúlíng 1g dàhuáng 0g Sìnìtāng 5g bànxià 1g shēngjiāng 1g guìzhī 1g	
Alternative prescriptions:	
Sìnìtāng 5g bànxià 1g wúzhūyú 1g dàhuáng 0g Sìnìtāng 5g shēngjiāng 1g guìzhī 1g Guìzhītāng 5g báisháo 1g huángqín 1g dàhuáng 0g + acupuncture	
Indicated diseases:	
Unspecified cerebrovascular disease 437.9 (Cerebrovascular disease, unspecified I679); Unspecified condition of brain 348.9 (Disorder of brain, unspecified G939); Alexia 315.01 (Dyslexia and alexia R480); Cardiovascular disease, unspecified 429.2 (Atherosclerotic heart disease of native coronary artery without angina pectoris I2510); Unspecified disorders of nervous system 349.9 (Disorder of central nervous system, unspecified G969); Neoplasm of unspecified nature of brain 239.6 (Neoplasm of unspecified behavior of brain D496); Malignant neoplasm of nervous system, part unspecified 192.9 (Malignant neoplasm of central nervous system, unspecified C729); Epilepsy, unspecified 345.9	
Unspecified cerebrovascular disease 437.9/I679 with dyslexia, acquired D004411:	
Bǔyánghuánwǔtāng 5g dānshēn 1g shíchāngpú 1g yuǎnzhì 1g + acupuncture to ♀	Bǔyánghuánwǔtāng 5g dānshēn 1g shíchāngpú 1g yuǎnzhì 1g + acupuncture to ♂
Unspecified condition of brain 348.9/G939 with dyslexia, acquired D004411:	
Bǔyánghuánwǔtāng 5g dānshēn 1g shíchāngpú 1g yuǎnzhì 1g + acupuncture to ♀	Bǔyánghuánwǔtāng 5g dānshēn 1g shíchāngpú 1g yuǎnzhì 1g + acupuncture to ♂
Epilepsy, unspecified 345.9 with dyslexia, acquired D004411:	
Cháihújiālónggǔmǔlìtāng 5g wēndǎntāng 5g shíchāngpú 1g yuǎnzhì 1g to ♀	Cháihújiālónggǔmǔlìtāng 5g wēndǎntāng 5g shíchāngpú 1g yuǎnzhì 1g to ♂

12.10. Pure Alexia

Individuals with pure alexia, i.e., pure word blindness, cannot read but other language-related capabilities such as writing, naming and auditory comprehension are intact. Infarction to the left posterior cerebral artery due to stroke or trauma causes pure alexia.

A case of alexia was reported in an adult onset adrenoleukodystrophy (Rosebush et al., 1999), a metabolic disease with which a patient can present with any combination of adrenal, gonadal, neurological, and psychiatric disorders. We also observe a spectrum of formulas for pure alexia in the table.

Table 12.10. Herbal prescriptions for pure alexia

<table>
<tr><td colspan="2">Pure Alexia: https://meshb.nlm.nih.gov/record/ui?ui=D020237.</td></tr>
<tr><td colspan="2">Common prescriptions:</td></tr>
<tr><td colspan="2">Sháoyàogāncǎotāng 5g shūjīnghuóxuètāng 5g dāngguīniāntòngtāng 5g + acupuncture
Sháoyàogāncǎotāng 5g shūjīnghuóxuètāng 5g + acupuncture</td></tr>
<tr><td colspan="2">Alternative prescriptions:</td></tr>
<tr><td colspan="2">Bǔzhōngyìqìtāng 5g + acupuncture
Shūjīnghuóxuètāng 5g
Shūjīnghuóxuètāng 5g dāngguīniāntòngtāng 5g mòyào 0g rǔxiāng 0g
Liùwèidìhuángwán 5g jiāwèixiāoyáosǎn 5g + acupuncture
Dāngguīniāntòngtāng 5g shūjīnghuóxuètāng 4g niúxī 1g mòyào 1g rǔxiāng 1g yánhúsuǒ 1g fùzǐ 1g guìzhī 1g fúlíng 1g jīxuèténg 1g + acupuncture</td></tr>
<tr><td colspan="2">Indicated diseases:</td></tr>
<tr><td colspan="2">Unspecified condition of brain 348.9 (Disorder of brain, unspecified G939); Peroxisomal disorders 277.86 (Peroxisomal disorder, unspecified E7150, Zellweger syndrome E71510, Neonatal adrenoleukodystrophy E71511, Adrenomyeloneuropathy E71522, X-linked adrenoleukodystrophy, unspecified type E71529, Other peroxisomal disorders E71548); Unspecified diseases of blood and blood-forming organs 289.9 (Disease of blood and blood-forming organs, unspecified D759); Unspecified disorders of nervous system 349.9 (Disorder of central nervous system, unspecified G969); Unspecified disorder of metabolism 277.9 (Metabolic disorder, unspecified E889); Alcohol abuse 305.0; Cardiovascular disease, unspecified 429.2 (Atherosclerotic heart disease of native coronary artery without angina pectoris I2510); Multiple myeloma 203.0; Unspecified hemorrhagic conditions 287.9 (Hemorrhagic condition, unspecified D699); Alexia 315.01 (Dyslexia and alexia R480)</td></tr>
<tr><td colspan="2">Unspecified condition of brain 348.9/G939 with alexia, pure D020237:</td></tr>
<tr><td>Bǔyánghuánwǔtāng 5g dānshēn 1g tiānmá 1g shíchāngpú 1g yuǎnzhì 1g + acupuncture to ♀</td><td>Bǔyánghuánwǔtāng 5g dānshēn 1g tiānmá 1g shíchāngpú 1g yuǎnzhì 1g + acupuncture to ♂</td></tr>
<tr><td colspan="2">Unspecified disorders of nervous system 349.9/G969 with alexia, pure D020237:</td></tr>
<tr><td>Shūjīnghuóxuètāng 5g píngwèisǎn 2g mùguā 1g sāngzhī 1g jīxuèténg 1g to ♀</td><td>Shūjīnghuóxuètāng 5g píngwèisǎn 2g mùguā 1g sāngzhī 1g jīxuèténg 1g to ♂</td></tr>
<tr><td colspan="2">Cardiovascular disease, unspecified 429.2/I2510 with alexia, pure D020237:</td></tr>
<tr><td>Sìnìtāng 5g gānlùyǐn 5g mǔdānpí 1g zhīzǐ 1g huánglián 0g to ♀</td><td>Xuèfǔzhúyūtāng 5g zhìgāncǎotāng 5g dānshēn 1g to ♂</td></tr>
</table>

References

Lum, J. A. G., Ullman, M. T., & Conti-Ramsden, G. (2013). Procedural learning is impaired in dyslexia: Evidence from a meta-analysis of serial reaction time studies. *Research in Developmental Disabilities, 34*(10), 3460–3476. https://doi.org/10.1016/j.ridd.2013.07.017.

Marienfeld, C. B., DiCapua, D. B., Sze, G. K., & Goldstein, J. M. (2010). Expressive Aphasia as a Presentation of Encephalitis with Bartonella henselae Infection in an Immunocompetent Adult. *Yale J Biol Med, 83*(2), 67–71.

Rosebush, P. I., Garside, S., Levinson, A. J., & Mazurek, M. F. (1999). The Neuropsychiatry of Adult-Onset Adrenoleukodystrophy. *The Journal of Neuropsychiatry and Clinical Neurosciences*, *11*(3), 315–327. https://doi.org/10.1176/jnp.11.3.315.

Wang, S. C. (2019). *Clinical Herbal Prescriptions: Principles and Practices of Herbal Formulations from Deep Learning Health Insurance Herbal Prescription Big Data*. WSPC. https://doi.org/10.1142/11211.

Wang, S. C. (2020). *Veterinary Herbal Pharmacopoeia*. Nova Science Publishers. https://doi.org/10.52305/GHTR1903.

Chapter 13

Sleep Wake Disorders

On average, humans spend about one third of our lives sleeping, while some other animals spend even more time sleeping. The fact that sleep is ubiquitous in the animal kingdom, including birds and mammals, suggests that it confers evolutionary advantages. The brain likely receives the most benefits from sleep as we feel so refreshed and happy in the morning after a good night of sleep. In particular, wastes of aerobic metabolism such as reactive oxygen species are cleared from the brain during sleep. Memories, an integral component of cognition, that are newly encoded are stabilized during sleep. Dreams also serve as a source of inspiration for our creative thinking. Sleep also rejuvenates other systems including the skeletomuscular, immune, and endocrine systems. We feel sleepy so we go to bed, as we feel hungry, so we take in food. Dysfunction of this sleep regulation arising from within the body can give rise to the signs and symptoms shown in Figure 13.1.

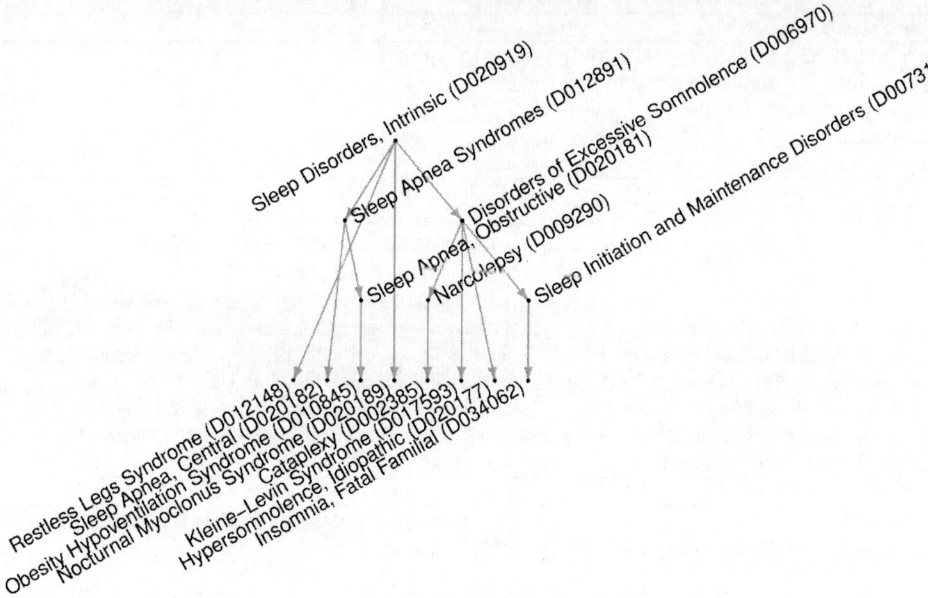

Figure 13.1. Hypersomnias or insomnias due to dysregulation of internal mechanisms or other sleep-related medical conditions.

The formulas and herbs that are commonly used for dyssomnia signs and symptoms include Sìnìtāng, Guìzhītāng, Shēngjiāng, Guìzhī, Dàhuáng, and Dānshēn. As needling has been shown to elicit autonomic nerve response, which varies across different sleep and wake stages, acupuncture is also frequently prescribed for the sleep-related signs and symptoms in this chapter.

The signs and symptoms can be indicative of or associated with various diseases, including unspecified disorders of the nervous system, unspecified cardiovascular disease, and unspecified condition of brain.

13.1. Restless Legs Syndrome

Restless legs syndrome, unlike habitual leg shaking, is an uncomfortable sensation in the legs and irresistible urge to move them in order to relieve the discomfort. Restless legs syndrome typically starts when one is at rest in the evening and worsens at night, disturbing the sleep. Causes of restless legs syndrome are unknown but changes in the dopamine pathway in the brain region controlling motion are involved. Risk factors for restless legs syndrome include nutrition deficiencies, kidney failure and Parkinson's disease.

Table 13.1. Herbal prescriptions for restless legs syndrome

Restless Legs Syndrome: https://meshb.nlm.nih.gov/record/ui?ui=D012148.	
Common prescriptions:	
Wūyàoshùnqìsǎn 5g huángqíwǔwùtāng 5g + acupuncture Wūyàoshùnqìsǎn 5g bǔyánghuánwǔtāng 5g + acupuncture	
Alternative prescriptions:	
Bǔyánghuánwǔtāng 5g dānshēn 1g shíchāngpú 1g yuǎnzhì 1g + acupuncture Bǔyánghuánwǔtāng 5g chuānqī 1g dānshēn 1g tiānmá 1g Wūyàoshùnqìsǎn 5g xuèfǔzhúyūtāng 3g + acupuncture Xiǎoxùmìngtāng 5g wūyàoshùnqìsǎn 5g bǔyánghuánwǔtāng 5g + acupuncture Wūyàoshùnqìsǎn 5g bǔyánghuánwǔtāng 5g dānshēn 1g	
Indicated diseases:	
Unspecified cerebrovascular disease 437.9 (Cerebrovascular disease, unspecified I679); Restless legs syndrome (RLS) 333.94 (Restless legs syndrome G2581); Cardiovascular disease, unspecified 429.2 (Atherosclerotic heart disease of native coronary artery without angina pectoris I2510); Unspecified condition of brain 348.9 (Disorder of brain, unspecified G939); Unspecified disorders of nervous system 349.9 (Disorder of central nervous system, unspecified G969); Congestive heart failure, unspecified 428.0 (Right heart failure due to left heart failure I50814, Heart failure, unspecified I509); Heart disease, unspecified 429.9 (Heart disease, unspecified I519); Multiple myeloma 203.0; Unspecified hemorrhagic conditions 287.9 (Hemorrhagic condition, unspecified D699); Unspecified diseases of blood and blood-forming organs 289.9 (Disease of blood and blood-forming organs, unspecified D759); Obsessive-compulsive disorders 300.3 (Mixed obsessional thoughts and acts F422, Hoarding disorder F423, Other obsessive-compulsive disorder F428, Obsessive-compulsive disorder, unspecified F429)	
Unspecified cerebrovascular disease 437.9/I679 with restless legs syndrome D012148:	
Bǔyánghuánwǔtāng 5g chuānqī 2g dānshēn 1g shíchāngpú 1g yuǎnzhì 1g + acupuncture to ♀	Bǔyánghuánwǔtāng 5g chuānqī 2g dānshēn 1g shíchāngpú 1g yuǎnzhì 1g + acupuncture to ♂
Congestive heart failure, unspecified 428.0/I50814,I509 with restless legs syndrome D012148:	
Shēngmàiyǐn 5g zhēnwǔtāng 5g to ♀	Shēngmàiyǐn 5g zhēnwǔtāng 5g dānshēn 1g to ♂
Cardiovascular disease, unspecified 429.2/I2510 with restless legs syndrome D012148:	
Sinìtāng 5g gānlùyǐn 5g mǔdānpí 1g zhīzǐ 1g huánglián 0g to ♀	Sinìtāng 5g gānlùyǐn 5g mǔdānpí 1g zhīzǐ 1g huánglián 0g to ♂
Restless legs syndrome (RLS) 333.94/G2581 with restless legs syndrome D012148:	
Sháoyàogāncǎotāng 5g huángqíwǔwùtāng 5g chuānxiōng 1g dānshēn 1g zhúrú 1g sāngzhī 1g dāngguī 1g jiānghuáng 1g to ♀	Sháoyàogāncǎotāng 5g huángqíwǔwùtāng 5g dānshēn 1g zhúrú 1g sāngzhī 1g jiānghuáng 1g to ♂

Wūyàoshùnqìsǎn is used in Section 5.3 for dyskinesia which involves involuntary repetitive movement of body parts including the legs and is used here for restless legs syndrome. A rising heart rate by periodic leg movements and sleep segmentation and deprivation due to restless leg syndrome raise the risk of cardiovascular diseases (Gottlieb et al., 2017).

13.2. Central Sleep Apnea

Central sleep apnea is repeated stops and restarts of breathing during sleep in the night, due to changes in the respiratory center in the brainstem. Brain infection, stroke and neck injury can cause central sleep apnea.

Table 13.2. Herbal prescriptions for central sleep apnea

Central Sleep Apnea: https://meshb.nlm.nih.gov/record/ui?ui=D020182.	
Common prescriptions:	
Guìzhītāng 5g shēngjiāng 1g báisháo 1g dàhuáng 0g Guìzhītāng 5g shēngjiāng 1g guìzhī 1g Máhuángfùzǐxìxīntāng 5g shēngjiāng 2g guìzhī 2g zhìgāncǎo 1g Guìzhītāng 5g shēngjiāng 1g báisháo 1g Máhuángfùzǐxìxīntāng 5g shēngjiāng 2g zhìgāncǎo 2g guìzhī 2g	
Alternative prescriptions:	
Sìnìtāng 5g bànxià 1g dàhuáng 0g Guìzhītāng 5g shēngjiāng 0g guìzhī 0g Máhuángfùzǐxìxīntāng 5g shēngjiāng 1g guìzhī 1g Sìnìtāng 5g bànxià 2g fúlíng 2g dàhuáng 0g	
Indicated and associated diseases:	
Congestive heart failure, unspecified 428.0 (Right heart failure due to left heart failure I50814, Heart failure, unspecified I509); Unspecified disorders of nervous system 349.9 (Disorder of central nervous system, unspecified G969); Unspecified sleep apnea 780.57 (Sleep apnea, unspecified G4730); Heart disease, unspecified 429.9 (Heart disease, unspecified I519); Cardiovascular disease, unspecified 429.2 (Atherosclerotic heart disease of native coronary artery without angina pectoris I2510); Hypertensive heart and chronic kidney disease 404; Secondary hypertension 405; Essential hypertension 401; Hypertensive chronic kidney disease 403; Hypertensive heart disease 402; Secondary cardiomyopathy, unspecified 425.9 (Cardiomyopathy due to drug and external agent I427); Congenital stenosis of aortic valve 746.3 (Congenital stenosis of aortic valve Q230)	
Congestive heart failure, unspecified 428.0/I50814,I509 with sleep apnea, central D020182:	
Shēngmàiyǐn 5g zhēnwǔtāng 5g dānshēn 1g huángqí 1g to ♀	Shēngmàiyǐn 5g xuèfǔzhúyūtāng 5g dānshēn 1g yùjīn 1g to ♂
Hypertensive heart and chronic kidney disease 404 with sleep apnea, central D020182:	
Bǔzhōngyìqìtāng 5g to ♀	Tiānmágōuténgyǐn 5g bǔyánghuánwǔtāng 5g to ♂
Secondary cardiomyopathy, unspecified 425.9/I427 with sleep apnea, central D020182:	
Xuèfǔzhúyūtāng 5g dānshēn 2g chuānqī 1g huángqí 1g rénshēn 1g guìzhī 1g guālóurén 1g xièbái 1g to ♀	Xuèfǔzhúyūtāng 5g dānshēn 2g chuānqī 1g huángqí 1g rénshēn 1g guìzhī 1g guālóurén 1g xièbái 1g to ♂

Guìzhītāng is used in Section 3.6 for hypoventilation and here for central sleep apnea which results in hypoventilation. Because of interactions between the cardiac and pulmonary systems, problems with one system can easily affect the other.

13.3. Obesity Hypoventilation Syndrome

Obesity hypoventilation syndrome is combination of a body mass index over 30 kg/m/m and an elevated daytime carbon dioxide level in the blood. The exact cause of obesity hypoventilation syndrome is unknown; however excessive weight in the chest wall makes it hard for the lung muscles to draw in air.

Table 13.3. Herbal prescriptions for obesity hypoventilation syndrome

<table>
<tr><td colspan="2">Obesity Hypoventilation Syndrome: https://meshb.nlm.nih.gov/record/ui?ui=D010845.</td></tr>
<tr><td colspan="2">Common prescriptions:</td></tr>
<tr><td colspan="2">Huángqíwǔwùtāng 5g dāngguīsìnìtāng 5g dānshēn 1g zhúrú 1g sāngzhī 1g jiānghuáng 1g
Huángqíwǔwùtāng 5g dāngguīsìnìtāng 5g dānshēn 2g zhúrú 2g sāngzhī 2g jiānghuáng 2g
Huángqíwǔwùtāng 5g dāngguīsìnìtāng 5g dānshēn 1g zhúrú 1g sāngzhī 1g jiānghuáng 1g + acupuncture
Xuèfǔzhúyūtāng 5g huángqíwǔwùtāng 5g dānshēn 1g zhúrú 1g sāngzhī 1g jiānghuáng 1g</td></tr>
<tr><td colspan="2">Alternative prescriptions:</td></tr>
<tr><td colspan="2">Dāngguīsìnìtāng 5g shēngjiāng 0g wúzhūyú 0g
Sìnìtāng 5g dāngguīsìnìtāng 5g shēngjiāng 1g wúzhūyú 1g
Sìnìtāng 5g huángqíwǔwùtāng 5g dānshēn 1g zhúrú 1g sāngzhī 1g jiānghuáng 1g
Guìzhītāng 5g gégēn 1g dàhuáng 0g
Huángqíwǔwùtāng 5g dānshēn 1g zhúrú 1g sāngzhī 1g huángqín 1g jiānghuáng 1g</td></tr>
<tr><td colspan="2">Indicated diseases:</td></tr>
<tr><td colspan="2">Obstructive sleep apnea (adult)(pediatric) 327.23 (Obstructive sleep apnea (adult) (pediatric) G4733); Obesity, unspecified 278.00 (Obesity, unspecified E669); Unspecified sleep apnea 780.57 (Sleep apnea, unspecified G4730); Unspecified disorders of nervous system 349.9 (Disorder of central nervous system, unspecified G969); Congestive heart failure, unspecified 428.0 (Right heart failure due to left heart failure I50814, Heart failure, unspecified I509); Heart disease, unspecified 429.9 (Heart disease, unspecified I519); Cardiovascular disease, unspecified 429.2 (Atherosclerotic heart disease of native coronary artery without angina pectoris I2510); Unspecified condition of brain 348.9 (Disorder of brain, unspecified G939)</td></tr>
<tr><td colspan="2">Congestive heart failure, unspecified 428.0/I50814,I509 with obesity hypoventilation syndrome D010845:</td></tr>
<tr><td>Shēngmàiyǐn 5g zhēnwǔtāng 5g dānshēn 1g to ♀</td><td>Shēngmàiyǐn 5g zhēnwǔtāng 5g dānshēn 1g to ♂</td></tr>
<tr><td colspan="2">Cardiovascular disease, unspecified 429.2/I2510 with obesity hypoventilation syndrome D010845:</td></tr>
<tr><td>Yùzhú 5g sìnìtāng 5g mǔdānpí 1g zhīzǐ 1g huánglián 0g to ♀</td><td>Yùzhú 5g sìnìtāng 5g zhìgāncǎotāng 5g to ♂</td></tr>
</table>

The modern uses of Huángqíwǔwùtāng are for chronic bronchitis, chronic sinusitis, and essential hypertension (Wang, 2019). It is thought to be used here to help the breathing of obesity hypoventilation syndrome patients. Note that obstructive sleep apnea patients are prone to acquiring obesity hypoventilation syndrome (Liu et al., 2017).

13.4. Nocturnal Myoclonus Syndrome

Nocturnal myoclonus syndrome, also known as periodic limb movement disorder, is characterized by involuntary and periodic movements of the lower extremities–unilateral or bilateral toes, ankles, knees and hips–during non-REM sleep. The exact cause of nocturnal myoclonus syndrome is unknown but psychopharmacologic medications and iron deficiency raise the risk of nocturnal myoclonus syndrome.

Table 13.4. Herbal prescriptions for nocturnal myoclonus syndrome

Nocturnal Myoclonus Syndrome: https://meshb.nlm.nih.gov/record/ui?ui=D020189.	
Common prescriptions:	
Guìzhītāng 5g shēngjiāng 1g báisháo 1g dàhuáng 0g Guìzhītāng 5g shēngjiāng 1g guìzhī 1g Guìzhītāng 5g shēngjiāng 1g guìzhī 1g dàhuáng 0g Guìzhītāng 5g shēngjiāng 1g báisháo 1g Guìzhītāng 5g shēngjiāng 1g báisháo 1g guìzhī 1g	
Alternative prescriptions:	
Guìzhītāng 5g shēngjiāng 1g guìzhī 1g + acupuncture Sìnìtāng 5g rénshēn 1g dàhuáng 0g Sìnìtāng 5g dāngguīsìnìtāng 5g shēngjiāng 1g wúzhūyú 1g	
Indicated diseases:	
Hypertensive heart and chronic kidney disease 404; Periodic limb movement disorder 327.51 (Periodic limb movement disorder G4761); Secondary hypertension 405; Essential hypertension 401; Hypertensive chronic kidney disease 403; Hypertensive heart disease 402; Cardiovascular disease, unspecified 429.2 (Atherosclerotic heart disease of native coronary artery without angina pectoris I2510); Unspecified disorders of nervous system 349.9 (Disorder of central nervous system, unspecified G969); Congestive heart failure, unspecified 428.0 (Right heart failure due to left heart failure I50814, Heart failure, unspecified I509); Heart disease, unspecified 429.9 (Heart disease, unspecified I519); Unspecified cerebrovascular disease 437.9 (Cerebrovascular disease, unspecified I679); Unspecified condition of brain 348.9 (Disorder of brain, unspecified G939)	
Hypertensive heart and chronic kidney disease 404 with nocturnal myoclonus syndrome D020189:	
Huángqíwǔwùtāng 5g chuānxiōng 1g dānshēn 1g zhúrú 1g sāngzhī 1g dāngguī 1g jiānghuáng 1g to ♀	Huángqíwǔwùtāng 5g dānshēn 1g zhúrú 1g sāngzhī 1g jiānghuáng 1g to ♂
Congestive heart failure, unspecified 428.0/I50814,I509 with nocturnal myoclonus syndrome D020189:	
Sìnìtāng 5g gānlùyǐn 5g mǔdānpí 1g zhīzǐ 1g huánglián 0g to ♀	Shēngmàiyǐn 5g zhēnwǔtāng 5g dānshēn 1g to ♂
Unspecified cerebrovascular disease 437.9/I679 with nocturnal myoclonus syndrome D020189:	
Bǔyánghuánwǔtāng 5g dānshēn 1g shíchāngpú 1g yuǎnzhì 1g + acupuncture to ♀	Bǔyánghuánwǔtāng 5g dānshēn 1g shíchāngpú 1g yuǎnzhì 1g + acupuncture to ♂

A major modern use of Guìzhī, the predominant herb in Guìzhītāng, is for other sleep disturbances (Wang, 2020). As nocturnal myoclonus syndrome disturbs sleep, it could be the reason behind the use of Guìzhītāng for nocturnal myoclonus syndrome. Nocturnal myoclonus syndrome prevails in patients with chronic kidney disease and increases their cardiovascular risk (Lindner et al., 2012).

13.5. Narcolepsy

Narcolepsy is a chronic condition of the brain that cannot regulate sleeping and waking cycles, resulting in excessive and irresistible sleepiness in the day regardless of whether sleep is adequate in the night. The exact cause of narcolepsy is unclear although autoimmune dysfunction is suspected.

Table 13.5. Herbal prescriptions for narcolepsy

Narcolepsy: https://meshb.nlm.nih.gov/record/ui?ui=D009290.
Common prescriptions:
Huángqíwǔwùtāng 5g dānshēn 1g zhúrú 1g sāngzhī 1g jiānghuáng 1g Huángqíwǔwùtāng 5g dānshēn 1g zhúrú 1g sāngzhī 1g jiānghuáng 1g + acupuncture Huángqíwǔwùtāng 5g dānshēn 1g zhúrú 1g sāngzhī 1g qínjiāo 1g jiānghuáng 1g Máhuángfùzǐxìxīntāng 5g shēngjiāng 2g guìzhī 2g zhìgāncǎo 1g
Alternative prescriptions:
Huángqíwǔwùtāng 5g dānshēn 2g zhúrú 2g sāngzhī 2g jiānghuáng 2g Máhuángfùzǐxìxīntāng 5g fùzǐ 3g guìzhī 3g dàzǎo 2g gānjiāng 2g zhìgāncǎotāng 2g Dāngguīsìnìtāng 5g shēngjiāng 1g wúzhūyú 1g Huángqíwǔwùtāng 5g dānshēn 1g zhúrú 1g sāngzhī 1g jiānghuáng 1g jīxuèténg 1g + acupuncture
Indicated diseases:
Narcolepsy 347.0; Recurrent hypersomnia 327.13 (Recurrent hypersomnia G4713); Epilepsy, unspecified 345.9; Unspecified condition of brain 348.9 (Disorder of brain, unspecified G939); Unspecified disorders of nervous system 349.9 (Disorder of central nervous system, unspecified G969); Schizoaffective disorder 295.7; Schizophreniform disorder 295.4; Multiple sclerosis 340 (Multiple sclerosis G35)

Huángqíwǔwùtāng 'benefits Qi, warms up meridians,' and 'harmonizes digestion, unlocks paralysis.' As Qi also helps regulate defense (i.e., immunity) in traditional Chinese medicine, the prescription is thought to help normalize the autoimmunity in narcolepsy.

13.6. Cataplexy

Cataplexy is transient and sudden loss of muscle strength triggered by strong emotions such as laughing, crying, terror and excitement. Patients with narcolepsy most likely experience cataplexy. The cause of cataplexy without narcolepsy is unknown.

Table 13.6. Herbal prescriptions for cataplexy

Cataplexy: https://meshb.nlm.nih.gov/record/ui?ui=D002385.
Common prescriptions:
Sìnìtāng 5g bànxià 1g dàhuáng 0g Sìnìtāng 5g shēngjiāng 1g guìzhī 1g Sìnìtāng 5g shēngjiāng 1g guìzhī 1g dàhuáng 0g Sìnìtāng 5g shēngjiāng 1g guìzhī 1g máhuáng 1g
Alternative prescriptions:
Sìnìtāng 5g rénshēn 1g dàhuáng 0g Sìnìtāng 5g guìzhī 1g máhuáng 1g xìxīn 1g Sìnìtāng 5g guìzhī 1g máhuáng 1g xìxīn 0g Sìnìtāng 5g bànxià 2g dàhuáng 0g
Indicated diseases:
Narcolepsy 347.0; Other disorders of lipoid metabolism 272.8 (Lipoid dermatoarthritis E7881, Other lipoprotein metabolism disorders E7889, Other specified metabolic disorders E8889); Recurrent hypersomnia 327.13 (Recurrent hypersomnia G4713); Unspecified condition of brain 348.9 (Disorder of brain, unspecified G939); Unspecified disorders of nervous system 349.9 (Disorder of central nervous system, unspecified G969); Unspecified disorder of metabolism 277.9 (Metabolic disorder, unspecified E889); Epilepsy, unspecified 345.9; Multiple sclerosis 340 (Multiple sclerosis G35)

Sìnìtāng is prescribed in Section 5.15 for catalepsy which can be considered a severe form of cataplexy.

13.7. Kleine-Levin Syndrome

Kleine-Levin syndrome is characterized by recurrent episodes of severe hypersomnia (up to 20 hours a day) accompanied by other cognitive and behavioral disturbances such as derealisation, overeating, hypersexuality and depression. Changes in the hypothalamic and thalamic areas of the brain which regulate appetite and sleep are suspected to cause Kleine-Levin syndrome.

Bŭzhōngyìqìtāng 'regulates the Spleen and Stomach' and is believed to help digestion, so is Xiăochάihútāng. Gāncăoxiăomàidàzăotāng and Cháihújiālónggŭmŭlìtāng are today used for anxiety state (Wang, 2019). Cháihújiālónggŭmŭlìtāng is also for neurasthenia, and nonpsychotic mental disorder (Wang, 2019). Guìzhījiālónggŭmŭlìtāng is nowadays used for unspecified insomnia (Wang, 2019). Their uses in the prescriptions are believe to counteract the diverse symptoms in Kleine-Levin syndrome.

Table 13.7. Herbal prescriptions for Kleine-Levin syndrome

Kleine-Levin Syndrome: https://meshb.nlm.nih.gov/record/ui?ui=D017593.	
Common prescriptions:	
Bŭzhōngyìqìtāng 5g + acupuncture Bŭzhōngyìqìtāng 5g	
Alternative prescriptions:	
Gāncăoxiăomàidàzăotāng 5g cháihújiālónggŭmŭlìtāng 5g băihé 2g bózĭrén 2g xiāngfù 2g yuănzhì 2g yùjīn 2g băihégùjīntāng 2g Xiăocháihútāng 5g língguìshùgāntāng 5g shíchāngpú 1g yuănzhì 1g Bŭzhōngyìqìtāng 5g chuānxiōng 1g shíchāngpú 1g xiāngfù 1g yuănzhì 1g Guìzhījiālónggŭmŭlìtāng 5g gāncăoxiăomàidàzăotāng 3g băihé 1g fúshén 1g yuănzhì 1g	
Indicated diseases:	
Recurrent hypersomnia 327.13 (Recurrent hypersomnia G4713); Eating disorder, unspecified 307.50 (Eating disorder, unspecified F509); Unspecified disorders of nervous system 349.9 (Disorder of central nervous system, unspecified G969); Stereotypic movement disorder 307.3 (Stereotyped movement disorders F984); Schizoaffective disorder 295.7; Schizophreniform disorder 295.4	
Recurrent hypersomnia 327.13/G4713 with Kleine-Levin syndrome D017593:	
Jiāwèixiāoyáosăn 5g gāncăoxiăomàidàzăotāng 5g héhuānpí 1g yèjiāoténg 1g to ♀	Xuèfŭzhúyūtāng 5g sháoyàogāncăotāng 5g shūjīnghuóxuètāng 5g + acupuncture to ♂

13.8. Idiopathic Hypersomnolence

Idiopathic hypersomnolence is characterized by prolonged nighttime sleep and daytime sleepiness. Patients with idiopathic hypersomnolence do not feel refreshed after sleep, nor do they wake up easily from sleep. The exact cause of idiopathic hypersomnolence is unknown.

Although Sháoyàogāncăotāng and Shūjīnghuóxuètāng are used for pains, a modern use of Báisháo and Gāncăo, which compose Sháoyàogāncăotāng and Shūjīnghuóxuètāng, is for other sleep disturbances (Wang, 2020). Systemic inflammation may promote excessive daytime sleepiness, increasing the risk of cardiovascular disease (Bock et al., 2022).

Table 13.8. Herbal prescriptions for idiopathic hypersomnolence

Idiopathic Hypersomnolence: https://meshb.nlm.nih.gov/record/ui?ui=D020177.	
Common prescriptions:	
Sháoyàogāncǎotāng 5g shūjīnghuóxuètāng 5g dāngguīniāntòngtāng 5g + acupuncture Sháoyàogāncǎotāng 5g shūjīnghuóxuètāng 5g + acupuncture	
Alternative prescriptions:	
Jiāwèixiāoyáosǎn 5g cháihúshūgāntāng 5g yèjiāoténg 2g dānshēn 1g shíchāngpú 1g yuǎnzhì 1g Shūjīnghuóxuètāng 5g sháoyàogāncǎotāng 4g mòyào 1g rǔxiāng 1g Shūjīnghuóxuètāng 5g dāngguīniāntòngtāng 5g niúxī 1g mòyào 1g rǔxiāng 1g yánhúsuǒ 1g fùzǐ 1g guìzhī 1g jīxuèténg 1g fùzǐ 1g + acupuncture Jiāwèixiāoyáosǎn 5g xiāngshāliùjūnzǐtāng 5g chuānxiōngchádiàosǎn 2g dānshēn 1g héhuānpí 1g Bǔzhōngyìqìtāng 5g	
Indicated diseases:	
Cardiovascular disease, unspecified 429.2 (Atherosclerotic heart disease of native coronary artery without angina pectoris I2510); Multiple myeloma 203.0; Unspecified hemorrhagic conditions 287.9 (Hemorrhagic condition, unspecified D699); Unspecified diseases of blood and blood-forming organs 289.9 (Disease of blood and blood-forming organs, unspecified D759); Unspecified condition of brain 348.9 (Disorder of brain, unspecified G939); Unspecified disorders of nervous system 349.9 (Disorder of central nervous system, unspecified G969); Unspecified disorder of metabolism 277.9 (Metabolic disorder, unspecified E889)	
Cardiovascular disease, unspecified 429.2/I2510 with hypersomnolence, idiopathic D020177:	
Sìnìtāng 5g gānlùyǐn 5g mǔdānpí 1g zhīzǐ 1g huánglián 0g to ♀	Xuèfǔzhúyūtāng 5g zhìgāncǎotāng 5g to ♂
Unspecified condition of brain 348.9/G939 with hypersomnolence, idiopathic D020177:	
Bǔyánghuánwǔtāng 5g dānshēn 1g tiānmá 1g shíchāngpú 1g yuǎnzhì 1g + acupuncture to ♀	Bǔyánghuánwǔtāng 5g shíchāngpú 1g yuǎnzhì 1g + acupuncture to ♂
Unspecified disorder of metabolism 277.9/E889 with hypersomnolence, idiopathic D020177:	
Rénshēnbàidúsǎn 5g xiǎocháihútāngqùrénshēn 5g yīnchénhāotāng 2g mùxiāng 1g yùjīn 1g to ♀	Dānshēn 5g tiānmágōuténgyǐn 5g sǎnzhǒngkuìjiāntāng 5g bǔyánghuánwǔtāng 5g to ♂

13.9. Sleep Initiation and Maintenance Disorders

Sleep initiation and maintenance disorders are unable to fall asleep or stay asleep. Causes of insomnia include pain, breathing problems, digestive problems, nocturia, stress, anxiety, trauma, caffeine and chemotherapy.

Table 13.9. Herbal prescriptions for sleep initiation and maintenance disorders

Sleep Initiation and Maintenance Disorders: https://meshb.nlm.nih.gov/record/ui?ui=D007319.
Common prescriptions:
Guìzhītāng 5g huángqí 1g dāngguī 1g Guìzhītāng 5g huángqí 2g báizhú 1g fùzǐ 1g fúlíng 1g Guìzhītāng 5g huángqí 2g báizhú 1g fúlíng 1g Guìzhītāng 5g huángqí 2g báizhú 1g fùzǐ 1g
Alternative prescriptions:
Guìzhītāng 5g wúzhūyútāng 3g fùzǐ 1g gānjiāng 1g Guìzhītāng 5g shēngjiāng 0g guìzhī 0g Sìnìtāng 5g guìzhī 1g máhuáng 1g xìxīn 0g Sìnìtāng 5g rénshēn 1g wúzhūyú 1g dàhuáng 0g Sìnìtāng 5g guìzhī 1g xìxīn 1g máhuáng 1g

Sleep Initiation and Maintenance Disorders: https://meshb.nlm.nih.gov/record/ui?ui=D007319.	
Indicated diseases:	
Other dermatoses 702; Unspecified disorders of nervous system 349.9 (Disorder of central nervous system, unspecified G969); Deformity and disproportion of reconstructed breast 612; Other disorders of breast 611; Benign mammary dysplasias 610; Posttraumatic stress disorder 309.81 (Post-traumatic stress disorder, unspecified F4310, Post-traumatic stress disorder, chronic F4312); Cardiovascular disease, unspecified 429.2 (Atherosclerotic heart disease of native coronary artery without angina pectoris I2510); Diabetes mellitus 250; Unspecified endocrine disorder 259.9 (Endocrine disorder, unspecified E349); Unspecified disorder of metabolism 277.9 (Metabolic disorder, unspecified E889); Dysmetabolic syndrome X 277.7 (Metabolic syndrome E8881); Phobia, unspecified 300.20 (Phobic anxiety disorder, unspecified F409)	
Other dermatoses 702 with sleep initiation and maintenance disorders D007319:	
Dāngguīsìnìtāng 5g wúzhūyú 1g fùzǐ 1g gānjiāng 1g to ♀	Dāngguīsìnìtāng 5g wúzhūyú 1g fùzǐ 1g gānjiāng 1g to ♂
Unspecified disorders of nervous system 349.9/G969 with sleep initiation and maintenance disorders D007319:	
Huángqíwǔwùtāng 5g chuānxiōng 1g dānshēn 1g zhúrú 1g sāngzhī 1g dāngguī 1g jiānghuáng 1g to ♀	Huángqíwǔwùtāng 5g chuānxiōng 1g dānshēn 1g zhúrú 1g sāngzhī 1g dāngguī 1g jiānghuáng 1g to ♂
Cardiovascular disease, unspecified 429.2/I2510 with sleep initiation and maintenance disorders D007319:	
Sìnìtāng 5g gānlùyǐn 5g mǔdānpí 1g zhīzǐ 1g huánglián 0g to ♀	Sìnìtāng 5g gānlùyǐn 5g mǔdānpí 1g zhīzǐ 1g huánglián 0g to ♂

Guìzhī in Guìzhītāng is today used for other sleep disturbances, among other conditions (Wang, 2020). Insomnia increases the risk of cardiovascular diseases, likely through a dysregulated hypothalamic-pituitary axis and increased inflammation (Javaheri and Redline, 2017).

13.10. Sleep Deprivation

Sleep deprivation, or sleeplessness, is inadequate quantity or quality of sleep to maintain decent alertness, performance and health. In contrast to insomnia, sleep deprived individuals are able to fall asleep. Sleep apnea, restless legs syndrome, working late, excessive caffeine consumption, anxiety and aging can cause sleep deprivation.

Table 13.10. Herbal prescriptions for sleep deprivation

Sleep Deprivation: https://meshb.nlm.nih.gov/record/ui?ui=D012892.
Common prescriptions:
Sìnìtāng 5g shēngjiāng 1g guìzhī 1g Sìnìtāng 5g guìzhī 1g máhuáng 1g xìxīn 1g Sìnìtāng 5g guìzhī 1g máhuáng 1g xìxīn 0g Sìnìtāng 5g guìzhī 2g máhuáng 2g xìxīn 1g Sìnìtāng 5g shēngjiāng 1g guìzhī 1g xìxīn 1g
Alternative prescriptions:
Sìnìtāng 5g guìzhī 1g máhuáng 0g Sìnìtāng 5g ròuguì 1g wúzhūyú 1g Bǔzhōngyìqìtāng 5g sìnìtāng 2g Sìnìtāng 5g máhuángfùzǐxìxīntāng 5g wúzhūyú 1g
Indicated diseases:
Unspecified disorders of nervous system 349.9 (Disorder of central nervous system, unspecified G969); Alcohol abuse 305.0; Cardiovascular disease, unspecified 429.2 (Atherosclerotic heart disease of native coronary artery without angina pectoris I2510); Dysmetabolic syndrome X 277.7 (Metabolic syndrome E8881); Unspecified disorder of metabolism 277.9 (Metabolic disorder, unspecified E889); Heart disease, unspecified 429.9 (Heart disease, unspecified I519)

Table 13.10. (Continued)

Sleep Deprivation: https://meshb.nlm.nih.gov/record/ui?ui=D012892.	
Unspecified disorders of nervous system 349.9/G969 with sleep deprivation D012892:	
Huángqíwǔwùtāng 5g chuānxiōng 1g dānshēn 1g zhúrú 1g sāngzhī 1g dāngguī 1g jiānghuáng 1g to ♀	Huángqíwǔwùtāng 5g chuānxiōng 1g dānshēn 1g zhúrú 1g sāngzhī 1g dāngguī 1g jiānghuáng 1g to ♂
Cardiovascular disease, unspecified 429.2/I2510 with sleep deprivation D012892:	
Yùzhú 5g sìnìtāng 5g mǔdānpí 1g zhīzǐ 1g to ♀	Yùzhú 5g sìnìtāng 5g mǔdānpí 1g zhīzǐ 1g to ♂
Heart disease, unspecified 429.9/I519 with sleep deprivation D012892:	
Sìnìtāng 5g gānlùyǐn 5g mǔdānpí 1g zhīzǐ 1g huánglián 0g to ♀	Sìnìtāng 5g gānlùyǐn 5g mǔdānpí 1g zhīzǐ 1g huánglián 0g to ♂

Sìnìtāng is supposed here to counteract the daytime sleepiness and tiredness complications of sleep deprivation. Sleep deprivation is associated with immune deregulation (Garbarino et al., 2021). Guìzhī's and Máhuáng's modern uses include allergic rhinitis (Wang, 2019). In addition, Guìzhī is also used for chronic pharyngitis and nasopharyngitis (Wang, 2019). Their incorporation in the prescriptions is therefore believed to help the immunity of sleep deprived patients.

13.11. Sleep Bruxism

Sleep bruxism is involuntary, repetitive clenching or grinding of the teeth during sleep. Causes of sleep bruxism are not well known but stress, anxiety, frustration, certain personality traits, and medications are risk factors.

Table 13.11. Herbal prescriptions for sleep bruxism

Sleep Bruxism: https://meshb.nlm.nih.gov/record/ui?ui=D020186.	
Common prescriptions:	
Guìzhītāng 5g báisháo 1g dàhuáng 0g Guìzhītāng 5g gégēn 1g Guìzhītāng 5g báisháo 1g dàhuáng 0g + acupuncture Guìzhītāng 5g gégēn 1g + acupuncture	
Alternative prescriptions:	
Guìzhītāng 5g shēngjiāng 0g guìzhī 0g Guìzhītāng 5g bànxià 1g dàhuáng 0g Guìzhītāng 5g shēngjiāng 1g báisháo 1g Guìzhītāng 5g máhuángfùzǐxìxīntāng 5g shēngjiāng 1g guìzhī 1g Máhuángfùzǐxìxīntāng 5g shēngjiāng 1g guìzhī 1g	
Indicated diseases:	
Sleep related bruxism 327.53 (Sleep related bruxism G4763); Unspecified disorder of joint, site unspecified 719.90 (Joint disorder, unspecified M259); Myopathy, unspecified 359.9 (Myopathy, unspecified G729); Unspecified disorders of nervous system 349.9 (Disorder of central nervous system, unspecified G969); Unspecified condition of brain 348.9 (Disorder of brain, unspecified G939)	
Sleep related bruxism 327.53/G4763 with sleep bruxism D020186:	
Guìzhītāng 5g báizhú 1g fùzǐ 1g to ♀	Guìzhītāng 5g báizhú 2g fùzǐ 2g báisháo 2g fúlíng 2g dǎngshēn 1g shēngjiāng 1g gānjiāng 1g dàhuáng 0g to ♂

Both Báisháo and Gégēn are today used for such general symptoms as unspecified sleep disturbance (Wang, 2019).

13.12. Somnambulism

Somnambulism, also known as sleepwalking, is getting up, walking and even performing complex tasks while in a state of sleep. Sleepwalking can last up to 30 minutes and sleepwalkers do not recall what happened after waking up in the morning. Causes of somnambulism are unknown.

Table 13.12. Herbal prescriptions for somnambulism

Somnambulism: https://meshb.nlm.nih.gov/record/ui?ui=D013009.	
Common prescriptions:	
Sìnìtāng 5g guìzhī 1g máhuáng 1g xìxīn 1g Sìnìtāng 5g guìzhī 1g máhuáng 1g xìxīn 0g Sìnìtāng 5g guìzhī 1g máhuáng 1g xìxīn 1g dàhuáng 0g	
Alternative prescriptions:	
Bǔzhōngyìqìtāng 5g + acupuncture Guìzhītāng 5g gégēn 2g dàhuáng 0g Sìnìtāng 5g shēngjiāng 1g guìzhī 1g Sìnìtāng 5g lǐzhōngtāng 5g ròuguì 1g yánhúsuǒ 1g zhìgāncǎotāng 1g + acupuncture Guìzhītāng 5g huángqí 2g dāngguī 1g + acupuncture	
Indicated diseases:	
Epilepsy, unspecified 345.9; Unspecified condition of brain 348.9 (Disorder of brain, unspecified G939); Unspecified disorders of nervous system 349.9 (Disorder of central nervous system, unspecified G969); Anorexia nervosa 307.1 (Anorexia nervosa, unspecified F5000); Eating disorder, unspecified 307.50 (Eating disorder, unspecified F509)	
Epilepsy, unspecified 345.9 with somnambulism D013009:	
Tiānwángbǔxīndān 5g cháihújiālónggǔmǔlìtāng 5g hǎipiāoxiāo 1g mùguā 1g báizhú 1g dìgǔpí 1g chuānxiōng 1g dìhuáng 1g to ♀	Wēndǎntāng 5g cháihújiālónggǔmǔlìtāng 4g tiānmá 1g shíchāngpú 1g yuǎnzhì 1g gōuténg 1g to ♂
Unspecified disorders of nervous system 349.9/G969 with somnambulism D013009:	
Huángqíwǔwùtāng 5g chuānxiōng 1g dānshēn 1g zhúrú 1g sāngzhī 1g dāngguī 1g jiānghuáng 1g to ♀	Huángqíwǔwùtāng 5g chuānxiōng 1g dānshēn 1g zhúrú 1g sāngzhī 1g dāngguī 1g jiānghuáng 1g to ♂

As Sìnìtāng is used in previous sections for sleep initiation and maintenance disorders as well as sleep deprivation, it is used here for sleepwalking, which is a problem with sleep maintenance and can contribute to sleep deprivation. Patients with sleep-related eating disorder are likely to be anorexics and share many clinical commonalities with sleepwalkers (Brion et al., 2012).

13.13. Jet Lag Syndrome

Jet lag syndrome occurs after one travels across over two timezones in a short time. Symptoms of jet lag vary and include sleep disturbance, cognitive deficits, daytime fatigue, headache, and gastrointestinal disturbances. Jet lag is caused by a mismatch of sleep-wake cycle between the body and the local environment.

Table 13.13. Herbal prescriptions for jet lag syndrome

Jet Lag Syndrome: https://meshb.nlm.nih.gov/record/ui?ui=D020179.	
Common prescriptions:	
Bǔzhōngyìqìtāng 5g + acupuncture Bǔzhōngyìqìtāng 5g	
Alternative prescriptions:	
Bǔzhōngyìqìtāng 5g shēngmàiyǐn 4g shíchāngpú 1g yuǎnzhì 1g Cháihújiālónggǔmǔlìtāng 5g shíchāngpú 1g fúshén 1g yuǎnzhì 1g + acupuncture Cháihújiālónggǔmǔlìtāng 5g wēndǎntāng 5g zhúrú 1g yèjiāoténg 1g yuǎnzhì 1g Cháihúguìzhītāng 5g wēndǎntāng 5g bózǐrén 1g yuǎnzhì 1g Cháihújiālónggǔmǔlìtāng 5g shíchāngpú 1g yuǎnzhì 1g	
Indicated diseases:	
Unspecified cerebrovascular disease 437.9 (Cerebrovascular disease, unspecified I679); Unspecified condition of brain 348.9 (Disorder of brain, unspecified G939); Cardiovascular disease, unspecified 429.2 (Atherosclerotic heart disease of native coronary artery without angina pectoris I2510); Unspecified disorders of nervous system 349.9 (Disorder of central nervous system, unspecified G969); Epilepsy, unspecified 345.9	
Unspecified cerebrovascular disease 437.9/I679 with Jet lag syndrome D020179:	
Bǔyánghuánwǔtāng 5g chuānqī 2g dānshēn 1g shíchāngpú 1g yuǎnzhì 1g + acupuncture to ♀	Bǔyánghuánwǔtāng 5g chuānqī 2g dānshēn 1g shíchāngpú 1g yuǎnzhì 1g + acupuncture to ♂
Unspecified disorders of nervous system 349.9/G969 with jet lag syndrome D020179:	
Huángqíwǔwùtāng 5g chuānxiōng 1g dānshēn 1g zhúrú 1g sāngzhī 1g dāngguī 1g jiānghuáng 1g to ♀	Huángqíwǔwùtāng 5g chuānxiōng 1g dānshēn 1g zhúrú 1g sāngzhī 1g dāngguī 1g jiānghuáng 1g to ♂
Unspecified condition of brain 348.9/G939 with jet lag syndrome D020179:	
Gāncǎoxiǎomàidàzǎotāng 5g cháihújiālónggǔmǔlìtāng 5g zhúrú 1g yèjiāoténg 1g yuǎnzhì 1g gōuténg 1g to ♀	Gāncǎoxiǎomàidàzǎotāng 5g cháihújiālónggǔmǔlìtāng 5g zhúrú 1g yèjiāoténg 1g yuǎnzhì 1g to ♂
Epilepsy, unspecified 345.9 with jet lag syndrome D020179:	
Tiānwángbǔxīndān 5g cháihújiālónggǔmǔlìtāng 5g hǎipiāoxiāo 1g nǚzhēnzǐ 1g báizhú 1g dǎngshēn 1g dìhuáng 0g to ♀	Tiānwángbǔxīndān 5g cháihújiālónggǔmǔlìtāng 5g hǎipiāoxiāo 1g nǚzhēnzǐ 1g báizhú 1g dìhuáng 1g huángbò 1g to ♂

Bǔzhōngyìqìtāng traditionally helps digestion. Cháihújiālónggǔmǔlìtāng is today used for neurasthenia (Wang, 2019). They are used here to alleviate jet lag syndrome.

13.14. Circadian Rhythm Sleep Disorders

Circadian rhythm sleep disorders are characterized by desynchronization between the internal wake-sleep rhythm and external light-darkness cycle. Job, sleep habits, medications and aging can cause circadian rhythm sleep disorders.

Sìnìtāng is used for sleep initiation and maintenance disorders and sleep deprivation in previous sections, and for circadian rhythm sleep disorders here.

Table 13.14. Herbal prescriptions for circadian rhythm sleep disorders

<table>
<tr><td colspan="2">Circadian Rhythm Sleep Disorders: https://meshb.nlm.nih.gov/record/ui?ui=D020178.</td></tr>
<tr><td colspan="2">Common prescriptions:</td></tr>
<tr><td colspan="2">Sìnìtāng 5g shēngjiāng 1g guìzhī 1g
Sìnìtāng 5g guìzhī 1g máhuáng 1g xìxīn 1g
Sìnìtāng 5g guìzhī 1g máhuáng 1g xìxīn 0g
Sìnìtāng 5g shēngjiāng 1g guìzhī 1g xìxīn 1g</td></tr>
<tr><td colspan="2">Alternative prescriptions:</td></tr>
<tr><td colspan="2">Sìnìtāng 5g rénshēn 1g bànxià 1g dàhuáng 0g
Sìnìtāng 5g guìzhī 1g
Sìnìtāng 5g guìzhī 2g shēngjiāng 1g wúzhūyú 1g
Sìnìtāng 5g bǔzhōngyìqìtāng 5g ròuguì 1g zhìgāncǎotāng 1g</td></tr>
<tr><td colspan="2">Indicated diseases:</td></tr>
<tr><td colspan="2">Other dermatoses 702; Unspecified disorders of nervous system 349.9 (Disorder of central nervous system, unspecified G969); Deformity and disproportion of reconstructed breast 612; Other disorders of breast 611; Benign mammary dysplasias 610; Alcohol abuse 305.0; Cardiovascular disease, unspecified 429.2 (Atherosclerotic heart disease of native coronary artery without angina pectoris I2510); Dysmetabolic syndrome X 277.7 (Metabolic syndrome E8881); Unspecified disorder of metabolism 277.9 (Metabolic disorder, unspecified E889)</td></tr>
<tr><td colspan="2">Other dermatoses 702 with sleep disorders, circadian rhythm D020178:</td></tr>
<tr><td>Dāngguīsìnìtāng 5g wúzhūyú 1g fùzǐ 1g gānjiāng 1g to ♀</td><td>Dāngguīsìnìtāng 5g wúzhūyú 1g fùzǐ 1g gānjiāng 1g to ♂</td></tr>
<tr><td colspan="2">Unspecified disorders of nervous system 349.9/G969 with sleep disorders, circadian rhythm D020178:</td></tr>
<tr><td>Huángqíwǔwùtāng 5g chuānxiōng 1g dānshēn 1g zhúrú 1g sāngzhī 1g dāngguī 1g jiānghuáng 1g to ♀</td><td>Huángqíwǔwùtāng 5g chuānxiōng 1g dānshēn 1g zhúrú 1g sāngzhī 1g dāngguī 1g jiānghuáng 1g to ♂</td></tr>
<tr><td colspan="2">Cardiovascular disease, unspecified 429.2/I2510 with sleep disorders, circadian rhythm D020178:</td></tr>
<tr><td>Sìnìtāng 5g gānlùyǐn 5g mǔdānpí 1g zhīzǐ 1g huánglián 0g to ♀</td><td>Sìnìtāng 5g gānlùyǐn 5g mǔdānpí 1g zhīzǐ 1g huánglián 1g to ♂</td></tr>
</table>

References

Bock, J., Covassin, N., & Somers, V. (2022). Excessive daytime sleepiness: an emerging marker of cardiovascular risk. *Heart*, *108*(22), 1761–1766. https://doi.org/10.1136/heartjnl-2021-319596.

Brion, A., Flamand, M., Oudiette, D., Voillery, D., Golmard, J.-L., & Arnulf, I. (2012). Sleep-related eating disorder versus sleepwalking: A controlled study. *Sleep Medicine*, *13*(8), 1094–1101. https://doi.org/10.1016/j.sleep.2012.06.012.

Garbarino, S., Lanteri, P., Bragazzi, N. L., Magnavita, N., & Scoditti, E. (2021). Role of sleep deprivation in immune-related disease risk and outcomes. *Communications Biology*, *4*, 1304. https://doi.org/10.1038/s42003-021-02825-4.

Gottlieb, D. J., Somers, V. K., Punjabi, N. M., & Winkelman, J. W. (2017). Restless legs syndrome and cardiovascular disease: a research roadmap. *Sleep Medicine*, *31*, 10–17. https://doi.org/10.1016/j.sleep.2016.08.008.

Javaheri, S., & Redline, S. (2017). Insomnia and Risk of Cardiovascular Disease. *Chest*, *152*(2), 435–444. https://doi.org/10.1016/j.chest.2017.01.026.

Lindner, A., Fornadi, K., Lazar, A. S., Czira, M. E., Dunai, A., Zoller, R., Veber, O., Szentkiralyi, A., Kiss, Z., Toronyi, E., Mucsi, I., Novak, M., & Molnar, M. Z. (2012). Periodic limb movements in sleep are associated with stroke and cardiovascular risk factors in patients with renal failure. *Journal of Sleep Research*, *21*(3), 297–307. https://doi.org/10.1111/j.1365-2869.2011.00956.x.

Liu, C., Chen, M.-S., & Yu, H. (2017). The relationship between obstructive sleep apnea and obesity hypoventilation syndrome: a systematic review and meta-analysis. *Oncotarget*, *8*(54), 93168–93178. https://doi.org/10.18632/oncotarget.21450.

Wang, S. C. (2019). *Clinical Herbal Prescriptions: Principles and Practices of Herbal Formulations from Deep Learning Health Insurance Herbal Prescription Big Data*. WSPC. https://doi.org/10.1142/11211.

Wang, S. C. (2020). *Veterinary Herbal Pharmacopoeia*. Nova Science Publishers. https://doi.org/10.52305/GHTR1903.

Chapter 14

Perceptual Disorders

Perception is the process by which the brain acquires, identifies and interprets the information it receives from the sense organs in order to understand the nature of the presented information and environment. Perception may seem effortless subjectively. However, operation of the sense organs is metabolically expensive. Furthermore, perception involves over half of the brain, which consumes one fourth of one's total metabolic budget. Perception therefore must be of adaptive importance in animal evolution. For example, prey should be able to perceive a looming predator as the same threat, even if the predator's size and shape keep changing. Guided by its perception, the prey takes actions to escape the predation. Impaired perceptual capabilities in humans can give rise to the signs and symptoms shown in Figure 14.1.

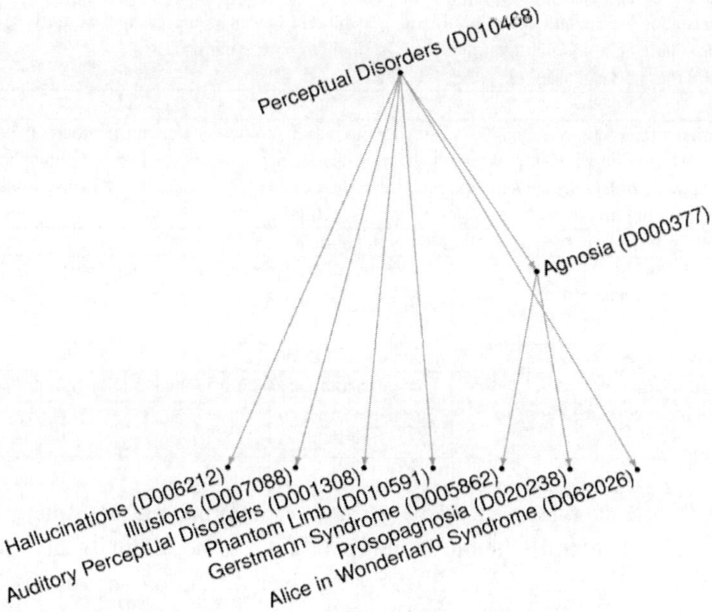

Figure 14.1. Signs and symptoms arising from impaired perceptual ability.

The formulas and herbs that are frequently used for the perceptual signs and symptoms include Sìnìtāng, Gāncǎoxiǎomàidàzǎotāng, Língguìshùgāntāng, Bǔzhōngyìqìtāng, Guìzhī, Shēngjiāng, Yuǎnzhì, Héhuānpí, and Shíchāngpú. Needling activates various regions of the brain, so acupuncture is also frequently prescribed, along with the herbal prescriptions, to the signs and symptoms of this chapter.

The diseases underlying the perceptual signs and symptoms include unspecified disorders of the nervous system, unspecified condition of brain, and neoplasm of unspecified nature of brain.

14.1. Hallucinations

Hallucinations are false perceptions in that the perceived external stimuli are actually absent. The wrongly sensed stimuli in hallucinations include light, sound, smell, taste, pressure, temperature and time duration. An example of auditory hallucination is hearing voices when no one has spoken. Causes of hallucinations include anxiety, substance dependence, medication side effect, lack of sleep, epilepsy, schizophrenia, depression, Alzheimer's disease and Parkinson's disease.

Table 14.1. Herbal prescriptions for hallucinations

Hallucinations: https://meshb.nlm.nih.gov/record/ui?ui=D006212.	
Common prescriptions:	
Gāncǎoxiǎomàidàzǎotāng 5g cháihújiālónggǔmǔlìtāng 5g shíchāngpú 1g yuǎnzhì 1g Gāncǎoxiǎomàidàzǎotāng 5g cháihújiālónggǔmǔlìtāng 5g Gāncǎoxiǎomàidàzǎotāng 5g cháihújiālónggǔmǔlìtāng 5g héhuānpí 1g yèjiāoténg 1g Gāncǎoxiǎomàidàzǎotāng 5g cháihújiālónggǔmǔlìtāng 5g héhuānpí 1g yèjiāoténg 1g fúshén 1g yuǎnzhì 1g Gāncǎoxiǎomàidàzǎotāng 5g cháihújiālónggǔmǔlìtāng 5g héhuānpí 1g yèjiāoténg 1g fúshén 1g	
Alternative prescriptions:	
Gāncǎoxiǎomàidàzǎotāng 5g guìzhījiālónggǔmǔlìtāng 5g Gāncǎoxiǎomàidàzǎotāng 5g cháihújiālónggǔmǔlìtāng 5g héhuānpí 1g yèjiāoténg 1g suānzǎorén 1g Gāncǎoxiǎomàidàzǎotāng 5g guìzhījiālónggǔmǔlìtāng 3g shíchāngpú 1g yuǎnzhì 1g Gāncǎoxiǎomàidàzǎotāng 5g yìgānsǎn 5g	
Indicated diseases:	
Unspecified disorders of nervous system 349.9 (Disorder of central nervous system, unspecified G969); Alcohol abuse 305.0; Depersonalization disorder 300.6 (Depersonalization-derealization syndrome F481); Schizophreniform disorder 295.4; Schizoaffective disorder 295.7; Dementia with Lewy bodies 331.82 (Dementia with Lewy bodies G3183); Unspecified condition of brain 348.9 (Disorder of brain, unspecified G939)	
Unspecified disorders of nervous system 349.9/G969 with hallucinations D006212:	
Huángqíwǔwùtāng 5g chuānxiōng 1g dānshēn 1g zhúrú 1g sāngzhī 1g dāngguī 1g jiānghuáng 1g to ♀	Xuèfǔzhúyūtāng 5g huángqíwǔwùtāng 5g dānshēn 1g zhúrú 1g sāngzhī 1g jiānghuáng 1g to ♂
Dementia with Lewy bodies 331.82/G3183 with hallucinations D006212:	
Gāncǎoxiǎomàidàzǎotāng 5g cháihújiālónggǔmǔlìtāng 5g shíchāngpú 1g yuǎnzhì 1g to ♀	Gāncǎoxiǎomàidàzǎotāng 5g cháihújiālónggǔmǔlìtāng 5g shíchāngpú 1g yuǎnzhì 1g to ♂

Today, both Gāncǎoxiǎomàidàzǎotāng and Cháihújiālónggǔmǔlìtāng are used for unspecified anxiety state and Cháihújiālónggǔmǔlìtāng is additionally used for unspecified nonpsychotic mental disorder (Wang, 2019). Moreover, Guìzhījiālónggǔmǔlìtāng is currently used for unspecified insomnia (Wang, 2019).

14.2. Illusions

Illusions are misperceptions in that the perceived external stimuli exist but are not what they actually are. Conflicting, insufficient or ambiguous sensory inputs make the brain to misinterpret. The distorted sensory stimuli can include any of the senses, but visual illusions are commonest as vision dominates over other senses. Examples of visual illusions are camouflage and magic performance. Stress, astigmatism, migraine, epilepsy, stroke, tumor, dementia and schizophrenia can cause illusions.

Huángqí and Rénshēn in Bǔzhōngyìqìtāng 'nourish Qi' while Bǔzhōngyìqìtāng is known to help digestion. Without changing the chemical composition of a food, the food's taste can change by changing the overlaying visual and olfactory information of the food, achieving taste illusions (Narumi et al., 2011). On the other hand, Wǔwèizǐ is today used for disorders of lacrimal system, and general symptoms including alteration of consciousness, hallucinations, syncope, convulsions, dizziness, sleep disturbance, fever, malaise, and excessive sweating, while Chuānxiōng is today used for migraine (Wang, 2019).

Table 14.2. Herbal prescriptions for illusions

<table>
<tr><td colspan="2">Illusions: https://meshb.nlm.nih.gov/record/ui?ui=D007088.</td></tr>
<tr><td colspan="2">Common prescriptions:</td></tr>
<tr><td colspan="2">Bǔzhōngyìqìtāng 5g</td></tr>
<tr><td colspan="2">Alternative prescriptions:</td></tr>
<tr><td colspan="2">Bǔzhōngyìqìtāng 5g fùzǐ 0g
Bǔzhōngyìqìtāng 5g wǔwèizǐ 1g ròudòukòu 1g wúzhūyú 1g bǔgǔzhī 1g
Bǔzhōngyìqìtāng 5g chuānxiōng 0g báizhǐ 0g
Sìnìtāng 5g shēngjiāng 1g guìzhī 1g xìxīn 0g</td></tr>
<tr><td colspan="2">Indicated diseases:</td></tr>
<tr><td colspan="2">Unspecified disorders of nervous system 349.9 (Disorder of central nervous system, unspecified G969); Posttraumatic stress disorder 309.81 (Post-traumatic stress disorder, unspecified F4310, Post-traumatic stress disorder, chronic F4312); Anorexia nervosa 307.1 (Anorexia nervosa, unspecified F5000); Eating disorder, unspecified 307.50 (Eating disorder, unspecified F509); Unspecified condition of brain 348.9 (Disorder of brain, unspecified G939); Neoplasm of unspecified nature of brain 239.6 (Neoplasm of unspecified behavior of brain D496); Malignant neoplasm of nervous system, part unspecified 192.9 (Malignant neoplasm of central nervous system, unspecified C729); Depersonalization disorder 300.6 (Depersonalization-derealization syndrome F481)</td></tr>
<tr><td colspan="2">Unspecified disorders of nervous system 349.9/G969 with illusions D007088:</td></tr>
<tr><td>Huángqíwǔwùtāng 5g chuānxiōng 1g dānshēn 1g zhúrú 1g sāngzhī 1g dāngguī 1g jiānghuáng 1g to ♀</td><td>Huángqíwǔwùtāng 5g chuānxiōng 1g dānshēn 1g zhúrú 1g sāngzhī 1g dāngguī 1g jiānghuáng 1g to ♂</td></tr>
<tr><td colspan="2">Unspecified condition of brain 348.9/G939 with illusions D007088:</td></tr>
<tr><td>Xiǎoxùmìngtāng 5g bǔyánghuánwǔtāng 5g tiānmá 1g shíchāngpú 1g yuǎnzhì 1g + acupuncture to ♀</td><td>Bǔyánghuánwǔtāng 5g dānshēn 1g shíchāngpú 1g yuǎnzhì 1g + acupuncture to ♂</td></tr>
</table>

14.3. Agnosia

Agnosia is inability to recognize and identify objects, shapes, persons, places, sounds and smells despite integrity of the sense organs. Agnosia can affect any senses but usually only one of the senses is affected. Causes of agnosia include traumatic brain injury, stroke, tumor, Alzheimer's disease and Parkinson's disease.

Table 14.3. Herbal prescriptions for agnosia

Agnosia: https://meshb.nlm.nih.gov/record/ui?ui=D000377.
Common prescriptions:
Bǔzhōngyìqìtāng 5g
Alternative prescriptions:
Bǔzhōngyìqìtāng 5g fùzǐ 0g Bǔzhōngyìqìtāng 5g dānshēn 0g Bǔzhōngyìqìtāng 5g dānshēn 1g Sìnìtāng 5g rénshēn 1g Sìnìtāng 5g bǔzhōngyìqìtāng 5g

Table 14.3. (Continued)

Agnosia: https://meshb.nlm.nih.gov/record/ui?ui=D000377.	
Indicated diseases:	
Unspecified condition of brain 348.9 (Disorder of brain, unspecified G939); Neoplasm of unspecified nature of brain 239.6 (Neoplasm of unspecified behavior of brain D496); Unspecified disorders of nervous system 349.9 (Disorder of central nervous system, unspecified G969); Malignant neoplasm of nervous system, part unspecified 192.9 (Malignant neoplasm of central nervous system, unspecified C729); Unspecified cerebrovascular disease 437.9 (Cerebrovascular disease, unspecified I679); Cardiovascular disease, unspecified 429.2 (Atherosclerotic heart disease of native coronary artery without angina pectoris I2510)	
Unspecified condition of brain 348.9/G939 with agnosia D000377:	
Bǔyánghuánwǔtāng 5g dānshēn 1g tiānmá 1g shíchāngpú 1g yuǎnzhì 1g gōuténg 1g + acupuncture to ♀	Bǔyánghuánwǔtāng 5g + acupuncture to ♂
Unspecified cerebrovascular disease 437.9/I679 with agnosia D000377:	
Bǔyánghuánwǔtāng 5g chuānqī 2g dānshēn 1g shíchāngpú 1g yuǎnzhì 1g + acupuncture to ♀	Bǔyánghuánwǔtāng 5g chuānqī 2g dānshēn 1g shíchāngpú 1g yuǎnzhì 1g + acupuncture to ♂

Bǔzhōngyìqìtāng is thought to alleviate olfactory agnosia and gustatory agnosia as Bǔzhōngyìqìtāng aids digestion.

14.4. Gerstmann Syndrome

Gerstmann syndrome is difficulty in writing, calculating, finger recognizing and left-right distinguishing. Gerstmann syndrome is caused by neurodegenerative or developmental changes to the temporal and parietal lobe junction on the left hemisphere of the brain.

Sìnìtāng is prescribed in Section 12.9 for acquired dyslexia, which is difficulty reading. In addition to the tetrad symptoms of pure Gerstmann syndrome, Gerstmann syndrome often has other symptoms including dyslexia (Kaufman, 2007, Chapter 8). The use of Sìnìtāng for Gerstmann syndrome is therefore understandable.

Table 14.4. Herbal prescriptions for Gerstmann syndrome

Gerstmann Syndrome: https://meshb.nlm.nih.gov/record/ui?ui=D005862.
Common prescriptions:
Sìnìtāng 5g shēngjiāng 1g guìzhī 1g Sìnìtāng 5g shēngjiāng 1g guìzhī 1g dàhuáng 0g Bǔzhōngyìqìtāng 5g Sìnìtāng 5g shēngjiāng 1g guìzhī 1g xìxīn 1g
Alternative prescriptions:
Sìnìtāng 5g guìzhī 1g máhuáng 1g xìxīn 1g Bǔzhōngyìqìtāng 5g + acupuncture Sìnìtāng 5g guìzhī 2g máhuáng 2g xìxīn 1g Máhuángfùzǐxìxīntāng 5g shēngjiāng 1g guìzhī 1g gāncǎo 1g
Indicated diseases:
Unspecified cerebrovascular disease 437.9 (Cerebrovascular disease, unspecified I679); Unspecified condition of brain 348.9 (Disorder of brain, unspecified G939); Cardiovascular disease, unspecified 429.2 (Atherosclerotic heart disease of native coronary artery without angina pectoris I2510); Unspecified disorders of nervous system 349.9 (Disorder of central nervous system, unspecified G969); Neoplasm of unspecified nature of brain 239.6 (Neoplasm of unspecified behavior of brain D496); Malignant neoplasm of nervous system, part unspecified 192.9 (Malignant neoplasm of central nervous system, unspecified C729); Epilepsy, unspecified 345.9

Gerstmann Syndrome: https://meshb.nlm.nih.gov/record/ui?ui=D005862.	
Unspecified cerebrovascular disease 437.9/I679 with Gerstmann syndrome D005862:	
Bǔyánghuánwǔtāng 5g chuānqī 2g dānshēn 1g shíchāngpú 1g yuǎnzhì 1g + acupuncture to ♀	Bǔyánghuánwǔtāng 5g chuānqī 2g dānshēn 1g shíchāngpú 1g yuǎnzhì 1g + acupuncture to ♂
Unspecified condition of brain 348.9/G939 with Gerstmann syndrome D005862:	
Bǔyánghuánwǔtāng 5g chuānqī 1g dānshēn 1g shíchāngpú 1g yuǎnzhì 1g + acupuncture to ♀	Bǔyánghuánwǔtāng 5g chuānqī 1g dānshēn 1g shíchāngpú 1g yuǎnzhì 1g + acupuncture to ♂
Epilepsy, unspecified 345.9 with Gerstmann syndrome D005862:	
Yìgānsǎn 5g guìzhījiālónggǔmǔlìtāng 5g xiōngqiōng 1g gǎoběn 1g to ♀	Wēndǎntāng 5g cháihújiālónggǔmǔlìtāng 4g shíchāngpú 1g yuǎnzhì 1g to ♂

14.5. Prosopagnosia

Prosopagnosia, or face blindness, is inability to recognize familiar faces including one's own face. Lesions to the brain areas responsible for face recognition cause prosopagnosia, including inheritance, encephalitis, stroke, tumor, Alzheimer's disease and Parkinson's disease.

Table 14.5. Herbal prescriptions for prosopagnosia

Prosopagnosia: https://meshb.nlm.nih.gov/record/ui?ui=D020238.	
Common prescriptions:	
Sìnìtāng 5g shēngjiāng 1g guìzhī 1g Máhuángfùzǐxìxīntāng 5g shēngjiāng 2g guìzhī 2g zhìgāncǎo 1g Máhuángfùzǐxìxīntāng 5g shēngjiāng 1g guìzhī 1g zhìgāncǎo 1g Máhuángfùzǐxìxīntāng 5g shēngjiāng 1g guìzhī 1g	
Alternative prescriptions:	
Sìnìtāng 5g shēngjiāng 1g guìzhī 1g bànxià 1g dàhuáng 0g Guìzhītāng 5g shēngjiāng 0g guìzhī 0g dàhuáng 0g Guìzhītāng 5g shēngjiāng 1g guìzhī 1g Sìnìtāng 5g bànxià 1g guìzhī 1g máhuáng 1g xìxīn 1g dàhuáng 0g	
Indicated diseases:	
Unspecified cerebrovascular disease 437.9 (Cerebrovascular disease, unspecified I679); Unspecified condition of brain 348.9 (Disorder of brain, unspecified G939); Cardiovascular disease, unspecified 429.2 (Atherosclerotic heart disease of native coronary artery without angina pectoris I2510); Unspecified disorders of nervous system 349.9 (Disorder of central nervous system, unspecified G969); Neoplasm of unspecified nature of brain 239.6 (Neoplasm of unspecified behavior of brain D496); Malignant neoplasm of nervous system, part unspecified 192.9 (Malignant neoplasm of central nervous system, unspecified C729); Epilepsy, unspecified 345.9	
Unspecified cerebrovascular disease 437.9/I679 with prosopagnosia D020238:	
Bǔyánghuánwǔtāng 5g sānqī 1g dānshēn 1g shíchāngpú 1g yuǎnzhì 1g + acupuncture to ♀	Bǔyánghuánwǔtāng 5g chuānqī 2g dānshēn 1g shíchāngpú 1g yuǎnzhì 1g + acupuncture to ♂
Unspecified condition of brain 348.9/G939 with prosopagnosia D020238:	
Bǔyánghuánwǔtāng 5g chuānqī 1g dānshēn 1g shíchāngpú 1g yuǎnzhì 1g + acupuncture to ♀	Bǔyánghuánwǔtāng 5g chuānqī 1g dānshēn 1g shíchāngpú 1g yuǎnzhì 1g + acupuncture to ♂
Epilepsy, unspecified 345.9 with prosopagnosia D020238:	
Tiānwángbǔxīndān 5g tiānmágōuténgyǐn 5g cháihújiālónggǔmǔlìtāng 5g to ♀	Tiānwángbǔxīndān 5g cháihújiālónggǔmǔlìtāng 5g hǎipiāoxiāo 1g mùguā 1g báizhú 1g dìgǔpí 1g chuānxiōng 1g dìhuáng 1g to ♂

Máhuángfùzǐxìxīntāng, in comparison with Sìnìtāng, orients more to the infection and inflammation of the underlying causes, as we pointed out earlier.

References

Kaufman, D. M. (2007). *Clinical neurology for psychiatrists* (6th edition). Saunders Elsevier.

Narumi, T., Nishizaka, S., Kajinami, T., Tanikawa, T., & Hirose, M. (2011). Meta Cookie+: An Illusion-Based Gustatory Display. *Virtual and Mixed Reality - New Trends,* 260–269. https://doi.org/10.1007/978-3-642-22021-0_29.

Wang, S. C. (2019). *Clinical Herbal Prescriptions: Principles and Practices of Herbal Formulations from Deep Learning Health Insurance Herbal Prescription Big Data.* WSPC. https://doi.org/10.1142/11211.

Chapter 15

Neuromuscular Diseases

Many of our daily activities, such as grocery shopping, grooming and housekeeping, require the use of our muscles. Muscle contractions consume energy which in the context of cells is adenosine triphosphate (ATP). Muscle cells only store a limited amount of ATP, which is quickly exhausted in the first few seconds of muscle contractions. If the activity requires movements over a couple of seconds, as in a 100-meter sprint, then high-energy compounds called creatine phosphate in muscle cells are anaerobically broken down to regenerate ATP to meet the muscular demand. If the activity requires to last longer than 10 seconds, as in a 100-meter swim, the ATP buffer depletes creatine phosphate soon and anaerobic glycolysis takes over to provide most of the ATP requirement. Glycolysis converts glycogen, which is a form of glucose storage in muscles, to ATP but glycogen in muscles would run out in a few minutes.

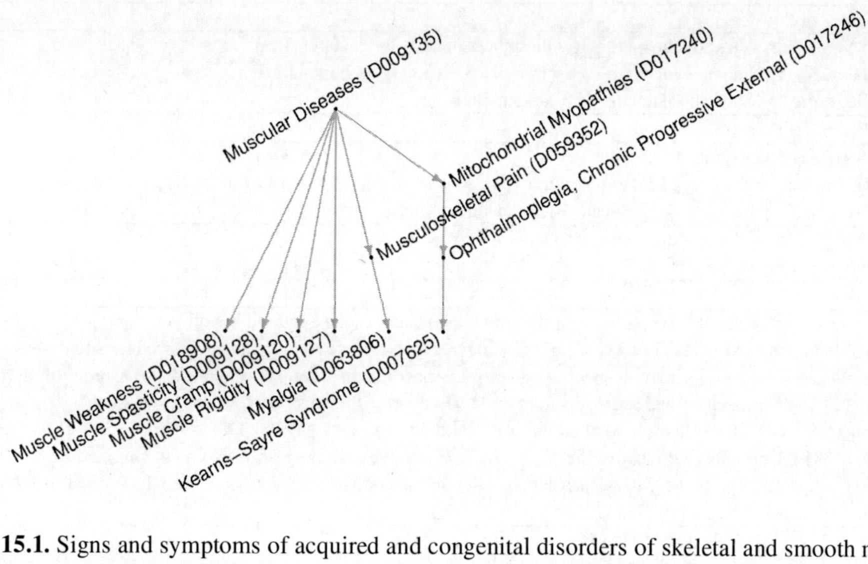

Figure 15.1. Signs and symptoms of acquired and congenital disorders of skeletal and smooth muscles.

If the physical activity requires continuous muscle movements for over a couple of minutes, as in a marathon, then oxygen from increased breathing and heartbeat arrives in muscles to fuel the mitochondrial respiration, taking over the glycolysis to meet the demand of ATP for sustained muscle movements. Mitochondrial respiration utilizes glucose and fatty acids from the blood, which is why exercise is effective in preventing metabolic disease such as obesity, diabetes and atherosclerosis. Abnormalities in the structure and metabolism of muscle cells give rise to muscular diseases which can present the signs and symptoms shown in Figure 15.1.

The formulas and herbs commonly used, together with acupuncture, for the muscular signs and symptoms are Huángqíwǔwùtāng, Dāngguīsìnìtāng, Xuèfǔzhúyūtāng, Dúhuójìshēngtāng, Dānshēn, Sāngzhī, Zhúrú, Jiānghuáng, Wúzhūyú, and Shēngjiāng.

The disease diagnoses commonly associated with the muscular signs and symptoms are unspecified disorders of nervous system, unspecified myopathy, and myoneural disorders.

15.1. Muscle Weakness

Muscle weakness is reduced strength in one or more muscles in contracting or moving the affected muscles. Causes of muscle weakness include lack of exercise, muscle injury, aging, infections, multiple sclerosis, chronic fatigue syndrome, stroke and diabetes.

Dúhuójìshēngtāng 'benefits the Liver and Kidney, nourishes Qi and Blood, expels Wind and Dampness, stops paralysis and pain.' Its modern uses are for lumbago, sciatica, and rheumatoid arthritis (Wang, 2019), all of which can induce muscle weakness.

Table 15.1. Herbal prescriptions for muscle weakness

Muscle Weakness: https://meshb.nlm.nih.gov/record/ui?ui=D018908.	
Common prescriptions:	
Dúhuójìshēngtāng 5g sháoyàogāncǎotāng 4g shūjīnghuóxuètāng 4g + acupuncture Dúhuójìshēngtāng 5g sháoyàogāncǎotāng 3g shūjīnghuóxuètāng 3g + acupuncture Dúhuójìshēngtāng 5g shūjīnghuóxuètāng 4g + acupuncture	
Alternative prescriptions:	
Dúhuójìshēngtāng 5g dùzhòng 1g xùduàn 1g Shūjīnghuóxuètāng 5g dúhuójìshēngtāng 5g niúxī 1g mòyào 1g rǔxiāng 1g fùzǐ 1g guìzhī 1g jīxuèténg 1g Dúhuójìshēngtāng 5g dùzhòng 1g yánhúsuǒ 1g jīxuèténg 1g xùduàn 1g	
Dúhuójìshēngtāng 5g sháoyàogāncǎotāng 3g dùzhòng 1g xùduàn 1g Dúhuójìshēngtāng 5g shūjīnghuóxuètāng 4g dùzhòng 1g mòyào 1g rǔxiāng 1g + acupuncture	
Indicated diseases:	
Myopathy, unspecified 359.9 (Myopathy, unspecified G729); Unspecified acquired hypothyroidism 244.9 (Hypothyroidism, unspecified E039); Myoneural disorders 358; Unspecified disorders of nervous system 349.9 (Disorder of central nervous system, unspecified G969); Unspecified disorder of thyroid 246.9 (Disorder of thyroid, unspecified E079); Unspecified endocrine disorder 259.9 (Endocrine disorder, unspecified E349); Other dermatoses 702; Dermatomyositis 710.3 (Juvenile dermatomyositis without myopathy M3303, Other dermatomyositis without myopathy M3313, Dermatopolymyositis, unspecified, organ involvement unspecified M3390, Dermatopolymyositis, unspecified without myopathy M3393); Disorders of calcium metabolism 275.4; Unspecified disorder of metabolism 277.9 (Metabolic disorder, unspecified E889)	
Myopathy, unspecified 359.9/G729 with muscle weakness D018908:	
Huángqíwǔwùtāng 5g dāngguīsìnìtāng 5g dānshēn 1g zhúrú 1g sāngzhī 1g jiānghuáng 1g to ♀	Huángqíwǔwùtāng 5g dāngguīsìnìtāng 5g dānshēn 1g zhúrú 1g sāngzhī 1g jiānghuáng 1g to ♂
Other dermatoses 702 with muscle weakness D018908:	
Jiědúsìwùtāng 5g xiāofēngsǎn 4g zhēnrénhuómìngyǐnqùchuānshānjiǎ 4g huángliánjiědútāng 4g to ♀	Jiědúsìwùtāng 5g xiāofēngsǎn 4g zhēnrénhuómìngyǐnqùchuānshānjiǎ 4g huángliánjiědútāng 4g to ♂

15.2. Muscle Hypotonia

Muscle tone is the tension in the relaxed muscle. It is the stiffness or resistance of the muscle. An adequate muscle tone enables one's body to behave like a spring so that a sudden push does not bend or overturn the body. Muscle hypotonia is decreased muscle tone. Damage to the brain, spinal cord, nerve or muscle can cause muscle hypotonia.

Huángqíwǔwùtāng 'benefits Qi, warms up meridians,' 'harmonizes digestion, unlocks paralysis,' and is used here to restore hypotonia. Muscle hypotonia is associated with congenital heart disease (Davison and Weiss, 1929).

Table 15.2. Herbal prescriptions for muscle hypotonia

Muscle Hypotonia: https://meshb.nlm.nih.gov/record/ui?ui=D009123.	
Common prescriptions:	
Huángqíwǔwùtāng 5g dānshēn 1g zhúrú 1g sāngzhī 1g jiānghuáng 1g Huángqíwǔwùtāng 5g dānshēn 1g zhúrú 1g sāngzhī 1g dāngguī 1g jiānghuáng 1g Huángqíwǔwùtāng 5g dānshēn 1g zhúrú 1g sāngzhī 1g jiānghuáng 1g jīxuèténg 1g Huángqíwǔwùtāng 5g dānshēn 1g zhúrú 1g sāngzhī 1g qínjiāo 1g jiānghuáng 1g	
Alternative prescriptions:	
Dāngguīsìnìtāng 5g shēngjiāng 1g wúzhūyú 1g fùzǐ 1g Dāngguīsìnìtāng 5g chuānwū 1g shēngjiāng 1g wúzhūyú 1g Máhuángfùzǐxìxīntāng 5g shēngjiāng 1g guìzhī 1g dàzǎo 1g gāncǎo 1g	
Indicated diseases:	
Heart disease, unspecified 429.9 (Heart disease, unspecified I519); Unspecified disorders of nervous system 349.9 (Disorder of central nervous system, unspecified G969); Digeorge's syndrome 279.11 (Di George's syndrome D821); Velo cardio facial syndrome 758.32 (Velo-cardio-facial syndrome Q9381), Cardiovascular disease, unspecified 429.2 (Atherosclerotic heart disease of native coronary artery without angina pectoris I2510); Hypoparathyroidism 252.1 (Hypoparathyroidism, unspecified E209); Unspecified disorder of parathyroid gland 252.9 (Disorder of parathyroid gland, unspecified E215); Unspecified endocrine disorder 259.9 (Endocrine disorder, unspecified E349); Unspecified congenital anomaly of heart 746.9 (Congenital malformation of cardiac chambers and connections, unspecified Q209, Congenital malformation of heart, unspecified Q249); Myopathy, unspecified 359.9 (Myopathy, unspecified G729); Unspecified disorder of metabolism 277.9 (Metabolic disorder, unspecified E889); Myoneural disorders 358; Unspecified condition of brain 348.9 (Disorder of brain, unspecified G939); Glycogenosis 271.0 (Glycogen storage disease, unspecified E7400, von Gierke disease E7401, McArdle disease E7404, Other glycogen storage disease E7409, Disorders of pyruvate metabolism and gluconeogenesis E744)	
Heart disease, unspecified 429.9/I519 with muscle hypotonia D009123:	
Sìnìtāng 5g gānlùyǐn 5g mǔdānpí 1g zhǐzǐ 1g huánglián 0g to ♀	Sìnìtāng 5g gānlùyǐn 5g mǔdānpí 1g zhǐzǐ 1g huánglián 0g to ♂
Myopathy, unspecified 359.9/G729 with muscle hypotonia D009123:	
Huángqíwǔwùtāng 5g dāngguīsìnìtāng 5g dānshēn 1g zhúrú 1g sāngzhī 1g jiānghuáng 1g to ♀	Huángqíwǔwùtāng 5g dāngguīsìnìtāng 5g dānshēn 1g zhúrú 1g sāngzhī 1g jiānghuáng 1g to ♂
Unspecified condition of brain 348.9/G939 with muscle hypotonia D009123:	
Bǔyánghuánwǔtāng 5g dānshēn 1g shíchāngpú 1g yuǎnzhì 1g + acupuncture to ♀	Bǔyánghuánwǔtāng 5g + acupuncture to ♂

15.3. Muscle Hypertonia

Muscle hypertonia is an abnormal increase in muscle tone. Damage to the neural pathway responsible for muscle tone by e.g., multiple sclerosis, Parkinson's disease, infection and stroke can cause muscle hypertonia.

Dāngguīsìnìtāng 'nourishes Blood, expels chills,' 'warms meridians, unclogs vessels,' and is used here for muscle hypertonia. Hypertonicity of intestinal smooth muscle can produce mucosal ischemia of the intestine in dogs (Parodi et al., 1987).

Table 15.3. Herbal prescriptions for muscle hypertonia

Muscle Hypertonia: https://meshb.nlm.nih.gov/record/ui?ui=D009122.	
Common prescriptions:	
Sháoyàogāncǎotāng 5g dāngguīniāntòngtāng 5g + acupuncture Sháoyàogāncǎotāng 5g dāngguīniāntòngtāng 5g	
Alternative prescriptions:	
Dāngguīsìnìtāng 5g shēngjiāng 0g wúzhūyú 0g Dāngguīsìnìtāng 5g shēngjiāng 1g wúzhūyú 1g Guizhītāng 5g chuānwū 1g Dāngguīsìnìtāng 5g huángqí 2g shēngjiāng 1g wúzhūyú 1g fùzǐ 1g Sháoyàogāncǎotāng 5g fùzǐ 0g dàhuáng 0g	
Indicated diseases:	
Myopathy, unspecified 359.9 (Myopathy, unspecified G729); Myoneural disorders 358; Unspecified disorders of nervous system 349.9 (Disorder of central nervous system, unspecified G969); Unspecified disorder of intestine 569.9 (Disease of intestine, unspecified K639); Diseases of the jaws 526; Bladder neck obstruction 596.0 (Bladder-neck obstruction N320); Unspecified disorder of bladder 596.9 (Bladder disorder, unspecified N329)	
Myopathy, unspecified 359.9/G729 with muscle hypertonia D009122:	
Huángqíwǔwùtāng 5g dāngguīsìnìtāng 5g dānshēn 1g zhúrú 1g sāngzhī 1g jiānghuáng 1g to ♀	Guīlùèrxiānjiāo 5g to ♂
Unspecified disorder of intestine 569.9/K639 with muscle hypertonia D009122:	
Xiāngshāliùjūnzǐtāng 5g cānlíngbáizhúsǎn 5g to ♀	Xiāngshāliùjūnzǐtāng 5g cānlíngbáizhúsǎn 5g to ♂
Unspecified disorders of nervous system 349.9/G969 with muscle hypertonia D009122:	
Huángqíwǔwùtāng 5g chuānxiōng 1g dānshēn 1g zhúrú 1g sāngzhī 1g dāngguī 1g jiānghuáng 1g to ♀	Huángqíwǔwùtāng 5g chuānxiōng 1g dānshēn 1g zhúrú 1g sāngzhī 1g dāngguī 1g jiānghuáng 1g to ♂

15.4. Muscular Atrophy

Muscular atrophy is wasting or thinning of the muscle mass. Damage by e.g., polio to the muscle or nerve connecting to the affected muscle can cause muscular atrophy. On the other hand, muscular atrophy due to muscle disuse is reversible.

Juānbìtāng 'benefits Qi, activates Blood,' 'expels Wind, dehumidifies,' and is today used for rheumatoid arthritis (Wang, 2019).

Table 15.4. Herbal prescriptions for muscular atrophy

Muscular Atrophy: https://meshb.nlm.nih.gov/record/ui?ui=D009133.
Common prescriptions:
Huángqíwǔwùtāng 5g juānbìtāng 5g dānshēn 1g zhúrú 1g sāngzhī 1g jiānghuáng 1g Huángqíwǔwùtāng 5g juānbìtāng 5g dānshēn 1g zhúrú 1g sāngzhī 1g jiānghuáng 1g + acupuncture Huángqíwǔwùtāng 5g juānbìtāng 5g dānshēn 1g zhúrú 1g sāngzhī 1g qínjiāo 1g jiānghuáng 1g
Alternative prescriptions:
Juānbìtāng 5g jīxuèténg 1g + acupuncture Juānbìtāng 5g huángqíwǔwùtāng 4g dānshēn 1g zhúrú 1g sāngzhī 1g jiānghuáng 1g Huángqíwǔwùtāng 5g juānbìtāng 5g dānshēn 1g zhúrú 1g sāngzhī 1g dāngguī 1g jiānghuáng 1g Juānbìtāng 5g jīxuèténg 0g xùduàn 0g Juānbìtāng 5g huángqíwǔwùtāng 4g yánhúsuǒ 1g jīxuèténg 1g + acupuncture

Muscular Atrophy: https://meshb.nlm.nih.gov/record/ui?ui=D009133.	
Indicated diseases:	
Primary lateral sclerosis 335.24 (Primary lateral sclerosis G1223); Unspecified disorder of metabolism 277.9 (Metabolic disorder, unspecified E889); Motor neuron disease 335.2; Anterior horn cell disease 335; Unspecified disease of spinal cord 336.9 (Disease of spinal cord, unspecified G959); Myoneural disorders 358; Unspecified disorders of nervous system 349.9 (Disorder of central nervous system, unspecified G969); Unspecified disorder of joint, site unspecified 719.90 (Joint disorder, unspecified M259); Myopathy, unspecified 359.9 (Myopathy, unspecified G729); Unspecified condition of brain 348.9 (Disorder of brain, unspecified G939)	
Primary lateral sclerosis 335.24/G1223 with muscular atrophy D009133:	
Huángqíwǔwùtāng 5g juānbìtāng 5g dānshēn 1g zhúrú 1g sāngzhī 1g jiānghuáng 1g to ♀	Huángqíwǔwùtāng 5g juānbìtāng 5g dānshēn 1g zhúrú 1g sāngzhī 1g jiānghuáng 1g to ♂
Unspecified disorders of nervous system 349.9/G969 with muscular atrophy D009133:	
Huángqíwǔwùtāng 5g chuānxiōng 1g dānshēn 1g zhúrú 1g sāngzhī 1g dāngguī 1g jiānghuáng 1g to ♀	Huángqíwǔwùtāng 5g chuānxiōng 1g dānshēn 1g zhúrú 1g sāngzhī 1g dāngguī 1g jiānghuáng 1g to ♂
Myopathy, unspecified 359.9/G729 with muscular atrophy D009133:	
Huángqíwǔwùtāng 5g juānbìtāng 5g sāngzhī 1g jīxuèténg 1g + acupuncture to ♀	Huángqíwǔwùtāng 5g juānbìtāng 5g dānshēn 1g zhúrú 1g sāngzhī 1g jiānghuáng 1g to ♂

15.5. Sarcopenia

Sarcopenia, a type of muscle atrophy, is progressive loss of the mass, function and strength of skeletal muscles associated with aging. Age related changes in hormones, cellular metabolism, inflammation, physical activity, and dietary intake can cause sarcopenia.

Zhēnwǔtāng 'warms up the Yang of the Kidney and Spleen,' and is thought to help the metabolism and digestion of the patient with sarcopenia. Note that Zhēnwǔtāng already contains Fùzǐ. Addition of Fùzǐ to the prescriptions is believed to enhance the effect of Yang warming up on the patient. Note that accumulation of advanced glycation end-products in the skin is associated with sarcopenia (Waqas et al., 2022).

Table 15.5. Herbal prescriptions for sarcopenia

Sarcopenia: https://meshb.nlm.nih.gov/record/ui?ui=D055948.
Common prescriptions:
Zhēnwǔtāng 5g fùzǐ 1g gānjiāng 1g Zhēnwǔtāng 5g fùzǐ 1g xìxīn 1g Zhēnwǔtāng 5g fùzǐ 1g gānjiāng 1g xìxīn 1g Zhēnwǔtāng 5g fùzǐ 1g Zhēnwǔtāng 5g fùzǐ 1g gānjiāng 1g tiáowèichéngqìtāng 1g
Alternative prescriptions:
Zhēnwǔtāng 5g fùzǐ 1g gānjiāng 1g xìxīn 1g mázǐrénwán 1g dàhuáng 0g Zhēnwǔtāng 5g fùzǐ 1g wǔwèizǐ 1g gānjiāng 1g xìxīn 1g Zhēnwǔtāng 5g fùzǐ 0g gānjiāng 0g xìxīn 0g Zhēnwǔtāng 5g shēngmàiyǐn 4g dānshēn 1g xiāngfù 1g yùjīn 1g Zhēnwǔtāng 5g fùzǐ 2g xìxīn 1g xiǎochéngqìtāng 0g
Indicated diseases:
Other dermatoses 702; Unspecified disorders of nervous system 349.9 (Disorder of central nervous system, unspecified G969); Deformity and disproportion of reconstructed breast 612; Other disorders of breast 611; Benign mammary dysplasias 610; Cardiovascular disease, unspecified 429.2 (Atherosclerotic heart disease of native coronary artery without angina pectoris I2510); Diabetes mellitus 250; Unspecified endocrine disorder 259.9 (Endocrine disorder, unspecified E349); Unspecified disorder of metabolism 277.9 (Metabolic disorder, unspecified E889); Diseases of the jaws 526; Malignant neoplasm of thorax 195.1 (Malignant neoplasm of thorax C761); Osteoporosis 733.0

Table 15.5. (Continued)

Sarcopenia: https://meshb.nlm.nih.gov/record/ui?ui=D055948.	
Other dermatoses 702 with sarcopenia D055948:	
Bàidúsǎn 5g zhēnrénhuómìngyǐnqùchuānshānjiǎ 4g huángliánjiědútāng 4g to ♀	Bàidúsǎn 5g zhēnrénhuómìngyǐnqùchuānshānjiǎ 4g huángliánjiědútāng 4g to ♂
Cardiovascular disease, unspecified 429.2/I2510 with sarcopenia D055948:	
Yùzhú 5g sìnìtāng 5g mǔdānpí 1g zhīzǐ 1g huánglián 0g to ♀	Sìnìtāng 5g gānlùyǐn 5g mǔdānpí 1g zhīzǐ 1g huánglián 0g to ♂
Diseases of the jaws 526 with sarcopenia D055948:	
Guìzhītāng 5g báisháo 1g dàhuáng 0g to ♀	Guìzhītāng 5g báisháo 1g dàhuáng 0g to ♂
Unspecified disorders of nervous system 349.9/G969 with sarcopenia D055948:	
Huángqíwǔwùtāng 5g chuānxiōng 1g dānshēn 1g zhúrú 1g sāngzhī 1g dāngguī 1g jiānghuáng 1g to ♀	Huángqíwǔwùtāng 5g chuānxiōng 1g dānshēn 1g zhúrú 1g sāngzhī 1g dāngguī 1g jiānghuáng 1g to ♂

15.6. Spasm

Spasm is involuntary contraction or tensing of a muscle or a group of muscles, including skeletal and smooth muscles. Overuse and straining of the muscle can cause muscle spasms.

Table 15.6. Herbal prescriptions for spasm

Spasm: https://meshb.nlm.nih.gov/record/ui?ui=D013035.	
Common prescriptions:	
Sháoyàogāncǎotāng 5g shūjīnghuóxuètāng 5g dāngguīniāntòngtāng 5g + acupuncture Sháoyàogāncǎotāng 5g shūjīnghuóxuètāng 5g + acupuncture	
Alternative prescriptions:	
Sháoyàogāncǎotāng 5g mùguā 1g niúxī 1g yánhúsuǒ 1g + acupuncture Sháoyàogāncǎotāng 5g shūjīnghuóxuètāng 5g niúxī 1g mòyào 1g rǔxiāng 1g + acupuncture Sháoyàogāncǎotāng 5g gégēntāng 5g Sháoyàogāncǎotāng 5g dāngguīniāntòngtāng 5g mòyào 1g rǔxiāng 1g Sháoyàogāncǎotāng 5g shūjīnghuóxuètāng 5g mòyào 1g rǔxiāng 1g wēilíngxiān 1g	
Indicated and associated diseases:	
Unspecified cerebrovascular disease 437.9 (Cerebrovascular disease, unspecified I679); Migraine 346; Cardiovascular disease, unspecified 429.2 (Atherosclerotic heart disease of native coronary artery without angina pectoris I2510); Unspecified condition of brain 348.9 (Disorder of brain, unspecified G939); Unspecified disorders of nervous system 349.9 (Disorder of central nervous system, unspecified G969); Unspecified disease of pharynx 478.20 (Other diseases of pharynx J392); Unspecified disorder of esophagus 530.9 (Disease of esophagus, unspecified K229); Conversion disorder 300.11 (Conversion disorder with motor symptom or deficit F444, Conversion disorder with sensory symptom or deficit F446); Somatization disorder 300.81 (Somatization disorder F450)	
Unspecified cerebrovascular disease 437.9/I679 with spasm D013035:	
Huángqíwǔwùtāng 5g bǔyánghuánwǔtāng 5g dānshēn 1g sāngzhī 1g jīxuèténg 1g + acupuncture to ♀	Bǔyánghuánwǔtāng 5g dānshēn 1g shíchāngpú 1g yuǎnzhì 1g + acupuncture to ♂
Unspecified disease of pharynx 478.20/J392 with spasm D013035:	
Guìzhītāng 5g bànxià 1g jiégěng 1g dàhuáng 0g to ♀	Guìzhītāng 5g jiégěng 1g liánqiáo 1g zhīzǐ 0g to ♂
Unspecified disorders of nervous system 349.9/G969 with spasm D013035:	
Huángqíwǔwùtāng 5g chuānxiōng 1g dānshēn 1g zhúrú 1g sāngzhī 1g dāngguī 1g jiānghuáng 1g to ♀	Huángqíwǔwùtāng 5g chuānxiōng 1g dānshēn 1g zhúrú 1g sāngzhī 1g dāngguī 1g jiānghuáng 1g to ♂

Sháoyàogāncǎotāng has long been used in traditional Chinese medicine for spasms. Note that an arterial spasm can cause vasoconstriction, leading to tissue ischemia and tissue death.

15.7. Hemifacial Spasm

Hemifacial spasm is frequent involuntary muscle spasms on one side of the face. Irritation or compression, by nearby blood vessels or tumor, of the facial nerve can cause hemifacial spasms.

Table 15.7. Herbal prescriptions for hemifacial spasm

Hemifacial Spasm: https://meshb.nlm.nih.gov/record/ui?ui=D019569.	
Common prescriptions:	
Wūyàoshùnqìsǎn 5g gégēntāng 5g + acupuncture Wūyàoshùnqìsǎn 5g huángqíwǔwùtāng 5g + acupuncture	
Alternative prescriptions:	
Gégēntāng 5g qínjiāo 1g gōuténg 1g Gégēntāng 5g báijiāngcán 1g qínjiāo 1g chántuì 1g gōuténg 1g Wūyàoshùnqìsǎn 5g gégēntāng 5g Wūyàoshùnqìsǎn 5g báizhǐ 1g gǎoběn 1g Wūyàoshùnqìsǎn 5g báizhǐ 0g báijiāngcán 0g dìlóng 0g chántuì 0g	
Indicated diseases:	
Trigeminal neuralgia 350.1 (Trigeminal neuralgia G500); Geniculate ganglionitis 351.1 (Geniculate ganglionitis G511); Facial nerve disorders 351; Unspecified disorder of cranial nerves 352.9 (Cranial nerve disorder, unspecified G529); Unspecified disorders of nervous system 349.9 (Disorder of central nervous system, unspecified G969); Blepharospasm 333.81 (Blepharospasm G245); Unspecified disorder of eyelid 374.9 (Unspecified disorder of eyelid H029); Disorder of eye, unspecified 379.90 (Unspecified disorder of eye and adnexa H579); Myoneural disorders 358; Unspecified condition of brain 348.9 (Disorder of brain, unspecified G939); Malignant neoplasm of cerebellum nos 191.6 (Malignant neoplasm of cerebellum C716); Neoplasm of unspecified nature of brain 239.6 (Neoplasm of unspecified behavior of brain D496); Malignant neoplasm of nervous system, part unspecified 192.9 (Malignant neoplasm of central nervous system, unspecified C729)	
Trigeminal neuralgia 350.1/G500 with hemifacial spasm D019569:	
Gégēntāng 5g báizhǐ 1g báijiāngcán 1g qínjiāo 1g chántuì 1g gōuténg 1g + acupuncture to ♀	Wūyàoshùnqìsǎn 5g báizhǐ 1g báijiāngcán 1g dìlóng 1g + acupuncture to ♂
Blepharospasm 333.81/G245 with hemifacial spasm D019569:	
Wūyàoshùnqìsǎn 5g báijiāngcán 1g dìlóng 1g qínjiāo 1g chántuì 1g gōuténg 1g + acupuncture to ♀	Wūyàoshùnqìsǎn 5g báijiāngcán 1g dìlóng 1g chántuì 1g + acupuncture to ♂
Unspecified condition of brain 348.9/G939 with hemifacial spasm D019569:	
Xiǎoxùmìngtāng 5g + acupuncture to ♀	Bǔyánghuánwǔtāng 5g dānshēn 1g shíchāngpú 1g yuǎnzhì 1g + acupuncture to ♂

A modern use of Wūyàoshùnqìsǎn is for unspecified neuralgia, neuritis and radiculitis (Wang, 2019). Its use here for facial spasms is believed to be due to the pharmacokinetic properties of Wūyàoshùnqìsǎn, which enable the distribution of its active ingredients to the face.

15.8. Muscle Spasticity

Muscle spasticity is prolonged contraction of one or more muscles when one tries to move or is at rest. Lesions to the areas of the brain and spinal cord controlling voluntary muscle stretch cause muscle spasticity, including traumatic brain or spinal cord injury, stroke, multiple sclerosis, and cerebral palsy.

Table 15.8. Herbal prescriptions for muscle spasticity

Muscle Spasticity: https://meshb.nlm.nih.gov/record/ui?ui=D009128.	
Common prescriptions:	
Huángqíwǔwùtāng 5g dānshēn 1g zhúrú 1g sāngzhī 1g jiānghuáng 1g Huángqíwǔwùtāng 5g dānshēn 1g zhúrú 1g sāngzhī 1g jiānghuáng 1g + acupuncture Huángqíwǔwùtāng 5g dānshēn 1g zhúrú 1g sāngzhī 1g dāngguī 1g jiānghuáng 1g Huángqíwǔwùtāng 5g dānshēn 1g zhúrú 1g sāngzhī 1g jiānghuáng 1g jīxuèténg 1g	
Alternative prescriptions:	
Huángqíwǔwùtāng 5g juānbìtāng 5g dānshēn 1g zhúrú 1g sāngzhī 1g jiānghuáng 1g + acupuncture Huángqíwǔwùtāng 5g dānshēn 1g zhúrú 1g sāngzhī 1g qínjiāo 1g jiānghuáng 1g Shūjīnghuóxuètāng 5g huángqíwǔwùtāng 5g dānshēn 1g sāngzhī 1g jīxuèténg 1g + acupuncture Huángqíwǔwùtāng 5g dānshēn 1g zhúrú 1g sāngzhī 1g jīxuèténg 1g gōuténg 1g Shēntòngzhúyūtāng 5g dāngguīsìnìtāng 5g	
Indicated diseases:	
Primary lateral sclerosis 335.24 (Primary lateral sclerosis G1223); Motor neuron disease 335.2; Anterior horn cell disease 335; Myopathy, unspecified 359.9 (Myopathy, unspecified G729); Myoneural disorders 358; Unspecified disorders of nervous system 349.9 (Disorder of central nervous system, unspecified G969); Primary cerebellar degeneration 334.2 (Congenital nonprogressive ataxia G110, Late-onset cerebellar ataxia G112); Unspecified disease of spinal cord 336.9 (Disease of spinal cord, unspecified G959); Unspecified condition of brain 348.9 (Disorder of brain, unspecified G939); Hereditary spastic paraplegia 334.1 (Hereditary spastic paraplegia G114); Critical illness polyneuropathy 357.82 (Critical illness polyneuropathy G6281)	
Primary lateral sclerosis 335.24/G1223 with muscle spasticity D009128:	
Huángqíwǔwùtāng 5g juānbìtāng 5g + acupuncture to ♀	Huángqíwǔwùtāng 5g bǔyánghuánwǔtāng 5g + acupuncture to ♂
Primary cerebellar degeneration 334.2/G110,G112 with muscle spasticity D009128:	
Bǔyánghuánwǔtāng 5g dúhuójìshēngtāng 5g to ♀	Bǔyánghuánwǔtāng 5g dānshēn 1g niúxī 1g shíchāngpú 1g yuǎnzhì 1g + acupuncture to ♂
Hereditary spastic paraplegia 334.1/G114 with muscle spasticity D009128:	
Bǔyánghuánwǔtāng 5g dānshēn 1g shíchāngpú 1g yuǎnzhì 1g + acupuncture to ♀	Bǔyánghuánwǔtāng 5g jìshēngshènqìwán 5g dānshēn 1g shíchāngpú 1g yuǎnzhì 1g + acupuncture to ♂

Huángqíwǔwùtāng is used for muscle hypotonia and is used here to relax spastic muscles.

15.9. Muscle Cramp

Muscle cramp is a sudden and usually painful contraction of the muscle. Muscle overuse, muscle strain, dehydration, restricted blood supply, and electrolyte imbalance can cause muscle cramps.

Table 15.9. Herbal prescriptions for muscle cramp

Muscle Cramp: https://meshb.nlm.nih.gov/record/ui?ui=D009120.	
Common prescriptions:	
Dāngguīsìnìtāng 5g shēngjiāng 1g wúzhūyú 1g Dāngguīsìnìtāng 5g shēngjiāng 1g wúzhūyú 1g fùzǐ 1g Dāngguīsìnìtāng 5g sìnìtāng 4g shēngjiāng 1g wúzhūyú 1g Dāngguīsìnìtāng 5g shēngjiāng 1g wúzhūyú 1g jīxuèténg 1g	
Alternative prescriptions:	
Huángqíwǔwùtāng 5g dānshēn 1g zhúrú 1g sāngzhī 1g jiānghuáng 1g Dāngguīsìnìtāng 5g fùzǐ 2g shēngjiāng 1g wúzhūyú 1g Huángqíwǔwùtāng 5g dāngguīsìnìtāng 5g dānshēn 2g zhúrú 2g sāngzhī 2g jiānghuáng 2g Dāngguīsìnìtāng 5g shēngjiāng 0g wúzhūyú 0g	
Indicated diseases:	
Myopathy, unspecified 359.9 (Myopathy, unspecified G729); Unspecified acquired hypothyroidism 244.9 (Hypothyroidism, unspecified E039); Myoneural disorders 358; Unspecified disorders of nervous system 349.9 (Disorder of central nervous system, unspecified G969); Unspecified disorder of thyroid 246.9 (Disorder of thyroid, unspecified E079); Unspecified endocrine disorder 259.9 (Endocrine disorder, unspecified E349); Unspecified disorder of joint, site unspecified 719.90 (Joint disorder, unspecified M259); Unspecified disorder of metabolism 277.9 (Metabolic disorder, unspecified E889); Other dermatoses 702	
Myopathy, unspecified 359.9/G729 with muscle cramp D009120:	
Huángqíwǔwùtāng 5g dāngguīsìnìtāng 5g dānshēn 1g zhúrú 1g sāngzhī 1g jiānghuáng 1g to ♀	Huángqíwǔwùtāng 5g dāngguīsìnìtāng 5g dānshēn 1g zhúrú 1g sāngzhī 1g jiānghuáng 1g to ♂
Other dermatoses 702 with muscle cramp D009120:	
Dāngguīsìnìtāng 5g shēngjiāng 1g wúzhūyú 1g to ♀	Xiāofēngsǎn 5g dāngguīyǐnzǐ 5g tǔfúlíng 1g báixiānpí 1g dìfūzǐ 1g to ♂

As Dāngguīsìnìtāng 'enriches Blood, expels chills' and 'warms meridians, unblocks vessels,' it is used to relieve muscle cramps. Hypothyroidism can develop hypothyroid myopathy including muscle weakness and muscle cramps (Fariduddin and Bansal, 2022).

15.10. Muscle Rigidity

Muscle rigidity or stiffness is tightness of the muscle so that one feels difficult to move the affected muscle. Muscle overuse, exercise, dehydration, electrolyte imbalance, infection, multiple sclerosis, toxins and medication can cause muscle rigidity.

Table 15.10. Herbal prescriptions for muscle rigidity

Muscle Rigidity: https://meshb.nlm.nih.gov/record/ui?ui=D009127.
Common prescriptions:
Sìnìtāng 5g dāngguīsìnìtāng 5g shēngjiāng 1g wúzhūyú 1g Máhuángfùzǐxìxīntāng 5g dāngguīsìnìtāng 5g shēngjiāng 1g wúzhūyú 1g fùzǐ 1g Máhuángfùzǐxìxīntāng 5g dāngguīsìnìtāng 5g shēngjiāng 1g wúzhūyú 1g Máhuángfùzǐxìxīntāng 5g dāngguīsìnìtāng 5g shēngjiāng 1g wúzhūyú 1g fùzǐ 1g guìzhī 1g Sìnìtāng 5g dāngguīsìnìtāng 5g wúzhūyú 1g gānjiāng 1g
Alternative prescriptions:
Sìnìtāng 5g guìzhī 1g máhuáng 1g xìxīn 0g Sìnìtāng 5g shēngjiāng 1g guìzhī 1g dàhuáng 0g Dāngguīsìnìtāng 5g shēngjiāng 1g wúzhūyú 1g Sìnìtāng 5g bànxià 1g dàhuáng 0g

Table 15.10. (Continued)

Muscle Rigidity: https://meshb.nlm.nih.gov/record/ui?ui=D009127.	
Indicated diseases:	
Neuroleptic malignant syndrome 333.92 (Malignant neuroleptic syndrome G210); Myopathy, unspecified 359.9 (Myopathy, unspecified G729); Unspecified condition of brain 348.9 (Disorder of brain, unspecified G939); Unspecified disorders of nervous system 349.9 (Disorder of central nervous system, unspecified G969); Myoneural disorders 358; Unspecified disorder of joint, site unspecified 719.90 (Joint disorder, unspecified M259)	
Neuroleptic malignant syndrome 333.92/G210 with muscle rigidity D009127:	
Huángqíwǔwùtāng 5g dāngguīsìnìtāng 5g dānshēn 1g sāngzhī 1g jīxuèténg 1g to ♀	Sháoyàogāncǎotāng 5g shūjīnghuóxuètāng 5g mùguā 1g niúxī 1g to ♂
Myopathy, unspecified 359.9/G729 with muscle rigidity D009127:	
Guìzhīsháoyàozhīmǔtāng 5g shūjīnghuóxuètāng 5g dúhuójìshēngtāng 5g to ♀	Guīlùèrxiānjiāo 5g to ♂

Máhuángfùzǐxìxīntāng is today used for chronic sinusitis, and allergic rhinitis (Wang, 2019), and therefore here for infection related muscle rigidity.

15.11. Dysarthria

Dysarthria is difficulty talking because of weakness or damage of the speech producing muscles including the lips, tongue, throat and lungs.

Table 15.11. Herbal prescriptions for dysarthria

Dysarthria: https://meshb.nlm.nih.gov/record/ui?ui=D004401.	
Common prescriptions:	
Sìnìtāng 5g bànxià 1g dàhuáng 0g Máhuángfùzǐxìxīntāng 5g shēngjiāng 1g guìzhī 1g Máhuángfùzǐxìxīntāng 5g shēngjiāng 1g guìzhī 1g zhìgāncǎo 1g Máhuángfùzǐxìxīntāng 5g shēngjiāng 1g guìzhī 1g gāncǎo 1g Sìnìtāng 5g bànxià 1g shēngjiāng 1g guìzhī 1g	
Alternative prescriptions:	
Sìnìtāng 5g bànxià 2g dàhuáng 0g Máhuángfùzǐxìxīntāng 5g fùzǐ 3g guìzhī 3g dàzǎo 2g zhìgāncǎo 2g gānjiāng 2g Guìzhītāng 5g shēngjiāng 0g guìzhī 0g Guìzhītāng 5g shēngjiāng 1g guìzhī 1g	
Indicated diseases:	
Unspecified disease of pharynx 478.20 (Other diseases of pharynx J392); Unspecified disorder of esophagus 530.9 (Disease of esophagus, unspecified K229); Myasthenia gravis without (acute) exacerbation 358.00 (Myasthenia gravis without (acute) exacerbation G7000); Unspecified cerebrovascular disease 437.9 (Cerebrovascular disease, unspecified I679); Primary lateral sclerosis 335.24 (Primary lateral sclerosis G1223); Disorders of hypoglossal [12th] nerve 352.5 (Disorders of hypoglossal nerve G523); Unspecified disorder of cranial nerves 352.9 (Cranial nerve disorder, unspecified G529); Unspecified disorders of nervous system 349.9 (Disorder of central nervous system, unspecified G969); Unspecified condition of brain 348.9 (Disorder of brain, unspecified G939)	
Unspecified disease of pharynx 478.20/J392 with dysarthria D004401:	
Qīngyānlìgétāng 5g màiméndōngtāng 5g yínqiàosǎn 5g to ♀	Bànxiàhòupòtāng 5g màiméndōngtāng 5g to ♂
Unspecified cerebrovascular disease 437.9/I679 with dysarthria D004401:	
Bǔyánghuánwǔtāng 5g sānqī 1g dānshēn 1g shíchāngpú 1g yuǎnzhì 1g + acupuncture to ♀	Bǔyánghuánwǔtāng 5g chuānqī 2g dānshēn 1g shíchāngpú 1g yuǎnzhì 1g + acupuncture to ♂
Disorders of hypoglossal [12th] nerve 352.5/G523 with dysarthria D004401:	
Guìzhītāng 5g bànxià 1g dàhuáng 0g to ♀	Guìzhītāng 5g bànxià 1g dàhuáng 0g to ♂

Máhuángfùzǐxìxīntāng is used for muscle hypotonia. Its use here for dysarthria could be attributed to its effects on the upper respiratory tract as its modern uses are for upper respiratory tract infections (Wang, 2019).

15.12. Fasciculation

Fasciculation is involuntary, intermittent contraction of muscle fibers, which is too weak to move a limb. Fasciculation results from over-activity of a motor neuron and its innervated muscle fibers. The cause of fasciculation is unknown, but anxiety is a risk factor.

Table 15.12. Herbal prescriptions for fasciculation

Fasciculation: https://meshb.nlm.nih.gov/record/ui?ui=D005207.	
Common prescriptions:	
Guìzhītāng 5g báisháo 1g dàhuáng 0g Máhuángfùzǐxìxīntāng 5g dāngguīsìnìtāng 5g shēngjiāng 1g wúzhūyú 1g fùzǐ 1g Guìzhītāng 5g gégēn 1g + acupuncture	
Alternative prescriptions:	
Sháoyàogāncǎotāng 5g dāngguīniāntòngtāng 5g dúhuójìshēngtāng 5g shūjīnghuóxuètāng 3g gégēntāng 3g guīlùèrxiānjiāo 3g niúxī 2g guìzhīsháoyàozhīmǔtāng 2g Dāngguīsìnìtāng 5g fùzǐ 1g + acupuncture Huángqíwǔwùtāng 5g gégēn 1g Guìzhītāng 5g fùzǐ 1g gégēn 1g	
Indicated diseases:	
Primary lateral sclerosis 335.24 (Primary lateral sclerosis G1223); Unspecified disorder of metabolism 277.9 (Metabolic disorder, unspecified E889); Motor neuron disease 335.2; Anterior horn cell disease 335; Unspecified disease of spinal cord 336.9 (Disease of spinal cord, unspecified G959); Myoneural disorders 358; Unspecified disorders of nervous system 349.9 (Disorder of central nervous system, unspecified G969); Myasthenia gravis without (acute) exacerbation 358.00 (Myasthenia gravis without (acute) exacerbation G7000); Myopathy, unspecified 359.9 (Myopathy, unspecified G729); Malignant neoplasm of thymus 164.0 (Malignant neoplasm of thymus C37); Malignant neoplasm of thorax 195.1 (Malignant neoplasm of thorax C761)	
Primary lateral sclerosis 335.24/G1223 with fasciculation D005207:	
Huángqíwǔwùtāng 5g bǔyánghuánwǔtāng 5g dānshēn 1g sāngzhī 1g jīxuèténg 1g + acupuncture to ♀	Shūjīnghuóxuètāng 5g huángqíwǔwùtāng 5g dānshēn 1g sāngzhī 1g jīxuèténg 1g + acupuncture to ♂
Myasthenia gravis without (acute) exacerbation 358.00/G7000 with fasciculation D005207:	
Bǔzhōngyìqìtāng 5g dúhuójìshēngtāng 5g to ♀	Bǔzhōngyìqìtāng 5g jìshēngshènqìwán 5g dùzhòng 1g xùduàn 1g to ♂
Myopathy, unspecified 359.9/G729 with fasciculation D005207:	
Sháoyàogāncǎotāng 5g huángqíwǔwùtāng 5g dānshēn 1g mùguā 1g niúxī 1g sāngzhī 1g to ♀	Guīlùèrxiānjiāo 5g to ♂
Unspecified disorders of nervous system 349.9/G969 with fasciculation D005207:	
Huángqíwǔwùtāng 5g chuānxiōng 1g dānshēn 1g zhúrú 1g sāngzhī 1g dāngguī 1g jiānghuáng 1g to ♀	Huángqíwǔwùtāng 5g chuānxiōng 1g dānshēn 1g zhúrú 1g sāngzhī 1g dāngguī 1g jiānghuáng 1g to ♂

Acute onset fasciculation was found to follow a viral infection (Blexrud et al., 1993). We see the prescription of Guìzhītāng or Máhuángfùzǐxìxīntāng, whose modern uses consist of upper respiratory tract infections (Wang, 2019).

15.13. Myotonia

Myotonia is delayed relaxation, due to over-excitability of the muscle fibers, after voluntary contraction of the muscle. Myotonia is a characteristic symptom of channelopathies which are caused by mutations in a gene encoding ion channel.

Table 15.13. Herbal prescriptions for myotonia

Myotonia: https://meshb.nlm.nih.gov/record/ui?ui=D009222.	
Common prescriptions:	
Huángqíwǔwùtāng 5g dānshēn 1g zhúrú 1g sāngzhī 1g jiānghuáng 1g Huángqíwǔwùtāng 5g dāngguīsìnìtāng 5g dānshēn 1g zhúrú 1g sāngzhī 1g jiānghuáng 1g Huángqíwǔwùtāng 5g dānshēn 1g zhúrú 1g sāngzhī 1g jiānghuáng 1g + acupuncture Huángqíwǔwùtāng 5g dāngguīsìnìtāng 5g dānshēn 2g zhúrú 2g sāngzhī 2g jiānghuáng 2g Huángqíwǔwùtāng 5g dāngguīsìnìtāng 5g dānshēn 1g zhúrú 1g sāngzhī 1g jiānghuáng 1g + acupuncture	
Alternative prescriptions:	
Huángqíwǔwùtāng 5g dānshēn 1g zhúrú 1g sāngzhī 1g jiānghuáng 1g jīxuèténg 1g + acupuncture Dāngguīsìnìtāng 5g sháoyàogāncǎotāng 2g jīxuèténg 1g + acupuncture Huángqíwǔwùtāng 5g dāngguīsìnìtāng 5g niúxī 1g sāngzhī 1g jīxuèténg 1g Dāngguīsìnìtāng 5g huángqí 2g shēngjiāng 1g wúzhūyú 1g	
Indicated diseases:	
Unspecified disorders of nervous system 349.9 (Disorder of central nervous system, unspecified G969); Unspecified acquired hypothyroidism 244.9 (Hypothyroidism, unspecified E039); Unspecified disorder of thyroid 246.9 (Disorder of thyroid, unspecified E079); Unspecified endocrine disorder 259.9 (Endocrine disorder, unspecified E349); Other dermatoses 702; Myopathy, unspecified 359.9 (Myopathy, unspecified G729); Dermatomyositis 710.3 (Juvenile dermatomyositis without myopathy M3303, Other dermatomyositis without myopathy M3313, Dermatopolymyositis, unspecified, organ involvement unspecified M3390, Dermatopolymyositis, unspecified without myopathy M3393); Myoneural disorders 358; Myotonic disorders 359.2; Myasthenia gravis without (acute) exacerbation 358.00 (Myasthenia gravis without (acute) exacerbation G7000)	
Unspecified disorders of nervous system 349.9/G969 with myotonia D009222:	
Huángqíwǔwùtāng 5g chuānxiōng 1g dānshēn 1g zhúrú 1g sāngzhī 1g dāngguī 1g jiānghuáng 1g to ♀	Huángqíwǔwùtāng 5g chuānxiōng 1g dānshēn 1g zhúrú 1g sāngzhī 1g dāngguī 1g jiānghuáng 1g to ♂
Other dermatoses 702 with myotonia D009222:	
Jiědúsìwùtāng 5g xiāofēngsǎn 4g zhēnrénhuómìngyǐnqùchuānshānjiǎ 4g huángliánjiědútāng 4g to ♀	Xiāofēngsǎn 5g jiědúsìwùtāng 5g zhēnrénhuómìngyǐnqùchuānshānjiǎ 4g huángliánjiědútāng 4g to ♂
Myotonic disorders 359.2 with myotonia D009222:	
Huángqíwǔwùtāng 5g dāngguīsìnìtāng 5g dānshēn 1g zhúrú 1g sāngzhī 1g jiānghuáng 1g to ♀	Huángqíwǔwùtāng 5g dāngguīsìnìtāng 5g dānshēn 1g zhúrú 1g sāngzhī 1g jiānghuáng 1g to ♂
Myasthenia gravis without (acute) exacerbation 358.00/G7000 with myotonia D009222:	
Bǔzhōngyìqìtāng 5g to ♀	Bāwèidìhuángwán 5g bǔzhōngyìqìtāng 5g to ♂
Myopathy, unspecified 359.9/G729 with myotonia D009222:	
Huángqíwǔwùtāng 5g dāngguīsìnìtāng 5g dānshēn 1g zhúrú 1g sāngzhī 1g jiānghuáng 1g to ♀	Huángqíwǔwùtāng 5g dāngguīsìnìtāng 5g dānshēn 1g zhúrú 1g sāngzhī 1g jiānghuáng 1g to ♂

Huángqíwǔwùtāng 'benefits Qi, warms meridians' and 'harmonizes digestion, unlocks paralysis.' Myotonia can be alleviated by warming up the contracted muscles. As Huángqíwǔwùtāng 'warms up meridians,' it is supposed to alleviate myotonia.

References

Blexrud, M. D., Windebank, A. J., & Daube, J. R. (1993). Long-term follow-up of 121 patients with benign fasciculations. *Annals of Neurology*, *34*(4), 622–625. https://doi.org/10.1002/ana.410340419.

Davison, C., & Weiss, M. M. (1929). Muscular Hypotonia Associated with Congenital Heart Disease. *Archives of Pediatrics & Adolescent Medicine*, *37*(2), 359–366. https://doi.org/10.1001/archpedi.1929.01930020129012.

Fariduddin, M. M., & Bansal, N. (2022). *Hypothyroid Myopathy*. In: StatPearls [Internet]. Treasure Island (FL), StatPearls Publishing. PMID: 30137798.

Parodi, J., Grisoni, E., Ferrario, C., Kramer, A., & Beven, E. (1987). Hypertonicity of intestinal smooth muscle as a factor of intestinal ischemia in necrotizing enterocolitis. *Journal of Pediatric Surgery*, *22*(8), 713–718. https://doi.org/10.1016/s0022-3468(87)80611-5.

Wang, S. C. (2019). *Clinical Herbal Prescriptions: Principles and Practices of Herbal Formulations from Deep Learning Health Insurance Herbal Prescription Big Data*. WSPC. https://doi.org/10.1142/11211.

Waqas, K., Chen, J., Trajanoska, K., Ikram, M. A., Uitterlinden, A. G., Rivadeneira, F., & Zillikens, M. C. (2022). Skin Autofluorescence, a Noninvasive Biomarker for Advanced Glycation End-products, Is Associated With Sarcopenia. *The Journal of Clinical Endocrinology & Metabolism*, *107*(2), e793–e803. https://doi.org/10.1210/clinem/dgab632.

Chapter 16

Immune System Diseases

Jawed vertebrates possess a pathogen-specific defense called the adaptive immune system that other organisms do not have. Development of vaccine and immunization exploits our knowledge of the adaptive immunity. The idea is that a substance, called antigen, is injected in small quantities into our body to elicit immune response against the substance. Later on, when larger amounts of the same substance enter into our body, our adaptive immune system is able to mount an immediate and massive attack against them because our immune system already recognizes and prepares for them. In traditional vaccines, the antigens are made of microbial proteins or inactive microbes. In mRNA vaccines, mRNA of the target microbial protein is injected into the upper arm. As mRNA is blueprint of protein, microbial proteins are synthesized inside the muscular cells of our body, eliciting the immune response. The advantages of mRNA vaccines are that their design is easier once the pathogen genomes are available and that their manufacture is easily scaled up, explaining the success of the mRNA COVID-19 vaccines. On the other hand, all organisms including plants and bacteria possess what is called innate immunity whose response is immediate but not pathogen specific. Moreover, the skin, cough reflex, gastric acid, and gut flora can be considered physical, mechanical, chemical and biological barriers, respectively, against foreign pathogens. Abnormalities in the immunological mechanisms can present the signs and symptoms shown in Figure 16.1. Note that many of them already appear in previous chapters.

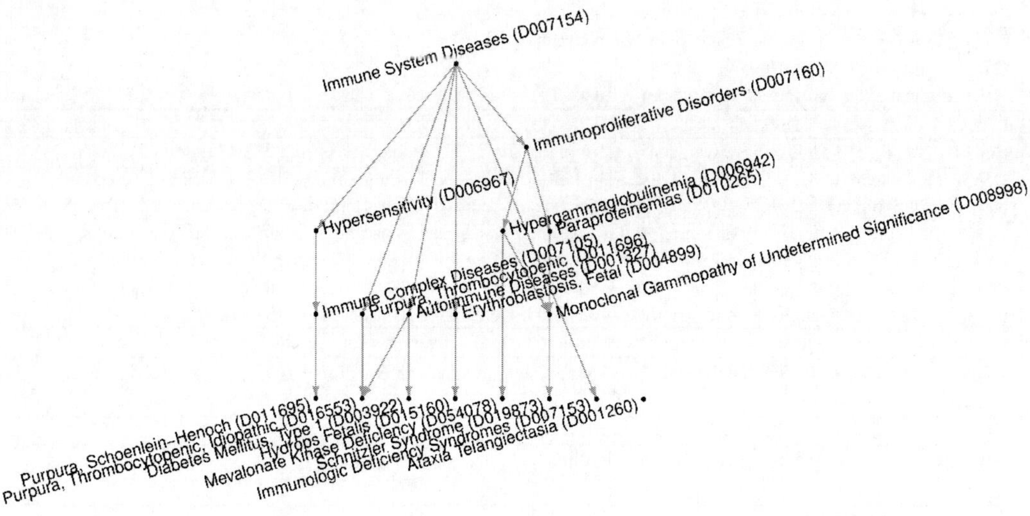

Figure 16.1. Congenital or acquired immune dysfunctions can affect different immune components and cause over- or underactive immune response.

The formulas and herbs commonly used for the immune signs and symptoms include Sháoyàogāncǎotāng, Xiāofēngsǎn, Shūjīnghuóxuètāng, Dāngguīniāntòngtāng, Guìzhīfúlíngwán, Niúxī, Yánhúsuǒ, Yìmǔcǎo, Xìxīn, and Huángqín.

The disease diagnoses that are associated with the signs and symptoms are unspecified cardiovascular disease, unspecified disorders of nervous system, unspecified disorder of metabolism, and unspecified diseases of blood and blood-forming organs.

16.1. Hydrops Fetalis

Hydrops fetalis is severe swelling in at least two body areas of an unborn or newborn baby. The immune etiology of hydrops fetalis is when the pregnant mother's blood type is Rh-negative while the baby's is Rh-positive, the mother's immune system then attacks the baby's red blood cells, causing fetal anemia. If the baby cannot overcome anemia, its heart may fail and lead to edema.

Table 16.1. Herbal prescriptions for hydrops fetalis

Hydrops Fetalis: https://meshb.nlm.nih.gov/record/ui?ui=D015160.	
Common prescriptions:	
Jiāwèixiāoyáosǎn 5g guìzhīfúlíngwán 5g dānshēn 1g xiāngfù 1g yìmǔcǎo 1g zélán 1g Guìzhīfúlíngwán 5g dāngguīsháoyàosǎn 5g dānshēn 1g xiāngfù 1g yìmǔcǎo 1g zélán 1g Guìzhīfúlíngwán 5g dāngguīsháoyàosǎn 5g dānshēn 1g xiāngfù 1g yìmǔcǎo 1g Jiāwèixiāoyáosǎn 5g guìzhīfúlíngwán 5g dānshēn 1g xiāngfù 1g yìmǔcǎo 1g Jiāwèixiāoyáosǎn 5g guìzhīfúlíngwán 5g dāngguīsháoyàosǎn 5g	
Alternative prescriptions:	
Táohóngsìwùtāng 5g dānshēn 1g éshù 1g gāncǎo 0g Wēnjīngtāng 5g dāngguīsháoyàosǎn 3g yìmǔcǎo 1g huángqí 1g shēngmá 1g mùtōng 1g fángfēng 1g cāngěrzǐ 1g xìxīn 0g Guìzhīfúlíngwán 5g wēnjīngtāng 5g dāngguīsháoyàosǎn 5g Guìzhīfúlíngwán 5g dāngguīsháoyàosǎn 5g Guìzhīfúlíngwán 5g xiāoyáosǎn 5g yìmǔcǎo 1g tùsīzǐ 1g	
Indicated and associated diseases:	
Hemolytic disease of fetus or newborn, due to isoimmunization 773; Alpha thalassemia 282.43 (Alpha thalassemia D560); Thalassemias 282.4; Unspecified diseases of blood and blood-forming organs 289.9 (Disease of blood and blood-forming organs, unspecified D759); Heart disease, unspecified 429.9 (Heart disease, unspecified I519); Unspecified congenital anomaly of heart 746.9 (Congenital malformation of cardiac chambers and connections, unspecified Q209, Congenital malformation of heart, unspecified Q249); Cardiovascular disease, unspecified 429.2 (Atherosclerotic heart disease of native coronary artery without angina pectoris I2510); Unspecified complication of pregnancy 646.9; Hemangioma of unspecified site 228.00 (Hemangioma unspecified site D1800)	
Hemolytic disease of fetus or newborn, due to isoimmunization 773 with hydrops fetalis D015160:	
Jiāwèixiāoyáosǎn 5g guīpítāng 5g dānshēn 1g xiāngfù 1g yìmǔcǎo 1g to ♀	Sǎnzhǒngkuìjiāntāng 5g bànzhīlián 2g báihuāshéshécǎo 2g to ♂
Heart disease, unspecified 429.9/I519 with hydrops fetalis D015160:	
Sìnìtāng 5g gānlùyǐn 5g mǔdānpí 1g zhīzǐ 1g huánglián 0g to ♀	Sìnìtāng 5g gānlùyǐn 5g mǔdānpí 1g zhīzǐ 1g huánglián 0g to ♂
Unspecified complication of pregnancy 646.9 with hydrops fetalis D015160:	
Dāngguīsháoyàosǎn 5g dùzhòng 1g sāngjìshēng 1g tùsīzǐ 1g xùduàn 1g to ♀	Dāngguīsháoyàosǎn 5g dùzhòng 1g sāngjìshēng 1g tùsīzǐ 1g xùduàn 1g to ♂

The modern uses of Jiāwèixiāoyáosǎn and Guìzhīfúlíngwán include unspecified chronic hepatitis (Wang, 2019). With fetal anemia, the fetus's liver overworks to replenish lost red blood cells, leading to hepatomegaly.

16.2. Schnitzler Syndrome

Schnitzler syndrome is characterized by repeated bouts of fever, urticarial rash, joint pain, joint inflammation, muscle pain, bone pain and headache. The exact cause of Schnitzler syndrome is unknown; however, cytokine interleukin-1 is suspected to play a role in the development of Schnitzler syndrome.

Both mevalonate kinase deficiency in Section 6.9 and Schnitzler syndrome are classified as autoinflammatory disorders, with the former being inborn and the latter acquired or late-onset. As both display similar symptoms, we see similar herbal prescriptions for them.

Table 16.2. Herbal prescriptions for Schnitzler syndrome

Schnitzler Syndrome: https://meshb.nlm.nih.gov/record/ui?ui=D019873.	
Common prescriptions:	
Sháoyàogāncǎotāng 5g shūjīnghuóxuètāng 5g dāngguīniāntòngtāng 5g + acupuncture Sháoyàogāncǎotāng 5g shūjīnghuóxuètāng 5g + acupuncture	
Alternative prescriptions:	
Zhènggǔzǐjīndān 5g dāngguīniāntòngtāng 5g yánhúsuǒ 2g dǎodìwúgōng 2g sháoyàogāncǎotāng 2g chuānwū 2g rǔxiāng 2g mòyào 1g xiǎoxiànxiōngtāng 1g + acupuncture Shūjīnghuóxuètāng 5g sháoyàogāncǎotāng 4g mòyào 1g rǔxiāng 1g yánhúsuǒ 1g + acupuncture Shūjīnghuóxuètāng 5g sháoyàogāncǎotāng 4g mòyào 1g rǔxiāng 1g + acupuncture Shēntòngzhúyūtāng 5g sháoyàogāncǎotāng 3g mòyào 1g rǔxiāng 1g + acupuncture Shūjīnghuóxuètāng 5g dāngguīniāntòngtāng 5g chuānqī 1g niúxī 1g yánhúsuǒ 1g qiānghuó 1g + acupuncture	
Indicated diseases:	
Cardiovascular disease, unspecified 429.2 (Atherosclerotic heart disease of native coronary artery without angina pectoris I2510); Multiple myeloma 203.0; Unspecified hemorrhagic conditions 287.9 (Hemorrhagic condition, unspecified D699); Unspecified diseases of blood and blood-forming organs 289.9 (Disease of blood and blood-forming organs, unspecified D759); Unspecified condition of brain 348.9 (Disorder of brain, unspecified G939); Unspecified disorder of metabolism 277.9 (Metabolic disorder, unspecified E889); Alexia 315.01 (Dyslexia and alexia R480); Unspecified disorders of nervous system 349.9 (Disorder of central nervous system, unspecified G969)	
Cardiovascular disease, unspecified 429.2/I2510 with Schnitzler syndrome D019873:	
Sìnìtāng 5g gānlùyǐn 5g mǔdānpí 1g zhīzǐ 1g huánglián 0g to ♀	Xuèfǔzhúyūtāng 5g zhìgāncǎotāng 5g to ♂
Unspecified condition of brain 348.9/G939 with Schnitzler syndrome D019873:	
Bǔyánghuánwǔtāng 5g + acupuncture to ♀	Bǔyánghuánwǔtāng 5g dānshēn 1g tiānmá 1g shíchāngpú 1g yuǎnzhì 1g + acupuncture to ♂

16.3. Hypergammaglobulinemia

Hypergammaglobulinemia, also known as polyclonal gammopathy, is too many antibodies in the blood serum. Chronic inflammation, autoimmune disorder, liver disease, and infection can cause hypergammaglobulinemia.

Xiāofēngsǎn and Dāngguīyǐnzǐ are today used for contact dermatitis and other eczema, and Xiāofēngsǎn is also used for unspecified urticaria (Wang, 2019). Skin disorders and hypergammaglobulinemia can be the result of immunodeficiencies (de Wit et al., 2018; Upton, 2015).

Table 16.3. Herbal prescriptions for hypergammaglobulinemia

<table>
<tr><td colspan="2">Hypergammaglobulinemia: https://meshb.nlm.nih.gov/record/ui?ui=D006942.</td></tr>
<tr><td colspan="2">Common prescriptions:</td></tr>
<tr><td colspan="2">Xiāofēngsǎn 5g dāngguīyǐnzǐ 5g tǔfúlíng 1g báixiānpí 1g dìfūzǐ 1g
Xiāofēngsǎn 5g dāngguīyǐnzǐ 5g báixiānpí 1g dìfūzǐ 1g
Xiāofēngsǎn 5g lóngdǎnxiègāntāng 5g tǔfúlíng 1g báixiānpí 1g dìfūzǐ 1g
Xiāofēngsǎn 5g dāngguīyǐnzǐ 5g báixiānpí 1g dìfūzǐ 1g mǔdānpí 1g chìsháo 1g
Xiāofēngsǎn 5g dāngguīyǐnzǐ 5g tǔfúlíng 1g báixiānpí 1g dìfūzǐ 1g mǔdānpí 1g chìsháo 1g</td></tr>
<tr><td colspan="2">Alternative prescriptions:</td></tr>
<tr><td colspan="2">Xiāofēngsǎn 5g zhēnrénhuómìngyǐnqùchuānshānjiǎ 2g báixiānpí 1g yúxīngcǎo 1g
Xiāofēngsǎn 5g zhēnrénhuómìngyǐnqùchuānshānjiǎ 5g báixiānpí 2g yúxīngcǎo 2g
Xiāofēngsǎn 5g jiāwèixiāoyáosǎn 3g báixiānpí 1g xuánshēn 1g mǔdānpí 1g jīnyínhuā 1g jílí 1g gāncǎo 0g
Jiědúsìwùtāng 5g báixiānpí 0g jīnchán 0g zǐsūyè 0g
Jīngfángbàidúsǎn 5g jiědúsìwùtāng 5g yìyǐrén 4g jīnyínhuā 1g gāncǎo 1g</td></tr>
<tr><td colspan="2">Indicated diseases:</td></tr>
<tr><td colspan="2">Cardiovascular disease, unspecified 429.2 (Atherosclerotic heart disease of native coronary artery without angina pectoris I2510); Other dermatoses 702; Multiple myeloma 203.0; Unspecified hemorrhagic conditions 287.9 (Hemorrhagic condition, unspecified D699); Unspecified diseases of blood and blood-forming organs 289.9 (Disease of blood and blood-forming organs, unspecified D759); Unspecified disorder of liver 573.9 (Liver disease, unspecified K769); Malignant neoplasm of liver, not specified as primary or secondary 155.2 (Malignant neoplasm of liver, not specified as primary or secondary C229); Diseases of the jaws 526</td></tr>
<tr><td colspan="2">Cardiovascular disease, unspecified 429.2/I2510 with hypergammaglobulinemia D006942:</td></tr>
<tr><td>Yùzhú 5g sìnìtāng 5g mǔdānpí 1g zhīzǐ 1g to ♀</td><td>Yùzhú 5g sìnìtāng 5g mǔdānpí 1g zhīzǐ 1g to ♂</td></tr>
<tr><td colspan="2">Unspecified disorder of liver 573.9/K769 with hypergammaglobulinemia D006942:</td></tr>
<tr><td>Jiāwèixiāoyáosǎn 5g cháihúshūgāntāng 5g dānshēn 1g bànzhīlián 1g báihuāshéshécǎo 1g to ♀</td><td>Xuèfǔzhúyūtāng 5g cháihúshūgāntāng 5g shānzhā 1g dānshēn 1g to ♂</td></tr>
</table>

References

de Wit, J., Brada, R. J. K., van Veldhuizen, J., Dalm, V. A. S. H., & Pasmans, S. G. M. A. (2018). Skin disorders are prominent features in primary immunodeficiency diseases: A systematic overview of current data. *Allergy*, *74*(3), 464–482. https://doi.org/10.1111/all.13681.

Upton, J. (2015). Immunodeficiencies with hypergammaglobulinemia: a review. *LymphoSign Journal*, *2*(2), 57–73. https://doi.org/10.14785/lpsn-2014-0019.

Wang, S. C. (2019). *Clinical Herbal Prescriptions: Principles and Practices of Herbal Formulations from Deep Learning Health Insurance Herbal Prescription Big Data*. WSPC. https://doi.org/10.1142/11211.

Chapter 17

Other Signs and Symptoms

Previous chapters have described signs and symptoms that are typically observed or experienced in a single organ or part of the body. This chapter discusses remaining signs and symptoms and in particular those that affect the entire body, such as fever and lethargy.

17.1. Seizures

Seizures are sudden, temporary excessive electrical discharges between the neurons in the brain, which change the movements, feelings, levels of consciousness, and behavior of the patient. Recurrent unprovoked seizures are a hallmark of epilepsy. Sleep deprivation, high fever, substance abuse, brain concussion and infection can cause seizures.

Table 17.1. Herbal prescriptions for seizures

Seizures: https://meshb.nlm.nih.gov/record/ui?ui=D012640.	
Common prescriptions:	
Tiānwángbǔxīndān 5g jiāwèixiāoyáosǎn 5g suānzǎoréntāng 5g Tiānwángbǔxīndān 5g jiāwèixiāoyáosǎn 5g Tiānwángbǔxīndān 5g jiāwèixiāoyáosǎn 5g gāncǎoxiǎomàidàzǎotāng 5g	
Alternative prescriptions:	
Gāncǎoxiǎomàidàzǎotāng 5g cháihúguìzhītāng 5g zhúrú 1g yèjiāoténg 1g yuǎnzhì 1g Tiānwángbǔxīndān 5g jiāwèixiāoyáosǎn 5g héhuānpí 1g yèjiāoténg 1g Tiānwángbǔxīndān 5g jiāwèixiāoyáosǎn 5g wēndǎntāng 5g héhuānpí 1g yèjiāoténg 1g fúshén 1g Guīpítāng 5g gāncǎoxiǎomàidàzǎotāng 4g héhuānpí 1g yèjiāoténg 1g fúshén 1g Tiānwángbǔxīndān 5g gāncǎoxiǎomàidàzǎotāng 2g mǔlì 1g lónggǔ 1g	
Indicated diseases:	
Unspecified cerebrovascular disease 437.9 (Cerebrovascular disease, unspecified I679); Unspecified condition of brain 348.9 (Disorder of brain, unspecified G939); Disorders of calcium metabolism 275.4; Cardiovascular disease, unspecified 429.2 (Atherosclerotic heart disease of native coronary artery without angina pectoris I2510); Unspecified disorders of nervous system 349.9 (Disorder of central nervous system, unspecified G969); Unspecified disorder of metabolism 277.9 (Metabolic disorder, unspecified E889); Heart disease, unspecified 429.9 (Heart disease, unspecified I519); Malignant neoplasm of heart 164.1 (Malignant neoplasm of heart C380); Tuberous sclerosis 759.5 (Tuberous sclerosis Q851); Malignant neoplasm of thorax 195.1 (Malignant neoplasm of thorax C761); Conversion disorder 300.11 (Conversion disorder with motor symptom or deficit F444, Conversion disorder with sensory symptom or deficit F446); Somatization disorder 300.81 (Somatization disorder F450)	
Unspecified cerebrovascular disease 437.9/I679 with seizures D012640:	
Bǔyánghuánwǔtāng 5g chuānqī 1g dānshēn 1g shíchāngpú 1g yuǎnzhì 1g + acupuncture to ♀	Bǔyánghuánwǔtāng 5g chuānqī 2g dānshēn 1g shíchāngpú 1g yuǎnzhì 1g + acupuncture to ♂
Heart disease, unspecified 429.9/I519 with seizures D012640:	
Sìnìtāng 5g gānlùyǐn 5g mǔdānpí 1g zhīzǐ 1g huánglián 0g to ♀	Sìnìtāng 5g gānlùyǐn 5g mǔdānpí 1g zhīzǐ 1g huánglián 0g to ♂
Unspecified disorders of nervous system 349.9/G969 with seizures D012640:	
Huángqíwǔwùtāng 5g chuānxiōng 1g dānshēn 1g zhúrú 1g sāngzhī 1g dāngguī 1g jiānghuáng 1g to ♀	Huángqíwǔwùtāng 5g chuānxiōng 1g dānshēn 1g zhúrú 1g sāngzhī 1g dāngguī 1g jiānghuáng 1g to ♂

Jiāwèixiāoyáosǎn 'softens the Liver, resolves depression,' and 'clears Heat, nourishes Blood.' Tiānwángbǔxīndān is currently mainly used for unspecified cardiac dysrhythmia (Wang, 2019). Cardiac arrhythmias usually occur during or after seizures and are implicated as the cause of death in epilepsy (van der Lende et al., 2016). On the other hand, Tiānwángbǔxīndān, Jiāwèixiāoyáosǎn and Suānzǎoréntāng are all tranquilizing in traditional Chinese medicine. The prescriptions are therefore thought to calm the brain activities and also address the potential cardiac complication.

17.2. Intellectual Disability

Intellectual disability is limitations in one's intellectual functioning and adaptive behaviors. Intellectual functioning includes learning, reasoning, problem solving, and decision making and is assessed by IQ test. Adaptive behaviors include feeding and dressing oneself, communicating and interacting with one's family, peers and others. Chromosome abnormalities and infections that impair brain development of children can cause intellectual disability.

Table 17.2. Herbal prescriptions for intellectual disability

<table>
<tr><td colspan="2">Intellectual Disability: https://meshb.nlm.nih.gov/record/ui?ui=D008607.</td></tr>
<tr><td colspan="2">Common prescriptions:</td></tr>
<tr><td colspan="2">Jiāwèixiāoyáosǎn 5g gāncǎoxiǎomàidàzǎotāng 5g héhuānpí 1g yèjiāoténg 1g
Jiāwèixiāoyáosǎn 5g gāncǎoxiǎomàidàzǎotāng 5g héhuānpí 1g yèjiāoténg 1g fúshén 1g
Jiāwèixiāoyáosǎn 5g gāncǎoxiǎomàidàzǎotāng 5g suānzǎoréntāng 5g
Jiāwèixiāoyáosǎn 5g gāncǎoxiǎomàidàzǎotāng 5g héhuānpí 1g bǎihé 1g yèjiāoténg 1g
Jiāwèixiāoyáosǎn 5g gāncǎoxiǎomàidàzǎotāng 5g héhuānpí 1g yèjiāoténg 1g bózǐrén 1g fúshén 1g</td></tr>
<tr><td colspan="2">Alternative prescriptions:</td></tr>
<tr><td colspan="2">Jiāwèixiāoyáosǎn 5g cháihúshūgāntāng 5g héhuānpí 4g shíchāngpú 1g yuǎnzhì 1g suānzǎorén 1g
Jiāwèixiāoyáosǎn 5g cháihúshūgāntāng 5g héhuānpí 3g shíchāngpú 1g yuǎnzhì 1g suānzǎorén 1g
Jiāwèixiāoyáosǎn 5g gāncǎoxiǎomàidàzǎotāng 2g chuānliànzǐ 1g dānshēn 1g yuǎnzhì 1g huángqín 1g
Jiāwèixiāoyáosǎn 5g suānzǎoréntāng 2g héhuānpí 1g yèjiāoténg 1g</td></tr>
<tr><td colspan="2">Indicated diseases:</td></tr>
<tr><td colspan="2">Heart disease, unspecified 429.9 (Heart disease, unspecified I519); Unspecified disorders of nervous system 349.9 (Disorder of central nervous system, unspecified G969); Unspecified endocrine disorder 259.9 (Endocrine disorder, unspecified E349); Gonadal dysgenesis 758.6 (Turner's syndrome, unspecified Q969); Cardiovascular disease, unspecified 429.2 (Atherosclerotic heart disease of native coronary artery without angina pectoris I2510); Indeterminate sex and pseudohermaphroditism 752.7 (Pseudohermaphroditism, unspecified Q563, Indeterminate sex, unspecified Q564); Unspecified congenital anomaly of heart 746.9 (Congenital malformation of cardiac chambers and connections, unspecified Q209, Congenital malformation of heart, unspecified Q249); Antisocial personality disorder 301.7 (Antisocial personality disorder F602); Narcissistic personality disorder 301.81 (Narcissistic personality disorder F6081); Avoidant personality disorder 301.82 (Avoidant personality disorder F606); Klinefelter's syndrome 758.7 (Klinefelter syndrome, unspecified Q984)</td></tr>
<tr><td colspan="2">Heart disease, unspecified 429.9/I519 with intellectual disability D008607:</td></tr>
<tr><td>Sìnìtāng 5g gānlùyǐn 5g mǔdānpí 1g zhīzǐ 1g huánglián 0g to ♀</td><td>Sìnìtāng 5g gānlùyǐn 5g mǔdānpí 1g zhīzǐ 1g huánglián 0g to ♂</td></tr>
<tr><td colspan="2">Unspecified disorders of nervous system 349.9/G969 with intellectual disability D008607:</td></tr>
<tr><td>Huángqíwǔwùtāng 5g chuānxiōng 1g dānshēn 1g zhúrú 1g sāngzhī 1g dāngguī 1g jiānghuáng 1g to ♀</td><td>Huángqíwǔwùtāng 5g chuānxiōng 1g dānshēn 1g zhúrú 1g sāngzhī 1g dāngguī 1g jiānghuáng 1g to ♂</td></tr>
</table>

Gāncǎoxiǎomàidàzǎotāng 'harmonizes interior, retards urgency, quiets spirits, settles anxiety,' and is currently used for unspecified anxiety state (Wang, 2019). Anxiety is very common in children with intellectual disability (Green et al., 2015). We therefore see both Jiāwèixiāoyáosǎn and Gāncǎoxiǎomàidàzǎotāng in the prescriptions for intellectual disability.

17.3. Learning Disorders

Learning disorders are conditions of the brain characterized by difficulties in reading, writing and numerical concepts. Factors that are associated with learning disorders include genetics, premature birth, low birth weight, toxic exposure, infection and malnutrition.

Table 17.3. Herbal prescriptions for learning disorders

Learning Disorders: https://meshb.nlm.nih.gov/record/ui?ui=D007859.	
Common prescriptions:	
Bǔyánghuánwǔtāng 5g chuānqī 1g dānshēn 1g shíchāngpú 1g yuǎnzhì 1g + acupuncture Bǔyánghuánwǔtāng 5g chuānqī 1g dānshēn 1g + acupuncture Bǔyánghuánwǔtāng 5g + acupuncture Bǔyánghuánwǔtāng 5g chuānqī 1g dānshēn 1g shíchāngpú 1g yuǎnzhì 1g	
Alternative prescriptions:	
Bǔyánghuánwǔtāng 5g dānshēn 1g shíchāngpú 1g yuǎnzhì 1g + acupuncture Bǔyánghuánwǔtāng 5g dānshēn 1g niúxī 1g sāngzhī 1g jīxuèténg 1g + acupuncture Bǔyánghuánwǔtāng 5g sānqī 1g Bǔyánghuánwǔtāng 5g niúxī 1g jīxuèténg 1g Bǔyánghuánwǔtāng 5g dānshēn 1g tiānmá 1g gōuténg 1g	
Indicated diseases:	
Heart disease, unspecified 429.9 (Heart disease, unspecified I519); Unspecified disorders of nervous system 349.9 (Disorder of central nervous system, unspecified G969); Digeorge's syndrome 279.11 (Di George's syndrome D821); Velo-cardio-facial syndrome 758.32 (Velo-cardio-facial syndrome Q9381); Cardiovascular disease, unspecified 429.2 (Atherosclerotic heart disease of native coronary artery without angina pectoris I2510); Hypoparathyroidism 252.1 (Hypoparathyroidism, unspecified E209); Unspecified disorder of parathyroid gland 252.9 (Disorder of parathyroid gland, unspecified E215); Unspecified endocrine disorder 259.9 (Endocrine disorder, unspecified E349); Unspecified congenital anomaly of heart 746.9 (Congenital malformation of cardiac chambers and connections, unspecified Q209, Congenital malformation of heart, unspecified Q249); Antisocial personality disorder 301.7 (Antisocial personality disorder F602); Narcissistic personality disorder 301.81 (Narcissistic personality disorder F6081); Avoidant personality disorder 301.82 (Avoidant personality disorder F606); Unspecified condition of brain 348.9 (Disorder of brain, unspecified G939); Tourette's disorder 307.23 (Tourette's disorder F952); Chronic motor or vocal tic disorder 307.22 (Chronic motor or vocal tic disorder F951); Transient tic disorder 307.21 (Transient tic disorder F950); Tic disorder, unspecified 307.20 (Tic disorder, unspecified F959); Klinefelter's syndrome 758.7 (Klinefelter syndrome, unspecified Q984); Indeterminate sex and pseudohermaphroditism 752.7 (Pseudohermaphroditism, unspecified Q563, Indeterminate sex, unspecified Q564); Gonadal dysgenesis 758.6 (Turner's syndrome, unspecified Q969)	
Heart disease, unspecified 429.9/I519 with learning disorders D007859:	
Sìnìtāng 5g gānlùyǐn 5g mǔdānpí 1g zhīzǐ 1g huánglián 0g to ♀	Sìnìtāng 5g gānlùyǐn 5g mǔdānpí 1g zhīzǐ 1g huánglián 0g to ♂
Unspecified disorders of nervous system 349.9/G969 with learning disorders D007859:	
Huángqíwǔwùtāng 5g chuānxiōng 1g dānshēn 1g zhúrú 1g sāngzhī 1g dāngguī 1g jiānghuáng 1g to ♀	Huángqíwǔwùtāng 5g chuānxiōng 1g dānshēn 1g zhúrú 1g sāngzhī 1g dāngguī 1g jiānghuáng 1g to ♂
Unspecified condition of brain 348.9/G939 with learning disorders D007859:	
Bǔyánghuánwǔtāng 5g dānshēn 1g tiānmá 1g shíchāngpú 1g yuǎnzhì 1g gōuténg 1g + acupuncture to ♀	Bǔyánghuánwǔtāng 5g chuānqī 1g dānshēn 1g shíchāngpú 1g yuǎnzhì 1g + acupuncture to ♂

Bŭyánghuánwŭtāng 'replenishes Qi, activates Blood, and opens collaterals.' Its modern uses are for unspecified essential hypertension, unspecified late effects of cerebrovascular disease, and unspecified anemia (Wang, 2019). It is believed to benefit the brain.

17.4. Fatigue

Fatigue is an overall feeling of tiredness and weakness, following a period of mental or physical exertion, that does not resolve after rest and sleep. Over-exercising, overwork, depression, chronic pain and chronic inflammation can lead to fatigue.

Table 17.4. Herbal prescriptions for fatigue

<table>
<tr><td colspan="2">Fatigue: https://meshb.nlm.nih.gov/record/ui?ui=D005221.</td></tr>
<tr><td colspan="2">Common prescriptions:</td></tr>
<tr><td colspan="2">Jiāwèixiāoyáosăn 5g zhìgāncăotāng 5g dānshēn 1g xiāngfù 1g yùjīn 1g
Jiāwèixiāoyáosăn 5g zhìgāncăotāng 5g dānshēn 1g bózĭrén 1g xiāngfù 1g yuănzhì 1g yùjīn 1g
Jiāwèixiāoyáosăn 5g zhìgāncăotāng 5g dānshēn 1g bózĭrén 1g xiāngfù 1g yùjīn 1g
Jiāwèixiāoyáosăn 5g zhìgāncăotāng 5g dānshēn 1g bózĭrén 1g yuănzhì 1g</td></tr>
<tr><td colspan="2">Alternative prescriptions:</td></tr>
<tr><td colspan="2">Jiāwèixiāoyáosăn 5g zhìgāncăotāng 5g dānshēn 2g xiāngfù 2g shénqū 2g yuănzhì 2g yùjīn 2g
Zhìgāncăotāng 5g jiāwèixiāoyáosăn 4g dānshēn 1g yánhúsuŏ 1g xiāngfù 1g yùjīn 1g
Jiāwèixiāoyáosăn 5g zhìgāncăotāng 5g cháihúshūgāntāng 5g dānshēn 1g
Zhìgāncăotāng 5g cháihúshūgāntāng 3g dānshēn 1g xiāngfù 1g yùjīn 1g
Zhìgāncăotāng 5g língguìshùgāntāng 5g bŭzhōngyìqìtāng 5g</td></tr>
<tr><td colspan="2">Indicated diseases:</td></tr>
<tr><td colspan="2">Cardiovascular disease, unspecified 429.2 (Atherosclerotic heart disease of native coronary artery without angina pectoris I2510); Vascular disorders of skin 709.1 (Vasculitis limited to the skin, unspecified L959); Panuveitis 360.12 (Panuveitis, unspecified eye H44119); Behcet's syndrome 136.1 (Behcet's disease M352); Other dermatoses 702; Disorder of eye, unspecified 379.90 (Unspecified disorder of eye and adnexa H579); Unspecified condition of brain 348.9 (Disorder of brain, unspecified G939); Unspecified endocrine disorder 259.9 (Endocrine disorder, unspecified E349); Malignant neoplasm of endocrine gland, site unspecified 194.9 (Malignant neoplasm of endocrine gland, unspecified C759); Unspecified disorders of nervous system 349.9 (Disorder of central nervous system, unspecified G969); Neoplasm of unspecified nature of brain 239.6 (Neoplasm of unspecified behavior of brain D496); Myopathy, unspecified 359.9 (Myopathy, unspecified G729); Unspecified acquired hypothyroidism 244.9 (Hypothyroidism, unspecified E039); Myoneural disorders 358; Unspecified disorder of thyroid 246.9 (Disorder of thyroid, unspecified E079); Malignant neoplasm of nervous system, part unspecified 192.9 (Malignant neoplasm of central nervous system, unspecified C729); Multiple myeloma 203.0; Unspecified hemorrhagic conditions 287.9 (Hemorrhagic condition, unspecified D699); Unspecified diseases of blood and blood-forming organs 289.9 (Disease of blood and blood-forming organs, unspecified D759)</td></tr>
<tr><td colspan="2">Cardiovascular disease, unspecified 429.2/I2510 with fatigue D005221:</td></tr>
<tr><td>Yùzhú 5g sìnìtāng 5g zhìgāncăotāng 2g to ♀</td><td>Yùzhú 5g sìnìtāng 5g zhìgāncăotāng 2g to ♂</td></tr>
<tr><td colspan="2">Unspecified condition of brain 348.9/G939 with fatigue D005221:</td></tr>
<tr><td>Bŭyánghuánwŭtāng 5g + acupuncture to ♀</td><td>Bŭyánghuánwŭtāng 5g + acupuncture to ♂</td></tr>
<tr><td colspan="2">Myopathy, unspecified 359.9/G729 with fatigue D005221:</td></tr>
<tr><td>Huángqíwŭwùtāng 5g dāngguīsìnìtāng 5g dānshēn 1g sāngzhī 1g jīxuèténg 1g to ♀</td><td>Huángqíwŭwùtāng 5g dāngguīsìnìtāng 5g dānshēn 1g zhúrú 1g sāngzhī 1g jiānghuáng 1g to ♂</td></tr>
</table>

Zhìgāncăotāng 'benefits Qi, tonifies Yin' and 'nourishes Blood, restores pulse.' Combining with Jiāwèixiāoyáosăn, the prescription is believed to relieve the physical and mental fatigue of the patient.

17.5. Mental Fatigue

Mental fatigue is mental exhaustion manifesting cognitive dulling. Mental fatigue usually follows prolonged cognitive activity or emotional stress. Perfectionism, procrastination and lack of sleep can result in mental fatigue.

Table 17.5. Herbal prescriptions for mental fatigue

Mental Fatigue: https://meshb.nlm.nih.gov/record/ui?ui=D005222.	
Common prescriptions:	
Sìnìtāng 5g rénshēn 1g bànxià 1g dàhuáng 0g Sìnìtāng 5g rénshēn 1g wúzhūyú 1g Sìnìtāng 5g lǐzhōngtāng 5g ròuguì 1g yánhúsuǒ 1g zhìgāncǎotāng 1g Sìnìtāng 5g rénshēn 1g	
Alternative prescriptions:	
Sìnìtāng 5g guìzhī 1g máhuáng 1g xìxīn 0g Sìnìtāng 5g guìzhī 1g máhuáng 1g xìxīn 1g Guìzhītāng 5g shēngjiāng 2g báisháo 2g dàhuáng 0g Sìnìtāng 5g guìzhī 1g máhuáng 0g	
Indicated diseases:	
Myopathy, unspecified 359.9 (Myopathy, unspecified G729); Chronic fatigue syndrome 780.71 (Chronic fatigue, unspecified R5382); Myoneural disorders 358; Unspecified disorders of nervous system 349.9 (Disorder of central nervous system, unspecified G969); Other dermatoses 702; Deformity and disproportion of reconstructed breast 612; Other disorders of breast 611; Benign mammary dysplasias 610; Heart disease, unspecified 429.9 (Heart disease, unspecified I519); Cardiovascular disease, unspecified 429.2 (Atherosclerotic heart disease of native coronary artery without angina pectoris I2510)	
Myopathy, unspecified 359.9/G729 with mental fatigue D005222:	
Huángqíwǔwùtāng 5g dāngguīsìnìtāng 5g dānshēn 1g zhúrú 1g sāngzhī 1g jiānghuáng 1g to ♀	Guīlùèrxiānjiāo 5g to ♂
Other dermatoses 702 with mental fatigue D005222:	
Dāngguīsìnìtāng 5g wúzhūyú 1g fùzǐ 1g gānjiāng 1g to ♀	Jiědúsìwùtāng 5g xiāofēngsǎn 4g zhēnrénhuómìngyǐnqùchuānshānjiǎ 1g huángliánjiědútāng 1g to ♂
Heart disease, unspecified 429.9/I519 with mental fatigue D005222:	
Sìnìtāng 5g gānlùyǐn 5g mǔdānpí 1g zhīzǐ 1g huánglián 0g to ♀	Sìnìtāng 5g gānlùyǐn 5g mǔdānpí 1g zhīzǐ 1g huánglián 0g to ♂

Cognitive functioning burns calories and mental fatigue sets in when the brain exhausts its energy. It is believed that Sìnìtāng is here trying to slow or relieve the exhaustion.

17.6. Fever

Fever is body temperature above its normal range. Fever is most often a result of one's immune response to infection.

Xīnyísǎn 'withstands Wind, expels chills', and is today used for unspecified sinusitis, while Xiǎoqīnglóngtāng is used for rhinitis, bronchitis and sinusitis (Wang, 2019). The prescriptions are therefore used for infection-related fevers. Note that adenoviruses that cause fever can also cause pink eye, i.e., conjunctivitis.

Table 17.6. Herbal prescriptions for fever

Fever: https://meshb.nlm.nih.gov/record/ui?ui=D005334.	
Common prescriptions:	
Xīnyísǎn 5g xiǎoqīnglóngtāng 2g xiāngshāliùjūnzǐtāng 2g Xīnyísǎn 5g xiǎoqīnglóngtāng 2g xiāngshāliùjūnzǐtāng 1g Xīnyísǎn 5g xiǎoqīnglóngtāng 3g xiāngshāliùjūnzǐtāng 2g	
Alternative prescriptions:	
Xīnyísǎn 5g xiāofēngsǎn 3g zhēnrénhuómìngyǐnqùchuānshānjiǎ 3g báixiānpí 1g yúxīngcǎo 1g xiǎoqīnglóngtāng 1g Cāngěrsǎn 5g máxìnggānshítāng 4g niúbàngzǐ 2g jiégěng 2g liánqiáo 2g yúxīngcǎo 2g qiánhú 1g Xīnyísǎn 5g xiǎoqīnglóngtāng 2g xiāngshāliùjūnzǐtāng 2g gégēntāng 2g Xīnyíqīngfèitāng 5g yínqiàosǎn 3g dìngchuǎntāng 2g bèimǔ 1g guālóurén 1g	
Indicated diseases:	
Cardiovascular disease, unspecified 429.2 (Atherosclerotic heart disease of native coronary artery without angina pectoris I2510); Vascular disorders of skin 709.1 (Vasculitis limited to the skin, unspecified L959); Panuveitis 360.12 (Panuveitis, unspecified eye H44119); Behcet's syndrome 136.1 (Behcet's disease M352); Other dermatoses 702; Disorder of eye, unspecified 379.90 (Unspecified disorder of eye and adnexa H579); Unspecified disorder of liver 573.9 (Liver disease, unspecified K769); Herpes simplex 054; Malignant neoplasm of liver, not specified as primary or secondary 155.2 (Malignant neoplasm of liver, not specified as primary or secondary C229); Diseases of the jaws 526; Heart disease, unspecified 429.9 (Heart disease, unspecified I519); Unspecified congenital anomaly of heart 746.9 (Congenital malformation of cardiac chambers and connections, unspecified Q209, Congenital malformation of heart, unspecified Q249)	
Cardiovascular disease, unspecified 429.2/I2510 with fever D005334:	
Yùzhú 5g sìnìtāng 5g mǔdānpí 1g zhīzǐ 1g huánglián 0g to ♀	Sìnìtāng 5g gānlùyǐn 5g mǔdānpí 1g zhīzǐ 1g huánglián 0g to ♂
Unspecified disorder of liver 573.9/K769 with fever D005334:	
Jiāwèixiāoyáosǎn 5g cháihúshūgāntāng 5g to ♀	Xuèfǔzhúyūtāng 5g cháihúshūgāntāng 5g to ♂
Heart disease, unspecified 429.9/I519 with fever D005334:	
Sìnìtāng 5g gānlùyǐn 5g mǔdānpí 1g zhīzǐ 1g huánglián 0g to ♀	Sìnìtāng 5g gānlùyǐn 5g mǔdānpí 1g zhīzǐ 1g huánglián 0g to ♂

17.7. Fever of Unknown Origin

Fever of unknown origin is fever for over three weeks without an explanation despite appropriate investigation. Although a cause has not been identified, infections, malignancies, and autoimmune conditions are still suspected to be responsible.

Table 17.7. Herbal prescriptions for fever of unknown origin

Fever of Unknown Origin: https://meshb.nlm.nih.gov/record/ui?ui=D005335.
Common prescriptions:
Shíshéntāng 5g zhǐsòusǎn 4g niúbàngzǐ 2g cāngěrzǐ 2g Shíshéntāng 5g zhǐsòusǎn 5g xīnyísǎn 5g Shíshéntāng 5g zhǐsòusǎn 4g niúbàngzǐ 1g cāngěrzǐ 1g Shíshéntāng 5g xīnyísǎn 5g
Alternative prescriptions:
Shíshéntāng 5g zhǐsòusǎn 2g xìngrén 1g cāngěrzǐ 1g Jiǔwèiqiānghuótāng 5g zhǐsòusǎn 4g shénqū 2g gégēn 2g Jiǔwèiqiānghuótāng 5g zhǐsòusǎn 4g niúbàngzǐ 1g shénqū 1g Xīnyíqīngfèitāng 5g máxìnggānshítāng 5g cāngěrsǎn 4g niúbàngzǐ 2g jiégěng 2g liánqiáo 2g yúxīngcǎo 2g Jiǔwèiqiānghuótāng 5g zhǐsòusǎn 2g gégēn 1g cāngěrzǐ 1g

Fever of Unknown Origin: https://meshb.nlm.nih.gov/record/ui?ui=D005335.	
Indicated diseases:	
Cardiovascular disease, unspecified 429.2 (Atherosclerotic heart disease of native coronary artery without angina pectoris I2510); Vascular disorders of skin 709.1 (Vasculitis limited to the skin, unspecified L959); Panuveitis 360.12 (Panuveitis, unspecified eye H44119); Behcet's syndrome 136.1 (Behcet's disease M352); Other dermatoses 702; Disorder of eye, unspecified 379.90 (Unspecified disorder of eye and adnexa H579); Diseases of the jaws 526; Neoplasm of unspecified nature of digestive system 239.0 (Neoplasm of unspecified behavior of digestive system D490); Diseases of the oral soft tissues, excluding lesions specific for gingiva and tongue 528; Multiple myeloma 203.0; Unspecified hemorrhagic conditions 287.9 (Hemorrhagic condition, unspecified D699); Unspecified diseases of blood and blood-forming organs 289.9 (Disease of blood and blood-forming organs, unspecified D759); Unspecified disorder of liver 573.9 (Liver disease, unspecified K769); Herpes simplex 054; Malignant neoplasm of liver, not specified as primary or secondary 155.2 (Malignant neoplasm of liver, not specified as primary or secondary C229)	
Cardiovascular disease, unspecified 429.2/I2510 with fever of unknown origin D005335:	
Yùzhú 5g sìnìtāng 5g zhìgāncǎotāng 5g to ♀	Sìnìtāng 5g gānlùyǐn 5g lóngdǎnxiègāntāng 5g to ♂
Diseases of the jaws 526 with fever of unknown origin D005335:	
Guìzhītāng 5g báisháo 1g dàhuáng 0g to ♀	Lǐzhōngtāng 5g bànxià 1g shārén 1g fúlíng 1g to ♂
Unspecified disorder of liver 573.9/K769 with fever of unknown origin D005335:	
Xuèfǔzhúyūtāng 5g cháihúshūgāntāng 5g dānshēn 1g yánhúsuǒ 1g xiāngfù 1g yùjīn 1g to ♀	Xuèfǔzhúyūtāng 5g cháihúshūgāntāng 5g lóngdǎnxiègāntāng 5g to ♂

Shíshéntāng is today used for unspecified sinusitis and Zhǐsòusǎn is today used for chronic bronchitis (Wang, 2019). The prescriptions therefore treat infection-related fever of unknown origin. Note that an ear or sinus infection can cause teeth or jaw pain.

17.8. Edema

Edema is accumulation of body fluid in the tissue. Common causes of edema include chronic heart failure, kidney diseases, liver cirrhosis, and medications.

Table 17.8. Herbal prescriptions for edema

Edema: https://meshb.nlm.nih.gov/record/ui?ui=D004487.
Common prescriptions:
Jiāwèixiāoyáosǎn 5g xiāngshāliùjūnzǐtāng 5g bànxiàxièxīntāng 2g héhuānpí 1g yánhúsuǒ 1g Jiāwèixiāoyáosǎn 5g dāngguīsháoyàosǎn 5g yánhúsuǒ 1g xiāngfù 1g yìmǔcǎo 1g Jiāwèixiāoyáosǎn 5g dāngguīsháoyàosǎn 5g xiāngfù 1g yìmǔcǎo 1g Jiāwèixiāoyáosǎn 5g dāngguīsháoyàosǎn 5g dānshēn 1g xiāngfù 1g yìmǔcǎo 1g zélán 1g
Alternative prescriptions:
Dāngguīsháoyàosǎn 5g yánhúsuǒ 0g xiāngfù 0g Wēnjīngtāng 5g dāngguīsháoyàosǎn 5g dānshēn 1g xiāngfù 1g yìmǔcǎo 1g Xiāoyáosǎn 5g guìzhīfúlíngwán 4g chuānliànzǐ 2g dānshēn 2g zélán 2g xiāngfù 1g Jiāwèixiāoyáosǎn 5g wēnjīngtāng 3g dāngguīsháoyàosǎn 3g xiāngfù 1g yìmǔcǎo 1g Jiāwèixiāoyáosǎn 5g xiāngshāliùjūnzǐtāng 5g bāwèidìhuángwán 4g héhuānpí 1g yánhúsuǒ 1g
Indicated diseases:
Exophthalmos, unspecified 376.30 (Unspecified exophthalmos H0520); Goiter, unspecified 240.9 (Iodine-deficiency related (endemic) goiter, unspecified E012, Nontoxic goiter, unspecified E049); Unspecified disorder of orbit 376.9 (Unspecified disorder of orbit H059); Disorder of eye, unspecified 379.90 (Unspecified disorder of eye and adnexa H579); Unspecified disorder of thyroid 246.9 (Disorder of thyroid, unspecified E079); Unspecified endocrine disorder 259.9 (Endocrine disorder, unspecified E349); Cardiovascular disease, unspecified 429.2 (Atherosclerotic heart disease of native coronary artery without angina pectoris I2510); Diabetic retinopathy 362.0; Diabetes with peripheral circulatory disorders 250.7; Unspecified retinal disorder 362.9 (Unspecified retinal disorder H359); Diabetes mellitus 250; Unspecified disorder of metabolism 277.9 (Metabolic disorder, unspecified E889); Unspecified acquired hypothyroidism 244.9 (Hypothyroidism, unspecified E039)

Table 17.8. (Continued)

Edema: https://meshb.nlm.nih.gov/record/ui?ui=D004487.	
Exophthalmos, unspecified 376.30/H0520 with edema D004487:	
Jiāwèixiāoyáosǎn 5g qǐjúdìhuángwán 5g nǚzhēnzǐ 1g héhuānpí 1g hànliáncǎo 1g yèjiāoténg 1g to ♀	Xīgānmíngmùtāng 5g zīshènmíngmùtāng 5g to ♂
Cardiovascular disease, unspecified 429.2/I2510 with edema D004487:	
Sìnìtāng 5g gānlùyǐn 5g mǔdānpí 1g zhīzǐ 1g huánglián 0g to ♀	Sìnìtāng 5g gānlùyǐn 5g to ♂

A modern use of Jiāwèixiāoyáosǎn is for unspecified chronic hepatitis and that of Dāngguīsháoyàosǎn is for unspecified disorders of menstruation (Wang, 2019). Edema in the face, breast and abdomen is among the premenstrual syndrome (Tacani et al., 2015). We thus see combination of Jiāwèixiāoyáosǎn and Dāngguīsháoyàosǎn among the prescriptions for edema.

17.9. Abnormal Reflex

Abnormal reflex refers to increased, decreased or absent response to a stimulus brought to the sensory system. An example of such reflex is vasoconstriction upon cold stimulation to the skin. Causes of abnormal reflexes include diabetic neuropathy, alcoholism, anemia, stroke, dementia, multiple sclerosis, and spinal cord injury.

Table 17.9. Herbal prescriptions for abnormal reflex

Abnormal Reflex: https://meshb.nlm.nih.gov/record/ui?ui=D012021.
Common prescriptions:
Bāwèidìhuángwán 5g sāngpiāoxiāosǎn 5g yìzhìrén 1g fùpénzǐ 1g Bāwèidìhuángwán 5g bǔzhōngyìqìtāng 5g Bāwèidìhuángwán 5g sāngpiāoxiāosǎn 5g bǔzhōngyìqìtāng 5g Bāwèidìhuángwán 5g sāngpiāoxiāosǎn 5g bǔzhōngyìqìtāng 5g fùpénzǐ 2g
Alternative prescriptions:
Bǔzhōngyìqìtāng 5g yìzhìrén 0g fùpénzǐ 0g Bǔzhōngyìqìtāng 5g shānyào 1g wūyào 1g yìzhìrén 1g Bǔzhōngyìqìtāng 5g bāwèidìhuángwán 2g Bǔzhōngyìqìtāng 5g yìzhìrén 0g Bāwèidìhuángwán 5g sāngpiāoxiāo 1g yìzhìrén 1g
Indicated diseases:
Polyneuropathy in diabetes 357.2 (Diabetes mellitus due to underlying condition with diabetic polyneuropathy E0842, Drug or chemical induced diabetes mellitus with neurological complications with diabetic polyneuropathy E0942, Type 1 diabetes mellitus with diabetic polyneuropathy E1042, Type 2 diabetes mellitus with diabetic polyneuropathy E1142, Other specified diabetes mellitus with diabetic polyneuropathy E1342); Diabetes with neurological manifestations 250.6; Myoneural disorders 358; Unspecified disorders of nervous system 349.9 (Disorder of central nervous system, unspecified G969); Diabetes mellitus 250; Unspecified endocrine disorder 259.9 (Endocrine disorder, unspecified E349); Heart disease, unspecified 429.9 (Heart disease, unspecified I519); Ptosis of eyelid 374.3; Unspecified congenital anomaly of heart 746.9 (Congenital malformation of cardiac chambers and connections, unspecified Q209, Congenital malformation of heart, unspecified Q249); Cardiovascular disease, unspecified 429.2 (Atherosclerotic heart disease of native coronary artery without angina pectoris I2510); Unspecified disorder of eyelid 374.9 (Unspecified disorder of eyelid H029); Disorder of eye, unspecified 379.90 (Unspecified disorder of eye and adnexa H579); Unspecified disorder of metabolism 277.9 (Metabolic disorder, unspecified E889); Unspecified condition of brain 348.9 (Disorder of brain, unspecified G939); Neoplasm of unspecified nature of brain 239.6 (Neoplasm of unspecified behavior of brain D496)

Abnormal Reflex: https://meshb.nlm.nih.gov/record/ui?ui=D012021.	
Polyneuropathy in diabetes 357.2/E0842,E0942,E1042,E1142,E1342 with reflex, abnormal D012021:	
Huángqíwǔwùtāng 5g dāngguīsìnìtāng 5g dānshēn 1g zhúrú 1g sāngzhī 1g jiānghuáng 1g to ♀	Bāwèidìhuángwán 5g báihǔjiārénshēntāng 5g dānshēn 1g tiānhuā 1g shíhú 1g to ♂
Heart disease, unspecified 429.9/I519 with reflex, abnormal D012021:	
Sìnìtāng 5g gānlùyǐn 5g mǔdānpí 1g zhīzǐ 1g huánglián 0g to ♀	Sìnìtāng 5g gānlùyǐn 5g mǔdānpí 1g zhīzǐ 1g huánglián 0g to ♂
Unspecified condition of brain 348.9/G939 with reflex, abnormal D012021:	
Xiǎoxùmìngtāng 5g bǔyánghuánwǔtāng 5g to ♀	Bǔyánghuánwǔtāng 5g dānshēn 1g shíchāngpú 1g yuǎnzhì 1g + acupuncture to ♂

A modern use of Bāwèidìhuángwán and Bǔzhōngyìqìtāng is for diabetes and anema, respectively (Wang, 2019). The prescriptions therefore target the underlying causes of abnormal reflexes.

17.10. Vertigo

Vertigo is the feeling that you, or the environment around you, are moving or spinning. Changes, by e.g., inflammation, in the inner ear apparatus which helps keep balance, can cause vertigo. Other causes include head or neck injury, stroke, tumor, migraine, and medication.

Língguìshùgāntāng is used in Section 2.1 for dizziness, which is a sense of disorientation. As vertigo is a subtype of dizziness, Língguìshùgāntāng is also used for vertigo.

Table 17.10. Herbal prescriptions for vertigo

Vertigo: https://meshb.nlm.nih.gov/record/ui?ui=D014717.	
Common prescriptions:	
Língguìshùgāntāng 5g shārén 1g xiǎohuíxiāng 1g fùzǐ 1g dàhuáng 0g Língguìshùgāntāng 5g fùzǐ 1g shārén 1g xìxīn 1g dàhuáng 0g Língguìshùgāntāng 5g bànxià 1g fùzǐ 1g shārén 1g xìxīn 1g dàhuáng 0g Língguìshùgāntāng 5g fùzǐ 1g shārén 1g dàhuáng 0g	
Alternative prescriptions:	
Língguìshùgāntāng 5g bànxià 1g shārén 1g fùzǐ 1g dàhuáng 0g Língguìshùgāntāng 5g shārén 2g fùzǐ 1g xìxīn 1g dàhuáng 0g Língguìshùgāntāng 5g shārén 1g dàhuáng 0g	
Indicated diseases:	
Visual deprivation nystagmus 379.53 (Visual deprivation nystagmus H5503); Dissociated nystagmus 379.55 (Dissociated nystagmus H5504); Nystagmus, unspecified 379.50 (Unspecified nystagmus H5500); Vertigo of central origin 386.2 (Vertigo of central origin, unspecified ear H8149); Brown's (tendon) sheath syndrome 378.61 (Brown's sheath syndrome, right eye H50611, Brown's sheath syndrome, left eye H50612); Internuclear ophthalmoplegia 378.86 (Internuclear ophthalmoplegia, unspecified eye H5120); Unspecified disorder of eye movements 378.9 (Unspecified disorder of binocular movement H519); Unspecified disorder of cranial nerves 352.9 (Cranial nerve disorder, unspecified G529); Unspecified disorder of ear 388.9 (Unspecified disorder of ear, bilateral H9393); Disorder of eye, unspecified 379.90 (Unspecified disorder of eye and adnexa H579); Unspecified disorders of nervous system 349.9 (Disorder of central nervous system, unspecified G969); Unspecified condition of brain 348.9 (Disorder of brain, unspecified G939)	
Visual deprivation nystagmus 379.53/H5503 with vertigo D014717:	
Qǐjúdìhuángwán 5g zīshènmíngmùtāng 5g to ♀	Qǐjúdìhuángwán 5g zīshènmíngmùtāng 5g to ♂

17.11. Syncope

Syncope, or fainting, is a sudden, temporary loss of consciousness and muscle strength with a quick recovery. Dizziness usually precedes syncope. Low blood pressure, low blood sugar, changes in blood volume or heart rate, intense pain, dehydration, carotid artery stenosis, and extreme stress can cause syncope.

Table 17.11. Herbal prescriptions for syncope

Syncope: https://meshb.nlm.nih.gov/record/ui?ui=D013575.	
Common prescriptions:	
Shēngmàiyǐn 5g bǔzhōngyìqìtāng 5g Shēngmàiyǐn 5g bǔzhōngyìqìtāng 5g dānshēn 1g Shēngmàiyǐn 5g zhìgāncǎotāng 5g bǔzhōngyìqìtāng 5g	
Alternative prescriptions:	
Shēngmàiyǐn 5g bǔzhōngyìqìtāng 5g chuānqī 1g dānshēn 1g Shēngmàiyǐn 5g bǔzhōngyìqìtāng 5g dānshēn 1g yùjīn 1g Sìnìtāng 5g shēngmàiyǐn 5g dānshēn 1g xiāngfù 1g yùjīn 1g Shēngmàiyǐn 5g língguìshùgāntāng 5g Bǔzhōngyìqìtāng 5g shēngmàiyǐn 4g	
Indicated diseases:	
Heart disease, unspecified 429.9 (Heart disease, unspecified I519); Unspecified disorders of nervous system 349.9 (Disorder of central nervous system, unspecified G969); Malignant neoplasm of heart 164.1 (Malignant neoplasm of heart C380); Cardiovascular disease, unspecified 429.2 (Atherosclerotic heart disease of native coronary artery without angina pectoris I2510); Malignant neoplasm of thorax 195.1 (Malignant neoplasm of thorax C761); Reticulosarcoma 200.0; Unspecified congenital anomaly of heart 746.9 (Congenital malformation of cardiac chambers and connections, unspecified Q209, Congenital malformation of heart, unspecified Q249)	
Heart disease, unspecified 429.9/I519 with syncope D013575:	
Sìnìtāng 5g gānlùyǐn 5g mǔdānpí 1g zhīzǐ 1g huánglián 0g to ♀	Sìnìtāng 5g gānlùyǐn 5g mǔdānpí 1g zhīzǐ 1g huánglián 0g to ♂

Shēngmàiyǐn 'benefits Qi, produces saliva' and 'conserves Yin, stops sweating.' Its modern uses are for palpitations, cardiac dysrhythmia, and heart disease (Wang, 2019). The prescriptions therefore target heart problem-related syncope.

17.12. Vasovagal Syncope

Vasovagal syncope, also called neurocardiogenic syncope, is fainting in response to an emotional trigger, such as the sight of blood, which causes the heartbeat and blood pressure to drop. One passes out as a result of sudden reduced oxygen-rich blood flow to the brain.

Table 17.12. Herbal prescriptions for vasovagal syncope

Vasovagal Syncope: https://meshb.nlm.nih.gov/record/ui?ui=D019462.
Common prescriptions:
Sìnìtāng 5g shēngmàiyǐn 5g bǔzhōngyìqìtāng 5g Sìnìtāng 5g shēngmàiyǐn 5g dānshēn 1g xiāngfù 1g yùjīn 1g Sìnìtāng 5g shēngmàiyǐn 5g dānshēn 1g xiāngfù 1g
Alternative prescriptions:
Sìnìtāng 5g bǔzhōngyìqìtāng 5g ròuguì 1g zhìgāncǎotāng 1g Sìnìtāng 5g rénshēn 1g Bǔzhōngyìqìtāng 5g shēngmàiyǐn 3g Sìnìtāng 5g rénshēn 1g bànxià 1g dàhuáng 0g Bǔzhōngyìqìtāng 5g sìnìtāng 4g

Vasovagal Syncope: https://meshb.nlm.nih.gov/record/ui?ui=D019462.	
Indicated diseases:	
Cardiac arrest 427.5 (Cardiac arrest, cause unspecified I469); Unspecified disorders of nervous system 349.9 (Disorder of central nervous system, unspecified G969); Heart disease, unspecified 429.9 (Heart disease, unspecified I519); Cardiovascular disease, unspecified 429.2 (Atherosclerotic heart disease of native coronary artery without angina pectoris I2510); Atrial fibrillation 427.31 (Unspecified atrial fibrillation I4891); Unspecified congenital anomaly of heart 746.9 (Congenital malformation of cardiac chambers and connections, unspecified Q209, Congenital malformation of heart, unspecified Q249)	
Cardiac arrest 427.5/I469 with syncope, vasovagal D019462:	
Tiānwángbǔxīndān 5g zhìgāncǎotāng 5g to ♀	Tiānwángbǔxīndān 5g zhìgāncǎotāng 5g dānshēn 1g to ♂
Atrial fibrillation 427.31/I4891 with syncope, vasovagal D019462:	
Shēngmàiyǐn 5g zhēnwǔtāng 5g to ♀	Shēngmàiyǐn 5g zhìgāncǎotāng 5g dānshēn 1g to ♂
Heart disease, unspecified 429.9/I519 with syncope, vasovagal D019462:	
Sìnìtāng 5g gānlùyǐn 5g mǔdānpí 1g zhīzǐ 1g huánglián 0g to ♀	Sìnìtāng 5g gānlùyǐn 5g mǔdānpí 1g zhīzǐ 1g huánglián 0g to ♂

The Chinse character *xīn* in Tiānwángbǔxīndān means "the heart," and the character *bǔ* means "to enhance." The formula was designed to strengthen the heart.

17.13. Coma

Coma, or persistent vegetative state, is a prolonged state of unconsciousness during which the patient is alive but cannot be awakened. Common causes of coma are drug overdose, cardiac arrest, stroke and trauma.

Table 17.13. Herbal prescriptions for coma

Coma: https://meshb.nlm.nih.gov/record/ui?ui=D003128	
Common prescriptions:	
Sìnìtāng 5g bànxià 1g dàhuáng 0g Sìnìtāng 5g shēngjiāng 1g guìzhī 1g Sìnìtāng 5g rénshēn 1g bànxià 1g dàhuáng 0g Sìnìtāng 5g rénshēn 1g wúzhūyú 1g Sìnìtāng 5g rénshēn 1g	
Alternative prescriptions:	
Sìnìtāng 5g rénshēn 1g dàhuáng 0g Sìnìtāng 5g rénshēn 2g bànxià 2g dàhuáng 0g Sìnìtāng 5g bànxià 2g dàhuáng 0g Sìnìtāng 5g rénshēn 1g bànxià 1g	
Indicated diseases:	
Unspecified disorders of nervous system 349.9 (Disorder of central nervous system, unspecified G969); Hypoglycemia, unspecified 251.2 (Hypoglycemia, unspecified E162); Schizophreniform disorder 295.4; Unspecified disorder of metabolism 277.9 (Metabolic disorder, unspecified E889); Schizoaffective disorder 295.7; Diabetes mellitus 250; Unspecified endocrine disorder 259.9 (Endocrine disorder, unspecified E349); Alcohol abuse 305.0	
Unspecified disorders of nervous system 349.9/G969 with coma D003128:	
Huángqíwǔwùtāng 5g chuānxiōng 1g dānshēn 1g zhúrú 1g sāngzhī 1g dāngguī 1g jiānghuáng 1g to ♀	Huángqíwǔwùtāng 5g chuānxiōng 1g dānshēn 1g zhúrú 1g sāngzhī 1g dāngguī 1g jiānghuáng 1g to ♂

If we consider consciousness as Yang, then Sìnìtāng 'restores Yang and rescues adversity.' Note also that a modern use of Bànxià and Dàhuáng is for essential hypertension (Wang, 2019).

17.14. Orthostatic Hypotension

Orthostatic hypotension, also known as postural hypotension, is a drop in blood pressure when one stands up after sitting or lying down. When a healthy individual stands up from sitting, as the blood pools in the legs, his body reacts to increase the heart rate and constrict the blood vessels in the legs in order to maintain a constant oxygenated blood flow to the brain. Failure to do so causes orthostatic hypotension.

Table 17.14. Herbal prescriptions for orthostatic hypotension

Orthostatic Hypotension: https://meshb.nlm.nih.gov/record/ui?ui=D007024.	
Common prescriptions:	
Sìnìtāng 5g rénshēn 1g wúzhūyú 1g Sìnìtāng 5g rénshēn 1g bànxià 1g dàhuáng 0g Sìnìtāng 5g rénshēn 1g Sìnìtāng 5g rénshēn 1g bànxià 1g Sìnìtāng 5g rénshēn 1g bànxià 1g gānjiāng 1g	
Alternative prescriptions:	
Sìnìtāng 5g rénshēn 2g bànxià 1g dàhuáng 0g Sìnìtāng 5g bànxià 1g guìzhī 1g xìxīn 1g máhuáng 1g dàhuáng 0g Sìnìtāng 5g shēngjiāng 1g guìzhī 1g Sìnìtāng 5g rénshēn 1g bànxià 1g jiégěng 1g dàhuáng 0g	
Indicated diseases:	
Hypertensive heart and chronic kidney disease 404; Unspecified disorders of nervous system 349.9 (Disorder of central nervous system, unspecified G969); Secondary hypertension 405; Essential hypertension 401; Hypertensive chronic kidney disease 403; Hypertensive heart disease 402; Cardiovascular disease, unspecified 429.2 (Atherosclerotic heart disease of native coronary artery without angina pectoris I2510); Hereditary sensory neuropathy 356.2 (Hereditary motor and sensory neuropathy G600); Critical illness polyneuropathy 357.82 (Critical illness polyneuropathy G6281); Myoneural disorders 358; Diabetes mellitus 250; Unspecified endocrine disorder 259.9 (Endocrine disorder, unspecified E349); Unspecified disorder of metabolism 277.9 (Metabolic disorder, unspecified E889)	
Hypertensive heart and chronic kidney disease 404 with hypotension, orthostatic D007024:	
Zhēnwǔtāng 5g wúzhūyútāng 3g fùzǐ 1g to ♀	Zhēnwǔtāng 5g fùzǐ 1g gānjiāng 1g to ♂
Cardiovascular disease, unspecified 429.2/I2510 with hypotension, orthostatic D007024:	
Yùzhú 5g sìnìtāng 5g mǔdānpí 1g zhīzǐ 1g huánglián 0g to ♀	Sìnìtāng 5g gānlùyǐn 5g mǔdānpí 1g zhīzǐ 1g huánglián 0g to ♂

The modern uses of Rénshēn include unspecified vertiginous syndromes and labyrinthine disorders, unspecified heart disease, and palpitations (Wang, 2020).

17.15. Cyanosis

Cyanosis is bluish discoloration of the skin and mucous membranes, such as the lips, mouth and nailbeds, due to circulation of deoxygenated blood through them. Causes of cyanosis include asthma, pneumonia, chronic obstructive pulmonary disease, heart failure, anemia and cold exposure.

Table 17.15. Herbal prescriptions for cyanosis

Cyanosis: https://meshb.nlm.nih.gov/record/ui?ui=D003490.	
Common prescriptions:	
Sìnìtāng 5g rénshēn 1g bànxià 1g dàhuáng 0g Sìnìtāng 5g rénshēn 1g wúzhūyú 1g Sìnìtāng 5g rénshēn 1g Sìnìtāng 5g rénshēn 1g bànxià 1g	
Alternative prescriptions:	
Shíquándàbǔtāng 5g sìnìtāng 5g chuānxiōng 1g ròuguì 1g yánhúsuǒ 1g zhìgāncǎotāng 1g Sìnìtāng 5g rénshēn 2g rénshēn 1g bànxià 1g dàhuáng 0g Xiǎojiànzhōngtāng 5g huángqí 1g dāngguī 1g	
Indicated diseases:	
Heart disease, unspecified 429.9 (Heart disease, unspecified I519); Tetralogy of fallot 745.2 (Tetralogy of Fallot Q213); Cardiovascular disease, unspecified 429.2 (Atherosclerotic heart disease of native coronary artery without angina pectoris I2510); Unspecified congenital anomaly of heart 746.9 (Congenital malformation of cardiac chambers and connections, unspecified Q209, Congenital malformation of heart, unspecified Q249); Patent ductus arteriosus 747.0 (Patent ductus arteriosus Q250); Malignant neoplasm of heart 164.1 (Malignant neoplasm of heart C380); Malignant neoplasm of thorax 195.1 (Malignant neoplasm of thorax C761); Unspecified diseases of blood and blood-forming organs 289.9 (Disease of blood and blood-forming organs, unspecified D759)	
Heart disease, unspecified 429.9/I519 with cyanosis D003490:	
Sìnìtāng 5g gānlùyǐn 5g mǔdānpí 1g zhīzǐ 1g huánglián 0g to ♀	Sìnìtāng 5g gānlùyǐn 5g mǔdānpí 1g zhīzǐ 1g huánglián 0g to ♂

Shíquándàbǔtāng is today used solely for anemia (Wang, 2019). Other the other hand, Xiǎojiànzhōngtāng's modern uses include dyspepsia and other specified disorders of function of stomach (Wang, 2019). Herbal prescription compositions differ depending on the cause of cyanosis.

17.16. Hypothermia

Hypothermia occurs when one's core body temperature falls below 35 degrees Celsius or 95 degrees Fahrenheit. Hypothermia is caused by decreased heat production or increased heat loss in such a way that heat loss is faster than heat production. Lengthy exposure to low temperatures such as being trapped in a car during a blizzard or immersion in cold water can cause hypothermia and severe hypothermia is fatal.

Table 17.16. Herbal prescriptions for hypothermia

Hypothermia: https://meshb.nlm.nih.gov/record/ui?ui=D007035.
Common prescriptions:
Sìnìtāng 5g bànxià 1g dàhuáng 0g Sìnìtāng 5g rénshēn 1g dàhuáng 0g Sìnìtāng 5g rénshēn 1g bànxià 1g dàhuáng 0g Sìnìtāng 5g guìzhī 1g máhuáng 1g xìxīn 1g Sìnìtāng 5g rénshēn 1g
Alternative prescriptions:
Sìnìtāng 5g dàhuáng 0g Sìnìtāng 5g bànxià 2g dàhuáng 0g Sìnìtāng 5g guìzhī 1g máhuáng 1g xìxīn 1g dàhuáng 0g Sìnìtāng 5g rénshēn 2g bànxià 1g dàhuáng 0g Sìnìtāng 5g bànxià 1g shēngjiāng 1g dàhuáng 0g

Table 17.16. (Continued)

Hypothermia: https://meshb.nlm.nih.gov/record/ui?ui=D007035.	
Indicated and associated diseases:	
Unspecified cerebrovascular disease 437.9 (Cerebrovascular disease, unspecified I679); Unspecified condition of brain 348.9 (Disorder of brain, unspecified G939); Cardiovascular disease, unspecified 429.2 (Atherosclerotic heart disease of native coronary artery without angina pectoris I2510); Unspecified disorders of nervous system 349.9 (Disorder of central nervous system, unspecified G969); Heart disease, unspecified 429.9 (Heart disease, unspecified I519); Ventricular septal defect 745.4 (Eisenmenger's syndrome I2783, Ventricular septal defect Q210); Unspecified congenital anomaly of heart 746.9 (Congenital malformation of cardiac chambers and connections, unspecified Q209, Congenital malformation of heart, unspecified Q249); Tetralogy of fallot 745.2 (Tetralogy of Fallot Q213)	
Unspecified cerebrovascular disease 437.9/I679 with hypothermia D007035:	
Bǔyánghuánwǔtāng 5g chuānqī 1g dānshēn 1g shíchāngpú 1g yuǎnzhì 1g + acupuncture to ♀	Bǔyánghuánwǔtāng 5g chuānqī 1g dānshēn 1g shíchāngpú 1g yuǎnzhì 1g + acupuncture to ♂
Heart disease, unspecified 429.9/I519 with hypothermia D007035:	
Sìnìtāng 5g gānlùyǐn 5g mǔdānpí 1g zhīzǐ 1g huánglián 0g to ♀	Sìnìtāng 5g gānlùyǐn 5g mǔdānpí 1g zhīzǐ 1g huánglián 0g to ♂

Since warmth is associated with the Yang element, Sìnìtāng is here believed to have the ability to internally warm up a hypothermic patient.

17.17. Asthenia

Asthenia is lack of strength or energy in all or parts of the body. Causes of asthenia include malnutrition, anemia, depression, lack of exercise, heart disease, chronic obstructive pulmonary disease, sleep apnea and aging.

Table 17.17. Herbal prescriptions for asthenia

Asthenia: https://meshb.nlm.nih.gov/record/ui?ui=D001247.
Common prescriptions:
Jiāwèixiāoyáosǎn 5g zhìgāncǎotāng 5g dānshēn 1g xiāngfù 1g yùjīn 1g Jiāwèixiāoyáosǎn 5g zhìgāncǎotāng 5g dānshēn 2g bózǐrén 2g xiāngfù 2g yuǎnzhì 2g yùjīn 2g Jiāwèixiāoyáosǎn 5g zhìgāncǎotāng 5g dānshēn 1g bózǐrén 1g xiāngfù 1g yuǎnzhì 1g yùjīn 1g Jiāwèixiāoyáosǎn 5g zhìgāncǎotāng 5g dānshēn 1g bózǐrén 1g xiāngfù 1g yùjīn 1g
Alternative prescriptions:
Sìnìtāng 5g rénshēn 1g bànxià 1g dàhuáng 0g Zhìgāncǎotāng 5g shēngmàiyǐn 3g mǔlì 1g lónggǔ 1g Sìnìtāng 5g zhìgāncǎotāng 5g dānshēn 1g bànxià 1g guālóurén 1g xièbái 1g Sìnìtāng 5g zhìgāncǎotāng 5g bǔzhōngyìqìtāng 5g dānshēn 1g Jiāwèixiāoyáosǎn 5g zhìgāncǎotāng 4g gāncǎoxiǎomàidàzǎotāng 2g xiāngfù 1g yùjīn 1g
Indicated diseases:
Cardiovascular disease, unspecified 429.2 (Atherosclerotic heart disease of native coronary artery without angina pectoris I2510); Vascular disorders of skin 709.1 (Vasculitis limited to the skin, unspecified L959); Panuveitis 360.12 (Panuveitis, unspecified eye H44119); Behcet's syndrome 136.1 (Behcet's disease M352); Other dermatoses 702; Disorder of eye, unspecified 379.90 (Unspecified disorder of eye and adnexa H579); Multiple myeloma 203.0; Unspecified hemorrhagic conditions 287.9 (Hemorrhagic condition, unspecified D699); Unspecified diseases of blood and blood-forming organs 289.9 (Disease of blood and blood-forming organs, unspecified D759); Unspecified disorder of liver 573.9 (Liver disease, unspecified K769); Malignant neoplasm of liver, not specified as primary or secondary 155.2 (Malignant neoplasm of liver, not specified as primary or secondary C229); Diseases of the jaws 526

Asthenia: https://meshb.nlm.nih.gov/record/ui?ui=D001247.	
Cardiovascular disease, unspecified 429.2/I2510 with asthenia D001247:	
Yùzhú 5g sìnìtāng 5g zhìgāncǎotāng 2g to ♀	Sìnìtāng 5g gānlùyǐn 5g mǔdānpí 1g zhīzǐ 1g huánglián 1g to ♂
Unspecified disorder of liver 573.9/K769 with asthenia D001247:	
Jiāwèixiāoyáosǎn 5g xuèfǔzhúyūtāng 5g dānshēn 1g xiāngfù 1g yùjīn 1g to ♀	Xuèfǔzhúyūtāng 5g cháihúshūgāntāng 5g to ♂

Asthenia is fatigue without prior exertion. Jiāwèixiāoyáosǎn and Zhìgāncǎotāng are used for fatigue. However, we also see Sìnìtāng in some of the alternative prescriptions for asthenia, as asthenia is considered more serious.

17.18. Apraxias

Apraxias are loss of ability to carry out gestures and tasks that require sequences of movements, despite mental willingness and physical ability. Examples of apraxias are unable to smile, take a bath, or type the keyboard. Lesions, due e.g., to stroke, tumor or dementia, in the hemispheric area of the brain responsible for motor planning cause apraxias.

Table 17.18. Herbal prescriptions for apraxias

Apraxias: https://meshb.nlm.nih.gov/record/ui?ui=D001072.	
Common prescriptions:	
Bǔzhōngyìqìtāng 5g + acupuncture Bǔzhōngyìqìtāng 5g	
Alternative prescriptions:	
Sìnìtāng 5g bànxià 1g dàhuáng 0g Máhuángfùzǐxìxīntāng 5g fùzǐ 2g guìzhī 2g gānjiāng 2g dàzǎo 1g zhìgāncǎo 1g Guìzhītāng 5g shēngjiāng 0g guìzhī 0g Bǔzhōngyìqìtāng 5g fùzǐ 1g Sìnìtāng 5g bǔzhōngyìqìtāng 5g chuānxiōng 1g ròuguì 1g zhìgāncǎotāng 1g	
Indicated diseases:	
Cardiovascular disease, unspecified 429.2 (Atherosclerotic heart disease of native coronary artery without angina pectoris I2510); Disorders of acoustic nerve 388.5 (Disorders of unspecified acoustic nerve H933X9); Unspecified disorder of cranial nerves 352.9 (Cranial nerve disorder, unspecified G529); Disorder of eye, unspecified 379.90 (Unspecified disorder of eye and adnexa H579); Unspecified disorders of nervous system 349.9 (Disorder of central nervous system, unspecified G969); Brown's (tendon) sheath syndrome 378.61 (Brown's sheath syndrome, right eye H50611, Brown's sheath syndrome, left eye H50612); Internuclear ophthalmoplegia 378.86 (Internuclear ophthalmoplegia, unspecified eye H5120); Unspecified disorder of eye movements 378.9 (Unspecified disorder of binocular movement H519); Keratitis 370; Unspecified corneal disorder 371.9 (Unspecified disorder of cornea H189); Unspecified cerebrovascular disease 437.9 (Cerebrovascular disease, unspecified I679); Unspecified condition of brain 348.9 (Disorder of brain, unspecified G939); Developmental coordination disorder 315.4 (Specific developmental disorder of motor function F82)	
Cardiovascular disease, unspecified 429.2/I2510 with apraxias D001072:	
Yùzhú 5g sìnìtāng 5g zhìgāncǎotāng 5g to ♀	Yùzhú 5g sìnìtāng 5g zhìgāncǎotāng 5g to ♂
Brown's (tendon) sheath syndrome 378.61/H50611,H50612 with apraxias D001072:	
Wūyàoshùnqìsǎn 5g to ♀	Wūyàoshùnqìsǎn 5g to ♂
Unspecified cerebrovascular disease 437.9/I679 with apraxias D001072:	
Bǔyánghuánwǔtāng 5g chuānqī 1g dānshēn 1g shíchāngpú 1g yuǎnzhì 1g + acupuncture to ♀	Bǔyánghuánwǔtāng 5g chuānqī 2g dānshēn 1g shíchāngpú 1g yuǎnzhì 1g + acupuncture to ♂

Verbal apraxias are speech impairments and aphasias (cf. Section 12.7) are language impairments. They are different disorders but have similar causes. We therefore see similar herbal prescriptions for them.

17.19. Mobility Limitation

Mobility limitation is limitation in one's ability to move around his or her environment with ease. Examples of mobility limitation are difficulty walking three blocks, climbing ten flights of stairs, or rolling over in bed. Aging, physical inactivity, obesity, arthritis, diabetes and heart disease can cause mobility limitation.

Table 17.19. Herbal prescriptions for mobility limitation

<table>
<tr><td colspan="2">Mobility Limitation: https://meshb.nlm.nih.gov/record/ui?ui=D051346.</td></tr>
<tr><td colspan="2">Common prescriptions:</td></tr>
<tr><td colspan="2">Sìnìtāng 5g wúzhūyútāng 5g máhuángfùzǐxìxīntāng 5g
Sìnìtāng 5g máhuángfùzǐxìxīntāng 5g dāngguīsìnìtāng 5g
Sìnìtāng 5g wúzhūyútāng 5g
Sìnìtāng 5g máhuángfùzǐxìxīntāng 5g</td></tr>
<tr><td colspan="2">Alternative prescriptions:</td></tr>
<tr><td colspan="2">Sìnìtāng 5g rénshēn 2g bànxià 2g gānjiāng 2g dàhuáng 0g
Sìnìtāng 5g guìzhī 1g máhuáng 1g xìxīn 1g
Sìnìtāng 5g guìzhī 2g máhuáng 2g xìxīn 1g dàhuáng 0g
Sìnìtāng 5g shēngjiāng 1g guìzhī 1g rénshēn 1g dàhuáng 0g
Sìnìtāng 5g rénshēn 2g mùguā 2g yánhúsuǒ 1g</td></tr>
<tr><td colspan="2">Indicated diseases:</td></tr>
<tr><td colspan="2">Unspecified disease of spinal cord 336.9 (Disease of spinal cord, unspecified G959); Acute poliomyelitis 045; Myoneural disorders 358; Unspecified disorders of nervous system 349.9 (Disorder of central nervous system, unspecified G969); Cardiovascular disease, unspecified 429.2 (Atherosclerotic heart disease of native coronary artery without angina pectoris I2510); Other dermatoses 702; Polyneuropathy in diabetes 357.2 (Diabetes mellitus due to underlying condition with diabetic polyneuropathy E0842, Drug or chemical induced diabetes mellitus with neurological complications with diabetic polyneuropathy E0942, Type 1 diabetes mellitus with diabetic polyneuropathy E1042, Type 2 diabetes mellitus with diabetic polyneuropathy E1142, Other specified diabetes mellitus with diabetic polyneuropathy E1342); Diabetes with neurological manifestations 250.6; Diabetes with peripheral circulatory disorders 250.7; Diabetes mellitus 250; Unspecified endocrine disorder 259.9 (Endocrine disorder, unspecified E349); Unspecified disorder of metabolism 277.9 (Metabolic disorder, unspecified E889); Unspecified cerebrovascular disease 437.9 (Cerebrovascular disease, unspecified I679); Unspecified condition of brain 348.9 (Disorder of brain, unspecified G939)</td></tr>
<tr><td colspan="2">Unspecified disease of spinal cord 336.9/G959 with mobility limitation D051346:</td></tr>
<tr><td>Shūjīnghuóxuètāng 5g dāngguīniāntòngtāng 5g dúhuójìshēngtāng 5g to ♀</td><td>Guīlùèrxiānjiāo 5g to ♂</td></tr>
<tr><td colspan="2">Cardiovascular disease, unspecified 429.2/I2510 with mobility limitation D051346:</td></tr>
<tr><td>Sìnìtāng 5g gānlùyǐn 5g mǔdānpí 1g zhīzǐ 1g huánglián 0g to ♀</td><td>Sìnìtāng 5g gānlùyǐn 5g mǔdānpí 1g zhīzǐ 1g huánglián 1g to ♂</td></tr>
<tr><td colspan="2">Unspecified cerebrovascular disease 437.9/I679 with mobility limitation D051346:</td></tr>
<tr><td>Bǔyánghuánwǔtāng 5g chuānqī 1g dānshēn 1g shíchāngpú 1g yuǎnzhì 1g + acupuncture to ♀</td><td>Bǔyánghuánwǔtāng 5g chuānqī 1g dānshēn 1g shíchāngpú 1g yuǎnzhì 1g + acupuncture to ♂</td></tr>
</table>

Mobility is Yang and Sìnìtāng comes to the help. Wúzhūyútāng is today used for migraine (Wang, 2019), which usually accompanies unsteadiness. Patients with atopic dermatitis have more problems with mobility (Hsieh et al., 2022).

17.20. Failure to Thrive

Failure to thrive is insufficient weight or weight gain in pediatric-aged patients. Causes of failure to thrive include insufficient calorie intake due to e.g., poverty or picky eating, malabsorption due to e.g., inborn errors of metabolism, increased basal metabolism due to hyperthyroidism, and chronic infection and inflammation.

Table 17.20. Herbal prescriptions for failure to thrive

<table>
<tr><td colspan="2">Failure to Thrive: https://meshb.nlm.nih.gov/record/ui?ui=D005183.</td></tr>
<tr><td colspan="2">Common prescriptions:</td></tr>
<tr><td colspan="2">Guìzhītāng 5g báisháo 1g dàhuáng 0g
Guìzhītāng 5g shēngjiāng 1g báisháo 1g dàhuáng 0g
Guìzhītāng 5g shēngjiāng 1g guìzhī 1g
Guìzhītāng 5g wúzhūyútāng 3g fùzǐ 1g gānjiāng 1g
Guìzhītāng 5g shēngjiāng 1g báisháo 1g</td></tr>
<tr><td colspan="2">Alternative prescriptions:</td></tr>
<tr><td colspan="2">Guìzhītāng 5g shēngjiāng 1g guìzhī 1g dàhuáng 0g
Guìzhītāng 5g shēngjiāng 0g guìzhī 0g
Guìzhītāng 5g jiégěng 1g dàhuáng 0g
Guìzhītāng 5g gāncǎo 1g báisháo 1g dàhuáng 0g</td></tr>
<tr><td colspan="2">Indicated diseases:</td></tr>
<tr><td colspan="2">Heart disease, unspecified 429.9 (Heart disease, unspecified I519); Other dermatoses 702; Congenital ectodermal dysplasia 757.31 (Ectodermal dysplasia (anhidrotic) Q824); Cardiovascular disease, unspecified 429.2 (Atherosclerotic heart disease of native coronary artery without angina pectoris I2510); Unspecified congenital anomaly of heart 746.9 (Congenital malformation of cardiac chambers and connections, unspecified Q209, Congenital malformation of heart, unspecified Q249); Unspecified condition of brain 348.9 (Disorder of brain, unspecified G939); Neoplasm of unspecified nature of brain 239.6 (Neoplasm of unspecified behavior of brain D496); Unspecified disorders of nervous system 349.9 (Disorder of central nervous system, unspecified G969); Malignant neoplasm of nervous system, part unspecified 192.9 (Malignant neoplasm of central nervous system, unspecified C729); Unspecified disorder of intestine 569.9 (Disease of intestine, unspecified K639); Unspecified disorder of metabolism 277.9 (Metabolic disorder, unspecified E889); Diseases of the jaws 526</td></tr>
<tr><td colspan="2">Heart disease, unspecified 429.9/I519 with failure to thrive D005183:</td></tr>
<tr><td>Sìnìtāng 5g gānlùyǐn 5g mǔdānpí 1g zhīzǐ 1g huánglián 0g to ♀</td><td>Sìnìtāng 5g gānlùyǐn 5g mǔdānpí 1g zhīzǐ 1g huánglián 0g to ♂</td></tr>
<tr><td colspan="2">Unspecified condition of brain 348.9/G939 with failure to thrive D005183:</td></tr>
<tr><td>Bǔyánghuánwǔtāng 5g tiānmá 1g shíchāngpú 1g yuǎnzhì 1g gōuténg 1g + acupuncture to ♀</td><td>Bǔyánghuánwǔtāng 5g + acupuncture to ♂</td></tr>
<tr><td colspan="2">Unspecified disorder of intestine 569.9/K639 with failure to thrive D005183:</td></tr>
<tr><td>Lǐzhōngtāng 5g báisháo 1g guìzhī 1g to ♀</td><td>Lǐzhōngtāng 5g fùzǐ 1g to ♂</td></tr>
</table>

As Guìzhītāng treats upper respiratory tract infections, the prescriptions are thought to improve failure to thrive due to infections.

17.21. Lethargy

Lethargy is lack of energy, motivation, emotion and enthusiasm for mental or physical tasks. Inadequate sleep including insufficient or oversleeping, alcohol, chemotherapy, depression, anemia, chronic pain and brain injury can cause lethargy.

If lethargy is considered a manifestation of a decline in the Yang energy, then Sìnìtāng tries to counter the course.

Table 17.21. Herbal prescriptions for lethargy

Lethargy: https://meshb.nlm.nih.gov/record/ui?ui=D053609.	
Common prescriptions:	
Sìnìtāng 5g bànxià 1g dàhuáng 0g Sìnìtāng 5g shēngjiāng 1g guìzhī 1g Sìnìtāng 5g rénshēn 1g wúzhūyú 1g Sìnìtāng 5g rénshēn 1g Sìnìtāng 5g shēngjiāng 1g guìzhī 1g xìxīn 1g	
Alternative prescriptions:	
Sìnìtāng 5g rénshēn 1g dàhuáng 0g Sìnìtāng 5g ròuguì 1g wúzhūyú 1g dàhuáng 0g Sìnìtāng 5g rénshēn 1g bànxià 1g jiégěng 1g dàhuáng 0g	
Indicated diseases:	
Unspecified cerebrovascular disease 437.9 (Cerebrovascular disease, unspecified I679); Unspecified condition of brain 348.9 (Disorder of brain, unspecified G939); Cardiovascular disease, unspecified 429.2 (Atherosclerotic heart disease of native coronary artery without angina pectoris I2510); Unspecified disorders of nervous system 349.9 (Disorder of central nervous system, unspecified G969); Unspecified endocrine disorder 259.9 (Endocrine disorder, unspecified E349); Unspecified disorder of metabolism 277.9 (Metabolic disorder, unspecified E889); Hypoglycemia, unspecified 251.2 (Hypoglycemia, unspecified E162)	
Unspecified cerebrovascular disease 437.9/I679 with lethargy D053609:	
Bǔyánghuánwǔtāng 5g dānshēn 1g shíchāngpú 1g yuǎnzhì 1g + acupuncture to ♀	Bǔyánghuánwǔtāng 5g dānshēn 1g shíchāngpú 1g yuǎnzhì 1g + acupuncture to ♂
Unspecified condition of brain 348.9/G939 with lethargy D053609:	
Bǔyánghuánwǔtāng 5g tiānmá 1g shíchāngpú 1g yuǎnzhì 1g gōuténg 1g + acupuncture to ♀	Bǔyánghuánwǔtāng 5g + acupuncture to ♂
Unspecified disorders of nervous system 349.9/G969 with lethargy D053609:	
Huángqíwǔwùtāng 5g chuānxiōng 1g dānshēn 1g zhúrú 1g sāngzhī 1g dāngguī 1g jiānghuáng 1g to ♀	Huángqíwǔwùtāng 5g chuānxiōng 1g dānshēn 1g zhúrú 1g sāngzhī 1g dāngguī 1g jiānghuáng 1g to ♂

17.22. Mutism

Mutism is a condition in which an individual is unable or unwilling to speak, despite having intact comprehension of speech. Damage of the areas of the brain responsible for speech production can cause mutism. Selective mutism is mainly caused by severe anxiety.

Table 17.22. Herbal prescriptions for mutism

Mutism: https://meshb.nlm.nih.gov/record/ui?ui=D009155.
Common prescriptions:
Bǔzhōngyìqìtāng 5g Sìnìtāng 5g bǔzhōngyìqìtāng 5g
Alternative prescriptions:
Bǔzhōngyìqìtāng 5g + acupuncture Xiǎojiànzhōngtāng 5g huángqí 1g chuānxiōng 1g dāngguī 1g Guìzhījiālónggǔmǔlìtāng 5g huángqí 1g fùzǐ 0g Guìzhījiālónggǔmǔlìtāng 5g bǔzhōngyìqìtāng 5g Sìnìtāng 5g bǔzhōngyìqìtāng 3g

Mutism: https://meshb.nlm.nih.gov/record/ui?ui=D009155.	
Indicated diseases:	
Unspecified condition of brain 348.9 (Disorder of brain, unspecified G939); Malignant neoplasm of cerebellum nos 191.6 (Malignant neoplasm of cerebellum C716); Unspecified disorders of nervous system 349.9 (Disorder of central nervous system, unspecified G969); Neoplasm of unspecified nature of brain 239.6 (Neoplasm of unspecified behavior of brain D496); Malignant neoplasm of nervous system, part unspecified 192.9 (Malignant neoplasm of central nervous system, unspecified C729); Unspecified cerebrovascular disease 437.9 (Cerebrovascular disease, unspecified I679); Cardiovascular disease, unspecified 429.2 (Atherosclerotic heart disease of native coronary artery without angina pectoris I2510)	
Unspecified condition of brain 348.9/G939 with mutism D009155:	
Bǔyánghuánwǔtāng 5g tiānmá 1g shíchāngpú 1g yuǎnzhì 1g gōuténg 1g + acupuncture to ♀	Bǔyánghuánwǔtāng 5g + acupuncture to ♂
Unspecified cerebrovascular disease 437.9/I679 with mutism D009155:	
Bǔyánghuánwǔtāng 5g dānshēn 1g shíchāngpú 1g yuǎnzhì 1g + acupuncture to ♀	Bǔyánghuánwǔtāng 5g dānshēn 1g shíchāngpú 1g yuǎnzhì 1g + acupuncture to ♂

Today, Bǔzhōngyìqìtāng is used for bronchitis and anemia; Sìnìtāng for hepatitis, irritable bowel syndrome, and bronchitis; Xiǎojiànzhōngtāng for allergic rhinitis, and dyspepsia and other specified disorders of function of stomach; and Guìzhījiālónggǔmǔlìtāng for allergic rhinitis and insomnia (Wang, 2019). The wide range of indications for the formulas in the prescriptions reflects the varied and often incoherent causes and patterns of mutism.

17.23. Catatonia

Catatonia is abnormal, usually lack of, movements and communications even though one is awake. Catatonia is often secondary to a psychiatric illness such as depression, bipolar disorder, schizophrenia and autism.

Table 17.23. Herbal prescriptions for catatonia

Catatonia: https://meshb.nlm.nih.gov/record/ui?ui=D002389.	
Common prescriptions:	
Sháoyàogāncǎotāng 5g shūjīnghuóxuètāng 5g dāngguīniāntòngtāng 5g + acupuncture Sháoyàogāncǎotāng 5g shūjīnghuóxuètāng 5g + acupuncture	
Alternative prescriptions:	
Sháoyàogāncǎotāng 5g niúxī 1g huángbò 1g cāngzhú 1g yìyǐrén 1g + acupuncture Sháoyàogāncǎotāng 5g shūjīnghuóxuètāng 5g mòyào 1g rǔxiāng 1g yánhúsuǒ 1g Sháoyàogāncǎotāng 5g mùguā 1g niúxī 1g dùzhòng 1g xùduàn 1g Sháoyàogāncǎotāng 5g cháihúguìzhītāng 4g yánhúsuǒ 1g + acupuncture Sháoyàogāncǎotāng 5g shūjīnghuóxuètāng 2g mùguā 1g jīxuèténg 1g + acupuncture	
Indicated diseases:	
Neuroleptic malignant syndrome 333.92 (Malignant neuroleptic syndrome G210); Schizophreniform disorder 295.4; Unspecified condition of brain 348.9 (Disorder of brain, unspecified G939); Unspecified disorders of nervous system 349.9 (Disorder of central nervous system, unspecified G969); Schizoaffective disorder 295.7; Schizophrenic disorders 295	
Neuroleptic malignant syndrome 333.92/G210 with catatonia D002389:	
Yìgānsǎn 5g sháoyàogāncǎotāng 5g mùguā 1g qínjiāo 1g gōuténg 1g to ♀	Yìgānsǎn 5g sháoyàogāncǎotāng 5g mùguā 1g niúxī 1g qínjiāo 1g gōuténg 1g to ♂
Unspecified condition of brain 348.9/G939 with catatonia D002389:	
Bǔyánghuánwǔtāng 5g tiānmá 1g shíchāngpú 1g yuǎnzhì 1g gōuténg 1g + acupuncture to ♀	Bǔyánghuánwǔtāng 5g dānshēn 1g shíchāngpú 1g yuǎnzhì 1g + acupuncture to ♂

Sháoyàogāncǎotāng, Shūjīnghuóxuètāng and Dāngguīniāntòngtāng are used for spasms and here for withdrawn or excited catatonia.

17.24. Trismus

Trismus, also known as lockjaw, is sustained spasm of the masticatory muscles so that jaw movements, and thus mouth opening, are limited. Infections, traumatic injury, head and neck tumor, radiotherapy and hysteria can cause trismus.

Table 17.24. Herbal prescriptions for trismus

Trismus: https://meshb.nlm.nih.gov/record/ui?ui=D014313.	
Common prescriptions:	
Sháoyàogāncǎotāng 5g shūjīnghuóxuètāng 5g dāngguīniāntòngtāng 5g + acupuncture Sháoyàogāncǎotāng 5g shūjīnghuóxuètāng 5g + acupuncture	
Alternative prescriptions:	
Sháoyàogāncǎotāng 5g shūjīnghuóxuètāng 5g yánhúsuǒ 1g + acupuncture Sháoyàogāncǎotāng 5g huángqíwǔwùtāng 5g dānshēn 2g zhúrú 2g yánhúsuǒ 2g sāngzhī 2g jīxuèténg 2g + acupuncture Sháoyàogāncǎotāng 5g shūjīnghuóxuètāng 5g yánhúsuǒ 1g gégēn 1g Shūjīnghuóxuètāng 5g sháoyàogāncǎotāng 3g mòyào 1g rǔxiāng 1g jīxuèténg 1g + acupuncture Sháoyàogāncǎotāng 5g gégēn 1g	
Indicated diseases:	
Myopathy, unspecified 359.9 (Myopathy, unspecified G729); Unspecified disorder of joint, site unspecified 719.90 (Joint disorder, unspecified M259); Unspecified disorders of nervous system 349.9 (Disorder of central nervous system, unspecified G969); Ankylosis of joint 718.5; Unspecified disease of pharynx 478.20 (Other diseases of pharynx J392); Malignant neoplasm of anterior wall of nasopharynx 147.3 (Malignant neoplasm of anterior wall of nasopharynx C113); Progressive myositis ossificans 728.11 (Myositis ossificans progressiva, unspecified site M6110)	
Myopathy, unspecified 359.9/G729 with trismus D014313:	
Sháoyàogāncǎotāng 5g huángqíwǔwùtāng 5g dānshēn 1g zhúrú 1g sāngzhī 1g jiānghuáng 1g to ♀	Guīlùèrxiānjiāo 5g to ♂
Unspecified disease of pharynx 478.20/J392 with trismus D014313:	
Guìzhītāng 5g báisháo 1g dàhuáng 0g to ♀	Bànxiàhòupòtāng 5g màiméndōngtāng 5g xuánshēn 1g jiégěng 1g to ♂

Guīlùèrxiānjiāo 'replenishes essence and marrow' and is today used for unspecified osteoporosis, and lumbago (Wang, 2019).

17.25. Prodromal Symptoms

Prodromal symptoms are clinical indicators, or subsymptoms, that occur days or hours before the onset of a disease such as migraine, epilepsy, and viral infection. Examples of prodromes include mood swings, irritability, malaise, low-grade fever, lack of appetite, and trouble sleeping.

Huòxiāngzhèngqìsǎn 'releases exterior, expels Dampness,' 'regulates Qi, harmonizes interior' and is today used for other and unspecified non-infectious gastroenteritis and colitis (Wang, 2019).

Table 17.25. Herbal prescriptions for prodromal symptoms

Prodromal Symptoms: https://meshb.nlm.nih.gov/record/ui?ui=D062706.	
Common prescriptions:	
Huòxiāngzhèngqìsǎn 5g Sìnìtāng 5g xuèfǔzhúyūtāng 5g Sìnìtāng 5g lǐzhōngtāng 5g	
Alternative prescriptions:	
Xiāoyáosǎn 5g cháihújiālónggǔmǔlìtāng 2g táohéchéngqìtāng 0g Huòxiāngzhèngqìsǎn 5g mùxiāng 0g shārén 0g huánglián 0g Sìnìtāng 5g xuèfǔzhúyūtāng 5g cháihúshūgāntāng 5g Sìnìtāng 5g wúzhūyútāng 5g zhēnwǔtāng 5g Sìnìtāng 5g gāncǎoxiǎomàidàzǎotāng 5g bǎihé 2g bózǐrén 2g yuǎnzhì 2g gōuténg 2g	
Indicated and associated diseases:	
Heart disease, unspecified 429.9 (Heart disease, unspecified I519); Digeorge's syndrome 279.11 (Di George's syndrome D821); Schizophrenic disorders 295; Velo-cardio-facial syndrome 758.32 (Velo-cardio-facial syndrome Q9381); Cardiovascular disease, unspecified 429.2 (Atherosclerotic heart disease of native coronary artery without angina pectoris I2510); Hypoparathyroidism 252.1 (Hypoparathyroidism, unspecified E209); Unspecified disorder of parathyroid gland 252.9 (Disorder of parathyroid gland, unspecified E215); Unspecified endocrine disorder 259.9 (Endocrine disorder, unspecified E349); Unspecified congenital anomaly of heart 746.9 (Congenital malformation of cardiac chambers and connections, unspecified Q209, Congenital malformation of heart, unspecified Q249); Schizophreniform disorder 295.4; Schizoaffective disorder 295.7; Schizotypal personality disorder 301.22 (Schizotypal disorder F21); Avoidant personality disorder 301.82 (Avoidant personality disorder F606); Narcissistic personality disorder 301.81 (Narcissistic personality disorder F6081)	
Heart disease, unspecified 429.9/I519 with prodromal symptoms D062706:	
Sìnìtāng 5g gānlùyǐn 5g mǔdānpí 1g zhīzǐ 1g huánglián 0g to ♀	Sìnìtāng 5g gānlùyǐn 5g mǔdānpí 1g zhīzǐ 1g huánglián 0g to ♂
Schizotypal personality disorder 301.22/F21 with prodromal symptoms D062706:	
Jiāwèixiāoyáosǎn 5g gāncǎoxiǎomàidàzǎotāng 5g héhuānpí 1g bǎihé 1g xiāngfù 1g yùjīn 1g to ♀	Gāncǎoxiǎomàidàzǎotāng 5g cháihújiālónggǔmǔlìtāng 5g wēndǎntāng 5g shíchāngpú 1g yuǎnzhì 1g to ♂

17.26. Motion Sickness

Motion sickness is feeling sick when one travels in a car, on a boat, train or airplane. Our vestibular system, which maintains balance and spatial orientation, senses motion while our visual system sees no or little movement. The two conflicting signals confuse our brain and make us feel sick.

A main symptom of motion sickness is cold sweats. This could be the reason Sìnìtāng is prescribed here.

Table 17.26. Herbal prescriptions for motion sickness

Motion Sickness: https://meshb.nlm.nih.gov/record/ui?ui=D009041.
Common prescriptions:
Sìnìtāng 5g rénshēn 1g bànxià 1g dàhuáng 0g Sìnìtāng 5g rénshēn 1g wúzhūyú 1g Sìnìtāng 5g rénshēn 1g bànxià 1g Sìnìtāng 5g rénshēn 1g Sìnìtāng 5g rénshēn 1g bànxià 1g gānjiāng 1g
Alternative prescriptions:
Sìnìtāng 5g rénshēn 2g bànxià 2g dàhuáng 0g Línggùishùgāntāng 5g bànxià 1g dàhuáng 0g

Table 17.26. (Continued)

Motion Sickness: https://meshb.nlm.nih.gov/record/ui?ui=D009041.	
Guìzhītāng 5g jiégěng 1g dàhuáng 0g Sìnìtāng 5g rénshēn 1g bànxià 1g yánhúsuǒ 1g dàhuáng 0g Sìnìtāng 5g rénshēn 2g yìzhìrén 1g fùpénzǐ 1g dàhuáng 0g	
Indicated diseases:	
Dissociated nystagmus 379.55 (Dissociated nystagmus H5504); Motion sickness 994.6 (Motion sickness, initial encounter T753XXA); Nystagmus, unspecified 379.50 (Unspecified nystagmus H5500); Visual deprivation nystagmus 379.53 (Visual deprivation nystagmus H5503); Brown's (tendon) sheath syndrome 378.61 (Brown's sheath syndrome, right eye H50611, Brown's sheath syndrome, left eye H50612); Internuclear ophthalmoplegia 378.86 (Internuclear ophthalmoplegia, unspecified eye H5120); Unspecified disorder of eye movements 378.9 (Unspecified disorder of binocular movement H519); Unspecified disorder of cranial nerves 352.9 (Cranial nerve disorder, unspecified G529); Disorder of eye, unspecified 379.90 (Unspecified disorder of eye and adnexa H579); Unspecified disorders of nervous system 349.9 (Disorder of central nervous system, unspecified G969); Migraine 346; Unspecified condition of brain 348.9 (Disorder of brain, unspecified G939); Unspecified disorder of ear 388.9 (Unspecified disorder of ear, bilateral H9393)	
Dissociated nystagmus 379.55/H5504 with motion sickness D009041:	
Qǐjúdìhuángwán 5g zīshènmíngmùtāng 5g to ♀	Qǐjúdìhuángwán 5g zīshènmíngmùtāng 5g to ♂
Migraine 346 with motion sickness D009041:	
Chuānxiōngchádiàosǎn 5g jiāwèixiāoyáosǎn 5g qīngshàngjuāntòngtāng 5g zhúrú 1g bózǐrén 1g yuǎnzhì 1g to ♀	Chuānxiōngchádiàosǎn 5g jiāwèixiāoyáosǎn 5g qīngshàngjuāntòngtāng 5g zhúrú 1g bózǐrén 1g yuǎnzhì 1g to ♂
Unspecified disorder of ear 388.9/H9393 with motion sickness D009041:	
Xiǎocháihútāng 5g língguìshùgāntāng 5g shíchāngpú 1g yuǎnzhì 1g to ♀	Xiǎocháihútāng 5g língguìshùgāntāng 5g shíchāngpú 1g yuǎnzhì 1g to ♂

17.27. Stuttering

Stuttering is involuntary repetition or prolongation of sounds, syllables or words. The cause of stuttering in children is not well understood, although genetics may contribute. Brain injury such as stroke can cause stuttering. Furthermore, it is now clear that psychogenic stuttering, i.e., stuttering related to emotional conditions such as anxiety, is rare.

Table 17.27. Herbal prescriptions for stuttering

Stuttering: https://meshb.nlm.nih.gov/record/ui?ui=D013342.
Common prescriptions:
Máhuángfùzǐxìxīntāng 5g shēngjiāng 1g guìzhī 1g zhìgāncǎo 1g Máhuángfùzǐxìxīntāng 5g shēngjiāng 2g guìzhī 2g zhìgāncǎo 1g Máhuángfùzǐxìxīntāng 5g shēngjiāng 1g guìzhī 1g Máhuángfùzǐxìxīntāng 5g shēngjiāng 2g zhìgāncǎo 2g guìzhī 2g Bǔzhōngyìqìtāng 5g
Alternative prescriptions:
Máhuángfùzǐxìxīntāng 5g shēngjiāng 2g guìzhī 2g gāncǎo 1g Bǔzhōngyìqìtāng 5g + acupuncture Sìnìtāng 5g shēngjiāng 0g guìzhī 0g
Indicated diseases:
Unspecified cerebrovascular disease 437.9 (Cerebrovascular disease, unspecified I679); Unspecified condition of brain 348.9 (Disorder of brain, unspecified G939); Cardiovascular disease, unspecified 429.2 (Atherosclerotic heart disease of native coronary artery without angina pectoris I2510); Unspecified disorders of nervous system 349.9 (Disorder of central nervous system, unspecified G969); Neoplasm of unspecified nature of brain 239.6 (Neoplasm of unspecified behavior of brain D496); Malignant neoplasm of nervous system, part unspecified 192.9 (Malignant neoplasm of central nervous system, unspecified C729); Epilepsy, unspecified 345.9; Phobia, unspecified 300.20 (Phobic anxiety disorder, unspecified F409)

Stuttering: https://meshb.nlm.nih.gov/record/ui?ui=D013342.	
Unspecified cerebrovascular disease 437.9/I679 with stuttering D013342:	
Bŭyánghuánwŭtāng 5g chuānqī 2g dānshēn 1g shíchāngpú 1g yuǎnzhì 1g + acupuncture to ♀	Bŭyánghuánwŭtāng 5g chuānqī 2g dānshēn 1g shíchāngpú 1g yuǎnzhì 1g + acupuncture to ♂
Unspecified condition of brain 348.9/G939 with stuttering D013342:	
Bŭyánghuánwŭtāng 5g dānshēn 1g tiānmá 1g shíchāngpú 1g yuǎnzhì 1g gōuténg 1g + acupuncture to ♀	Bŭyánghuánwŭtāng 5g chuānqī 1g dānshēn 1g shíchāngpú 1g yuǎnzhì 1g + acupuncture to ♂
Epilepsy, unspecified 345.9 with stuttering D013342:	
Yìgānsǎn 5g cháihújiālónggŭmŭlìtāng 5g dānshēn 1g tiānmá 1g gōuténg 1g to ♀	Yìgānsǎn 5g cháihújiālónggŭmŭlìtāng 5g dānshēn 1g shíchāngpú 1g yuǎnzhì 1g to ♂
Unspecified disorders of nervous system 349.9/G969 with stuttering D013342:	
Huángqíwŭwùtāng 5g chuānxiōng 1g dānshēn 1g zhúrú 1g sāngzhī 1g dāngguī 1g jiānghuáng 1g to ♀	Huángqíwŭwùtāng 5g chuānxiōng 1g dānshēn 1g zhúrú 1g sāngzhī 1g dāngguī 1g jiānghuáng 1g to ♂

Máhuángfùzǐxìxīntāng is used in Chapters 4 and 5 for hiccup, hyperkinesias, hypokinesias and ataxia, and here for stuttering, which affects coordination of the muscles involved in breathing, voicing and articulating.

17.28. Low Cardiac Output

Low cardiac output is decreased cardiac output at rest or during stress. Heart failure, severe sepsis, and severe blood loss can cause low cardiac output.

Table 17.28. Herbal prescriptions for low cardiac output

Low Cardiac Output: https://meshb.nlm.nih.gov/record/ui?ui=D002303.	
Common prescriptions:	
Sìnìtāng 5g bànxià 1g dàhuáng 0g Sìnìtāng 5g rénshēn 1g wúzhūyú 1g Sìnìtāng 5g rénshēn 1g bànxià 1g dàhuáng 0g Sìnìtāng 5g rénshēn 1g	
Alternative prescriptions:	
Sìnìtāng 5g shēngjiāng 0g guìzhī 0g Sìnìtāng 5g wúzhūyú 0g Sìnìtāng 5g rénshēn 1g wúzhūyú 1g dàhuáng 0g	
Indicated diseases:	
Congestive heart failure, unspecified 428.0 (Right heart failure due to left heart failure I50814, Heart failure, unspecified I509); Unspecified disorder of metabolism 277.9 (Metabolic disorder, unspecified E889); Heart disease, unspecified 429.9 (Heart disease, unspecified I519); Cardiovascular disease, unspecified 429.2 (Atherosclerotic heart disease of native coronary artery without angina pectoris I2510); Unspecified congenital anomaly of heart 746.9 (Congenital malformation of cardiac chambers and connections, unspecified Q209, Congenital malformation of heart, unspecified Q249); Malignant neoplasm of heart 164.1 (Malignant neoplasm of heart C380); Malignant neoplasm of thorax 195.1 (Malignant neoplasm of thorax C761); Congenital mitral insufficiency 746.6 (Congenital mitral insufficiency Q233)	
Congestive heart failure, unspecified 428.0/I50814,I509 with cardiac output, low D002303:	
Zhēnwŭtāng 5g fùzǐ 1g gānjiāng 1g xìxīn 1g to ♀	Shēngmàiyǐn 5g xuèfŭzhúyūtāng 5g dānshēn 1g yùjīn 1g to ♂
Heart disease, unspecified 429.9/I519 with cardiac output, low D002303:	
Sìnìtāng 5g gānlùyǐn 5g mŭdānpí 1g zhīzǐ 1g huánglián 0g to ♀	Sìnìtāng 5g gānlùyǐn 5g mŭdānpí 1g zhīzǐ 1g huánglián 0g to ♂

Pumping of the heart sends oxygen- and nutrient-rich blood to where it is needed including the brain, liver and muscles. When cardiac output is low, all psychophysiological activities, i.e., Yang, go down. Sìnìtāng is here supposed to rescue the collapsing Yang.

17.29. High Cardiac Output

Cardiac output goes up during exercise to meet the increased muscular demand. High cardiac output can also be caused by anemia, pregnancy, hypoxia, hyperthyroidism, sepsis and organ failure.

Table 17.29. Herbal prescriptions for high cardiac output

High Cardiac Output: https://meshb.nlm.nih.gov/record/ui?ui=D016534	
Common prescriptions:	
Sìnìtāng 5g bànxià 1g dàhuáng 0g Sìnìtāng 5g shēngjiāng 1g guìzhī 1g Sìnìtāng 5g rénshēn 1g bànxià 1g dàhuáng 0g Sìnìtāng 5g rénshēn 1g	
Alternative prescriptions:	
Sìnìtāng 5g rénshēn 1g dàhuáng 0g Sìnìtāng 5g rénshēn 2g bànxià 1g dàhuáng 0g Sìnìtāng 5g rénshēn 1g wúzhūyú 0g Sìnìtāng 5g shēngjiāng 2g guìzhī 2g dàhuáng 0g Sìnìtāng 5g fúlíng 2g bànxià 1g dàhuáng 0g	
Indicated diseases:	
Congestive heart failure, unspecified 428.0 (Right heart failure due to left heart failure I50814, Heart failure, unspecified I509); End stage renal disease 585.6 (End stage renal disease N186); Heart disease, unspecified 429.9 (Heart disease, unspecified I519); Cardiovascular disease, unspecified 429.2 (Atherosclerotic heart disease of native coronary artery without angina pectoris I2510); Renal failure, unspecified 586 (Unspecified kidney failure N19); Unspecified disorder of metabolism 277.9 (Metabolic disorder, unspecified E889)	
Congestive heart failure, unspecified 428.0/I50814,I509 with cardiac output, high D016534:	
Shēngmàiyǐn 5g zhēnwǔtāng 5g dānshēn 1g to ♀	Shēngmàiyǐn 5g xuèfǔzhúyūtāng 5g dānshēn 1g yùjīn 1g to ♂
Heart disease, unspecified 429.9/I519 with cardiac output, high D016534:	
Sìnìtāng 5g gānlùyǐn 5g mǔdānpí 1g zhīzǐ 1g huánglián 0g to ♀	Sìnìtāng 5g gānlùyǐn 5g mǔdānpí 1g zhīzǐ 1g huánglián 0g to ♂

Compensatory changes of the heart can cause high cardiac output, leading to eventual heart failure, which is prescribed by Sìnìtāng.

17.30. Heart Murmurs

Heart murmurs are extra and unusual sounds heard with a stethoscope when blood flows through the chambers and valves of the heart. Heart murmurs can signal a heart problem. Anemia which changes the viscosity of the blood can also cause heart murmurs. Other causes include high blood pressure, overactive thyroid and infections.

Zhēnwǔtāng is today used for unspecified essential hypertension (Wang, 2019) and is here to alleviate heart murmurs.

Table 17.30. Herbal prescriptions for heart murmurs

Heart Murmurs: https://meshb.nlm.nih.gov/record/ui?ui=D006337.	
Common prescriptions:	
Zhēnwǔtāng 5g fùzǐ 1g gānjiāng 1g Zhēnwǔtāng 5g fùzǐ 1g xìxīn 1g Zhēnwǔtāng 5g fùzǐ 1g gānjiāng 1g xìxīn 1g	
Zhēnwǔtāng 5g fùzǐ 1g xìxīn 1g tiáowèichéngqìtāng 1g Zhēnwǔtāng 5g fùzǐ 1g	
Alternative prescriptions:	
Zhēnwǔtāng 5g wǔwèizǐ 0g gānjiāng 0g xìxīn 0g Zhēnwǔtāng 5g fùzǐ 1g xìxīn 1g mázǐrénwán 1g dàhuáng 0g Zhēnwǔtāng 5g wǔwèizǐ 1g gānjiāng 1g xìxīn 1g Sìnìtāng 5g gānlùyǐn 5g	
Indicated diseases:	
Heart disease, unspecified 429.9 (Heart disease, unspecified I519); Malignant neoplasm of heart 164.1 (Malignant neoplasm of heart C380); Cardiovascular disease, unspecified 429.2 (Atherosclerotic heart disease of native coronary artery without angina pectoris I2510); Malignant neoplasm of thorax 195.1 (Malignant neoplasm of thorax C761); Ventricular septal defect 745.4 (Eisenmenger's syndrome I2783, Ventricular septal defect Q210); Unspecified congenital anomaly of heart 746.9 (Congenital malformation of cardiac chambers and connections, unspecified Q209, Congenital malformation of heart, unspecified Q249); Congenital heart block 746.86 (Congenital heart block Q246); Congenital stenosis of aortic valve 746.3 (Congenital stenosis of aortic valve Q230)	
Heart disease, unspecified 429.9/I519 with heart murmurs D006337:	
Sìnìtāng 5g gānlùyǐn 5g mǔdānpí 1g zhīzǐ 1g huánglián 0g to ♀	Sìnìtāng 5g gānlùyǐn 5g mǔdānpí 1g zhīzǐ 1g huánglián 0g to ♂

17.31. Mydriasis

Mydriasis is excessive widening of the pupils, which collect light for image formation in the retina. Control of the pupillary size is autonomic so that pupils constrict in bright light and dilate in dim light conditions. Damage to the oculomotor nerve which resizes the pupillary aperture can cause mydriasis. Eye care medication and drug use can also cause mydriasis. High levels of oxytocin hormone are also known to dilate the pupils.

Table 17.31. Herbal prescriptions for mydriasis

Mydriasis: https://meshb.nlm.nih.gov/record/ui?ui=D015878.
Common prescriptions:
Guìzhītāng 5g wúzhūyútāng 3g fùzǐ 1g gānjiāng 1g Guìzhītāng 5g wúzhūyútāng 3g fùzǐ 1g Guìzhītāng 5g wúzhūyútāng 3g fùzǐ 2g gānjiāng 2g Guìzhītāng 5g wúzhūyútāng 3g fùzǐ 1g xìxīn 1g Guìzhītāng 5g wúzhūyútāng 3g fùzǐ 2g gānjiāng 1g
Alternative prescriptions:
Guìzhītāng 5g bànxià 1g báisháo 1g dàhuáng 0g Guìzhītāng 5g wúzhūyútāng 3g fùzǐ 1g gānjiāng 1g xìxīn 1g Sìnìtāng 5g gǒuqǐzǐ 1g júhuā 1g Sìnìtāng 5g bànxià 2g yánhúsuǒ 1g dàhuáng 0g Guìzhītāng 5g shēngjiāng 1g guìzhī 1g
Indicated diseases:
Primary open angle glaucoma 365.11 (Primary open-angle glaucoma, right eye, stage unspecified H401110, Primary open-angle glaucoma, right eye, mild stage H401111, Primary open-angle glaucoma, right eye, moderate stage H401112, Primary open-angle glaucoma, right eye, severe stage H401113, Primary open-angle glaucoma, right eye, indeterminate stage H401114, Primary open-angle glaucoma, left eye, stage unspecified H401120, Primary open-angle

Table 17.31. (Continued)

Mydriasis: https://meshb.nlm.nih.gov/record/ui?ui=D015878.	
glaucoma, left eye, mild stage H401121, Primary open-angle glaucoma, left eye, moderate stage H401122, Primary open-angle glaucoma, left eye, severe stage H401123, Primary open-angle glaucoma, left eye, indeterminate stage H401124, Primary open-angle glaucoma, bilateral, stage unspecified H401130, Primary open-angle glaucoma, bilateral, mild stage H401131, Primary open-angle glaucoma, bilateral, moderate stage H401132, Primary open-angle glaucoma, bilateral, severe stage H401133, Primary open-angle glaucoma, bilateral, indeterminate stage H401134, Primary open-angle glaucoma, unspecified eye, stage unspecified H401190, Primary open-angle glaucoma, unspecified eye, mild stage H401191, Primary open-angle glaucoma, unspecified eye, moderate stage H401192, Primary open-angle glaucoma, unspecified eye, severe stage H401193, Primary open-angle glaucoma, unspecified eye, indeterminate stage H401194); Open-angle glaucoma 365.1; Glaucoma 365; Ocular hypertension 365.04 (Ocular hypertension, unspecified eye H40059); Disorder of eye, unspecified 379.90 (Unspecified disorder of eye and adnexa H579); Cardiovascular disease, unspecified 429.2 (Atherosclerotic heart disease of native coronary artery without angina pectoris I2510); Diabetic retinopathy 362.0; Diabetes with peripheral circulatory disorders 250.7; Unspecified retinal disorder 362.9 (Unspecified retinal disorder H359); Diabetes mellitus 250; Unspecified endocrine disorder 259.9 (Endocrine disorder, unspecified E349); Unspecified disorder of metabolism 277.9 (Metabolic disorder, unspecified E889); Heart disease, unspecified 429.9 (Heart disease, unspecified I519); Patent ductus arteriosus 747.0 (Patent ductus arteriosus Q250); Unspecified congenital anomaly of heart 746.9 (Congenital malformation of cardiac chambers and connections, unspecified Q209, Congenital malformation of heart, unspecified Q249)	
Primary open angle glaucoma 365.11/H401110,H401111,H401112,H401113,H401114,H401120,H401121,H401122, H401123,H401124,H401130,H401131,H401132,H401133,H401134,H401190,H401191, H401192,H401193,H401194 with Mydriasis D015878:	
Qǐjúdìhuángwán 5g xǐgānmíngmùtāng 5g zīshènmíngmùtāng 5g to ♀	Qǐjúdìhuángwán 5g xǐgānmíngmùtāng 5g zīshènmíngmùtāng 5g to ♂
Cardiovascular disease, unspecified 429.2/I2510 with mydriasis D015878:	
Yùzhú 5g sìnìtāng 5g mǔdānpí 1g zhīzǐ 1g huánglián 1g to ♀	Sìnìtāng 5g gānlùyǐn 5g mǔdānpí 1g zhīzǐ 1g huánglián 1g to ♂
Heart disease, unspecified 429.9/I519 with mydriasis D015878:	
Sìnìtāng 5g gānlùyǐn 5g mǔdānpí 1g zhīzǐ 1g huánglián 0g to ♀	Sìnìtāng 5g gānlùyǐn 5g mǔdānpí 1g zhīzǐ 1g huánglián 0g to ♂

Guìzhītāng is used in Chapter 1 for headache. Wúzhūyútāng's modern uses include migraine (Wang, 2019). Episodic unilateral mydriasis was reported to be associated with migraine (Skeik and Jabr, 2011). Use of the formulas in the prescriptions is therefore thought to target the comorbidities of mydriasis.

17.32. Miosis

Miosis, opposite of mydriasis, is excessive constriction of the pupils. Aging, smoking, iris inflammation, opioid drug use, and head injury can cause miosis.

Table 17.32. Herbal prescriptions for miosis

Miosis: https://meshb.nlm.nih.gov/record/ui?ui=D015877.
Common prescriptions:
Sìnìtāng 5g shēngjiāng 1g guìzhī 1g Máhuángfùzǐxìxīntāng 5g shēngjiāng 2g guìzhī 2g zhìgāncǎo 1g Máhuángfùzǐxìxīntāng 5g shēngjiāng 1g guìzhī 1g zhìgāncǎo 1g Máhuángfùzǐxìxīntāng 5g shēngjiāng 1g guìzhī 1g Máhuángfùzǐxìxīntāng 5g shēngjiāng 2g zhìgāncǎo 2g guìzhī 2g dàzǎo 1g

Miosis: https://meshb.nlm.nih.gov/record/ui?ui=D015877.	
Alternative prescriptions:	
Máhuángfùzǐxìxīntāng 5g fùzǐ 3g guìzhī 3g báizhú 2g wúzhūyú 2g gānjiāng 2g zhìgāncǎotāng 2g Guìzhītāng 5g shēngjiāng 1g guìzhī 1g dàhuáng 0g Guìzhītāng 5g shēngjiāng 1g báisháo 1g Máhuángfùzǐxìxīntāng 5g fùzǐ 3g guìzhī 3g dàzǎo 2g gānjiāng 2g zhìgāncǎotāng 2g Guìzhītāng 5g shēngjiāng 0g báisháo 0g dàhuáng 0g	
Indicated diseases:	
Primary open angle glaucoma 365.11 (Primary open-angle glaucoma, right eye, stage unspecified H401110, Primary open-angle glaucoma, right eye, mild stage H401111, Primary open-angle glaucoma, right eye, moderate stage H401112, Primary open-angle glaucoma, right eye, severe stage H401113, Primary open-angle glaucoma, right eye, indeterminate stage H401114, Primary open-angle glaucoma, left eye, stage unspecified H401120, Primary open-angle glaucoma, left eye, mild stage H401121, Primary open-angle glaucoma, left eye, moderate stage H401122, Primary open-angle glaucoma, left eye, severe stage H401123, Primary open-angle glaucoma, left eye, indeterminate stage H401124, Primary open-angle glaucoma, bilateral, stage unspecified H401130, Primary open-angle glaucoma, bilateral, mild stage H401131, Primary open-angle glaucoma, bilateral, moderate stage H401132, Primary open-angle glaucoma, bilateral, severe stage H401133, Primary open-angle glaucoma, bilateral, indeterminate stage H401134, Primary open-angle glaucoma, unspecified eye, stage unspecified H401190, Primary open-angle glaucoma, unspecified eye, mild stage H401191, Primary open-angle glaucoma, unspecified eye, moderate stage H401192, Primary open-angle glaucoma, unspecified eye, severe stage H401193, Primary open-angle glaucoma, unspecified eye, indeterminate stage H401194); Open-angle glaucoma 365.1; Glaucoma 365; Ocular hypertension 365.04 (Ocular hypertension, unspecified eye H40059); Disorder of eye, unspecified 379.90 (Unspecified disorder of eye and adnexa H579); Unspecified disorders of nervous system 349.9 (Disorder of central nervous system, unspecified G969); Unspecified retinal disorder 362.9 (Unspecified retinal disorder H359); Cardiovascular disease, unspecified 429.2 (Atherosclerotic heart disease of native coronary artery without angina pectoris I2510); Diabetic retinopathy 362.0; Diabetes with peripheral circulatory disorders 250.7; Diabetes mellitus 250; Unspecified endocrine disorder 259.9 (Endocrine disorder, unspecified E349); Unspecified disorder of metabolism 277.9 (Metabolic disorder, unspecified E889)	
Primary open angle glaucoma 365.11/H401110,H401111,H401112,H401113,H401114,H401120,H401121,H401122, H401123,H401124,H401130,H401131,H401132,H401133,H401134,H401190,H401191, H401192,H401193,H401194 with Miosis D015877:	
Qǐjúdìhuángwán 5g xǐgānmíngmùtāng 5g zīshènmíngmùtāng 5g to ♀	Xǐgānmíngmùtāng 5g zīshènmíngmùtāng 5g to ♂
Unspecified retinal disorder 362.9/H359 with miosis D015877:	
Qǐjúdìhuángwán 5g zīshènmíngmùtāng 4g xuèfǔzhúyūtāng 2g to ♀	Qǐjúdìhuángwán 5g zīshènmíngmùtāng 3g xuèfǔzhúyūtāng 2g to ♂
Cardiovascular disease, unspecified 429.2/I2510 with miosis D015877:	
Yùzhú 5g sìnìtāng 5g mǔdānpí 1g zhīzǐ 1g huánglián 1g to ♀	Sìnìtāng 5g gānlùyǐn 5g lóngdǎnxiègāntāng 5g to ♂

Modern uses of Máhuángfùzǐxìxīntāng include unspecified sinusitis (Wang, 2019). A case of Horner Syndrome—an oculosympathetic palsy which causes miosis—as complication of bacterial sphenoid sinusitis was reported (Kacker et al., 2019).

17.33. Anisocoria

Anisocoria is unequal pupil size. Migraine, oculomotor nerve palsy, multiple sclerosis, eye injury, brain tumor, and topical ophthalmic drug use can cause anisocoria.

Horner Syndrome that affects one side of the face causes anisocoria of the affected side. We see Máhuángfùzǐxìxīntāng's use for miosis and anisocoria.

Table 17.33. Herbal prescriptions for anisocoria

Anisocoria: https://meshb.nlm.nih.gov/record/ui?ui=D015875.	
Common prescriptions:	
Máhuángfùzǐxìxīntāng 5g shēngjiāng 2g guìzhī 2g zhìgāncǎo 1g Máhuángfùzǐxìxīntāng 5g shēngjiāng 1g guìzhī 1g zhìgāncǎo 1g Máhuángfùzǐxìxīntāng 5g shēngjiāng 1g guìzhī 1g Máhuángfùzǐxìxīntāng 5g shēngjiāng 2g zhìgāncǎo 2g guìzhī 2g Máhuángfùzǐxìxīntāng 5g shēngjiāng 2g zhìgāncǎo 2g guìzhī 2g dàzǎo 1g	
Alternative prescriptions:	
Dāngguīsìnìtāng 5g shēngjiāng 0g wúzhūyú 0g Sìnìtāng 5g shēngjiāng 1g guìzhī 1g Máhuángfùzǐxìxīntāng 5g shēngjiāng 2g fùzǐ 2g guìzhī 2g dàzǎo 2g zhìgāncǎo 2g	
Indicated diseases:	
Primary open angle glaucoma 365.11 (Primary open-angle glaucoma, right eye, stage unspecified H401110, Primary open-angle glaucoma, right eye, mild stage H401111, Primary open-angle glaucoma, right eye, moderate stage H401112, Primary open-angle glaucoma, right eye, severe stage H401113, Primary open-angle glaucoma, right eye, indeterminate stage H401114, Primary open-angle glaucoma, left eye, stage unspecified H401120, Primary open-angle glaucoma, left eye, mild stage H401121, Primary open-angle glaucoma, left eye, moderate stage H401122, Primary open-angle glaucoma, left eye, severe stage H401123, Primary open-angle glaucoma, left eye, indeterminate stage H401124, Primary open-angle glaucoma, bilateral, stage unspecified H401130, Primary open-angle glaucoma, bilateral, mild stage H401131, Primary open-angle glaucoma, bilateral, moderate stage H401132, Primary open-angle glaucoma, bilateral, severe stage H401133, Primary open-angle glaucoma, bilateral, indeterminate stage H401134, Primary open-angle glaucoma, unspecified eye, stage unspecified H401190, Primary open-angle glaucoma, unspecified eye, mild stage H401191, Primary open-angle glaucoma, unspecified eye, moderate stage H401192, Primary open-angle glaucoma, unspecified eye, severe stage H401193, Primary open-angle glaucoma, unspecified eye, indeterminate stage H401194); Open-angle glaucoma 365.1; Glaucoma 365; Ocular hypertension 365.04 (Ocular hypertension, unspecified eye H40059); Disorder of eye, unspecified 379.90 (Unspecified disorder of eye and adnexa H579); Unspecified disorders of nervous system 349.9 (Disorder of central nervous system, unspecified G969); Unspecified cerebrovascular disease 437.9 (Cerebrovascular disease, unspecified I679); Cardiovascular disease, unspecified 429.2 (Atherosclerotic heart disease of native coronary artery without angina pectoris I2510); Unspecified condition of brain 348.9 (Disorder of brain, unspecified G939); Diabetic retinopathy 362.0; Diabetes with peripheral circulatory disorders 250.7; Unspecified retinal disorder 362.9 (Unspecified retinal disorder H359); Diabetes mellitus 250; Unspecified endocrine disorder 259.9 (Endocrine disorder, unspecified E349); Unspecified disorder of metabolism 277.9 (Metabolic disorder, unspecified E889)	
Primary open angle glaucoma 365.11/H401110,H401111,H401112,H401113,H401114,H401120,H401121,H401122, H401123,H401124,H401130,H401131,H401132,H401133,H401134,H401190,H401191, H401192,H401193,H401194 with anisocoria D015875:	
Qǐjúdìhuángwán 5g xǐgānmíngmùtāng 5g zīshènmíngmùtāng 5g to ♀	Qǐjúdìhuángwán 5g xǐgānmíngmùtāng 5g zīshènmíngmùtāng 5g to ♂
Unspecified cerebrovascular disease 437.9/I679 with anisocoria D015875:	
Bǔyánghuánwǔtāng 5g dānshēn 1g shíchāngpú 1g yuǎnzhì 1g + acupuncture to ♀	Bǔyánghuánwǔtāng 5g dānshēn 1g shíchāngpú 1g yuǎnzhì 1g + acupuncture to ♂
Cardiovascular disease, unspecified 429.2/I2510 with anisocoria D015875:	
Yùzhú 5g sìnìtāng 5g mǔdānpí 1g zhīzǐ 1g huánglián 1g to ♀	Sìnìtāng 5g gānlùyǐn 5g mǔdānpí 1g zhīzǐ 1g huánglián 1g to ♂
Disorder of eye, unspecified 379.90/H579 with anisocoria D015875:	
Qǐjúdìhuángwán 5g xǐgānmíngmùtāng 5g zīshènmíngmùtāng 5g to ♀	Qǐjúdìhuángwán 5g xǐgānmíngmùtāng 5g zīshènmíngmùtāng 5g to ♂

17.34. Hot Flashes

Hot flashes are sudden flares of heat, flush and sweating. The cause of hot flashes is not well known but hormone changes are suggested as hot flashes typically occur during menopausal transitions.

Table 17.34. Herbal prescriptions for hot flashes

Hot Flashes: https://meshb.nlm.nih.gov/record/ui?ui=D019584.	
Common prescriptions:	
Shíliùwèiliúqìyǐn 5g jiāwèixiāoyáosǎn 5g sǎnzhǒngkuìjiāntāng 5g xuánshēn 1g mǔlì 1g bèimǔ 1g xiàkūcǎo 1g Shíliùwèiliúqìyǐn 5g jiāwèixiāoyáosǎn 5g sǎnzhǒngkuìjiāntāng 5g Shíliùwèiliúqìyǐn 5g jiāwèixiāoyáosǎn 5g sǎnzhǒngkuìjiāntāng 5g xuánshēn 1g mǔlì 1g bèimǔ 1g Shíliùwèiliúqìyǐn 5g sǎnzhǒngkuìjiāntāng 5g	
Alternative prescriptions:	
Xiǎocháihútāng 5g màiyá 3g xiāngfù 1g dàhuáng 0g Shíliùwèiliúqìyǐn 5g cháihúshūgāntāng 5g sǎnzhǒngkuìjiāntāng 5g Jiāwèixiāoyáosǎn 5g màiyá 1g xiāngfù 1g Xuèfǔzhúyūtāng 5g cháihúshūgāntāng 5g chuānliànzǐ 1g yánhúsuǒ 1g Jiāwèixiāoyáosǎn 5g gāncǎoxiǎomàidàzǎotāng 5g dānshēn 1g xiāngfù 1g yìmǔcǎo 1g yùjīn 1g	
Indicated diseases:	
Other dermatoses 702; Premature menopause 256.31 (Symptomatic premature menopause E28310, Asymptomatic premature menopause E28319); Malignant neoplasm of uterus, part unspecified 179 (Malignant neoplasm of uterus, part unspecified C55); Unspecified disorder of uterus 621.9 (Noninflammatory disorder of uterus, unspecified N859); Malignant neoplasm of other and unspecified female genital organs 184; Deformity and disproportion of reconstructed breast 612; Other disorders of breast 611; Benign mammary dysplasias 610; Unspecified disorder of female genital organs 629.9 (Unspecified condition associated with female genital organs and menstrual cycle N949); Osteoporosis 733.0; Unspecified disorder of metabolism 277.9 (Metabolic disorder, unspecified E889)	
Other dermatoses 702 with hot flashes D019584:	
Jiědúsìwùtāng 5g xiāofēngsǎn 4g zhēnrénhuómìngyǐnqùchuānshānjiǎ 4g huángliánjiědútāng 4g to ♀	Jiědúsìwùtāng 5g xiāofēngsǎn 4g zhēnrénhuómìngyǐnqùchuānshānjiǎ 4g huángliánjiědútāng 4g to ♂
Premature menopause 256.31/E28310,E28319 with hot flashes D019584:	
Guìzhīfúlíngwán 5g màiyá 2g hónghuā 1g táorén 1g to ♀	Guìzhīfúlíngwán 5g shānyào 2g hónghuā 2g táorén 2g kǔshēngēn 1g to ♂

Shíliùwèiliúqìyǐn ‘regulates Qi, activates Blood,’ ‘benefits Qi, opens meridians,’ and ‘removes lumps, excludes carbuncles.’ Sǎnzhǒngkuìjiāntāng literally reads ‘decoction to dissolve lumps and destruct hardening.’ As hot flashes are prevalent in patients with cancer (Fisher et al., 2013), the prescriptions are believed to focus on cancer patients presenting with hot flashes.

17.35. Cerebrospinal Fluid Leak

Cerebrospinal fluid is a clear liquid, within the membranes covering the brain and spinal cord, that protects and cushions the delicate brain and spinal cord. A tear or a hole in the layers of the membranes can cause cerebrospinal fluid leak. Closed head injury, brain tumor, sinus surgery, and spinal injury and surgery can cause cerebrospinal fluid leak.

As cranial cerebrospinal fluid often leaks through the nose and can manifest digestive symptoms such as loss of appetite, nausea and vomiting, Bǔzhōngyìqìtāng is prescribed. Cerebrospinal fluid rhinorrhoea is associated with rhinitis and sinusitis (Ozdogan et al., 2015), which are what Huángqíwǔwùtāng, Dāngguīsìnìtāng and Máhuángfùzǐxìxīntāng are used for today.

Table 17.35. Herbal prescriptions for cerebrospinal fluid leak

Cerebrospinal Fluid Leak: https://meshb.nlm.nih.gov/record/ui?ui=D065634.	
Common prescriptions:	
Bǔzhōngyìqìtāng 5g + acupuncture Bǔzhōngyìqìtāng 5g	
Alternative prescriptions:	
Huángqíwǔwùtāng 5g dānshēn 1g zhúrú 1g sāngzhī 1g dāngguī 1g jiānghuáng 1g Dāngguīsìnìtāng 5g shēngjiāng 1g wúzhūyú 1g Bǔzhōngyìqìtāng 5g fùzǐ 0g Dāngguīsìnìtāng 5g shēngjiāng 1g wúzhūyú 1g fùzǐ 1g Máhuángfùzǐxìxīntāng 5g fùzǐ 3g guìzhī 3g gānjiāng 3g dàzǎo 2g zhìgāncǎo 2g zhìgāncǎotāng 2g	
Indicated diseases:	
Unspecified condition of brain 348.9 (Disorder of brain, unspecified G939); Unspecified endocrine disorder 259.9 (Endocrine disorder, unspecified E349); Malignant neoplasm of endocrine gland, site unspecified 194.9 (Malignant neoplasm of endocrine gland, unspecified C759); Unspecified disorders of nervous system 349.9 (Disorder of central nervous system, unspecified G969); Neoplasm of unspecified nature of brain 239.6 (Neoplasm of unspecified behavior of brain D496); Unspecified cerebrovascular disease 437.9 (Cerebrovascular disease, unspecified I679); Cardiovascular disease, unspecified 429.2 (Atherosclerotic heart disease of native coronary artery without angina pectoris I2510); Malignant neoplasm of nervous system, part unspecified 192.9 (Malignant neoplasm of central nervous system, unspecified C729); Vaginal enterocele, congenital or acquired 618.6 (Vaginal enterocele N815)	
Unspecified condition of brain 348.9/G939 with cerebrospinal fluid leak D065634:	
Bǔyánghuánwǔtāng 5g chuānqī 1g dānshēn 1g shíchāngpú 1g yuǎnzhì 1g + acupuncture to ♀	Bǔyánghuánwǔtāng 5g chuānqī 1g dānshēn 1g shíchāngpú 1g yuǎnzhì 1g + acupuncture to ♂
Unspecified cerebrovascular disease 437.9/I679 with cerebrospinal fluid leak D065634:	
Bǔyánghuánwǔtāng 5g chuānqī 1g dānshēn 1g shíchāngpú 1g yuǎnzhì 1g + acupuncture to ♀	Bǔyánghuánwǔtāng 5g chuānqī 2g dānshēn 1g shíchāngpú 1g yuǎnzhì 1g + acupuncture to ♂
Unspecified disorders of nervous system 349.9/G969 with cerebrospinal fluid leak D065634:	
Huángqíwǔwùtāng 5g chuānxiōng 1g dānshēn 1g zhúrú 1g sāngzhī 1g dāngguī 1g jiānghuáng 1g to ♀	Huángqíwǔwùtāng 5g chuānxiōng 1g dānshēn 1g zhúrú 1g sāngzhī 1g dāngguī 1g jiānghuáng 1g to ♂

17.36. Stupor

Stupor is a state of greatly dulled responsiveness to stimuli and absence of spontaneous movements. Stupor can be caused by narcotics, intoxicants, heavy metal poisoning, brain injury, brain tumor, depression, and infectious diseases.

Table 17.36. Herbal prescriptions for stupor

Stupor: https://meshb.nlm.nih.gov/record/ui?ui=D053608.
Common prescriptions:
Guìzhītāng 5g shēngjiāng 1g báisháo 1g dàhuáng 0g Guìzhītāng 5g shēngjiāng 1g guìzhī 1g Guìzhītāng 5g shēngjiāng 1g báisháo 1g Guìzhītāng 5g shēngjiāng 1g guìzhī 1g dàhuáng 0g Guìzhītāng 5g shēngjiāng 1g báisháo 1g guìzhī 1g
Alternative prescriptions:
Dāngguīsìnìtāng 5g wúzhūyú 1g fùzǐ 1g gānjiāng 1g Sìnìtāng 5g huángqíwǔwùtāng 5g dānshēn 1g zhúrú 1g sāngzhī 1g jiānghuáng 1g Guìzhītāng 5g shēngjiāng 1g guìzhī 1g + acupuncture Guìzhītāng 5g fùzǐ 1g + acupuncture Guìzhītāng 5g huángqí 2g dāngguī 1g

Stupor: https://meshb.nlm.nih.gov/record/ui?ui=D053608.	
Indicated diseases:	
Epilepsy, unspecified 345.9; Unspecified condition of brain 348.9 (Disorder of brain, unspecified G939); Unspecified disorders of nervous system 349.9 (Disorder of central nervous system, unspecified G969); Schizophreniform disorder 295.4; Schizoaffective disorder 295.7; Hypoglycemia, unspecified 251.2 (Hypoglycemia, unspecified E162); Unspecified disorder of metabolism 277.9 (Metabolic disorder, unspecified E889)	
Epilepsy, unspecified 345.9 with stupor D053608:	
Tiānmágōuténgyǐn 5g jiāwèixiāoyáosǎn 5g cháihújiālónggǔmǔlìtāng 5g dúhuójìshēngtāng 5g shēntòngzhúyūtāng 4g dǎngshēn 2g to ♀	Wēndǎntāng 5g cháihújiālónggǔmǔlìtāng 4g dānshēn 1g shíchāngpú 1g yuǎnzhì 1g to ♂
Unspecified disorders of nervous system 349.9/G969 with stupor D053608:	
Huángqíwǔwùtāng 5g chuānxiōng 1g dānshēn 1g zhúrú 1g sāngzhī 1g dāngguī 1g jiānghuáng 1g to ♀	Huángqíwǔwùtāng 5g chuānxiōng 1g dānshēn 1g zhúrú 1g sāngzhī 1g dāngguī 1g jiānghuáng 1g to ♂

Guìzhītāng is used for upper respiratory tract infections (Wang, 2019) and headache, and is thought to be used here for infection-induced stupor.

17.37. Meningism

Meningism is characterized by stiff neck, photophobia and headache. Meningism is caused by nonmeningitic irritation of the membranes covering the central nervous system, called the meninges. Causes of meningism include influenza, malaria, pneumonia, septic shock and poisoning.

As the modern uses of Máhuángfùzǐxìxīntāng are for chronic sinusitis and allergic rhinitis (Wang, 2019), the prescriptions therefore target the infectious conditions underlying meningism.

Table 17.37. Herbal prescriptions for meningism

Meningism: https://meshb.nlm.nih.gov/record/ui?ui=D008580.
Common prescriptions:
Máhuángfùzǐxìxīntāng 5g fùzǐ 3g guìzhī 3g gānjiāng 3g dàzǎo 2g zhìgāncǎotāng 2g Máhuángfùzǐxìxīntāng 5g fùzǐ 3g guìzhī 3g dàzǎo 2g zhìgāncǎo 2g gānjiāng 2g Máhuángfùzǐxìxīntāng 5g fùzǐ 3g guìzhī 3g dàzǎo 2g gānjiāng 2g zhìgāncǎotāng 2g Máhuángfùzǐxìxīntāng 5g fùzǐ 3g guìzhī 3g gānjiāng 3g dàzǎo 2g zhìgāncǎo 2g wēilíngxiān 2g
Alternative prescriptions:
Máhuángfùzǐxìxīntāng 5g fùzǐ 3g guìzhī 3g dàzǎo 2g zhìgāncǎo 2g wēilíngxiān 2g gānjiāng 2g Dāngguīsìnìtāng 5g wúzhūyú 1g fùzǐ 1g gānjiāng 1g Máhuángfùzǐxìxīntāng 5g shēngjiāng 1g zhìgāncǎo 1g guìzhī 1g Máhuángfùzǐxìxīntāng 5g shēngjiāng 1g guìzhī 1g gāncǎo 0g
Indicated diseases:
Meningitis, unspecified 322.9 (Meningitis, unspecified G039); Unspecified viral meningitis 047.9 (Viral meningitis, unspecified A879); Unspecified disorders of nervous system 349.9 (Disorder of central nervous system, unspecified G969); Cryptococcosis 117.5 (Pulmonary cryptococcosis B450, Disseminated cryptococcosis B457, Cryptococcosis, unspecified B459); Candidiasis 112; Coccidioidomycosis 114; Histoplasmosis 115; Blastomycotic infection 116; Other mycoses 117; Opportunistic mycoses 118 (Other specified mycoses B488); Dermatophytosis 110; Human immunodeficiency virus [HIV] disease 042 (Human immunodeficiency virus [HIV] disease B20); Dermatomycosis, other and unspecified 111; Unspecified cerebrovascular disease 437.9 (Cerebrovascular disease, unspecified I679); Unspecified condition of brain 348.9 (Disorder of brain, unspecified G939); Cardiovascular disease, unspecified 429.2 (Atherosclerotic heart disease of native coronary artery without angina pectoris I2510)

Table 17.37. (Continued)

Meningism: https://meshb.nlm.nih.gov/record/ui?ui=D008580.	
Meningitis, unspecified 322.9/G039 with meningism D008580:	
Bǔzhōngyìqìtāng 5g guīpítāng 5g to ♀	Bǔyánghuánwǔtāng 5g + acupuncture to ♂
Unspecified cerebrovascular disease 437.9/I679 with meningism D008580:	
Bǔyánghuánwǔtāng 5g sānqī 1g dānshēn 1g shíchāngpú 1g yuǎnzhì 1g + acupuncture to ♀	Bǔyánghuánwǔtāng 5g dānshēn 1g shíchāngpú 1g yuǎnzhì 1g + acupuncture to ♂

17.38. Chills

Chills are the feeling of being cold. Low ambient temperature, low blood sugar, malaria, hangover, and infection can bring on chills.

Both Sìnìtāng and Máhuángfùzǐxìxīntāng contain Fùzǐ, which is known to be able to warm up the body. Tonsillitis can cause chills and jaw pain.

Table 17.38. Herbal prescriptions for chills

Chills: https://meshb.nlm.nih.gov/record/ui?ui=D023341.	
Common prescriptions:	
Sìnìtāng 5g bànxià 1g dàhuáng 0g Sìnìtāng 5g shēngjiāng 1g guìzhī 1g Máhuángfùzǐxìxīntāng 5g shēngjiāng 2g guìzhī 2g zhìgāncǎo 1g Máhuángfùzǐxìxīntāng 5g shēngjiāng 1g guìzhī 1g Máhuángfùzǐxìxīntāng 5g shēngjiāng 2g zhìgāncǎo 2g guìzhī 2g	
Alternative prescriptions:	
Sìnìtāng 5g rénshēn 2g bànxià 2g dàhuáng 0g Máhuángfùzǐxìxīntāng 5g shēngjiāng 1g guìzhī 1g zhìgāncǎo 1g Sìnìtāng 5g shēngjiāng 1g guìzhī 1g xìxīn 1g máhuáng 1g	
Indicated and associated diseases:	
Diseases of the jaws 526; Diseases of the oral soft tissues, excluding lesions specific for gingiva and tongue 528; Gastric ulcer 531; Unspecified disorder of liver 573.9 (Liver disease, unspecified K769); Malignant neoplasm of liver, not specified as primary or secondary 155.2 (Malignant neoplasm of liver, not specified as primary or secondary C229); Heart disease, unspecified 429.9 (Heart disease, unspecified I519); Cardiovascular disease, unspecified 429.2 (Atherosclerotic heart disease of native coronary artery without angina pectoris I2510); Unspecified disorder of metabolism 277.9 (Metabolic disorder, unspecified E889)	
Diseases of the jaws 526 with Chills D023341:	
Guìzhītāng 5g báisháo 1g dàhuáng 0g to ♀	Dāngguīsìnìtāng 5g wúzhūyú 1g fùzǐ 1g gānjiāng 1g to ♂
Unspecified disorder of liver 573.9/K769 with chills D023341:	
Jiāwèixiāoyáosǎn 5g cháihúshūgāntāng 5g to ♀	Xuèfǔzhúyūtāng 5g cháihúshūgāntāng 5g to ♂
Heart disease, unspecified 429.9/I519 with chills D023341:	
Sìnìtāng 5g gānlùyǐn 5g mǔdānpí 1g zhīzǐ 1g huánglián 0g to ♀	Sìnìtāng 5g gānlùyǐn 5g mǔdānpí 1g zhīzǐ 1g huánglián 0g to ♂
Unspecified disorder of metabolism 277.9/E889 with chills D023341:	
Dāngguīsìnìtāng 5g huángqí 2g shēngjiāng 1g wúzhūyú 1g to ♀	Liùwèidìhuángwán 5g bǔzhōngyìqìtāng 5g to ♂

17.39. Premature Aging

Premature aging occurs when biological aging is faster than chronological aging, which is caused by shortening of the DNA-protecting telomeres during cell division. Premature aging displays such signs as hyperpigmented spots, wrinkles, sagging skin, itchy skin, grey hair, hair loss, and memory problems. Causes of premature aging include smoking, stress, sleep problems, alcohol, and genetics.

Xuèfǔzhúyūtāng 'activates Blood, dissolves stasis' and 'moves Qi, stops pain.' Bǔyánghuánwǔtāng 'supplements Qi, activates Blood, and opens meridians.' A school of traditional Chinese medicine posits that aging is due to depletion in both Qi and Blood (Wang, 2013). We see here the use of Qi and Blood supplementing formulas to counteract premature aging. On the other hand, as cardiovascular and cerebrovascular diseases are the two leading debilitating conditions in modern societies, Xuèfǔzhúyūtāng and Bǔyánghuánwǔtāng are prescribed for them.

Table 17.39. Herbal prescriptions for premature aging

<table>
<tr><td colspan="2">Premature Aging: https://meshb.nlm.nih.gov/record/ui?ui=D019588.</td></tr>
<tr><td colspan="2">Common prescriptions:</td></tr>
<tr><td colspan="2">Xuèfǔzhúyūtāng 5g bǔyánghuánwǔtāng 5g
Xuèfǔzhúyūtāng 5g dānshēn 1g
Xuèfǔzhúyūtāng 5g dānshēn 1g yánhúsuǒ 1g xiāngfù 1g yùjīn 1g
Xuèfǔzhúyūtāng 5g bǔyánghuánwǔtāng 5g dānshēn 1g
Xuèfǔzhúyūtāng 5g dānshēn 1g yánhúsuǒ 1g</td></tr>
<tr><td colspan="2">Alternative prescriptions:</td></tr>
<tr><td colspan="2">Xuèfǔzhúyūtāng 5g dānshēn 0g
Xuèfǔzhúyūtāng 5g dānshēn 0g mòyào 0g rǔxiāng 0g
Xuèfǔzhúyūtāng 5g fùfāngdānshēnpiàn 5g + acupuncture
Xuèfǔzhúyūtāng 5g shānzhā 1g shénqū 1g màiyá 1g
Xuèfǔzhúyūtāng 5g sānqī 1g dānshēn 1g chìsháo 1g</td></tr>
<tr><td colspan="2">Indicated diseases:</td></tr>
<tr><td colspan="2">Unspecified cerebrovascular disease 437.9 (Cerebrovascular disease, unspecified I679); Unspecified condition of brain 348.9 (Disorder of brain, unspecified G939); Unspecified disorder of metabolism 277.9 (Metabolic disorder, unspecified E889); Cardiovascular disease, unspecified 429.2 (Atherosclerotic heart disease of native coronary artery without angina pectoris I2510); Unspecified disorders of nervous system 349.9 (Disorder of central nervous system, unspecified G969); Other dermatoses 702; Lipodystrophy 272.6 (Lipodystrophy, not elsewhere classified E881); Human immunodeficiency virus [HIV] disease 042 (Human immunodeficiency virus [HIV] disease B20)</td></tr>
<tr><td colspan="2">Unspecified cerebrovascular disease 437.9/I679 with aging, premature D019588:</td></tr>
<tr><td>Bǔyánghuánwǔtāng 5g sānqī 1g dānshēn 1g shíchāngpú 1g yuǎnzhì 1g + acupuncture to ♀</td><td>Bǔyánghuánwǔtāng 5g chuānqī 2g dānshēn 1g shíchāngpú 1g yuǎnzhì 1g + acupuncture to ♂</td></tr>
<tr><td colspan="2">Other dermatoses 702 with aging, premature D019588:</td></tr>
<tr><td>Yùnǚjiān 5g xuèfǔzhúyūtāng 3g dāngguīsháoyàosǎn 3g báijiāngcán 1g to ♀</td><td>Yùnǚjiān 5g xuèfǔzhúyūtāng 3g dāngguīsháoyàosǎn 3g báijiāngcán 1g to ♂</td></tr>
</table>

17.40. Feminization

Feminization is development of female secondary sex characteristics such as enlarged breasts. Feminization in the male is most likely caused by decreased androgen or increased estrogen levels in serum.

Huánshǎodān, which literally reads 'rejuvenating elixir,' 'nourishes Qi-Blood,' 'replenishes Yin, benefits the Kidney,' and is today used for osteoporosis (Wang, 2019). Modern uses of Yínyánghuò include impotence of organic origin, and unspecified disorder of male genital organs (Wang, 2020). Zuǒguīwán 'nourishes Yin, replenishes the Kidney,' 'refills semen, benefits marrow,' and is today used for osteoporosis (Wang, 2019). The prescriptions look to maintain or restore the sexual potency in aging males.

Table 17.40. Herbal prescriptions for feminization

<table>
<tr><td colspan="2">Feminization: https://meshb.nlm.nih.gov/record/ui?ui=D005262.</td></tr>
<tr><td colspan="2">Common prescriptions:</td></tr>
<tr><td colspan="2">Huánshǎodān 5g yínyánghuò 1g tùsīzǐ 1g
Huánshǎodān 5g yínyánghuò 1g
Huánshǎodān 5g yínyánghuò 1g shéchuángzǐ 1g tùsīzǐ 1g
Huánshǎodān 5g yínyánghuò 1g shéchuángzǐ 1g</td></tr>
<tr><td colspan="2">Alternative prescriptions:</td></tr>
<tr><td colspan="2">Liùwèidìhuángwán 5g jīnsuǒgùjīngwán 5g
Zuǒguīwán 5g bǔzhōngyìqìtāng 5g
Jīnsuǒgùjīngwán 5g huánshǎodān 5g ròucōngróng 2g yínyánghuò 2g bājǐtiān 1g
Huánshǎodān 5g bǔzhōngyìqìtāng 4g yínyánghuò 1g
Zuǒguīwán 5g yínyánghuò 1g shéchuángzǐ 1g tùsīzǐ 1g suǒyáng 1g</td></tr>
<tr><td colspan="2">Indicated diseases:</td></tr>
<tr><td colspan="2">Unspecified disorder of adrenal glands 255.9 (Disorder of adrenal gland, unspecified E279); Malignant neoplasm of adrenal gland 194.0 (Malignant neoplasm of unspecified part of unspecified adrenal gland C7490); Indeterminate sex and pseudohermaphroditism 752.7 (Pseudohermaphroditism, unspecified Q563, Indeterminate sex, unspecified Q564); Unspecified endocrine disorder 259.9 (Endocrine disorder, unspecified E349); Unspecified disorder of metabolism 277.9 (Metabolic disorder, unspecified E889); Malignant neoplasm of endocrine gland, site unspecified 194.9 (Malignant neoplasm of endocrine gland, unspecified C759); Gonadal dysgenesis 758.6 (Turner's syndrome, unspecified Q969); Unspecified disorder of liver 573.9 (Liver disease, unspecified K769); Malignant neoplasm of liver, not specified as primary or secondary 155.2 (Malignant neoplasm of liver, not specified as primary or secondary C229); Diseases of the jaws 526; Malignant neoplasm of male genital organ, site unspecified 187.9 (Malignant neoplasm of male genital organ, unspecified C639); Unspecified disorder of male genital organs 608.9 (Disorder of male genital organs, unspecified N509, Pelvic and perineal pain R102); Malignant neoplasm of testis 186</td></tr>
<tr><td colspan="2">Unspecified disorder of adrenal glands 255.9/E279 with feminization D005262:</td></tr>
<tr><td>Jiāwèixiāoyáosǎn 5g zuǒguīwán 5g nǚzhēnzǐ 1g hànliáncǎo 1g to ♀</td><td>Yòuguīwán 5g huánshǎodān 5g ròucōngróng 1g yínyánghuò 1g to ♂</td></tr>
<tr><td colspan="2">Unspecified endocrine disorder 259.9/E349 with feminization D005262:</td></tr>
<tr><td>Jiāwèixiāoyáosǎn 5g zuǒguīwán 5g nǚzhēnzǐ 1g hànliáncǎo 1g to ♀</td><td>Huánshǎodān 5g ròucōngróng 1g yínyánghuò 1g suǒyáng 1g to ♂</td></tr>
<tr><td colspan="2">Unspecified disorder of liver 573.9/K769 with feminization D005262:</td></tr>
<tr><td>Jiāwèixiāoyáosǎn 5g cháihúshūgāntāng 5g to ♀</td><td>Liùwèidìhuángwán 5g jīnsuǒgùjīngwán 5g cháihúshūgāntāng 5g to ♂</td></tr>
</table>

17.41. Virilism

Virilism is development of male secondary sex characteristics such as increased upper body muscle mass. Excessive adrenal androgen production and use of anabolic steroids can cause virilism in the female.

Yòuguīwán 'warms up Kidney-Yang' and 'refills semen, replenishes Blood.' Both Yòuguīwán and Zuǒguīwán benefit the Kidney. The difference between Yòuguīwán and Zuǒguīwán is that according to Chinese medical classics the former enhances Kidney-Yang while the latter Kidney-Yin. Bājǐtiān is today used for unspecified male infertility, and impotence of organic origin (Wang, 2020), while Nǚzhēnzǐ is today used for disorders of menstruation and other abnormal bleeding from female genital tract (Wang, 2019). The prescriptions for virilism look to improve either male sexuality or female fertility. Moreover, in the end of the table, the prescriptions for unspecified endocrine disorder with virilism look to restore the sex hormone balance in women and men.

Table 17.41. Herbal prescriptions for virilism

Virilism: https://meshb.nlm.nih.gov/record/ui?ui=D014770.	
Common prescriptions:	
Yòuguīwán 5g zuǒguīwán 5g bājǐtiān 1g ròucōngróng 1g yínyánghuò 1g tùsīzǐ 1g Yòuguīwán 5g zuǒguīwán 5g bājǐtiān 1g ròucōngróng 1g yínyánghuò 1g Yòuguīwán 5g zuǒguīwán 5g bājǐtiān 1g yínyánghuò 1g tùsīzǐ 1g Yòuguīwán 5g zuǒguīwán 5g bājǐtiān 1g ròucōngróng 1g tùsīzǐ 1g Jiāwèixiāoyáosǎn 5g yòuguīwán 5g zuǒguīwán 5g bājǐtiān 1g ròucōngróng 1g yínyánghuò 1g	
Alternative prescriptions:	
Zuǒguīwán 5g xiāoyáosǎn 5g nǚzhēnzǐ 1g hànliáncǎo 1g Yòuguīwán 5g bājǐtiān 1g yínyánghuò 1g shéchuángzǐ 1g tùsīzǐ 1g Zuǒguīwán 5g jiāwèixiāoyáosǎn 4g bājǐtiān 1g yínyánghuò 1g tùsīzǐ 1g fùpénzǐ 1g Zuǒguīwán 5g jiāwèixiāoyáosǎn 4g bājǐtiān 1g ròucōngróng 1g yínyánghuò 1g tùsīzǐ 1g Liùwèidìhuángwán 5g jiāwèixiāoyáosǎn 5g nǚzhēnzǐ 1g hànliáncǎo 1g ējiāo 1g tùsīzǐ 1g	
Indicated diseases:	
Unspecified disorder of adrenal glands 255.9 (Disorder of adrenal gland, unspecified E279); Malignant neoplasm of adrenal gland 194.0 (Malignant neoplasm of unspecified part of unspecified adrenal gland C7490); Unspecified disorder of male genital organs 608.9 (Disorder of male genital organs, unspecified N509, Pelvic and perineal pain R102); Indeterminate sex and pseudohermaphroditism 752.7 (Pseudohermaphroditism, unspecified Q563, Indeterminate sex, unspecified Q564); Unspecified endocrine disorder 259.9 (Endocrine disorder, unspecified E349); Unspecified disorder of metabolism 277.9 (Metabolic disorder, unspecified E889); Malignant neoplasm of ovary 183.0 (Malignant neoplasm of unspecified ovary C569); Malignant neoplasm of male genital organ, site unspecified 187.9 (Malignant neoplasm of male genital organ, unspecified C639); Malignant neoplasm of other and unspecified female genital organs 184; Malignant neoplasm of testis 186; Malignant neoplasm of endocrine gland, site unspecified 194.9 (Malignant neoplasm of endocrine gland, unspecified C759); Unspecified disorder of female genital organs 629.9 (Unspecified condition associated with female genital organs and menstrual cycle N949)	
Unspecified disorder of adrenal glands 255.9/E279 with virilism D014770:	
Jiāwèixiāoyáosǎn 5g zuǒguīwán 5g nǚzhēnzǐ 1g hànliáncǎo 1g to ♀	Yòuguīwán 5g huánshǎodān 5g ròucōngróng 1g yínyánghuò 1g to ♂
Unspecified endocrine disorder 259.9/E349 with virilism D014770:	
Jiāwèixiāoyáosǎn 5g zuǒguīwán 5g nǚzhēnzǐ 1g hànliáncǎo 1g to ♀	Huánshǎodān 5g ròucōngróng 1g yínyánghuò 1g suǒyáng 1g to ♂

17.42. Hirsutism

Hirsutism is excessive growth of dark, coarse hair in the areas of the body where hair is absent or fine such as the face, neck, chest, tummy, back and thighs. Problems related to endocrine that increase androgen production can cause hirsutism, so can medication side effects.

Both Zhēnrénhuómìngyǐn and Jīngfángbàidúsǎn are today used for contact dermatitis and other eczema (Wang, 2019). As hyperandrogenism also causes inflamed skin such as acne, the prescriptions mitigate the cutaneous symptoms of hyperandrogenism.

Table 17.42. Herbal prescriptions for hirsutism

<table>
<tr><td colspan="2">Hirsutism: https://meshb.nlm.nih.gov/record/ui?ui=D006628.</td></tr>
<tr><td colspan="2">Common prescriptions:</td></tr>
<tr><td colspan="2">Jiāwèixiāoyáosǎn 5g zhēnrénhuómìngyǐn 5g jīngfángbàidúsǎn 5g</td></tr>
<tr><td colspan="2">Alternative prescriptions:</td></tr>
<tr><td colspan="2">Jiāwèixiāoyáosǎn 5g cháihúshūgāntāng 5g báizhǐ 1g jīnyínhuā 1g liánqiáo 1g púgōngyīng 1g
Jiāwèixiāoyáosǎn 5g qīngshàngfángfēngtāng 5g zhēnrénhuómìngyǐnqùchuānshānjiǎ 4g jīnyínhuā 1g liánqiáo 1g
Jiāwèixiāoyáosǎn 5g zhēnrénhuómìngyǐn 5g dānshēn 2g xiāngfù 2g sāngbáipí 2g liánqiáo 2g púgōngyīng 2g
Jiāwèixiāoyáosǎn 5g qīngshàngfángfēngtāng 4g zhēnrénhuómìngyǐnqùchuānshānjiǎ 2g púgōngyīng 1g
Jiāwèixiāoyáosǎn 5g zhēnrénhuómìngyǐn 5g dānshēn 2g xiāngfù 2g xiàkūcǎo 2g liánqiáo 2g yìyǐrén 2g</td></tr>
<tr><td colspan="2">Indicated diseases:</td></tr>
<tr><td colspan="2">Other dermatoses 702; Polycystic ovaries 256.4 (Polycystic ovarian syndrome E282); Unspecified disorder of female genital organs 629.9 (Unspecified condition associated with female genital organs and menstrual cycle N949); Indeterminate sex and pseudohermaphroditism 752.7 (Pseudohermaphroditism, unspecified Q563, Indeterminate sex, unspecified Q564); Unspecified disorder of adrenal glands 255.9 (Disorder of adrenal gland, unspecified E279); Unspecified endocrine disorder 259.9 (Endocrine disorder, unspecified E349); Unspecified disorder of metabolism 277.9 (Metabolic disorder, unspecified E889); Acne varioliformis 706.0 (Acne varioliformis L702); Malignant neoplasm of adrenal gland 194.0 (Malignant neoplasm of unspecified part of unspecified adrenal gland C7490); Malignant neoplasm of endocrine gland, site unspecified 194.9 (Malignant neoplasm of endocrine gland, unspecified C759)</td></tr>
<tr><td colspan="2">Other dermatoses 702 with hirsutism D006628:</td></tr>
<tr><td>Jiāwèixiāoyáosǎn 5g zhēnrénhuómìngyǐn 5g dānshēn 1g sāngbáipí 1g liánqiáo 1g yìyǐrén 1g to ♀</td><td>Jiāwèixiāoyáosǎn 5g zhēnrénhuómìngyǐn 5g dānshēn 1g sāngbáipí 1g liánqiáo 1g yìyǐrén 1g to ♂</td></tr>
<tr><td colspan="2">Acne varioliformis 706.0/L702 with hirsutism D006628:</td></tr>
<tr><td>Zhēnrénhuómìngyǐnqùchuānshānjiǎ 5g tǔfúlíng 2g púgōngyīng 2g tǔfúlíng 1g zhībódìhuángwán 1g to ♀</td><td>Sǎnzhǒngkuìjiāntāng 5g zhībódìhuángwán 2g lóngdǎnxiègāntāng 2g púgōngyīng 1g liánqiáo 1g zǐhuādìdīng 1g to ♂</td></tr>
</table>

References

Fisher, W. I., Johnson, A. K., Elkins, G. R., Otte, J. L., Burns, D. S., Yu, M., & Carpenter, J. S. (2013). Risk Factors, Pathophysiology, and Treatment of Hot Flashes in Cancer. *CA: A Cancer Journal for Clinicians*, *63*(3), 167–192. https://doi.org/10.3322/caac.21171.

Green, S., Berkovits, L., & Baker, B. (2015). Symptoms and development of anxiety in children with or without intellectual disability. *J Clin Child Adolesc Psychol.*, *44*(1), 137–144. https://doi.org/10.1080/15374416.2013.873979.

Hsieh, B.-J., Shen, D., Hsu, C.-J., Chan, T. C., Cho, Y.-T., Tang, C.-H., & Chu, C.-Y. (2022). The impact of atopic dermatitis on health-related quality of life in Taiwan. *Journal of the Formosan Medical Association*, *121*(1), 269–277. https://doi.org/10.1016/j.jfma.2021.03.024.

Käcker, C., Wagner, F., Caversaccio, M., & Anschuetz, L. (2019). Horner Syndrome as Complication of Acute Sphenoid Sinusitis. *Case Reports in Neurology*, *11*(1), 112–116. https://doi.org/10.1159/000497742.

Ozdogan, S., Gergin, Y. E., Gergin, S., Tatarli, N., & Hicdonmez, T. (2015). Spontaneous Rhinorrhea mimicking sinusitis. *Pan African Medical Journal*, *20*, 97. https://doi.org/10.11604/pamj.2015.20.97.5748.

Skeik, N., & Jabr, F. (2011). Migraine with benign episodic unilateral mydriasis. *International Journal of General Medicine*, *4*, 501–503. https://doi.org/10.2147/ijgm.s18613.

Tacani, P., de Oliveira Ribeiro, D., Barros Guimarães, B. E., Perez Machado, A. F., & Tacani, R. E. (2015). Characterization of symptoms and edema distribution in premenstrual syndrome. *International Journal of Women's Health*, *7*, 297–303. https://doi.org/10.2147/ijwh.s74251.

van der Lende, M., Surges, R., Sander, J. W., & Thijs, R. D. (2016). Cardiac arrhythmias during or after epileptic seizures. *Journal of Neurology, Neurosurgery & Psychiatry*, *87*(1), 69–74. jnnp-2015-310559. https://doi.org/10.1136/jnnp-2015-310559.

Wang, S. C. (2013). *Western Biomedicine and Eastern Therapeutics: An Integrative Strategy for Personalized and Preventive Healthcare*. WSPC. https://doi.org/10.1142/8533.

Wang, S. C. (2019). *Clinical Herbal Prescriptions: Principles and Practices of Herbal Formulations from Deep Learning Health Insurance Herbal Prescription Big Data*. WSPC. https://doi.org/10.1142/11211.

Wang, S. C. (2020). *Veterinary Herbal Pharmacopoeia*. Nova Science Publishers. https://doi.org/10.52305/GHTR1903.

Part II. From Herbs to Signs and Symptoms

Chapter 18

Individual Formulas and Herbs

In Part I of the book, we provide prescriptions for various signs and symptoms. This presentation style is useful for herbalists and patients seeking herbal remedies. In Part II, we reverse the approach by presenting the indications for various formulas and herbs. In doing so, we record individual formulas and herbs that appear in the prescription tables in the first part of the book to compile a table in Section 18.1.

In Table 18.1, formulas and herbs are ordered alphabetically so that the reader can easily locate the interested formula and herb. Table 18.1 is conservative in the sense that the identified signs and symptoms are from the prescriptions in previous tables. In Section 18.2, we go a step further to show the relevant signs and symptoms of a formula or herb from the neighborhood of the vector representation of the formula or herb in the embedding space from the embedding layer of the trained multilingual transformer neural network model (cf. Appendix).

The results are presented in the form of a wordcloud, where a larger-sized sign or symptom indicates a higher relevance to the formula or herb. The information provided by the sign and symptom clouds is therefore more exploratory in nature than that presented in Table 18.1. The sign and symptom clouds (or symptom clouds for simplicity) are ordered according to the frequency of use of the formula or herb. The second part of the book is useful for herbalists who want to create new prescriptions or avoid using contraindicated herbs and formulas.

18.1. Signs and Symptoms of Formulas and Herbs

Table 18.1. Signs and symptoms of individual formulas and herbs

Formula or Herb	Signs and Symptoms
Bāwèidìhuángwán	Amblyopia, Color vision defects, Wolfram syndrome, Polyuria, Albuminuria, Urinary incontinence, stress, Urinary incontinence, urge, Urinary bladder, overactive, Quadriplegia, Brown-Sequard syndrome, Fetal weight, Urinary bladder, neurogenic, Reflex, abnormal
Bāzhèngsǎn	Flank pain, Colic, Proteinuria
Báixiānpí	Purpura fulminans, Purpura, thrombotic thrombocytopenic, Purpura, hyperglobulinemic, Purpura, Schoenlein-Henoch, Purpura, Hypergammaglobulinemia
Báihǔjiārénshēntāng	Fetal macrosomia
Báihǔtāng	Diplopia
Báisháo	Acute pain, Blindness, cortical, Snoring, Hypoventilation, Mouth breathing, Anorexia, Flatulence, Gagging, Aerophagy, Livedo reticularis, Cachexia, Emaciation, Sleep bruxism, Failure to thrive
Báizhǐ	Toothache
Báizhú	Flushing, Sleep initiation and maintenance disorders
Bǎnlángēn	Diplopia

Table 18.1. (Continued)

Formula or Herb	Signs and Symptoms
Bànxià	Renal colic, Glossalgia, Usher syndromes, Hearing loss, functional, Apnea, Hypercapnia, Cheyne-Stokes respiration, Hypocapnia, Hyperoxia, Anorexia, Dyspepsia, Hematemesis, Heartburn, Diarrhea, infantile, Menkes kinky hair syndrome, Choroid hemorrhage, Gastroparesis, Thinness, Consciousness disorders, Delirium, Amnesia, anterograde, Weight loss, Dyslexia, acquired, Coma, Hypotension, orthostatic, Cyanosis, Hypothermia, Lethargy, Cardiac output, low, Cardiac output, high, Motion sickness
Bànxiàxièxīntāng	Obesity
Bèimǔ	Cough, Sneezing, Vocal cord paralysis, Pseudobulbar palsy, Obesity, Fever, Hot flashes
Bózǐrén	Jet lag syndrome, Mutism
Bǔyánghuánwǔtāng	Kearns-Sayre syndrome, Brown-Sequard syndrome, Restless legs syndrome, Aging, premature, Learning disorders
Bǔzhōngyìqìtāng	Olfaction disorders, Wolfram syndrome, Hyperacusis, Hearing loss, functional, Cerebrospinal fluid rhinorrhea, Constipation, Encopresis, Tetany, Flushing, Pallor, Waterhouse-Friderichsen syndrome, Cafe-au-lait spots, Tinea pedis, Polyuria, Prostatism, Urinary bladder, overactive, Quadriplegia, Brown-Sequard syndrome, Kleine-Levin syndrome, Illusions, Gerstmann syndrome, Urinary bladder, neurogenic, Anomia, Jet lag syndrome, Agnosia, Reflex, abnormal, Syncope, Syncope, vasovagal, Mutism, Stuttering, Cerebrospinal fluid leak, Apraxias
Cāngzhú	Arthralgia, Chest pain
Cǎojuémíng	Photophobia, Vitreous hemorrhage, Obesity, morbid, Obesity, abdominal, Pediatric obesity
Cháihújiālónggǔmǔlìtāng	Hyperventilation, Hallucinations
Cháihúshūgāntāng	Angina, stable, Breakthrough pain, Menkes kinky hair syndrome, Primary progressive nonfluent aphasia, Jaundice, Intellectual disability, Prodromal symptoms
Chántuì	Hemifacial spasm
Chēqiánzǐ	Hearing loss, conductive, Fetal hypoxia, Hemiplegia, Auditory perceptual disorders, Proteinuria
Chuānliànzǐ	Machado-Joseph disease, Prodromal symptoms
Chuānqī	Kearns-Sayre syndrome, Restless legs syndrome, Learning disorders
Chuānwū	Neck pain
Chuānxiōng	Olfaction disorders
Chuānxiōngchádiàosǎn	Toothache, Facial paralysis
Dàzhēnjiāotāng	Gait ataxia, Huntington disease
Dàhuáng	Neck pain, Abdomen, acute, Toothache, Acute pain, Pain, referred, Renal colic, Glossalgia, Dizziness, Scotoma, Dysgeusia, Ageusia, Tinnitus, Hyperacusis, Hearing loss, high-frequency, Hearing loss, unilateral, Hearing loss, bilateral, Hearing loss, functional, Hearing loss, mixed conductive-sensorineural, Hearing loss, sudden, Presbycusis, Hearing loss, central, Hearing loss, noise-induced, Apnea, Snoring, Hypoventilation, Hypercapnia, Cheyne-Stokes respiration, Hypocapnia, Mouth breathing, Hyperoxia, Dyspnea, paroxysmal, Constipation, Anorexia, Dyspepsia, Postoperative nausea and vomiting, Hematemesis, Heartburn, Diarrhea, infantile, Gagging, Eructation, Encopresis, Aerophagy, Catalepsy, Huntington disease, Menkes kinky hair syndrome, Purpura, thrombotic thrombocytopenic, Choroid hemorrhage, Oliguria, Hypercalciuria, Gastroparesis, Pseudobulbar palsy, Cachexia, Thinness, Consciousness disorders, Delirium, Auditory perceptual disorders, Amnesia, anterograde, Amnesia, retrograde, Sleep apnea, central, Nocturnal myoclonus syndrome, Cataplexy, Purpura, Schoenlein-Henoch, Pain, postoperative, Pruritus vulvae, Weight loss, Emaciation, Dyslexia, acquired, Sleep bruxism, Dysarthria, Vertigo, Syncope, vasovagal, Coma, Hypotension, orthostatic, Hypothermia, Failure to thrive, Lethargy, Cardiac output, low, Cardiac output, high, Mydriasis, Stupor, Chills, Motion sickness

Formula or Herb	Signs and Symptoms
Dàzǎo	Gait ataxia, Meningism
Dānshēn	Pain threshold, Myalgia, Angina pectoris, variant, Angina, stable, Hypesthesia, Hyperesthesia, Paresthesia, Hyperalgesia, Photophobia, Hemianopsia, Kearns-Sayre syndrome, Tetany, Lesch-Nyhan syndrome, Mucopolysaccharidosis II, Hemiplegia, Supranuclear palsy, progressive, Primary progressive nonfluent aphasia, Restless legs syndrome, Obesity hypoventilation syndrome, Alice in Wonderland syndrome, Muscle spasticity, Hydrops fetalis, Chest pain, Intermittent claudication, Jaundice, Ophthalmoplegia, Narcolepsy, Muscle hypotonia, Muscular atrophy, Myotonia, Fatigue, Syncope, Asthenia, Hirsutism, Aging, premature, Learning disorders
Dāngguī	Prostatism
Dāngguīniāntòngtāng	Chronic pain, Labor pain, Metatarsalgia, Alice in Wonderland syndrome, Athetosis, Ataxia telangiectasia, Huntington disease, Adrenoleukodystrophy, Mevalonate kinase deficiency, Mucopolysaccharidosis II, Alexia, pure, Arthralgia, Paraplegia, Overweight, Muscle hypertonia
Dāngguīsháoyàosǎn	Dysmenorrhea, Lesch-Nyhan syndrome, Dysuria, Hydrops fetalis, Edema
Dāngguīsìnìtāng	Phantom limb, Scotoma, Hemianopsia, Amaurosis fugax, Ageusia, Hypocapnia, Tremor, Hyperkinesis, Dyskinesia, drug-induced, Hypokinesia, Tics, Alkalosis, respiratory, Insulin coma, Adrenoleukodystrophy, Nocturia, Ideal body weight, Amnesia, transient global, Obesity hypoventilation syndrome, Nocturnal myoclonus syndrome, Muscle cramp, Muscle rigidity, Dyslexia, acquired, Narcolepsy, Fasciculation, Myotonia, Miosis, Anisocoria, Cerebrospinal fluid leak
Dǐdāngtāng	Flank pain, Flatulence, Proteinuria
Dìfūzǐ	Purpura fulminans, Purpura, thrombotic thrombocytopenic, Purpura, hyperglobulinemic, Hemoglobinuria, Purpura, Schoenlein-Henoch, Purpura, Hypergammaglobulinemia
Dìlóng	Striae distensae
Dìhuáng	Abdomen, acute, Infantile apparent life-threatening event, Constipation, Ecchymosis
Dúhuójìshēngtāng	Low back pain, Muscle weakness, Back pain, Paraplegia, Paraparesis
Dùzhòng	Amblyopia, Chorea gravidarum, Muscle weakness, Paraplegia, Paraparesis
Éshù	Fetal weight
Èrshùtāng	Shoulder pain, Neuralgia, postherpetic, Respiratory paralysis, Neuralgia
Fángfēngtōngshèngsǎn	Obesity, morbid, Obesity, abdominal, Pediatric obesity
Fángjǐhuángqítāng	Obesity, morbid, Pediatric obesity
Fúshén	Intellectual disability
Fúlíng	Hypercapnia, Dyspepsia, Hematemesis, Heartburn, Diarrhea, infantile, Flushing, Gastroparesis, Pain, postoperative
Fùpénzǐ	Polyuria, Urinary incontinence, stress, Urinary incontinence, urge, Urinary bladder, overactive, Quadriplegia, Urinary bladder, neurogenic, Reflex, abnormal
Fùzǐ	Neck pain, Eye pain, Visceral pain, Dizziness, Amaurosis fugax, Tinnitus, Hyperacusis, Hearing loss, high-frequency, Hearing loss, unilateral, Hearing loss, bilateral, Usher syndromes, Hearing loss, mixed conductive-sensorineural, Hearing loss, sudden, Presbycusis, Hearing loss, noise-induced, Hiccup, Flatulence, Eructation, Tremor, Hyperkinesis, Dyskinesia, drug-induced, Hypokinesia, Gait ataxia, Synkinesis, Insulin coma, Cafe-au-lait spots, Oliguria, Obesity, morbid, Ideal body weight, Hypersomnolence, idiopathic, Illusions, Phantom limb, Pain, postoperative, Psychomotor agitation, Sleep initiation and maintenance disorders, Agnosia, Muscle hypertonia, Sarcopenia, Fasciculation, Vertigo, Meningism, Heart murmurs, Mydriasis, Cerebrospinal fluid leak, Apraxias
Gānlùyǐn	Fetal hypoxia, Halitosis, Ecchymosis, Gingival hemorrhage, Vocal cord paralysis
Gāncǎo	Brown-Sequard syndrome, Anomia
Gāncǎoxiǎomàidàzǎotāng	Hyperventilation, Kleine-Levin syndrome, Hallucinations, Intellectual disability

Table 18.1. (Continued)

Formula or Herb	Signs and Symptoms
Gānjiāng	Presbycusis, Dyskinesia, drug-induced, Synkinesis, Brown-Sequard syndrome, Phantom limb, Psychomotor agitation, Sarcopenia, Mobility limitation, Heart murmurs, Mydriasis, Apraxias
Gégēn	Renal colic, Hearing loss, central, Encopresis, Menkes kinky hair syndrome, Prostatism, Respiratory paralysis, Sleep bruxism
Gégēnhuángqínhuángliántāng	Dyspepsia, Hematemesis, Heartburn, Diarrhea, infantile, Aerophagy, Gastroparesis, Weight gain
Gégēntāng	Toothache, Ataxia telangiectasia, Hemifacial spasm
Gōuténg	Hemifacial spasm
Gǒuqǐzǐ	Eye pain, Amblyopia, Wolfram syndrome, Cafe-au-lait spots
Guālóurén	Angina pectoris, variant, Syncope
Guīpítāng	Tetany
Guìzhī	Chronic pain, Pain, intractable, Phantom limb, Neuralgia, postherpetic, Blindness, cortical, Amaurosis fugax, Dysgeusia, Ageusia, Cheyne-Stokes respiration, Dyspnea, paroxysmal, Cerebrospinal fluid rhinorrhea, Hiccup, Postoperative nausea and vomiting, Hypokinesia, Akathisia, drug-induced, Gait ataxia, Catalepsy, Kearns-Sayre syndrome, Pyruvate dehydrogenase complex deficiency disease, Livedo reticularis, Choroid hemorrhage, Hypercalciuria, Brown-Sequard syndrome, Amnesia, retrograde, Amnesia, transient global, Sleep apnea, central, Nocturnal myoclonus syndrome, Cataplexy, Gerstmann syndrome, Prosopagnosia, Muscle rigidity, Glossalgia, Psychomotor agitation, Pruritus vulvae, Aphasia, primary progressive, Anomia, Sleep deprivation, Somnambulism, Sleep disorders, circadian rhythm, Agnosia, Dysarthria, Mobility limitation, Meningism, Miosis, Anisocoria, Stupor, Stuttering, Chills, Apraxias
Guìzhīfúlíngwán	Dysmenorrhea, Lesch-Nyhan syndrome, Dysuria, Fetal weight, Hydrops fetalis
Guìzhītāng	Pain threshold, Neck pain, Pain, intractable, Acute pain, Visceral pain, Renal colic, Glossalgia, Headache, Hyperalgesia, Scotoma, Blindness, cortical, Dysgeusia, Ageusia, Hearing loss, central, Snoring, Hypoventilation, Hypercapnia, Sneezing, Mouth breathing, Dyspnea, paroxysmal, Anorexia, Gagging, Eructation, Encopresis, Aerophagy, Menkes kinky hair syndrome, Flushing, Livedo reticularis, Cafe-au-lait spots, Choroid hemorrhage, Prostatism, Hypercalciuria, Vocal cord paralysis, Pseudobulbar palsy, Cachexia, Thinness, Amnesia, anterograde, Sleep apnea, central, Nocturnal myoclonus syndrome, Prosopagnosia, Pruritus vulvae, Weight loss, Emaciation, Sleep initiation and maintenance disorders, Sleep bruxism, Fasciculation, Mental fatigue, Failure to thrive, Mutism, Mydriasis, Stupor, Motion sickness
Hǎipiāoxiāo	Facial paralysis, Fever
Héhuānpí	Pudendal neuralgia, Pelvic girdle pain, Piriformis muscle syndrome, Labor pain, Mastodynia, Breakthrough pain, Alice in Wonderland syndrome, Infantile apparent life-threatening event, Vomiting, anticipatory, Neuroacanthocytosis, Chorea gravidarum, Mevalonate kinase deficiency, Glycogen storage disease, type IIb, Primary progressive nonfluent aphasia, Hypertriglyceridemic waist, Necrolytic migratory erythema, Ophthalmoplegic migraine, Insomnia, fatal familial, Hallucinations, Seizures, Intellectual disability
Héshǒuwū	Adrenoleukodystrophy, Obesity, abdominal
Hòupò	Abdomen, acute, Huntington disease
Huánshǎodān	Color vision defects, Wolfram syndrome, Waterhouse-Friderichsen syndrome, Lower urinary tract symptoms, Feminization
Huángqíwǔwùtāng	Pain threshold, Neck pain, Pain, intractable, Myalgia, Hypesthesia, Hyperesthesia, Paresthesia, Hyperalgesia, Hemianopsia, Dyskinesia, drug-induced, Athetosis, Tics, Machado-Joseph disease, Synkinesis, Mucopolysaccharidosis II, Obesity hypoventilation syndrome, Muscle spasticity, Muscle cramp, Narcolepsy, Muscle hypotonia, Muscular atrophy, Myotonia

Formula or Herb	Signs and Symptoms
Huángqín	Diplopia, Cough, Flatulence, Purpura, thrombocytopenic, idiopathic, Purpura, thrombotic thrombocytopenic, Oliguria, Facial paralysis, Weight gain
Huángbò	Piriformis muscle syndrome, Torticollis, Opsoclonus-myoclonus syndrome, Weight gain, Arthralgia, Back pain
Huángliánjiědútāng	Purpura, thrombocytopenic, idiopathic, Purpura, Pruritus, Pruritus ani
Huángqí	Encopresis, Flushing, Hemoptysis, Albuminuria, Prostatism, Sleep initiation and maintenance disorders
Huòxiāngzhèngqìsǎn	Weight gain
Jīxuèténg	Failed back surgery syndrome, Paresthesia, Bulimia, Machado-Joseph disease, Neuralgia, Overweight
Jishēngshènqìwán	Urinary incontinence, stress
Jiāwèixiāoyáosǎn	Breakthrough pain, Hyperventilation, Infantile apparent life-threatening event, Chorea gravidarum, Menkes kinky hair syndrome, Retinal hemorrhage, Hemiplegia, Facial paralysis, Primary progressive nonfluent aphasia, Alice in Wonderland syndrome, Hydrops fetalis, Jaundice, Seizures, Intellectual disability, Fatigue, Edema, Asthenia, Hirsutism, Hot flashes
Jiānghuáng	Shoulder pain, Athetosis, Myalgia, Facial pain, Neuralgia
Jiégěng	Earache, Tinea pedis, Hemoptysis, Fever, Fever of unknown origin
Jiégěngtāng	Glossalgia, Hoarseness, Sneezing, Mouth breathing, Vocal cord paralysis, Pseudobulbar palsy
Jīnqiáncǎo	Colic
Jīnyínhuā	Purpura, Schoenlein-Henoch, Purpura, hyperglobulinemic, Purpura fulminans, Pruritus
Jīngfángbàidúsǎn	Purpura fulminans, Purpura, thrombocytopenic, idiopathic, Purpura, thrombotic thrombocytopenic, Purpura, Schoenlein-Henoch, Purpura, hyperglobulinemic, Purpura, Ophthalmoplegia
Júhuā	Amblyopia
Juānbìtāng	Myalgia, Muscular atrophy
Lǐzhōngtāng	Phantom limb, Hyperemesis gravidarum
Liánqiáo	Hoarseness, Purpura, Schoenlein-Henoch, Purpura, hyperglobulinemic, Purpura fulminans, Pruritus, Oral hemorrhage, Hirsutism
Língguìshùgāntāng	Earache, Dizziness, Tinnitus, Hyperacusis, Hearing loss, high-frequency, Hearing loss, unilateral, Hearing loss, bilateral, Usher syndromes, Hearing loss, mixed conductive-sensorineural, Hearing loss, conductive, Hearing loss, sudden, Presbycusis, Hearing loss, noise-induced, Auditory perceptual disorders, Vertigo
Liùwèidìhuángwán	Waterhouse-Friderichsen syndrome, Albuminuria, Virilism
Lóngdǎnxiègāntāng	Purpura, thrombotic thrombocytopenic, Hemoglobinuria, Jaundice
Máxìnggānshítāng	Cough, Supranuclear palsy, progressive, Dyspnea, Ophthalmoplegia
Máhuáng	Somnambulism
Máhuángfùzǐxìxīntāng	Blindness, cortical, Amaurosis fugax, Ageusia, Dyspnea, paroxysmal, Hiccup, Hyperkinesis, Hypokinesia, Akathisia, drug-induced, Gait ataxia, Pyruvate dehydrogenase complex deficiency disease, Flushing, Livedo reticularis, Hypercalciuria, Delirium, Sleep apnea, central, Gerstmann syndrome, Prosopagnosia, Muscle rigidity, Psychomotor agitation, Aphasia, primary progressive, Anomia, Narcolepsy, Muscle hypotonia, Dysarthria, Fasciculation, Mobility limitation, Meningism, Miosis, Anisocoria, Stuttering, Chills
Mázǐrénwán	Abdomen, acute, Constipation, Sarcopenia
Màiméndōng	Constipation, Abdomen, acute, Ecchymosis, Fetal macrosomia
Mòyào	Low back pain, Failed back surgery syndrome, Sciatica, Pelvic girdle pain, Labor pain, Breakthrough pain, Metatarsalgia, Alice in Wonderland syndrome, Transient tachypnea of the newborn, Infantile apparent life-threatening event, Vomiting, anticipatory, Chorea gravidarum, Opsoclonus-myoclonus syndrome, Hyperlactatemia, Primary progressive nonfluent aphasia, Striae distensae, Urinoma, Alexia, pure, Hypersomnolence, idiopathic, Muscle weakness, Mevalonate kinase deficiency, Schnitzler syndrome, Facial pain, Intermittent claudication, Spasm, Catatonia
Mǔdānpí	Diplopia

Table 18.1. (Continued)

Formula or Herb	Signs and Symptoms
Mŭlì	Hoarseness, Sneezing, Vocal cord paralysis, Pseudobulbar palsy, Hot flashes
Mùzéicăo	Vision, low, Photophobia, Hyphema, Vitreous hemorrhage, Retinal hemorrhage, Night blindness
Mùguā	Slit ventricle syndrome, Torticollis, Mevalonate kinase deficiency, Hypertriglyceridemic waist, Catatonia, Trismus
Mùxiāng	Jaundice, obstructive, Supranuclear palsy, progressive
Niúxī	Low back pain, Flank pain, Mastodynia, Slit ventricle syndrome, Hearing loss, conductive, Torticollis, Ataxia telangiectasia, Neuroacanthocytosis, Hypertriglyceridemic waist, Necrolytic migratory erythema, Auditory perceptual disorders, Arthralgia, Back pain, Paraplegia, Overweight, Trismus
Píngwèisăn	Jaundice, obstructive, Obesity
Púgōngyīng	Fetal weight, Pruritus, Proteinuria
Qĭjúdìhuángwán	Vision, low, Photophobia, Amblyopia, Kearns-Sayre syndrome, Hyphema, Vitreous hemorrhage, Retinal hemorrhage, Night blindness
Qínjiāo	Bulimia, Hemifacial spasm
Qīngwèisăn	Fetal hypoxia, Halitosis, Gingival hemorrhage, Oral hemorrhage
Rénshēn	Hearing loss, functional, Apnea, Hypocapnia, Hyperoxia, Alkalosis, respiratory, Nocturia, Consciousness disorders, Delirium, Amnesia, anterograde, Amnesia, retrograde, Postoperative nausea and vomiting, Mental fatigue, Syncope, vasovagal, Coma, Hypotension, orthostatic, Cyanosis, Hypothermia, Lethargy, Cardiac output, low, Cardiac output, high, Motion sickness
Rénshēnbàidúsăn	Supranuclear palsy, progressive, Ophthalmoplegia
Ròuguì	Phantom limb, Olfaction disorders, Cerebrospinal fluid rhinorrhea, Hyperemesis gravidarum, Insulin coma, Pallor, Nocturia, Mobility limitation
Rŭxiāng	Low back pain, Failed back surgery syndrome, Sciatica, Pelvic girdle pain, Labor pain, Metatarsalgia, Transient tachypnea of the newborn, Vomiting, anticipatory, Opsoclonus-myoclonus syndrome, Hyperlactatemia, Striae distensae, Urinoma, Alexia, pure, Hypersomnolence, idiopathic, Schnitzler syndrome, Spasm
Rùnchángwán	Abdomen, acute, Constipation
Sānbìtāng	Machado-Joseph disease, Paraparesis
Sānléng	Fetal weight
Sănzhŏngkuìjiāntāng	Supranuclear palsy, progressive, Fetal weight, Hot flashes
Sāngpiāoxiāosăn	Polyuria, Urinary incontinence, stress, Urinary incontinence, urge, Urinary bladder, overactive, Quadriplegia, Urinary bladder, neurogenic, Reflex, abnormal
Sāngzhī	Pain threshold, Chronic pain, Pain, intractable, Myalgia, Hypesthesia, Hyperesthesia, Paresthesia, Hyperalgesia, Hemianopsia, Athetosis, Respiratory paralysis, Obesity hypoventilation syndrome, Muscle spasticity, Narcolepsy, Muscle hypotonia, Muscular atrophy, Myotonia
Shārén	Dizziness, Tinnitus, Hearing loss, high-frequency, Hearing loss, unilateral, Hearing loss, bilateral, Usher syndromes, Hearing loss, mixed conductive-sensorineural, Hearing loss, sudden, Hearing loss, noise-induced, Jaundice, obstructive, Obesity, Vertigo
Shānzhā	Adrenoleukodystrophy, Obesity, morbid, Obesity, abdominal, Pediatric obesity
Sháoyàogāncăotāng	Failed back surgery syndrome, Eye pain, Visceral pain, Sciatica, Pudendal neuralgia, Pelvic girdle pain, Renal colic, Piriformis muscle syndrome, Mastodynia, Slit ventricle syndrome, Hypesthesia, Hyperesthesia, Alice in Wonderland syndrome, Diplopia, Transient tachypnea of the newborn, Infantile apparent life-threatening event, Bulimia, Vomiting, anticipatory, Torticollis, Akathisia, drug-induced, Ataxia telangiectasia, Neuroacanthocytosis, Huntington disease, Opsoclonus-myoclonus syndrome, Hyperlactatemia, Mevalonate kinase deficiency, Glycogen storage disease type IIb, Primary progressive nonfluent aphasia, Hypertriglyceridemic waist, Striae distensae, Necrolytic migratory erythema, Choroid hemorrhage, Urinoma,

Formula or Herb	Signs and Symptoms
	Ophthalmoplegic migraine, Hypersomnolence, idiopathic, Insomnia, fatal familial, Schnitzler syndrome, Facial pain, Back pain, Intermittent claudication, Pruritus vulvae, Muscle hypertonia, Spasm, Catatonia, Trismus
Shéchuángzǐ	Color vision defects, Hemoglobinuria, Lower urinary tract symptoms
Shēntòngzhúyūtāng	Muscle spasticity, Intermittent claudication, Pain, postoperative
Shénqū	Pediatric obesity
Shēngmàiyǐn	Hearing loss, functional, Encopresis, Tetany, Sarcopenia, Fatigue, Syncope, Syncope, vasovagal, Heart murmurs
Shēngjiāng	Acute pain, Glossalgia, Scotoma, Blindness, cortical, Amaurosis fugax, Ageusia, Hearing loss, central, Snoring, Hypoventilation, Mouth breathing, Dyspnea, paroxysmal, Hiccup, Gagging, Eructation, Aerophagy, Tremor, Hyperkinesis, Akathisia, drug-induced, Tics, Catalepsy, Alkalosis, respiratory, Pyruvate dehydrogenase complex deficiency disease, Pallor, Livedo reticularis, Cachexia, Thinness, Ideal body weight, Amnesia, transient global, Sleep apnea, central, Nocturnal myoclonus syndrome, Cataplexy, Gerstmann syndrome, Prosopagnosia, Muscle cramp, Muscle rigidity, Pruritus vulvae, Weight loss, Emaciation, Aphasia, primary progressive, Anomia, Dyslexia, acquired, Sleep deprivation, Sleep disorders, circadian rhythm, Muscle hypertonia, Dysarthria, Fasciculation, Failure to thrive, Miosis, Anisocoria, Stupor, Stuttering, Chills, Cerebrospinal fluid leak
Shíchāngpú	Earache, Primary progressive nonfluent aphasia, Jet lag syndrome, Learning disorders
Shūjīnghuóxuètāng	Chronic pain, Shoulder pain, Low back pain, Failed back surgery syndrome, Eye pain, Neuralgia, postherpetic, Sciatica, Pudendal neuralgia, Pelvic girdle pain, Piriformis muscle syndrome, Labor pain, Mastodynia, Metatarsalgia, Slit ventricle syndrome, Paresthesia, Alice in Wonderland syndrome, Transient tachypnea of the newborn, Bulimia, Vomiting, anticipatory, Torticollis, Athetosis, Akathisia, drug-induced, Machado-Joseph disease, Ataxia telangiectasia, Neuroacanthocytosis, Chorea gravidarum, Opsoclonus-myoclonus syndrome, Hyperlactatemia, Mevalonate kinase deficiency, Glycogen storage disease type IIb, Mucopolysaccharidosis II, Primary progressive nonfluent aphasia, Hypertriglyceridemic waist, Striae distensae, Necrolytic migratory erythema, Urinoma, Respiratory paralysis, Ophthalmoplegic migraine, Alexia, pure, Hypersomnolence, idiopathic, Insomnia, fatal familial, Muscle weakness, Schnitzler syndrome, Facial pain, Neuralgia, Pain, postoperative, Paraplegia, Paraparesis, Overweight, Spasm, Catatonia, Trismus
Sìnìtāng	Pain, intractable, Phantom limb, Pain, referred, Visceral pain, Renal colic, Glossalgia, Olfaction disorders, Scotoma, Dysgeusia, Hearing loss, functional, Presbycusis, Hearing loss, noise-induced, Apnea, Hypercapnia, Cheyne-Stokes respiration, Hypocapnia, Hyperoxia, Dyspnea, paroxysmal, Cerebrospinal fluid rhinorrhea, Hiccup, Postoperative nausea and vomiting, Hyperemesis gravidarum, Eructation, Tremor, Hyperkinesis, Hypokinesia, Tics, Catalepsy, Alkalosis, respiratory, Wolfram syndrome, Insulin coma, Pyruvate dehydrogenase complex deficiency disease, Pallor, Cafe-au-lait spots, Choroid hemorrhage, Prostatism, Nocturia, Hypercalciuria, Thinness, Ideal body weight, Consciousness disorders, Delirium, Auditory perceptual disorders, Amnesia, anterograde, Amnesia, retrograde, Amnesia, transient global, Sleep apnea, central, Obesity hypoventilation syndrome, Nocturnal myoclonus syndrome, Cataplexy, Illusions, Gerstmann syndrome, Prosopagnosia, Muscle cramp, Muscle rigidity, Psychomotor agitation, Pruritus vulvae, Aphasia, primary progressive, Anomia, Dyslexia, acquired, Sleep deprivation, Somnambulism, Sleep disorders, circadian rhythm, Agnosia, Dysarthria, Mental fatigue, Syncope, vasovagal, Coma, Hypotension, orthostatic, Cyanosis, Hypothermia, Mobility limitation, Lethargy, Cardiac output, low, Cardiac output, high, Heart murmurs, Mydriasis, Miosis, Anisocoria, Stupor, Chills, Cerebrospinal fluid leak, Motion sickness, Prodromal symptoms, Apraxias

Table 18.1. (Continued)

Formula or Herb	Signs and Symptoms
Tiānhuā	Purpura, thrombocytopenic, idiopathic, Fetal macrosomia, Gingival hemorrhage
Tiānmágōuténgyǐn	Hemiplegia
Tiáowèichéngqìtāng	Pain, referred, Dizziness, Hearing loss, mixed conductive-sensorineural, Hyperoxia, Flatulence
Tǔfúlíng	Purpura fulminans, Purpura, Schoenlein-Henoch, Purpura, thrombotic thrombocytopenic, Hemoglobinuria, Purpura, Hypergammaglobulinemia
Tùsīzǐ	Color vision defects, Wolfram syndrome, Waterhouse-Friderichsen syndrome, Feminization
Wēndǎntāng	Obesity, abdominal
Wēnjīngtāng	Dysmenorrhea, Lesch-Nyhan syndrome
Wūyàoshùnqìsǎn	Neuralgia, postherpetic, Dyskinesia, drug-induced, Synkinesis, Restless legs syndrome, Hemifacial spasm
Wúzhūyú	Phantom limb, Eye pain, Visceral pain, Scotoma, Wolfram syndrome, Hyperemesis gravidarum, Tremor, Hyperkinesis, Hypokinesia, Tics, Alkalosis, respiratory, Insulin coma, Pallor, Nocturia, Ideal body weight, Amnesia, transient global, Illusions, Muscle cramp, Muscle rigidity, Agnosia, Muscle hypertonia, Fasciculation, Mental fatigue, Syncope, vasovagal, Cyanosis, Cerebrospinal fluid leak
Wúzhūyútāng	Amaurosis fugax, Usher syndromes, Hearing loss, noise-induced, Hypercapnia, Mouth breathing, Eructation, Failure to thrive, Mydriasis
Wǔlínsǎn	Flank pain, Colic, Proteinuria
Wǔlíngsǎn	Usher syndromes, Flatulence, Oliguria, Kearns-Sayre syndrome, Weight gain, Meningism
Xǐgānmíngmùtāng	Eye pain, Vision, low, Photophobia, Hyphema, Vitreous hemorrhage, Night blindness
Xìxīn	Dysgeusia, Hyperacusis, Purpura, thrombocytopenic, idiopathic, Gerstmann syndrome, Sleep deprivation, Somnambulism, Sleep disorders, circadian rhythm, Sarcopenia, Mental fatigue, Heart murmurs
Xiāngfù	Pain, referred, Dysmenorrhea, Lesch-Nyhan syndrome, Dysuria, Facial paralysis, Weight gain, Kleine-Levin syndrome, Hydrops fetalis, Fatigue, Edema, Asthenia, Aging, premature
Xiāngshāliùjūnzǐtāng	Hemoptysis, Jaundice, obstructive, Fever, Edema
Xiāofēngsǎn	Purpura fulminans, Purpura, thrombocytopenic, idiopathic, Purpura, thrombotic thrombocytopenic, Purpura, Schoenlein-Henoch, Purpura, hyperglobulinemic, Purpura, Hypergammaglobulinemia
Xiǎocháihútāng	Earache, Pain, referred, Hearing loss, unilateral, Hearing loss, conductive, Jaundice, obstructive, Auditory perceptual disorders, Motion sickness
Xiǎoxùmìngtāng	Synkinesis
Xiǎoqīnglóngtāng	Hemoptysis, Tinea pedis, Fever
Xièbái	Angina pectoris, variant, Syncope
Xīnyísǎn	Hemoptysis, Fever, Fever of unknown origin
Xìngrén	Tinea pedis
Xùduàn	Neuralgia, postherpetic, Pudendal neuralgia, Muscle weakness, Paraparesis
Xuánshēn	Sneezing, Ecchymosis, Gingival hemorrhage, Fetal macrosomia, Oral hemorrhage, Ophthalmoplegia, Hot flashes
Xuèfǔzhúyūtāng	Myalgia, Angina pectoris, variant, Angina, stable, Kearns-Sayre syndrome, Adrenoleukodystrophy, Obesity, abdominal, Amnesia, transient global, Intermittent claudication, Syncope, Aging, premature, Prodromal symptoms
Yánhúsuǒ	Pain, intractable, Shoulder pain, Pain, referred, Flank pain, Visceral pain, Neuralgia, postherpetic, Sciatica, Piriformis muscle syndrome, Dysmenorrhea, Angina, stable, Mastodynia, Metatarsalgia, Slit ventricle syndrome, Olfaction disorders, Alice in Wonderland syndrome, Transient tachypnea of the newborn, Bulimia, Postoperative nausea and vomiting, Hyperemesis gravidarum, Halitosis, Machado-Joseph disease, Ataxia telangiectasia, Neuroacanthocytosis, Huntington disease, Hyperlactatemia, Mevalonate kinase deficiency, Glycogen

Formula or Herb	Signs and Symptoms
	storage disease type IIb, Mucopolysaccharidosis II, Primary progressive nonfluent aphasia, Jaundice, obstructive, Cafe-au-lait spots, Necrolytic migratory erythema, Dysuria, Urinoma, Respiratory paralysis, Ophthalmoplegic migraine, Alexia, pure, Insomnia, fatal familial, Schnitzler syndrome, Facial pain, Neuralgia, Chest pain, Intermittent claudication, Paraplegia, Paraparesis, Overweight, Obesity, Spasm, Edema, Catatonia, Aging, premature, Prodromal symptoms
Yèjiāoténg	Hyperventilation, Ophthalmoplegic migraine, Hallucinations, Seizures, Intellectual disability
Yìqìcōngmíngtāng	Earache, Hearing loss, conductive
Yìmǔcǎo	Dysmenorrhea, Lesch-Nyhan syndrome, Dysuria, Hydrops fetalis, Edema
Yìyǐrén	Dyspnea, Hirsutism
Yìzhìrén	Polyuria, Albuminuria, Urinary incontinence, stress, Urinary incontinence, urge, Urinary bladder, overactive, Quadriplegia, Urinary bladder, neurogenic, Reflex, abnormal
Yínqiàosǎn	Diplopia, Cough, Purpura, Schoenlein-Henoch, Facial paralysis
Yínyánghuò	Color vision defects, Wolfram syndrome, Waterhouse-Friderichsen syndrome, Urinary incontinence, urge, Lower urinary tract symptoms, Feminization, Virilism
Yùjīn	Angina, stable, Supranuclear palsy, progressive, Fatigue, Asthenia, Prodromal symptoms
Yùnǚjiān	Halitosis, Ecchymosis, Purpura fulminans, Purpura, hyperglobulinemic, Gingival hemorrhage, Oral hemorrhage
Yùquánwán	Albuminuria, Fetal macrosomia
Yuǎnzhì	Earache, Breakthrough pain, Hearing loss, conductive, Hyperventilation, Auditory perceptual disorders, Primary progressive nonfluent aphasia, Restless legs syndrome, Kleine-Levin syndrome, Hallucinations, Alice in Wonderland syndrome, Jaundice, Jet lag syndrome, Seizures, Mutism
Zéxiè	Adrenoleukodystrophy
Zhēnrénhuómìngyǐnqùchuānshānjiǎ	Hypergammaglobulinemia, Hirsutism
Zhēnwǔtāng	Hyperoxia, Hiccup, Oliguria, Postoperative nausea and vomiting, Sarcopenia, Heart murmurs
Zhènggǔzǐjīndān	Chest pain
Zhībódìhuángwán	Fetal hypoxia, Ecchymosis, Hemiplegia, Fetal macrosomia, Kearns-Sayre syndrome
Zhīzǐ	Cough, Hoarseness, Vocal cord paralysis
Zhìgāncǎo	Akathisia, drug-induced, Pyruvate dehydrogenase complex deficiency disease, Hypercalciuria, Prosopagnosia, Aphasia, primary progressive, Miosis, Anisocoria, Stuttering
Zhìgāncǎotāng	Olfaction disorders, Hyperemesis gravidarum, Gait ataxia, Insulin coma, Pallor, Nocturia, Consciousness disorders, Delirium, Phantom limb, Psychomotor agitation, Dysarthria, Fatigue, Mental fatigue, Asthenia, Mobility limitation, Meningism, Stuttering
Zhúrú	Pain threshold, Myalgia, Hypesthesia, Hyperesthesia, Hyperalgesia, Hemianopsia, Hyperventilation, Dyskinesia, drug-induced, Athetosis, Tics, Synkinesis, Glycogen storage disease type IIb, Mucopolysaccharidosis II, Obesity hypoventilation syndrome, Muscle spasticity, Muscle cramp, Narcolepsy, Muscle hypotonia, Muscular atrophy, Myotonia
Zīshènmíngmùtāng	Vision, low, Photophobia, Amblyopia, Hyphema, Vitreous hemorrhage, Retinal hemorrhage, Night blindness

18.2. Sign and Symptom Clouds of Formulas and Herbs

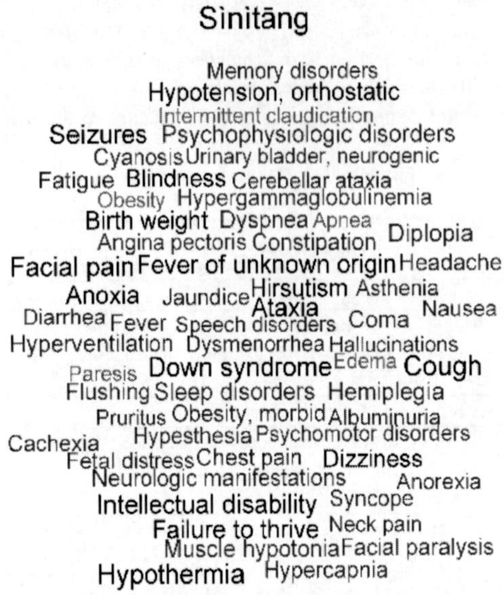

Figure 18.1. Sìnìtāng symptom cloud.

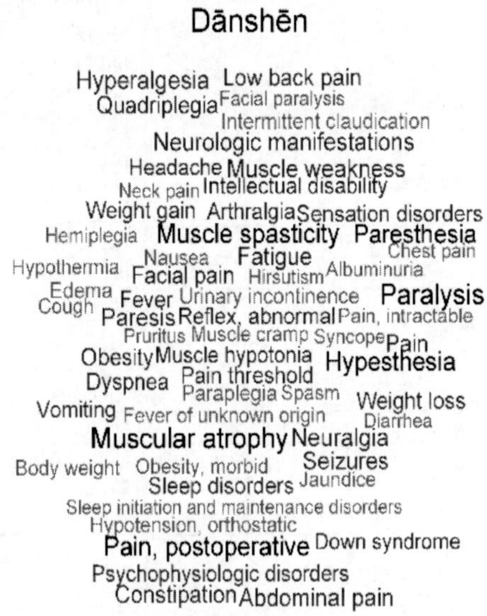

Figure 18.2. Dānshēn symptom cloud.

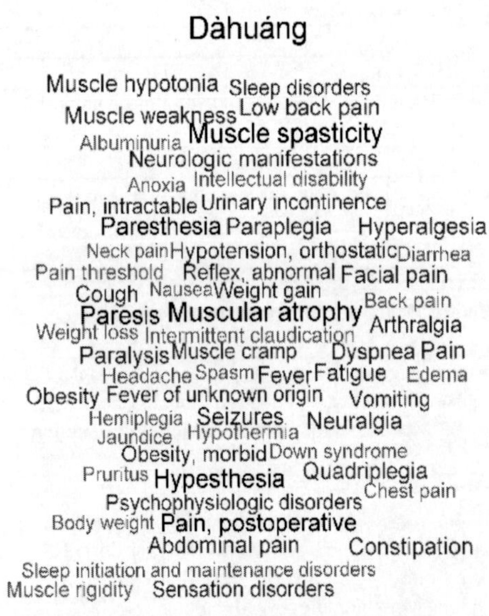

Figure 18.3. Dàhuáng symptom cloud.

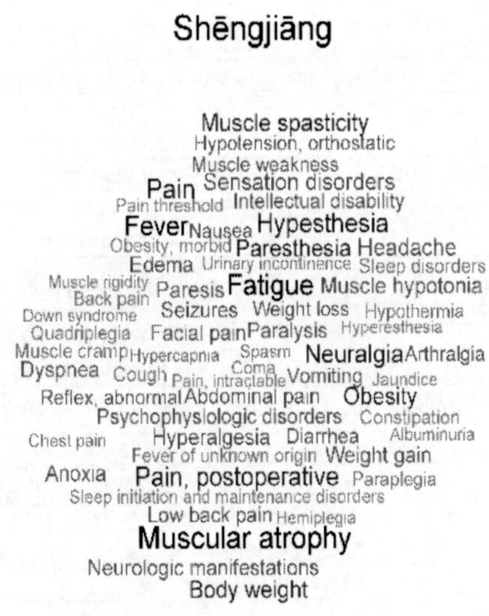

Figure 18.4. Shēngjiāng symptom cloud.

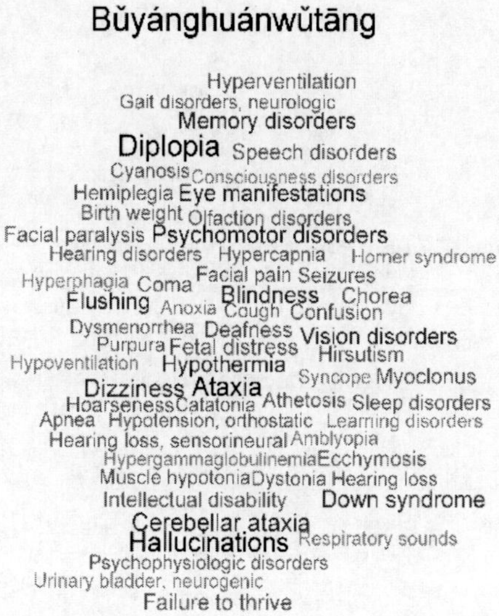

Figure 18.5. Bǔyánghuánwǔtāng symptom cloud.

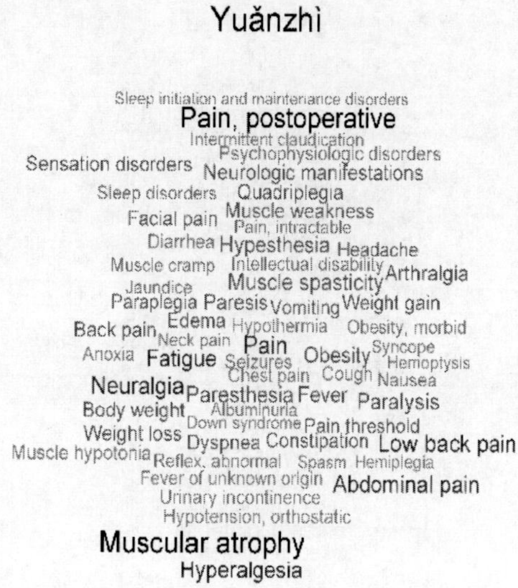

Figure18.6. Yuǎnzhì symptom cloud.

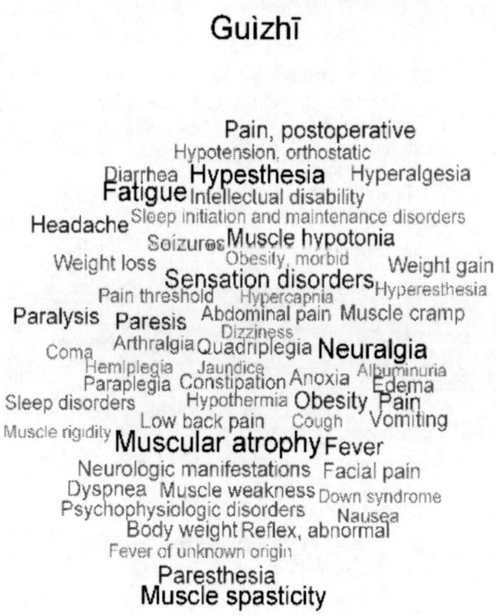

Figure 18.7. Guìzhī symptom cloud.

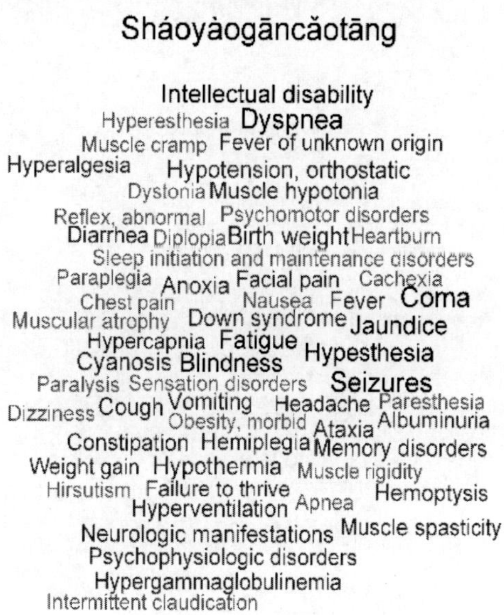

Figure 18.8. Sháoyàogāncǎotāng symptom cloud.

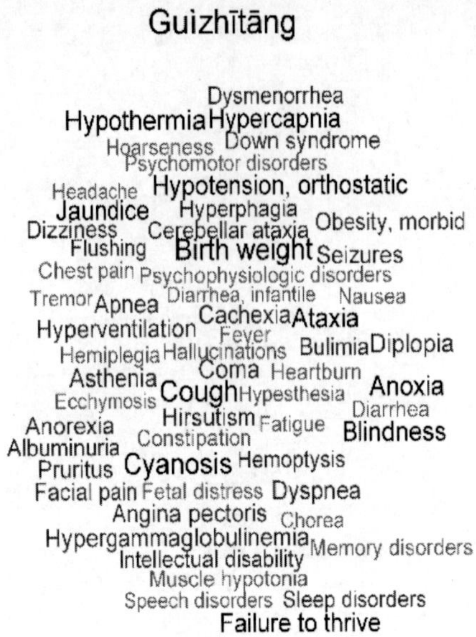

Figure 18.9. Guìzhītāng symptom cloud.

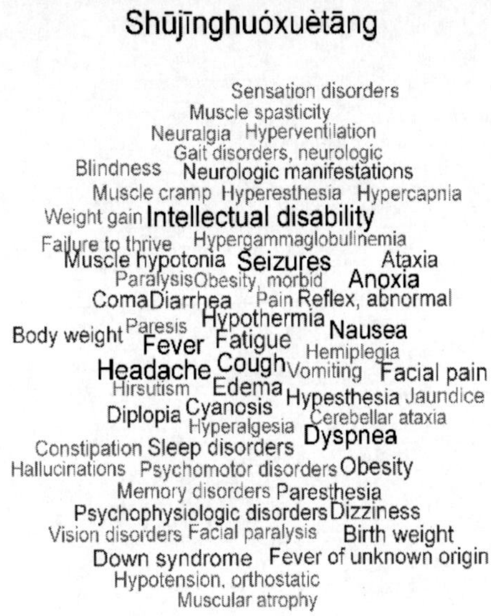

Figure 18.10. Shūjīnghuóxuètāng symptom cloud.

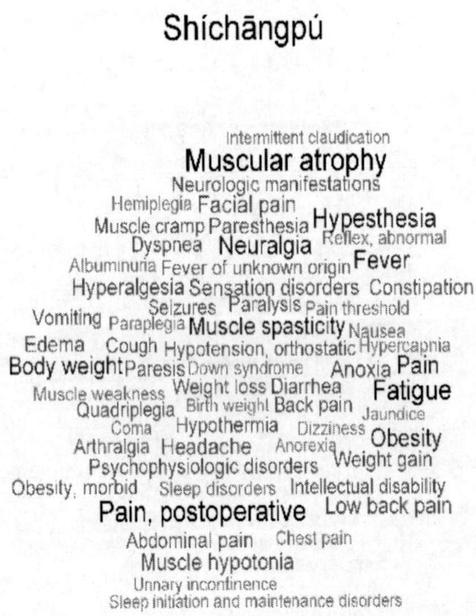

Figure 18.11. Shíchāngpú symptom cloud.

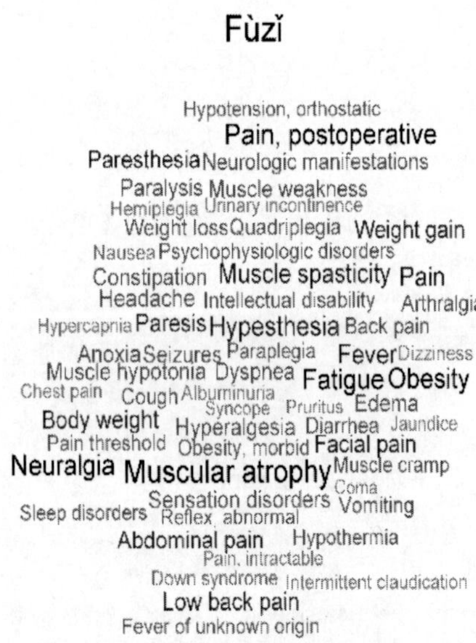

Figure 18.12. Fùzǐ symptom cloud.

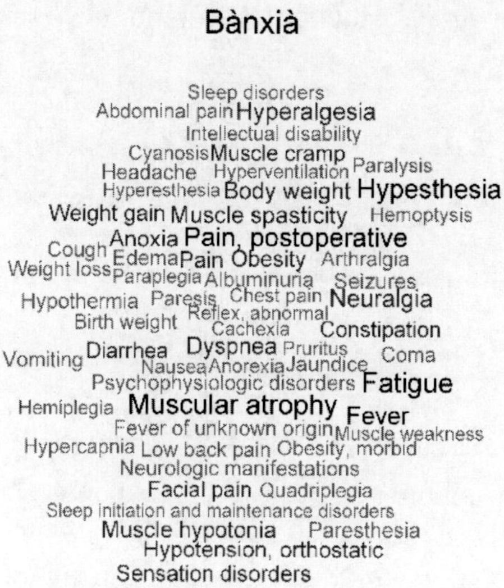

Figure 18.13. Bànxià symptom cloud.

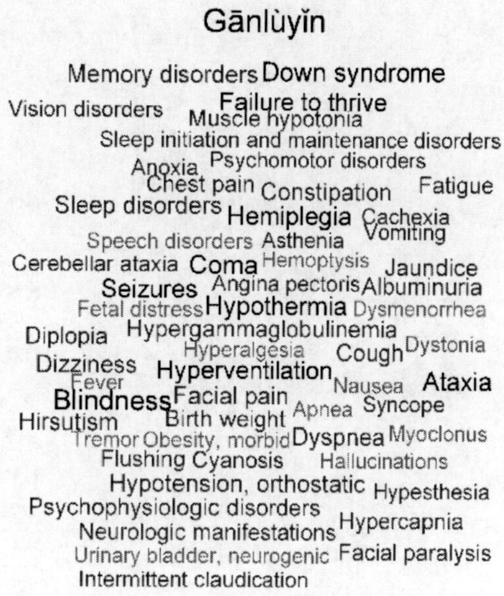

Figure 18.14. Gānlùyǐn symptom cloud.

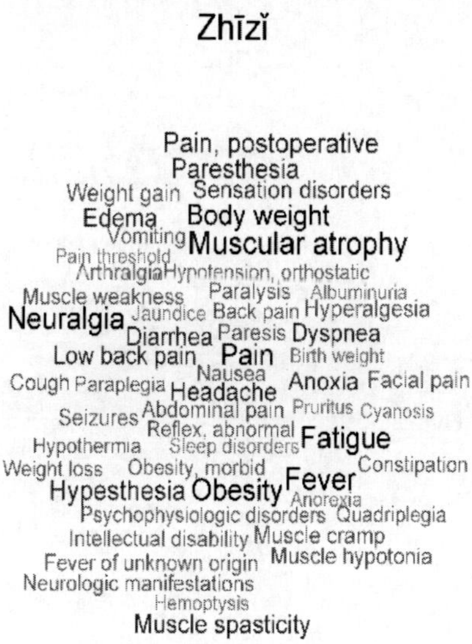

Figure 18.15. Zhīzǐ symptom cloud.

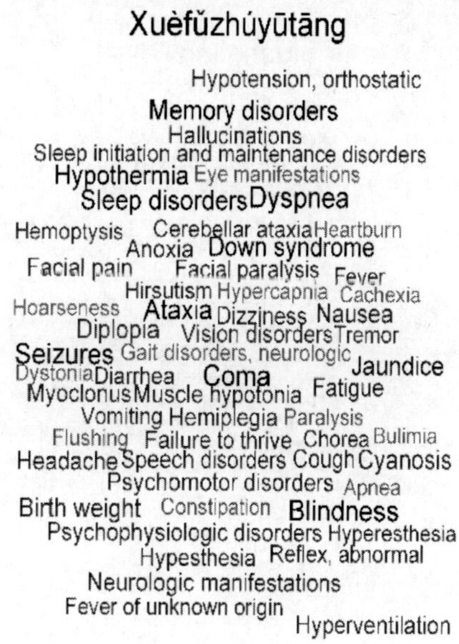

Figure 18.16. Xuèfǔzhúyūtāng symptom cloud.

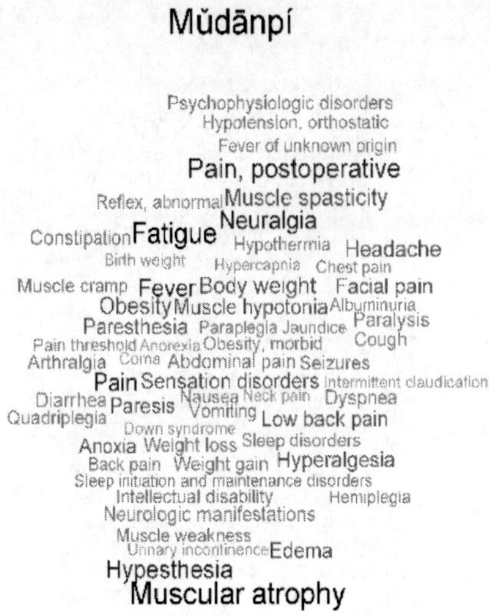

Figure 18.17. Mǔdānpí symptom cloud.

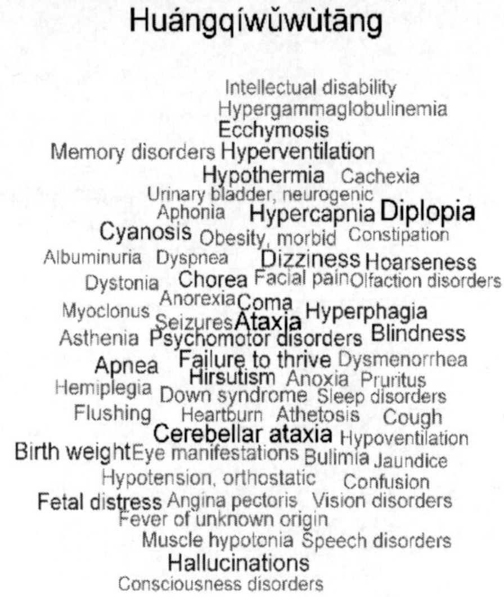

Figure 18.18. Huángqíwǔwùtāng symptom cloud.

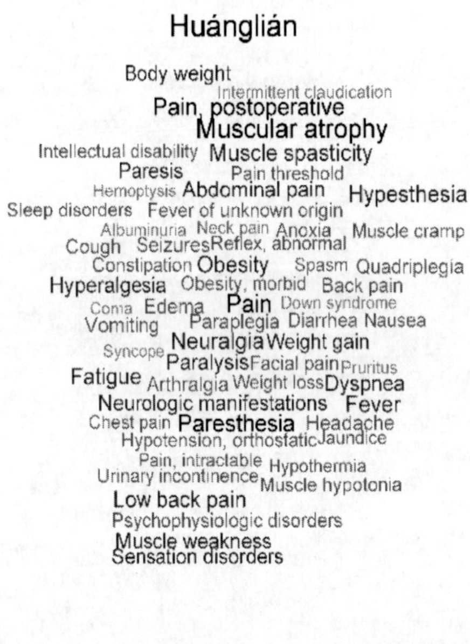

Figure 18.19. Huánglián symptom cloud.

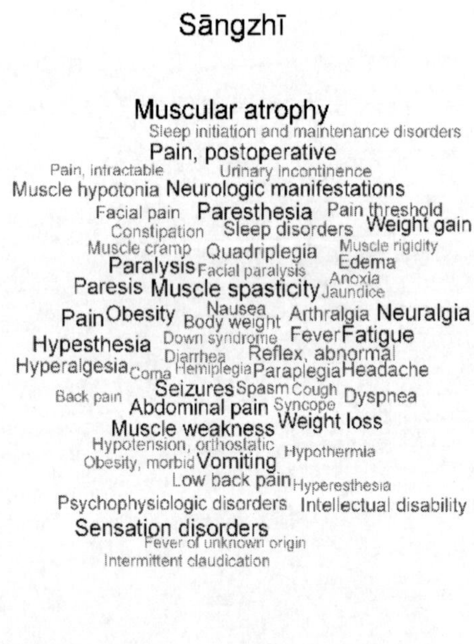

Figure 18.20. Sāngzhī symptom cloud.

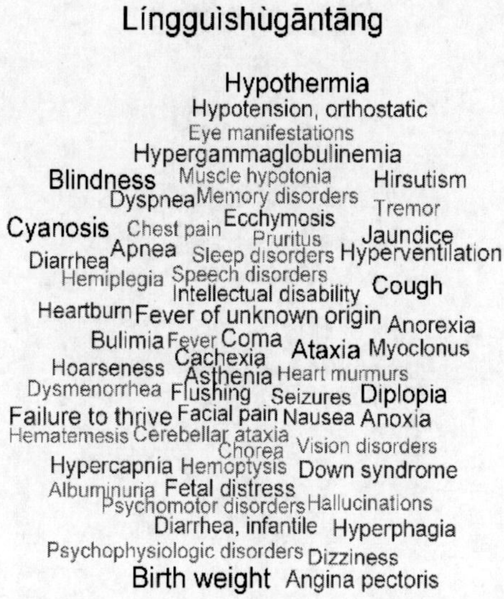

Figure 18.21. Língguìshùgāntāng symptom cloud.

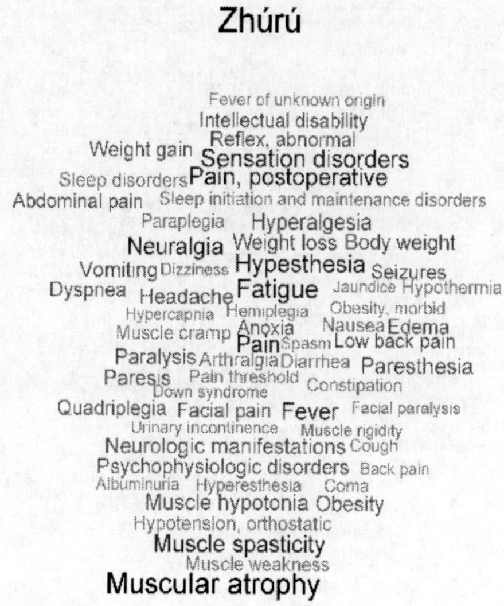

Figure 18.22. Zhúrú symptom cloud.

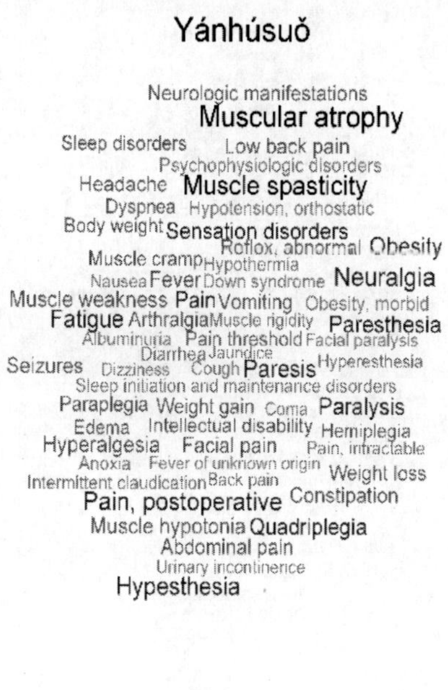

Figure 18.23. Yánhúsuǒ symptom cloud.

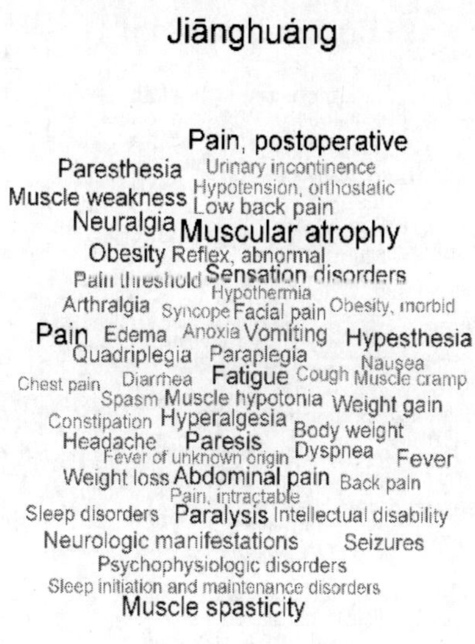

Figure 18.24. Jiānghuáng symptom cloud.

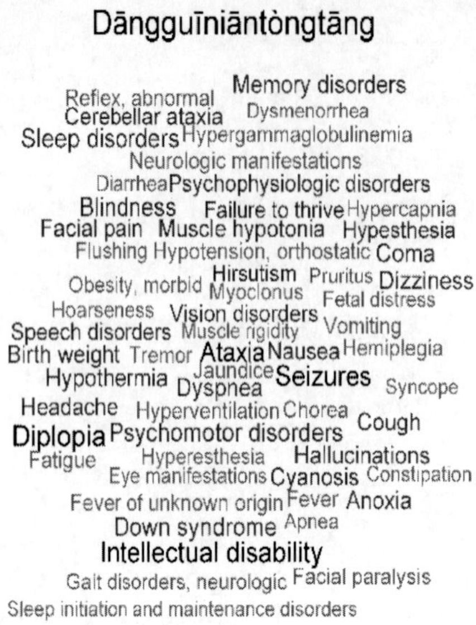

Figure 18.25. Dāngguīniāntòngtāng symptom cloud.

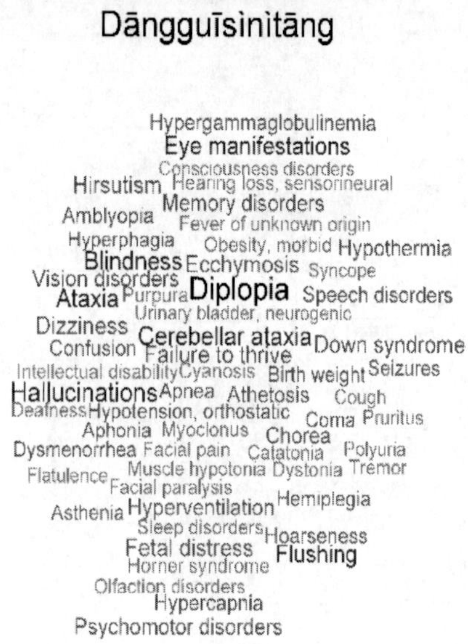

Figure 18.26. Dāngguīsìnìtāng symptom cloud.

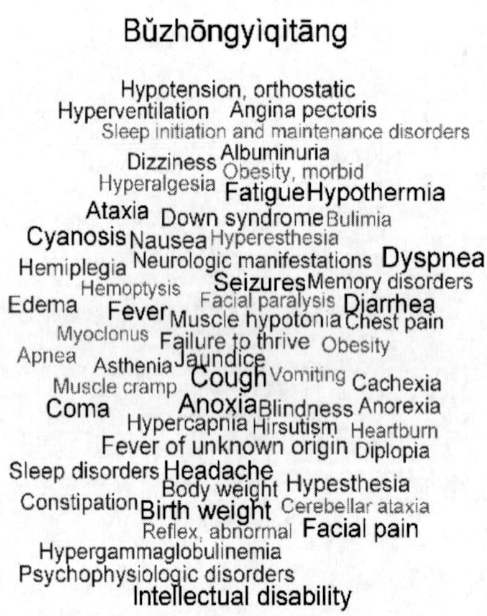

Figure 18.27. Bǔzhōngyìqìtāng symptom cloud.

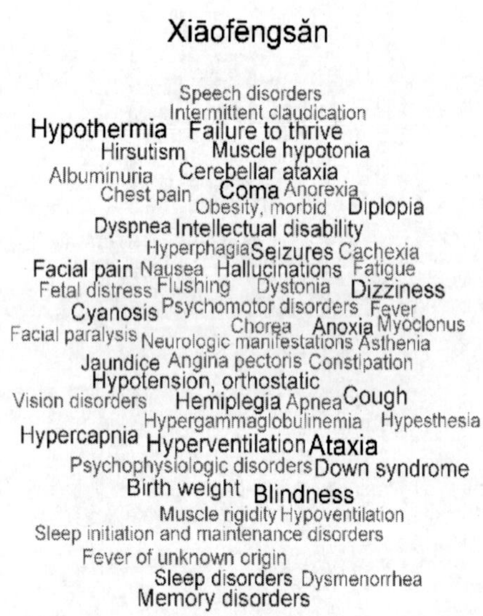

Figure 18.28. Xiāofēngsǎn symptom cloud.

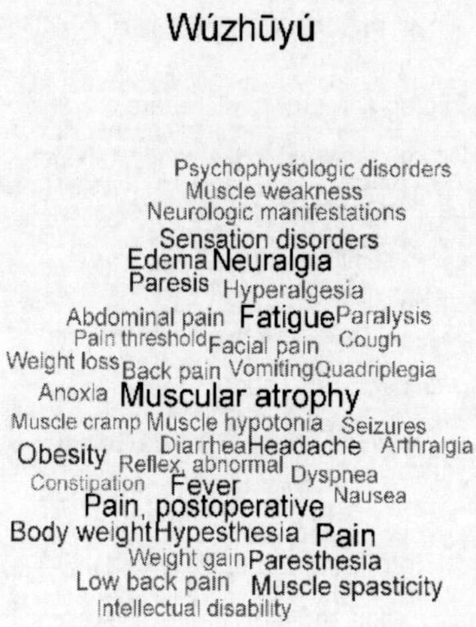

Figure 18.29. Wúzhūyú symptom cloud.

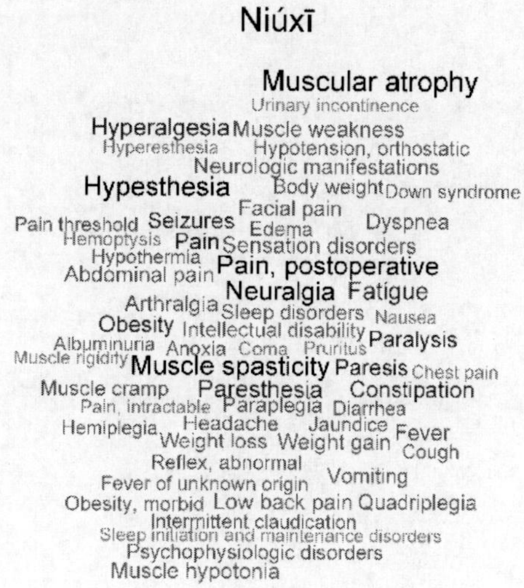

Figure 18.30. Niúxī symptom cloud.

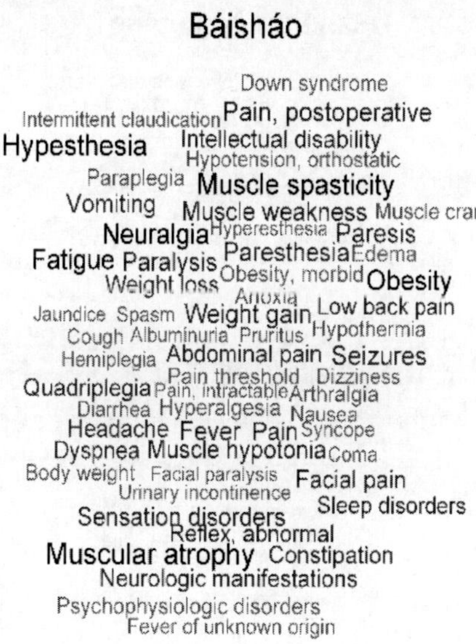

Figure 18.31. Báisháo symptom cloud.

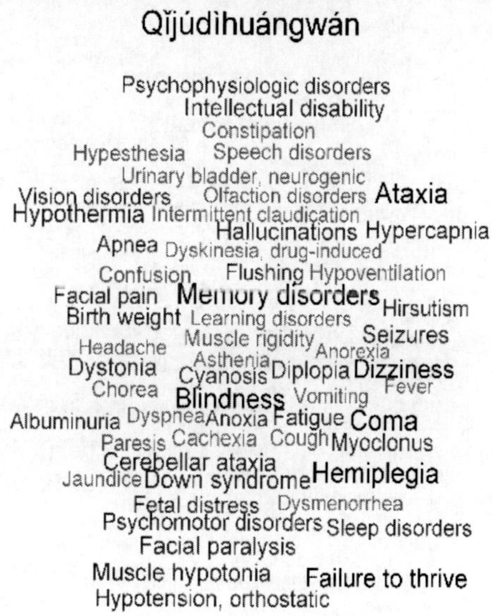

Figure 18.32. Qǐjúdìhuángwán symptom cloud.

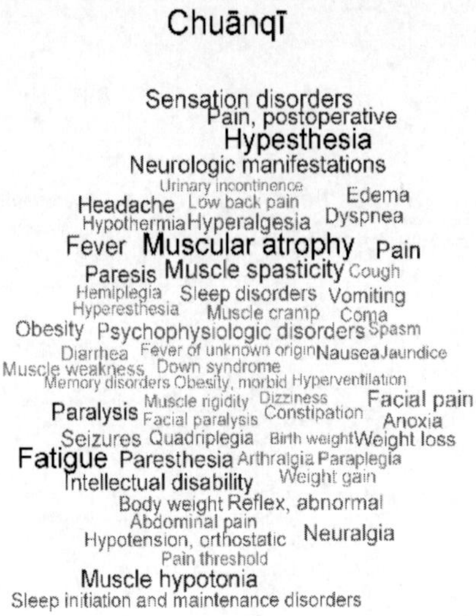

Figure 18.33. Chuānqī symptom cloud.

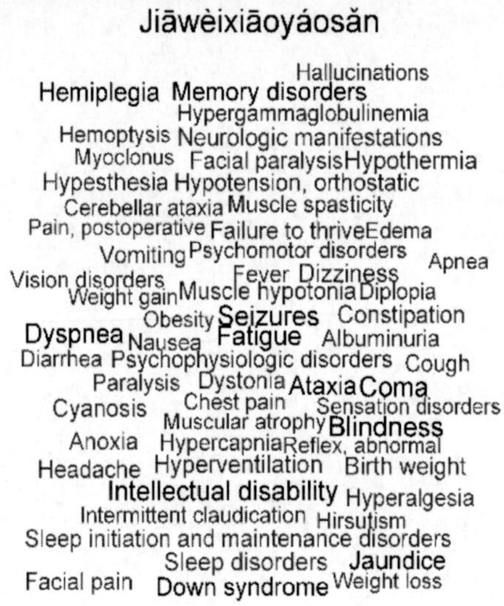

Figure 18.34. Jiāwèixiāoyáosǎn symptom cloud.

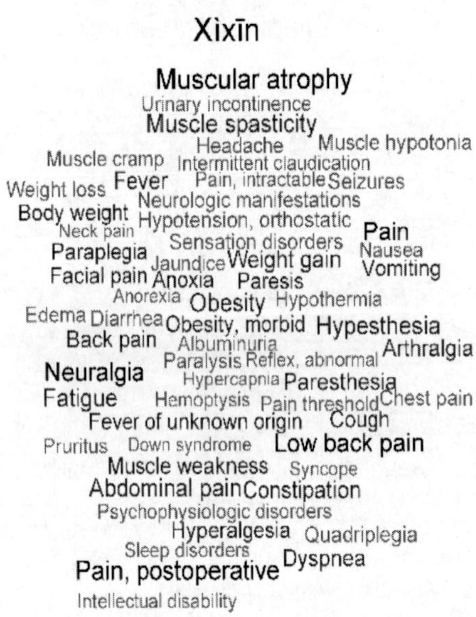

Figure 18.35. Xìxīn symptom cloud.

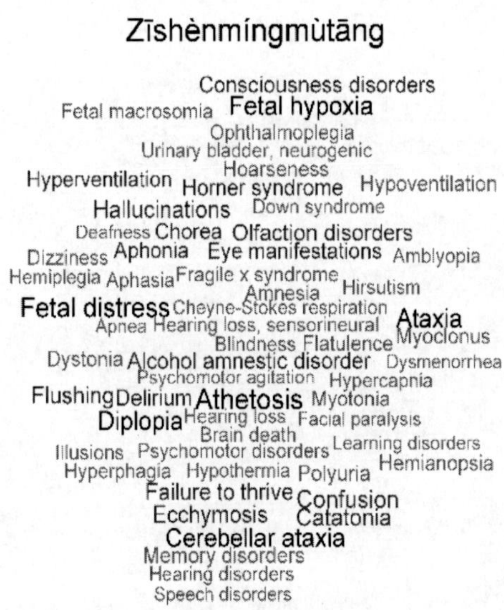

Figure 18.36. Zīshènmíngmùtāng symptom cloud.

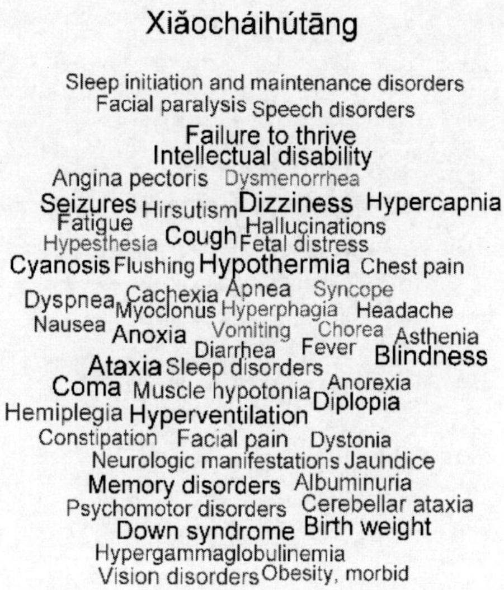

Figure 18.37. Xiǎocháihútāng symptom cloud.

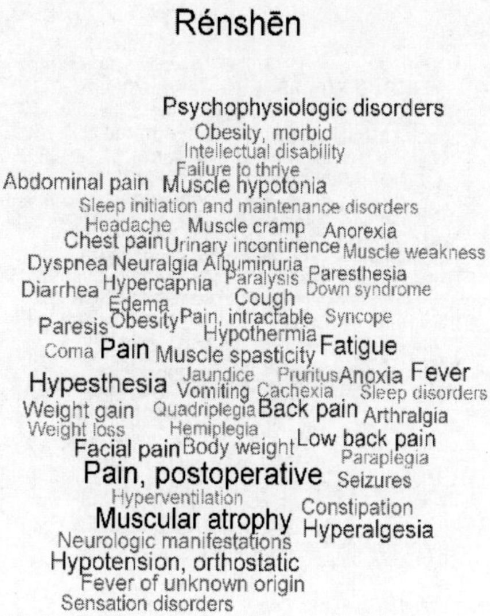

Figure 18.38. Rénshēn symptom cloud.

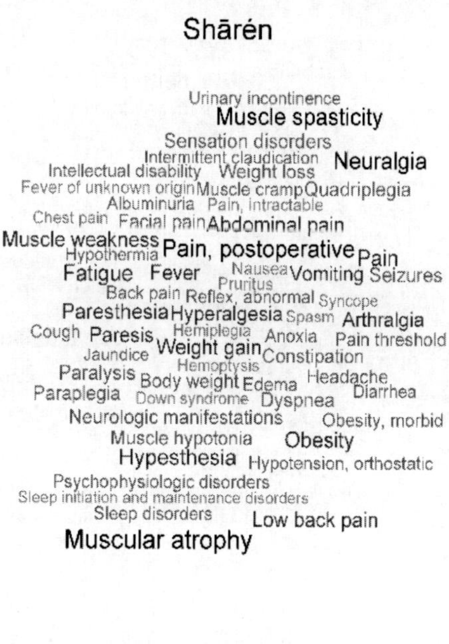

Figure 18.39. Shārén symptom cloud.

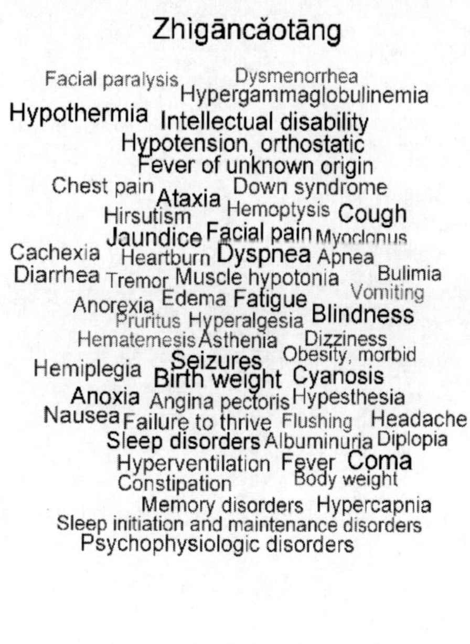

Figure 18.40. Zhìgāncǎotāng symptom cloud.

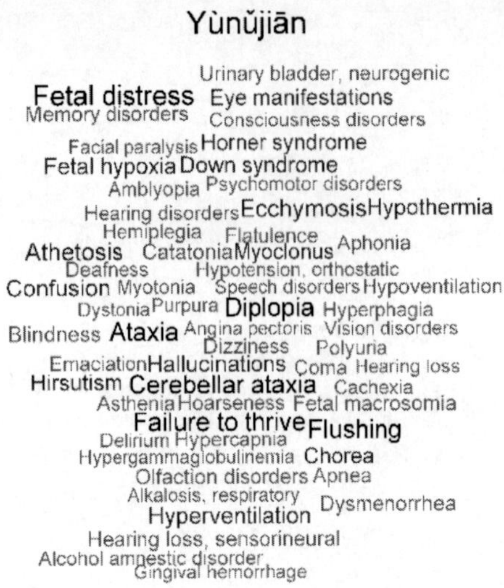

Figure 18.41. Yùnǚjiān symptom cloud.

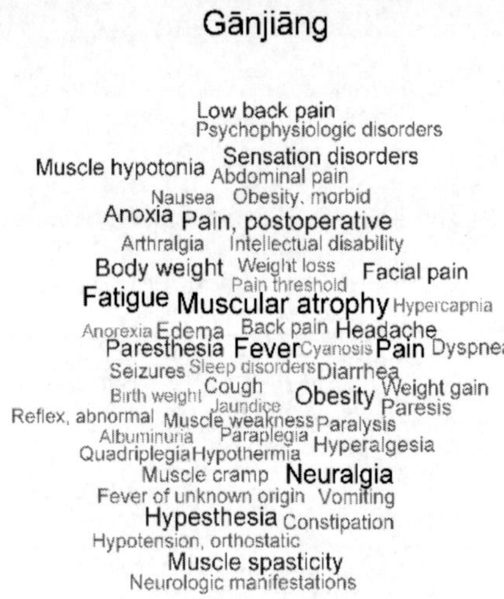

Figure 18.42. Gānjiāng symptom cloud.

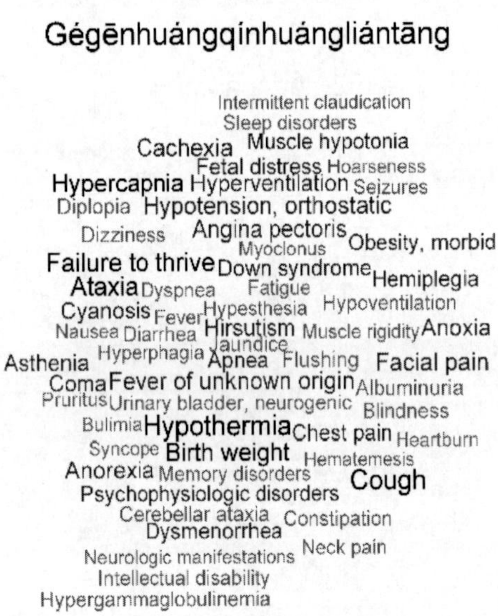

Figure 18.43. Gégēnhuángqínhuángliántāng symptom cloud.

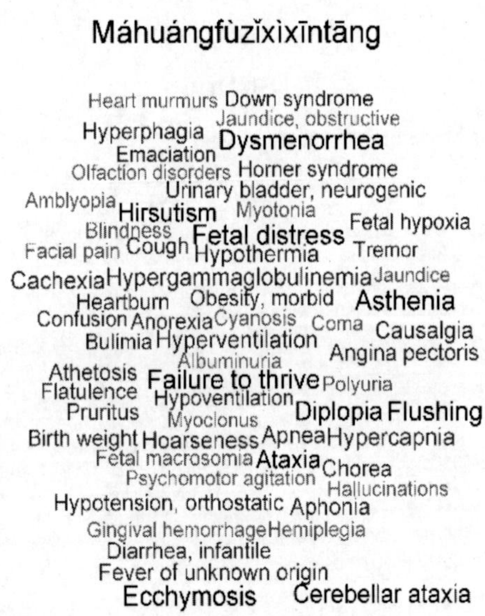

Figure 18.44. Máhuángfùzǐxìxīntāng symptom cloud.

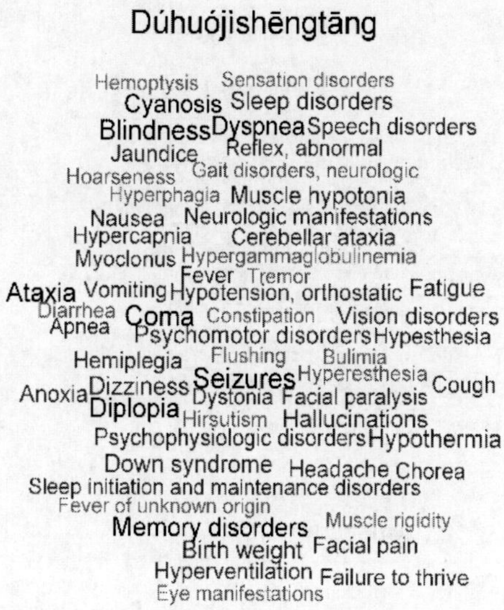

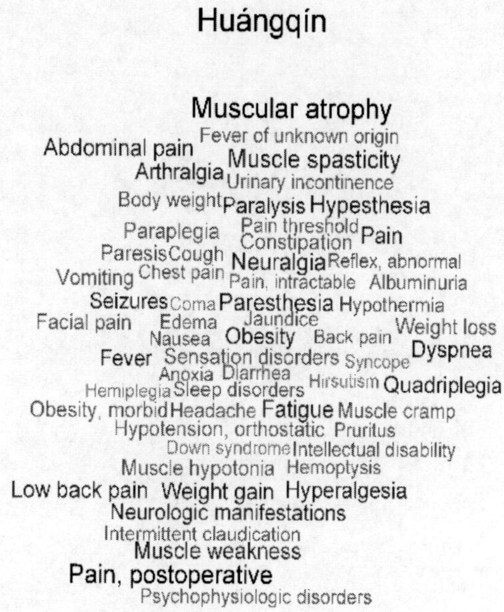

Figure 18.45. Dúhuójìshēngtāng symptom cloud. **Figure 18.46.** Huángqín symptom cloud.

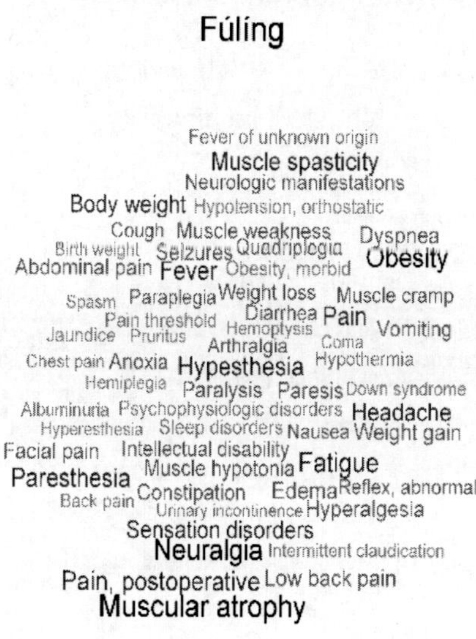

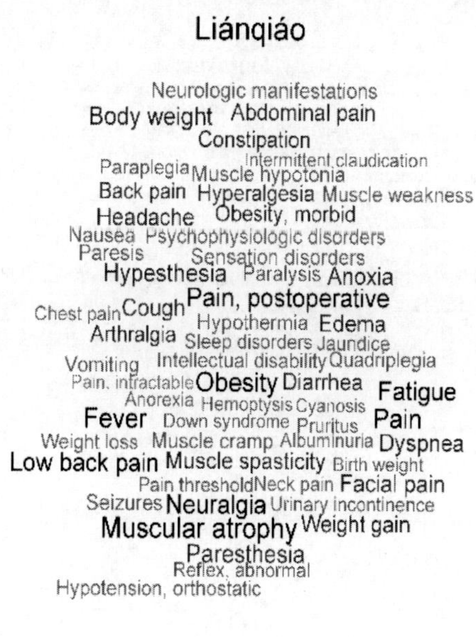

Figure 18.47. Fúlíng symptom cloud. **Figure 18.48.** Liánqiáo symptom cloud.

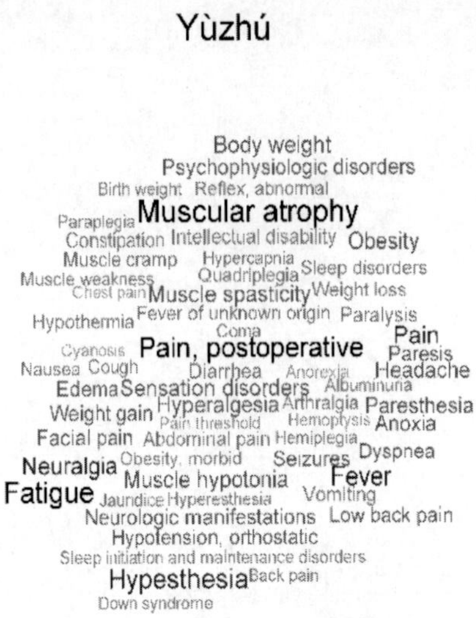

Figure 18.49. Yùzhú symptom cloud.

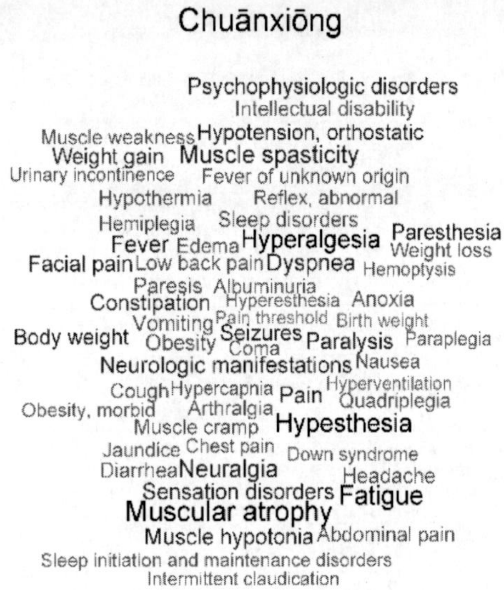

Figure 18.50. Chuānxiōng symptom cloud.

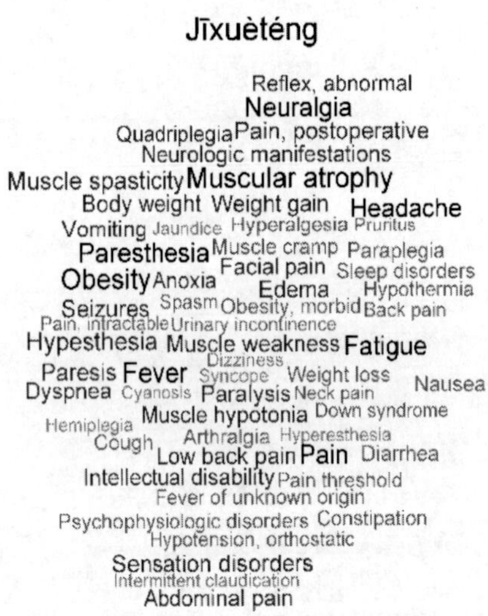

Figure 18.51. Jīxuèténg symptom cloud.

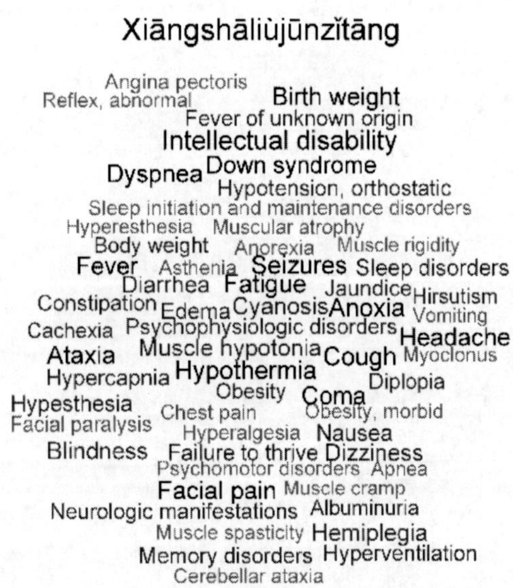

Figure 18.52. Xiāngshāliùjūnzǐtāng symptom cloud.

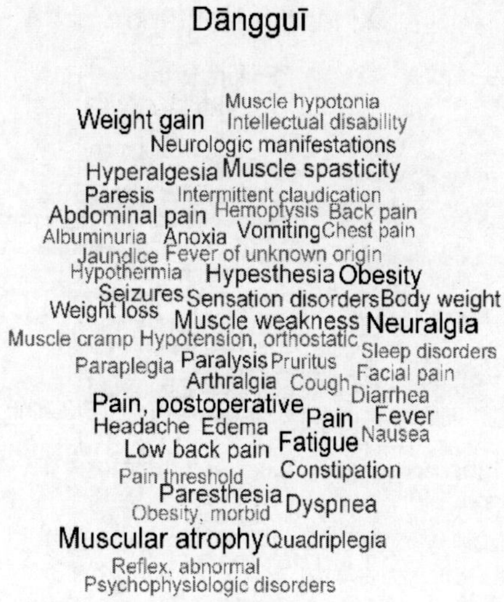

Figure 18.53. Dānguī symptom cloud.

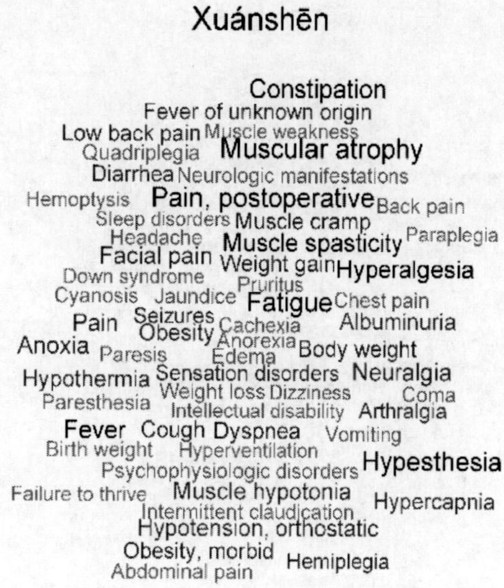

Figure 18.54. Xuánshēn symptom cloud.

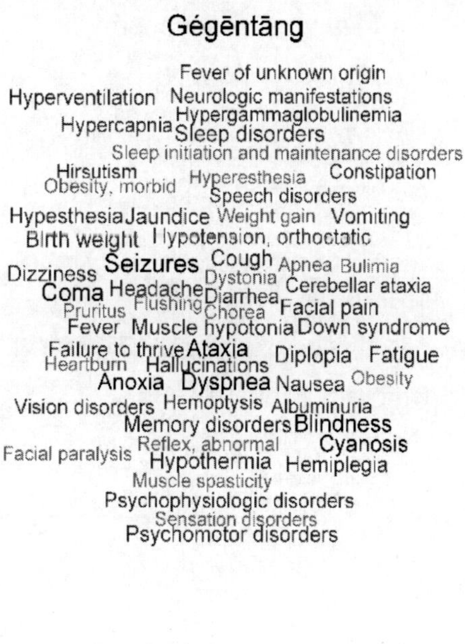

Figure 18.55. Gégēntāng symptom cloud.

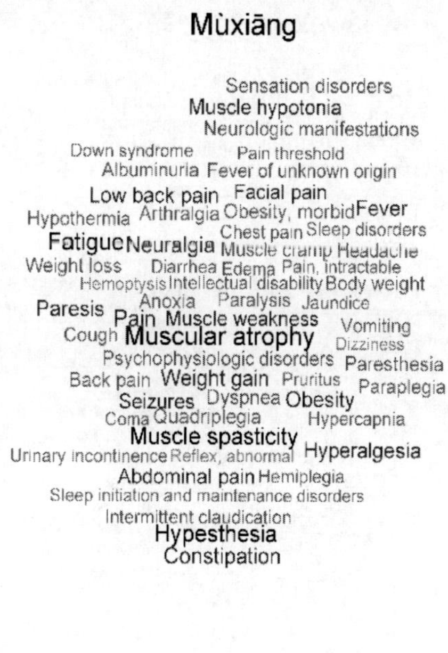

Figure 18.56. Mùxiāng symptom cloud.

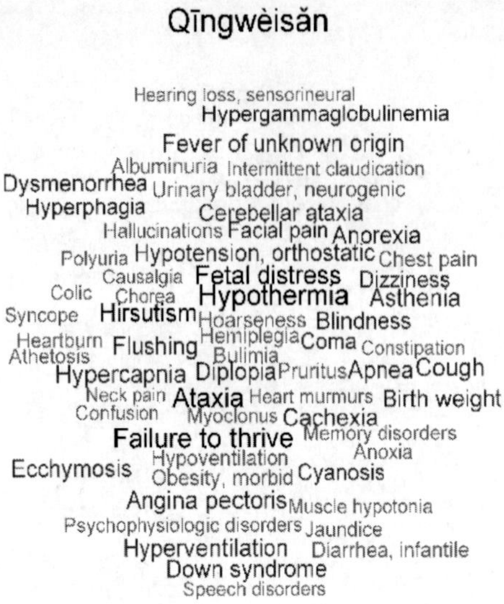

Figure 18.57. Qīngwèisǎn symptom cloud.

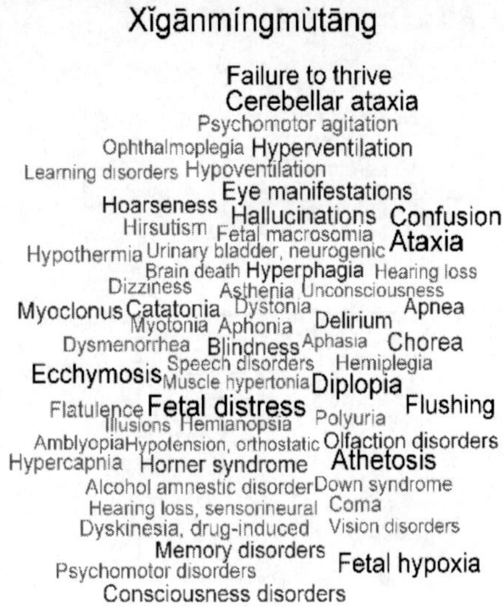

Figure 18.58. Xǐgānmíngmùtāng symptom cloud.

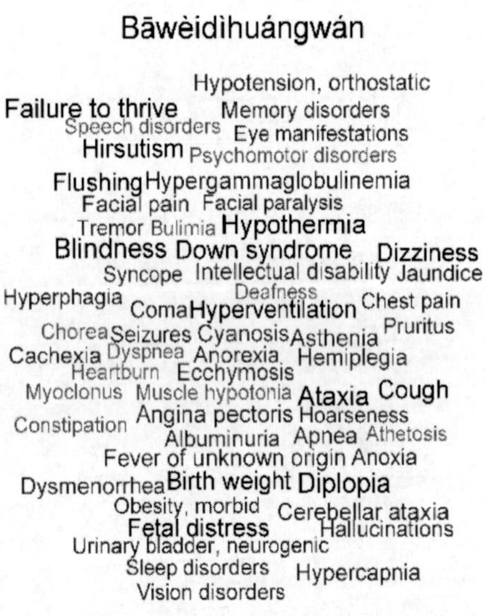

Figure 18.59. Bāwèidìhuángwán symptom cloud.

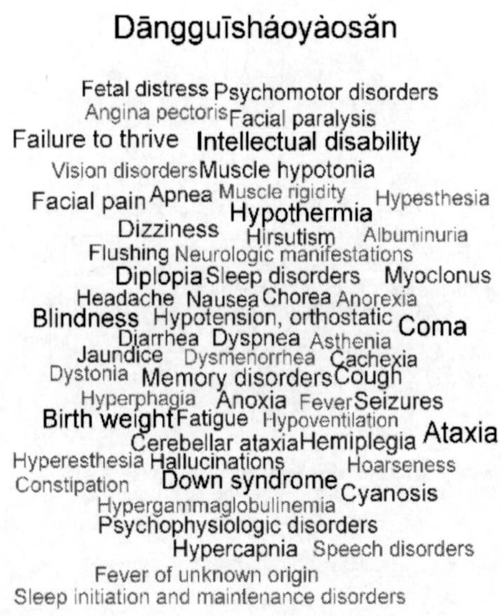

Figure 18.60. Dāngguīsháoyàosǎn symptom cloud.

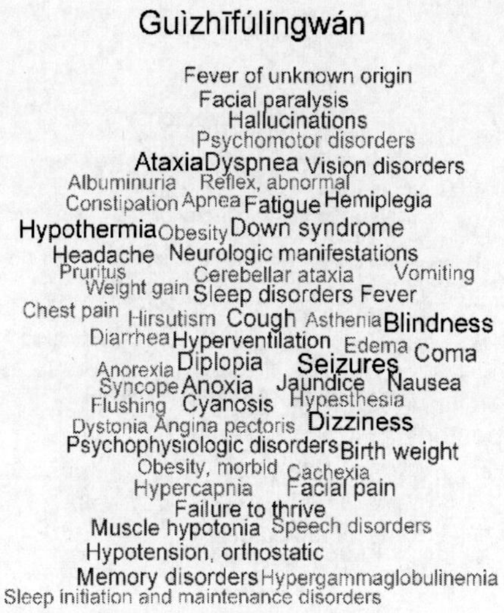

Figure 18.61. Guìzhīfúlíngwán symptom cloud.

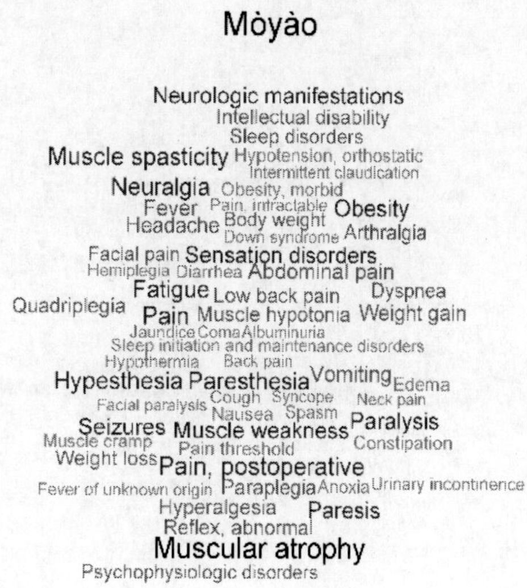

Figure 18.62. Mòyào symptom cloud.

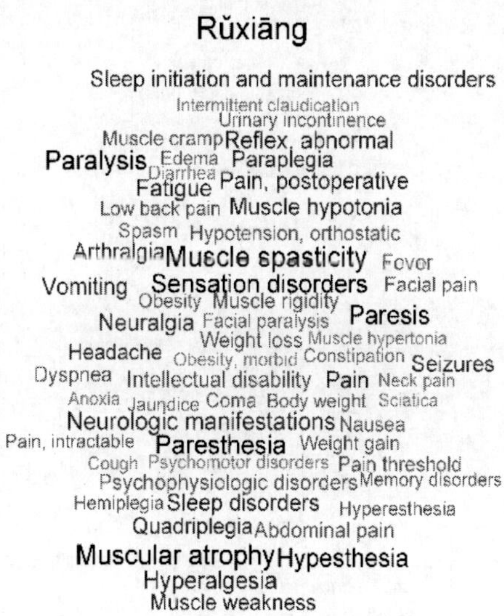

Figure 18.63. Rǔxiāng symptom cloud.

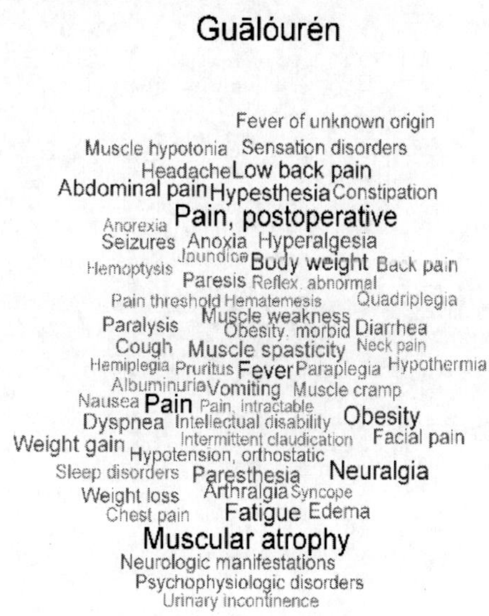

Figure 18.64. Guālóurén symptom cloud.

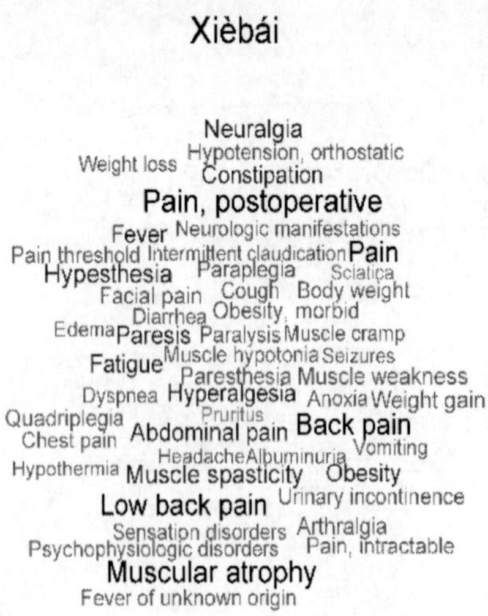

Figure 18.65. Xièbái symptom cloud.

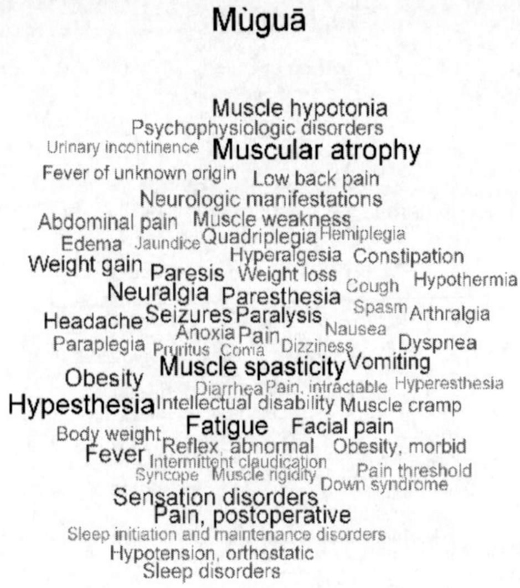

Figure 18.66. Mùguā symptom cloud.

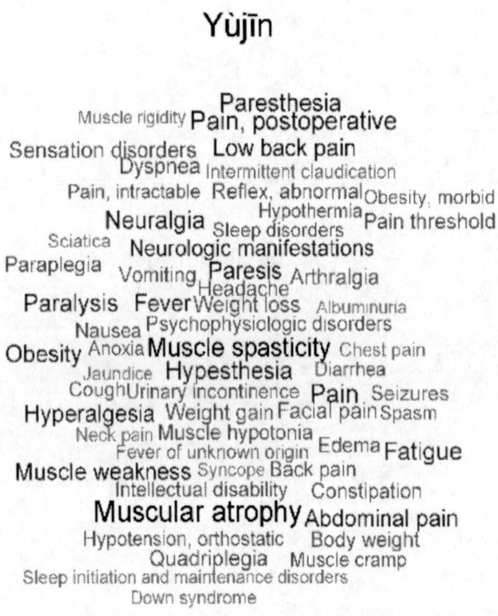

Figure 18.67. Yùjīn symptom cloud.

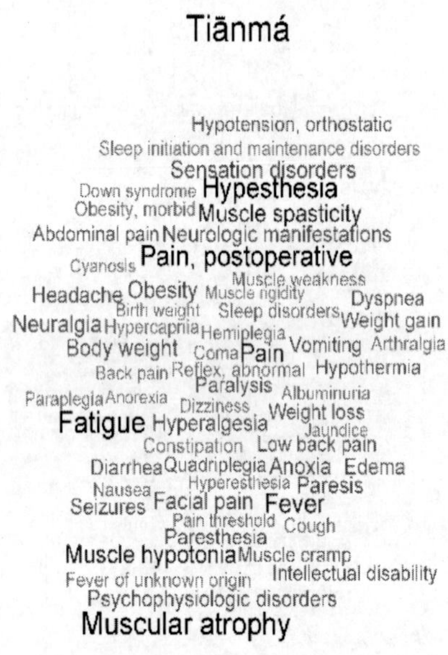

Figure 18.68. Tiānmá symptom cloud.

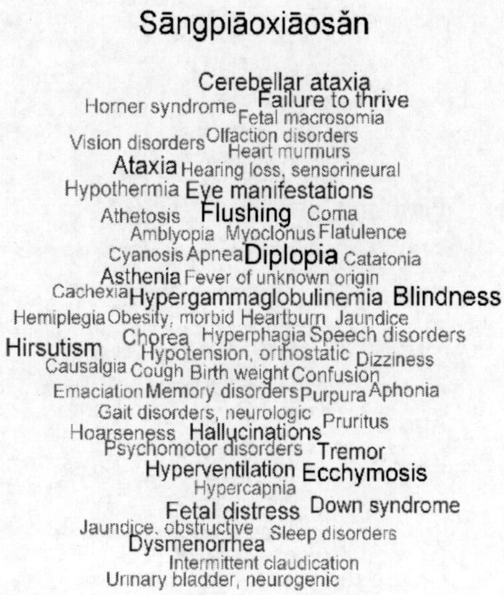

Figure 18.69. Sāngpiāoxiāosǎn symptom cloud.

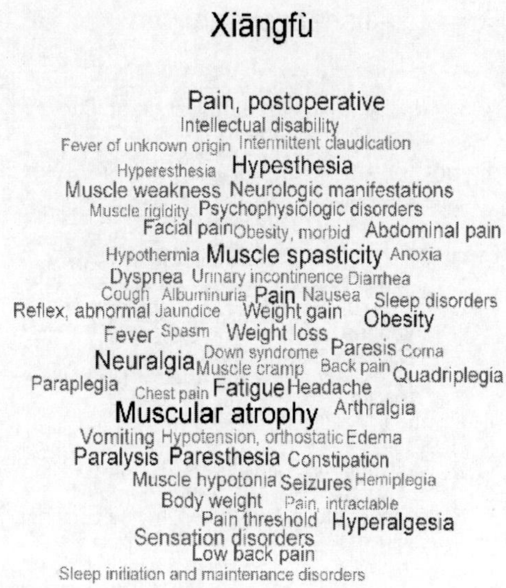

Figure 18.70. Xiāngfù symptom cloud.

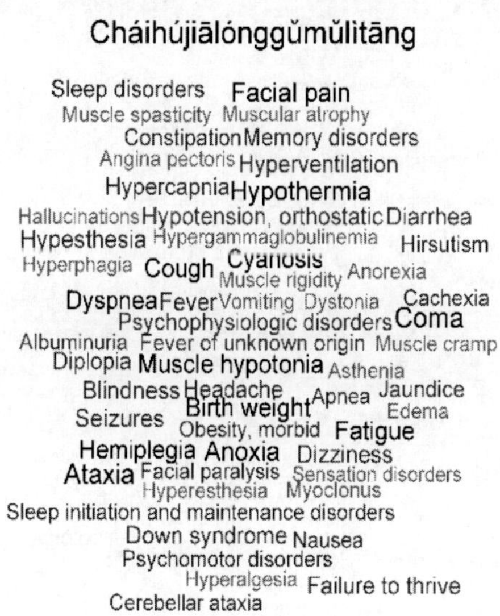

Figure 18.71. Cháihújiālónggǔmǔlìtāng symptom cloud.

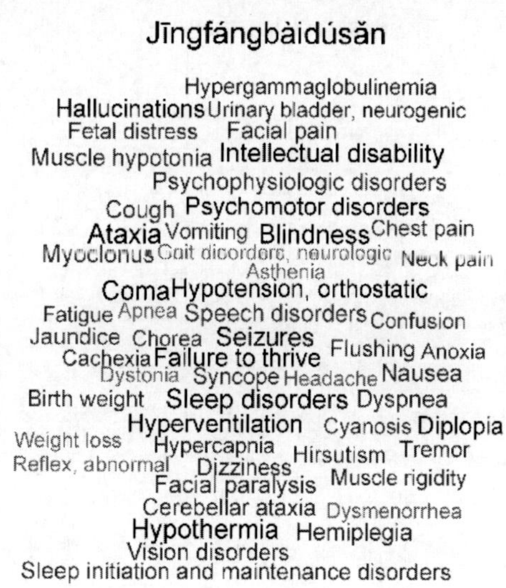

Figure 18.72. Jīngfángbàidúsǎn symptom cloud.

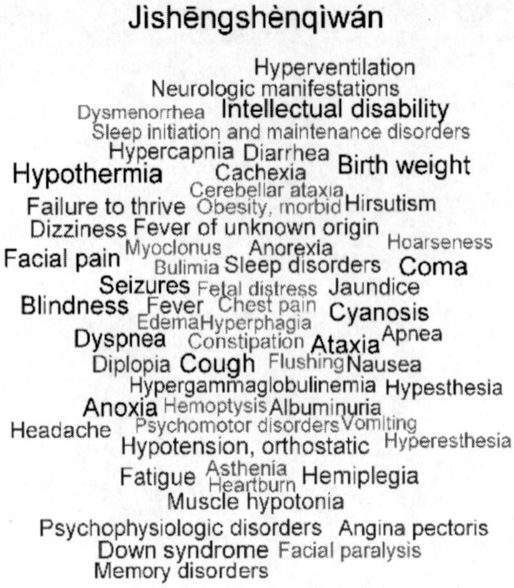

Figure 18.73. Jìshēngshènqìwán symptom cloud.

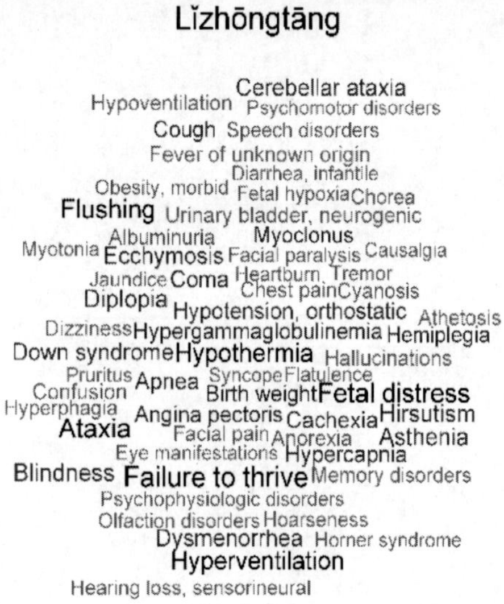

Figure 18.74. Lǐzhōngtāng symptom cloud.

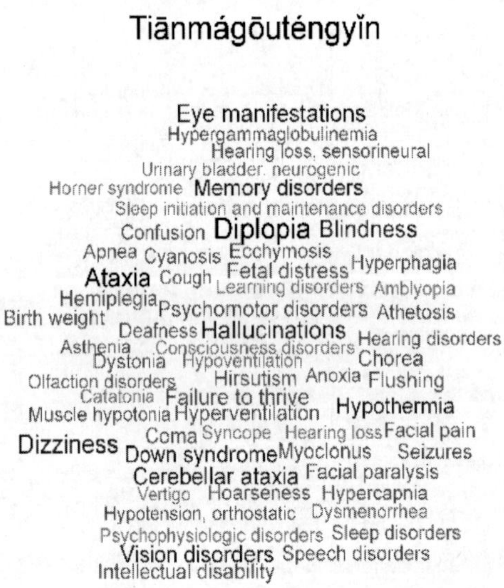

Figure 18.75. Tiānmágōuténgyǐn symptom cloud.

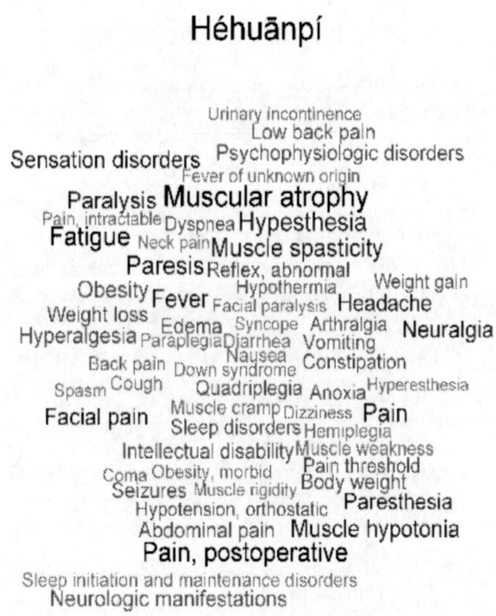

Figure 18.76. Héhuānpí symptom cloud.

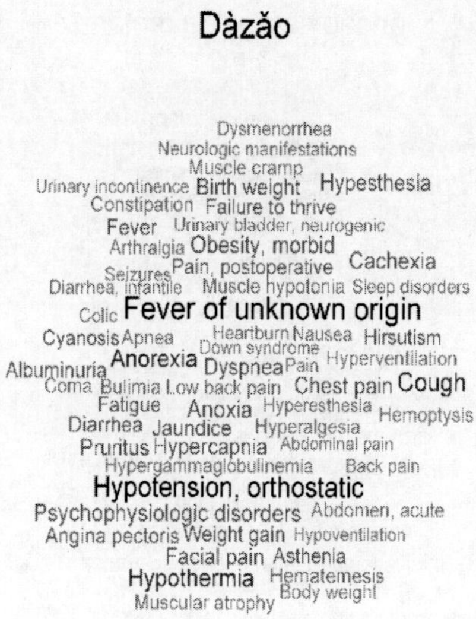

Figure 18.77. Dàzǎo symptom cloud.

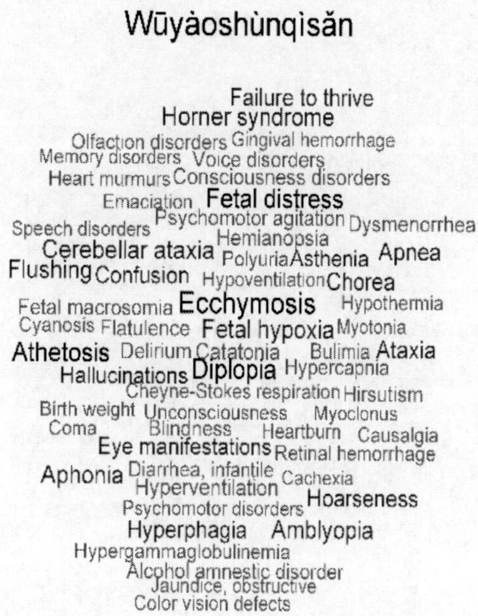

Figure 18.78. Wūyàoshùnqìsǎn symptom cloud.

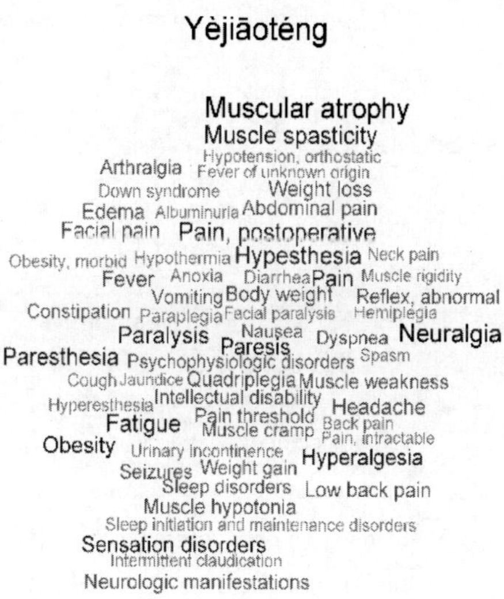

Figure 18.79. Yèjiāoténg symptom cloud.

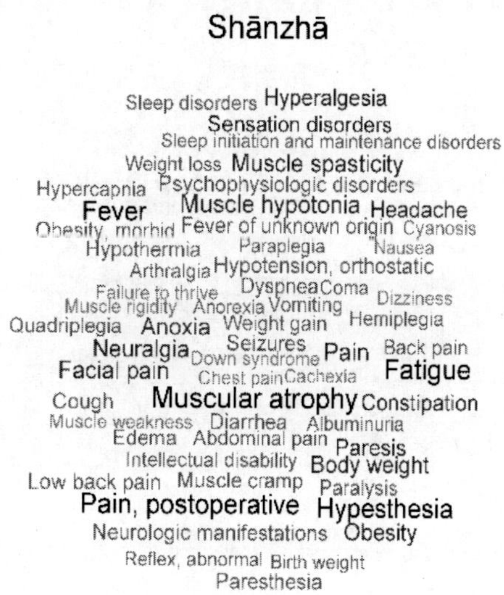

Figure 18.80. Shānzhā symptom cloud.

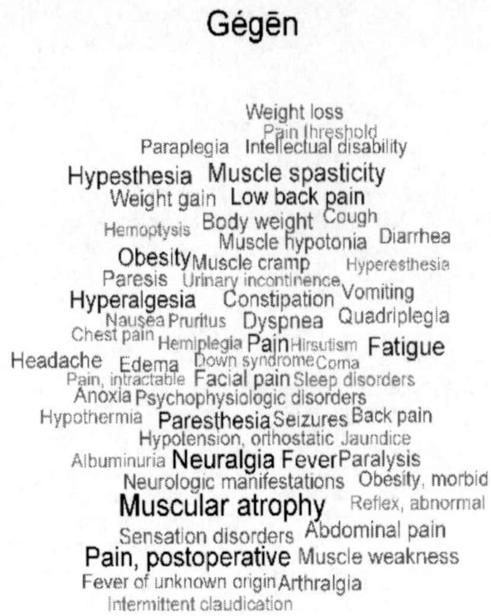

Figure 18.81. Gégēn symptom cloud.

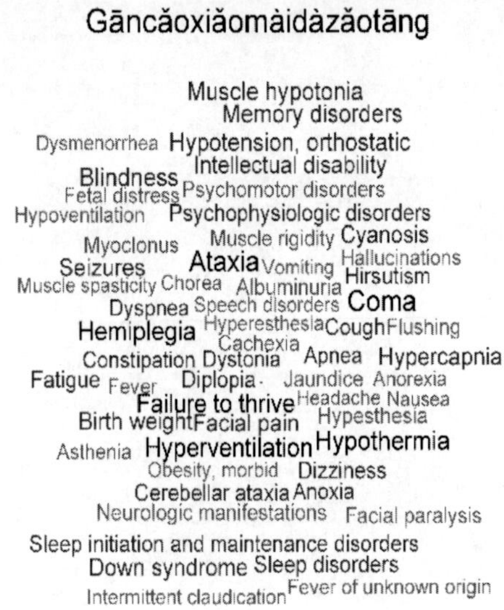

Figure 18.82. Gāncǎoxiǎomàidàzǎotāng symptom cloud.

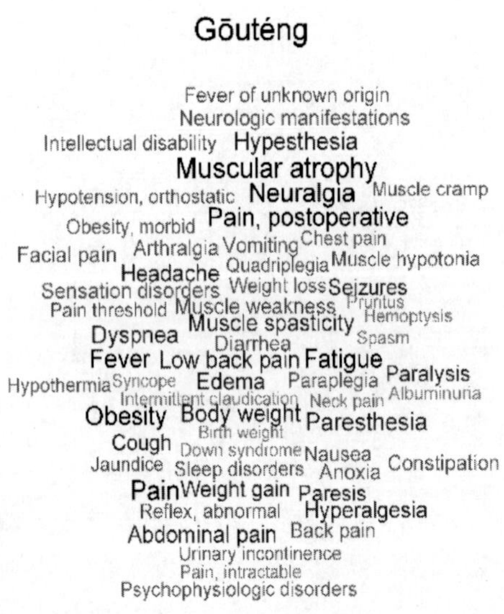

Figure 18.83. Gōuténg symptom cloud.

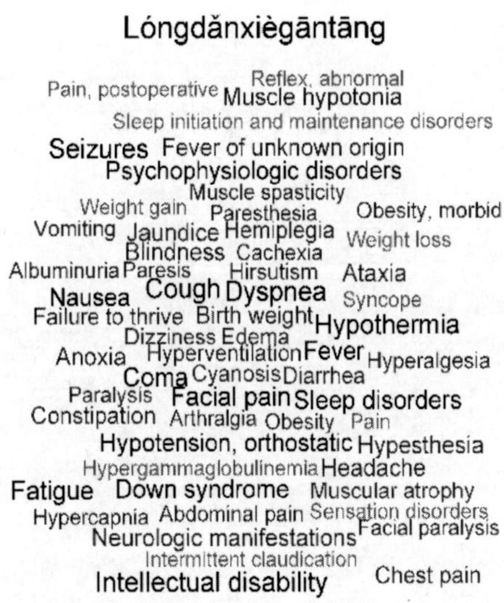

Figure 18.84. Lóngdǎnxiègāntāng symptom cloud.

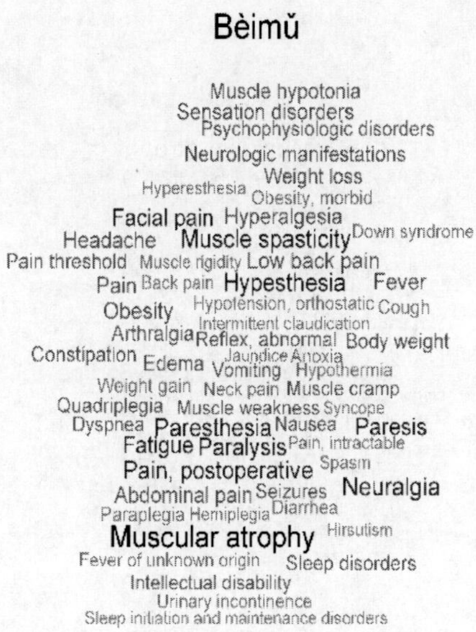

Figure 18.85. Bèimǔ symptom cloud.

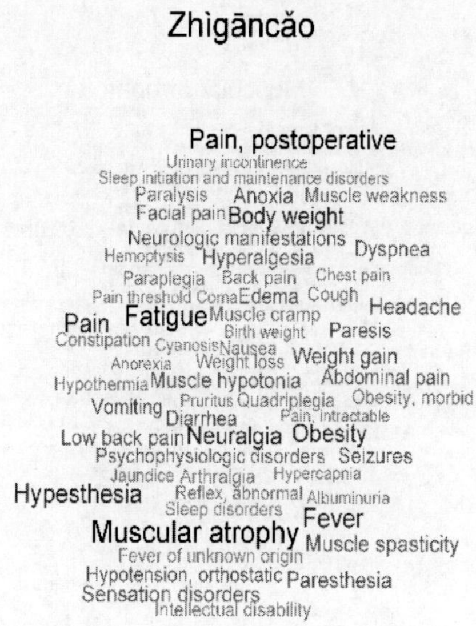

Figure 18.86. Zhìgāncǎo symptom cloud.

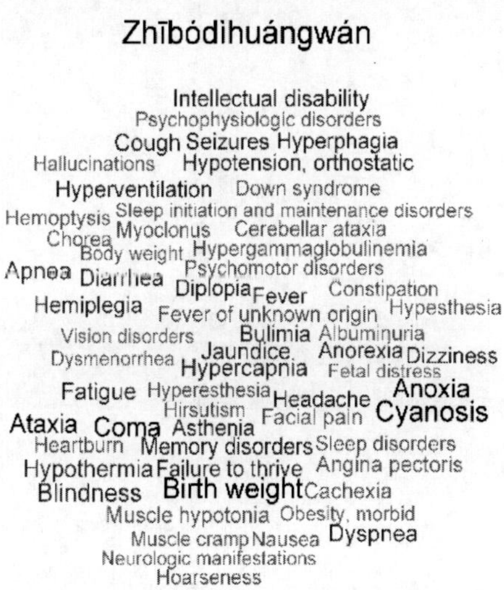

Figure 18.87. Zhībódìhuángwán symptom cloud.

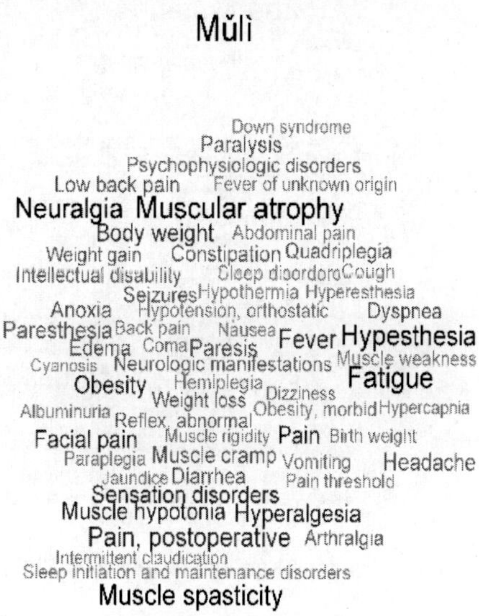

Figure 18.88. Mǔlì symptom cloud.

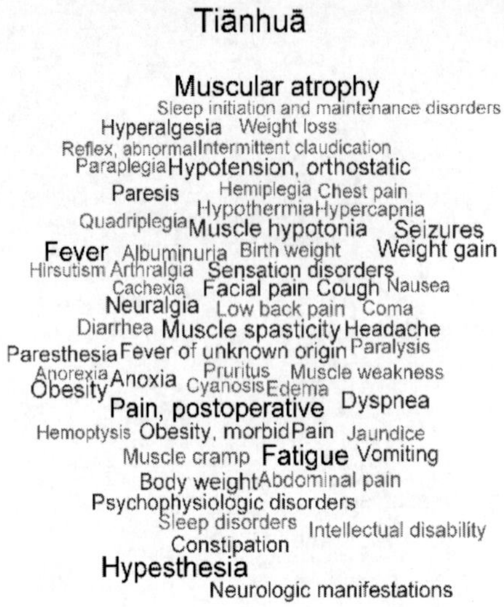

Figure 18.89. Tiānhuā symptom cloud.

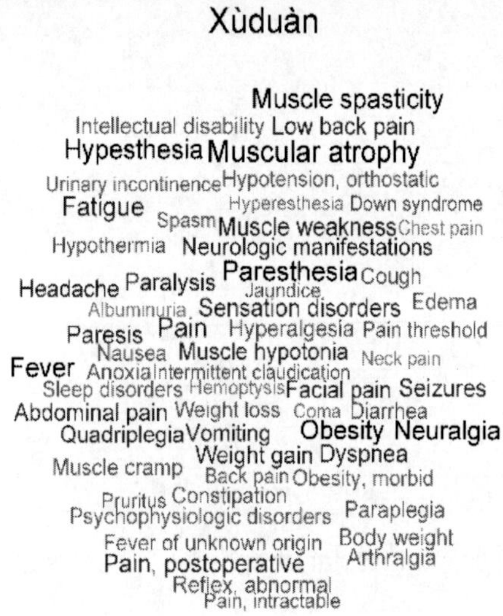

Figure 18.90. Xùduàn symptom cloud.

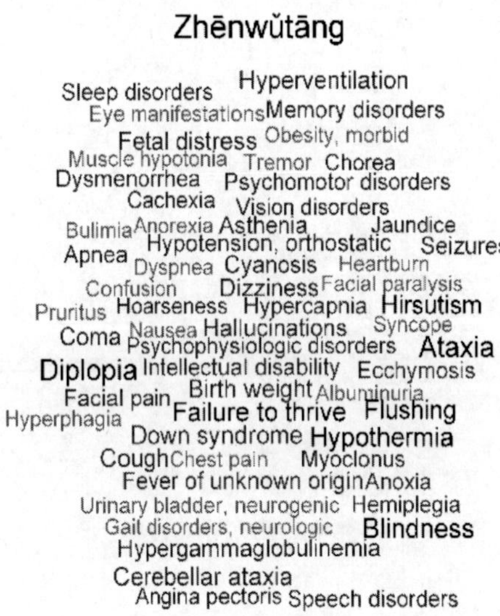

Figure 18.91. Zhēnwǔtāng symptom cloud.

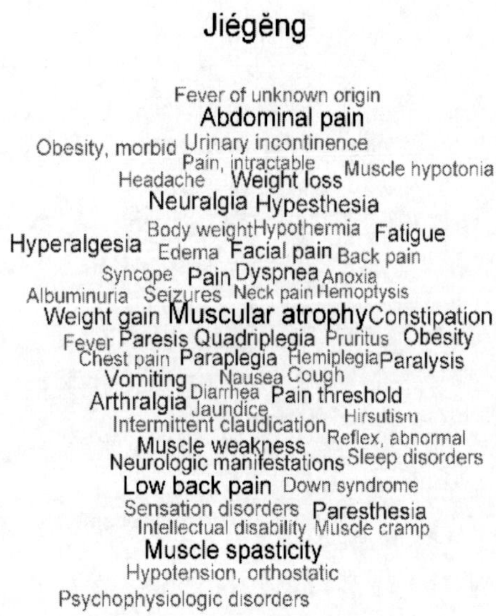

Figure 18.92. Jiégěng symptom cloud.

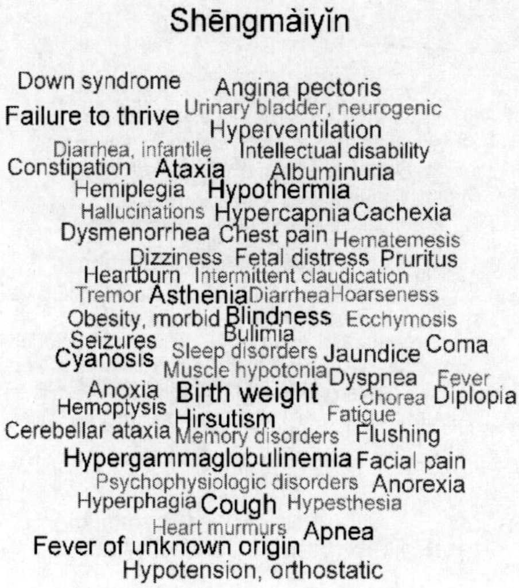

Figure 18.93. Shēngmàiyǐn symptom cloud.

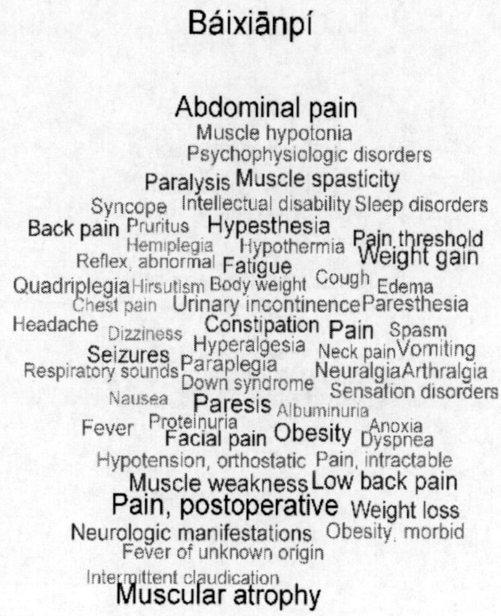

Figure 18.94. Báixiānpí symptom cloud.

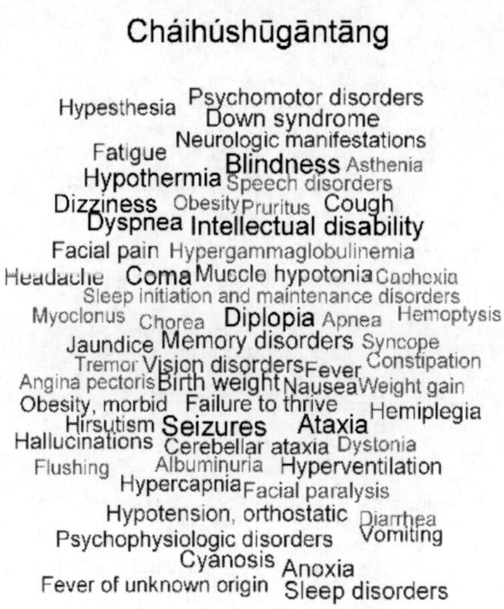

Figure 18.95. Cháihúshūgāntāng symptom cloud.

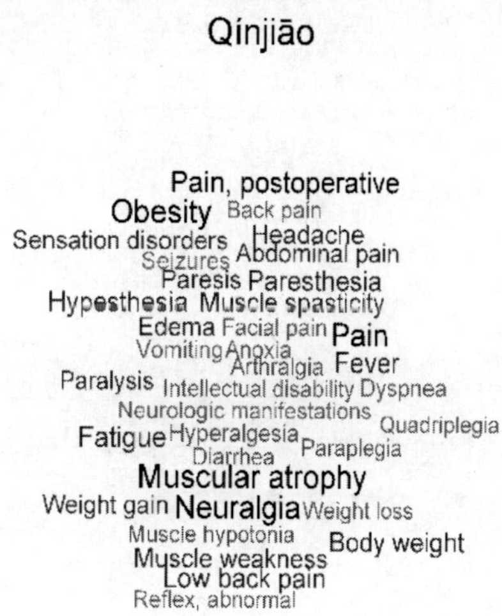

Figure 18.96. Qínjiāo symptom cloud.

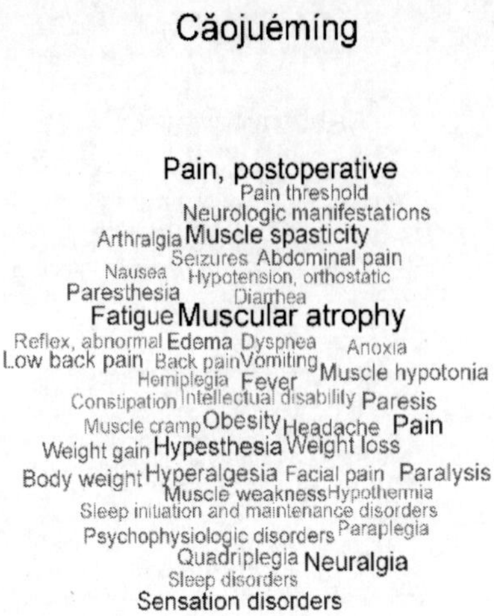

Figure 18.97. Cǎojuémíng symptom cloud.

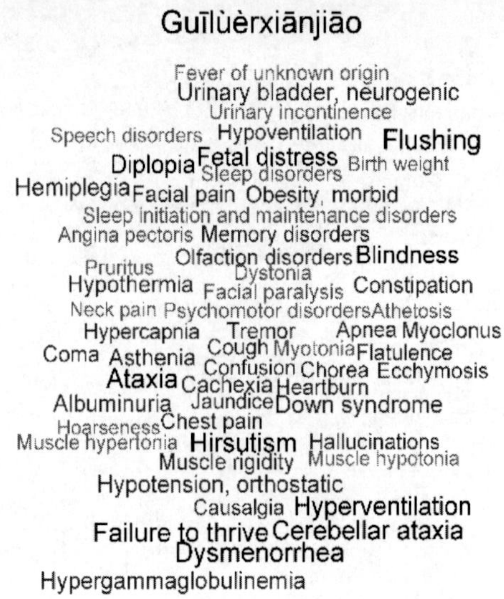

Figure 18.98. Guīlùèrxiānjiāo symptom cloud.

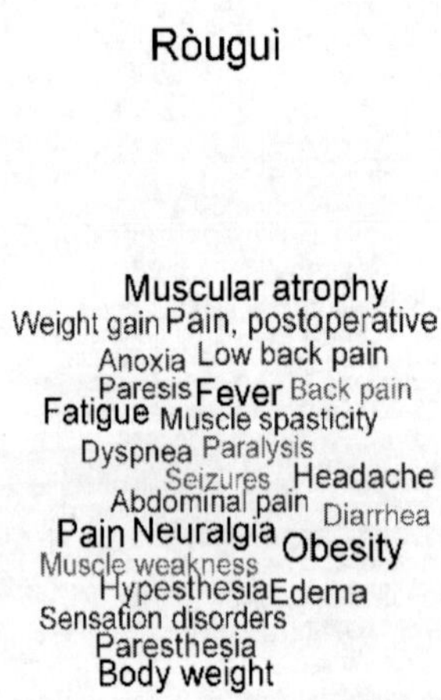

Figure 18.99. Ròuguì symptom cloud.

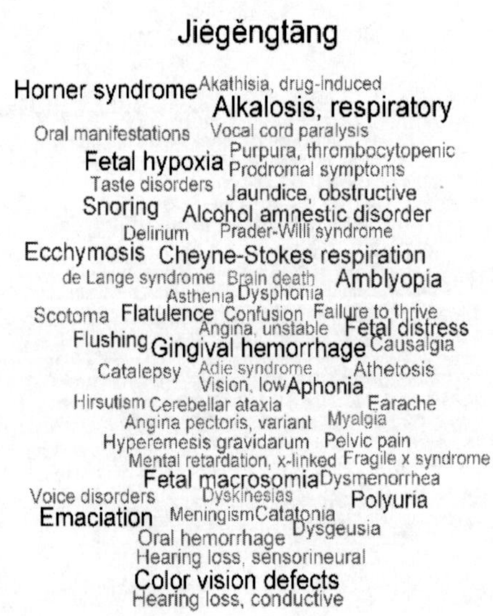

Figure 18.100. Jiégěngtāng symptom cloud.

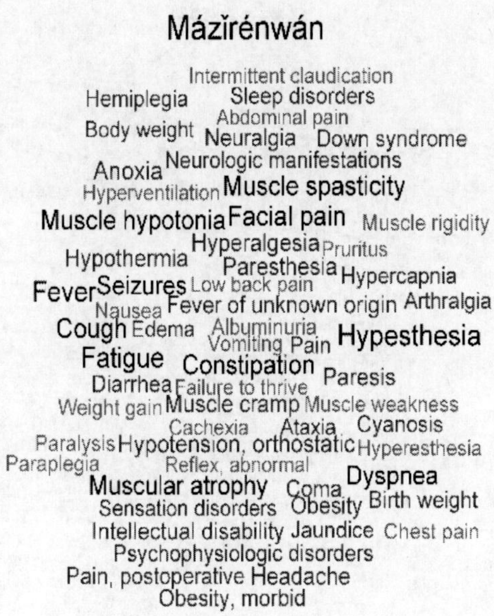

Figure 18.101. Mázǐrénwán symptom cloud.

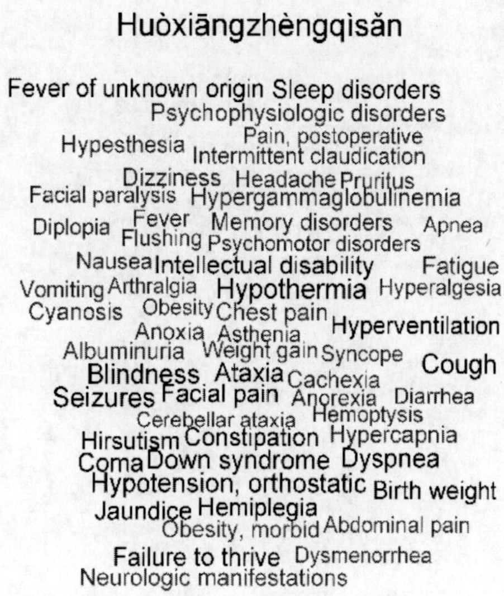

Figure 18.102. Huòxiāngzhèngqìsǎn symptom cloud.

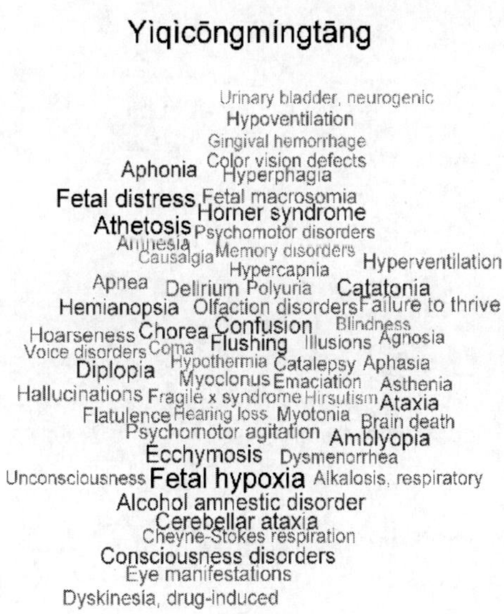

Figure 18.103. Yìqìcōngmíngtāng symptom cloud.

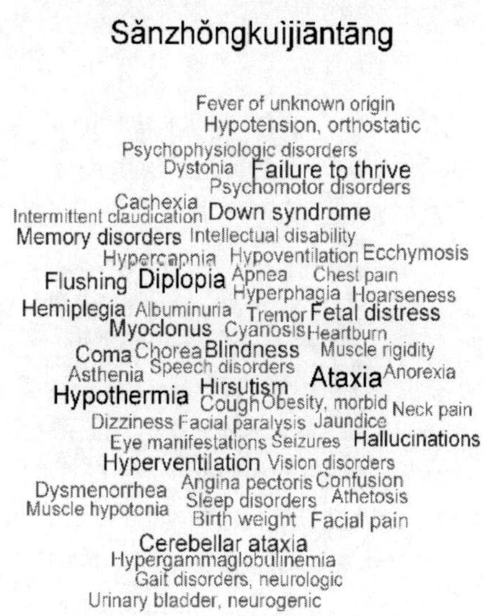

Figure 18.104. Sǎnzhǒngkuìjiāntāng symptom cloud.

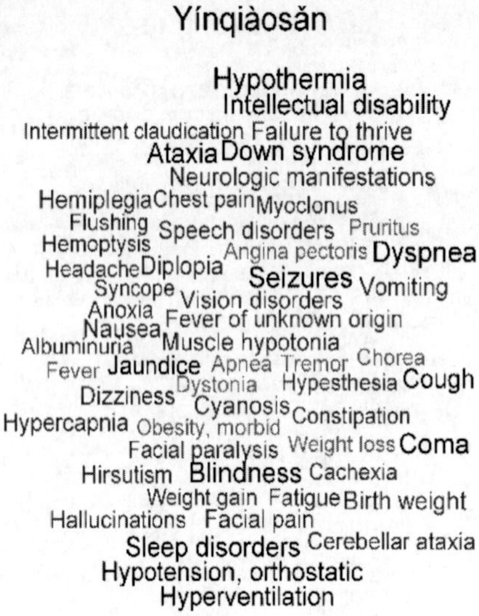

Figure 18.105. Yínqiàosǎn symptom cloud.

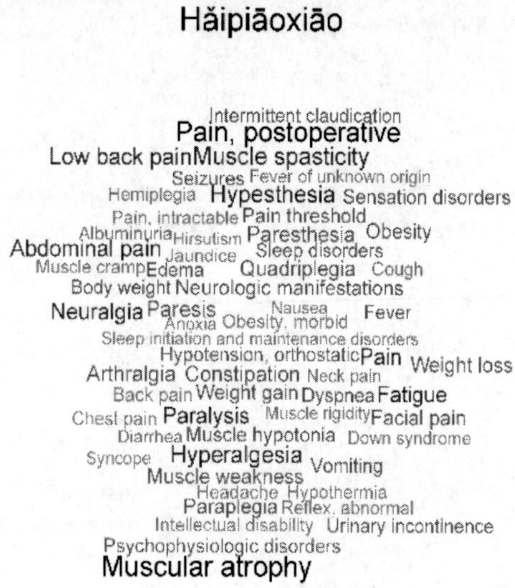

Figure 18.106 .Hǎipiāoxiāo symptom cloud.

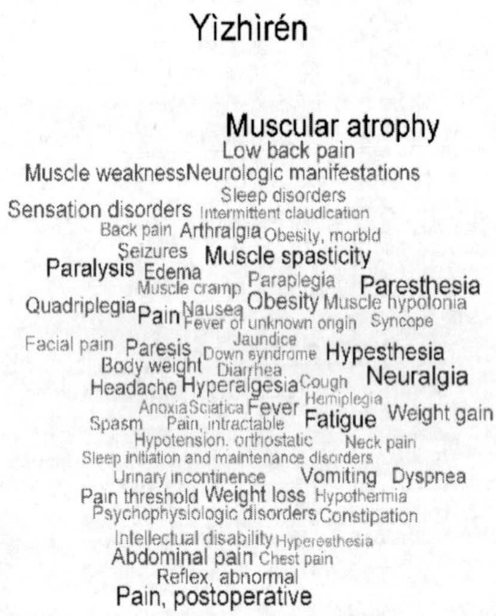

Figure 18.107. Yìzhìrén symptom cloud.

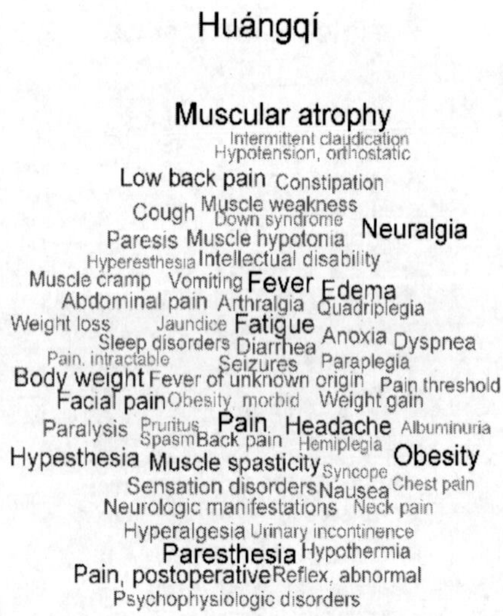

Figure 18.108. Huángqí symptom cloud.

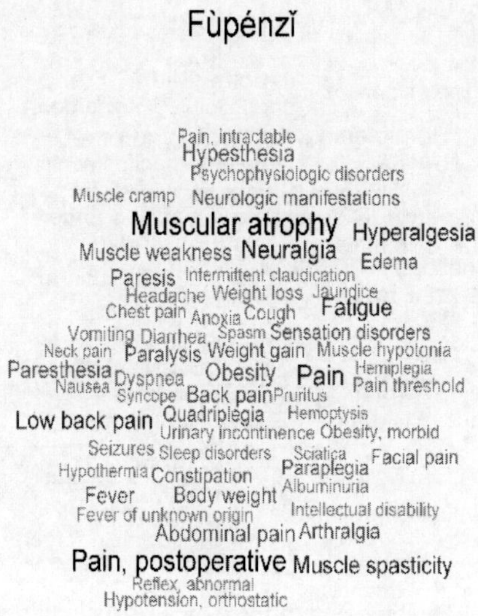

Figure 18.109. Fùpénzǐ symptom cloud.

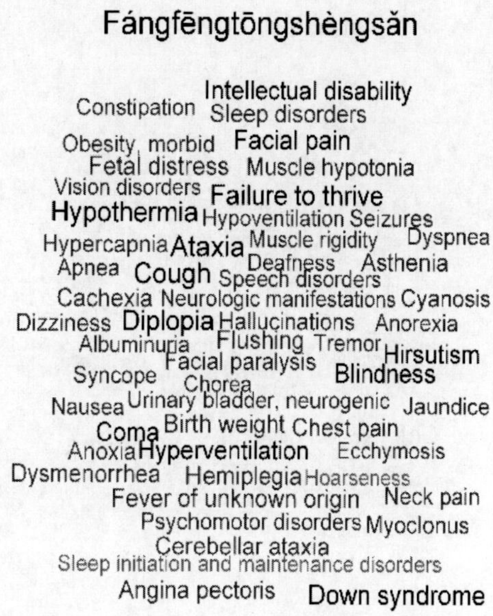

Figure 18.110. Fángfēngtōngshèngsǎn symptom cloud.

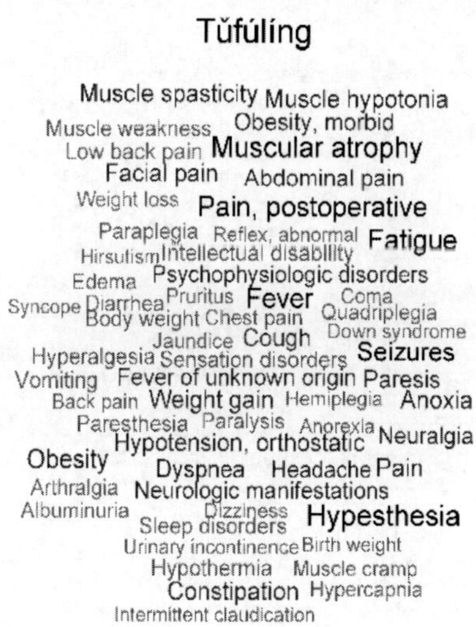

Figure 18.111. Tǔfúlíng symptom cloud.

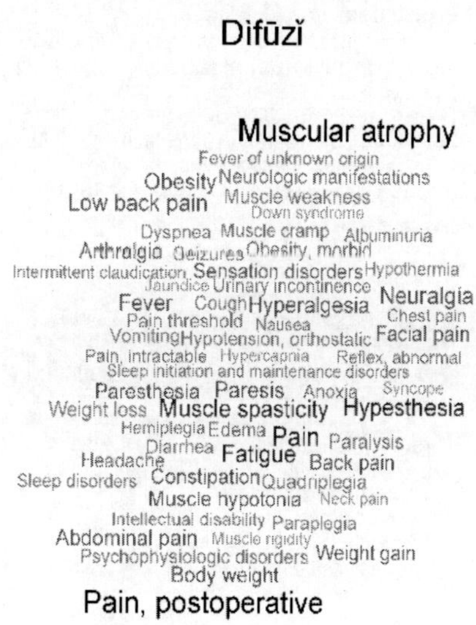

Figure 18.112. Dìfūzǐ symptom cloud.

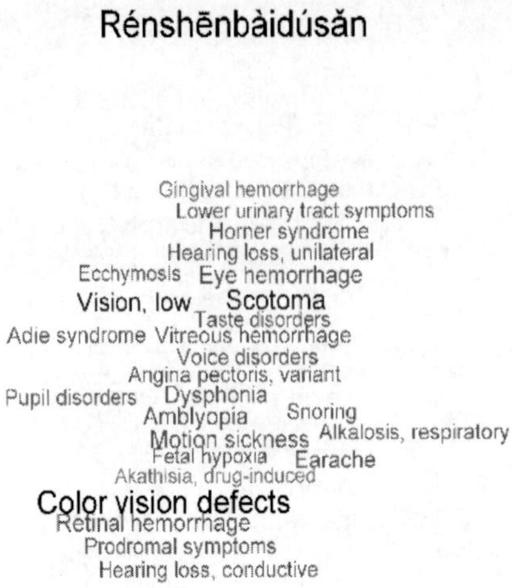

Figure 18.113. Rénshēnbàidúsǎn symptom cloud.

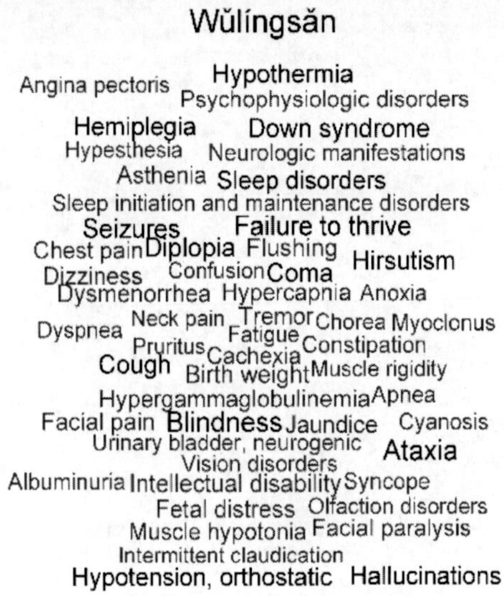

Figure 18.114. Wǔlíngsǎn symptom cloud.

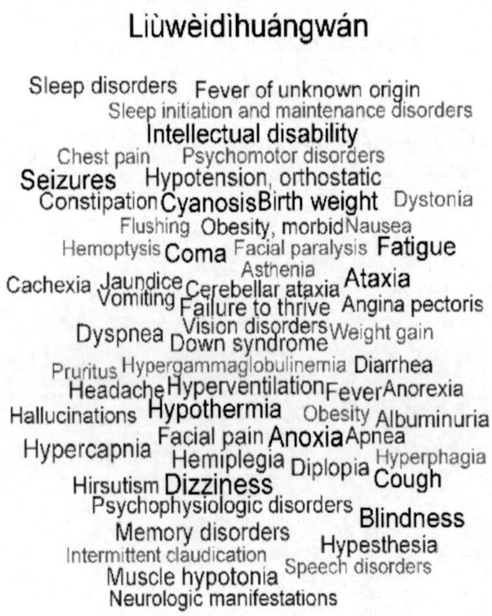

Figure 18.115. Liùwèidìhuángwán symptom cloud.

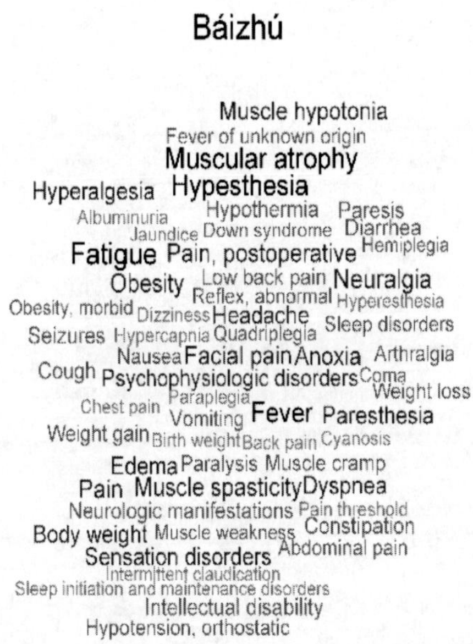

Figure 18.116. Báizhú symptom cloud.

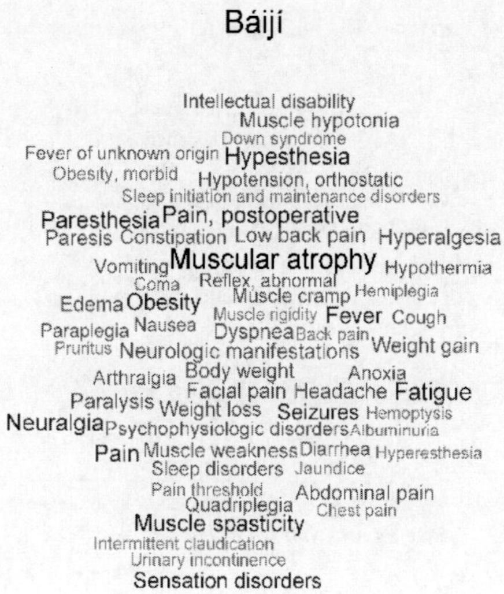

Figure 18.117. Báijí symptom cloud.

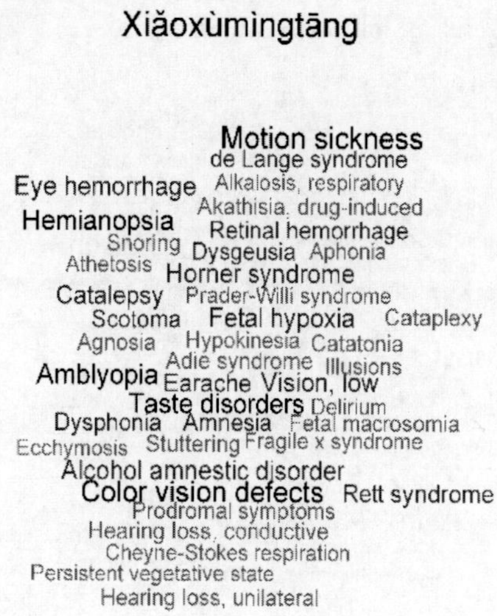

Figure 18.118 .Xiǎoxùmìngtāng symptom cloud.

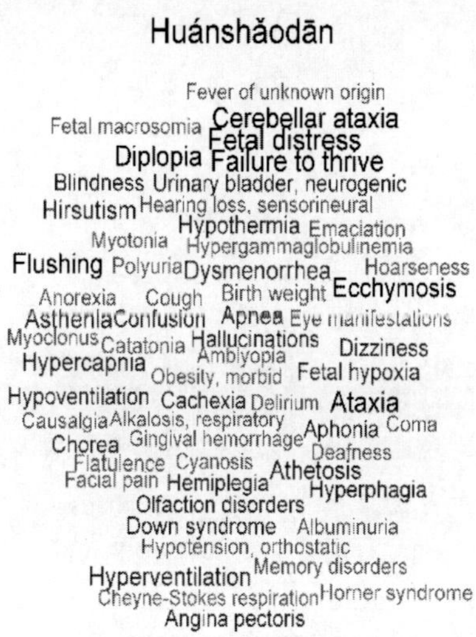

Figure 18.119. Huánshǎodān symptom cloud.

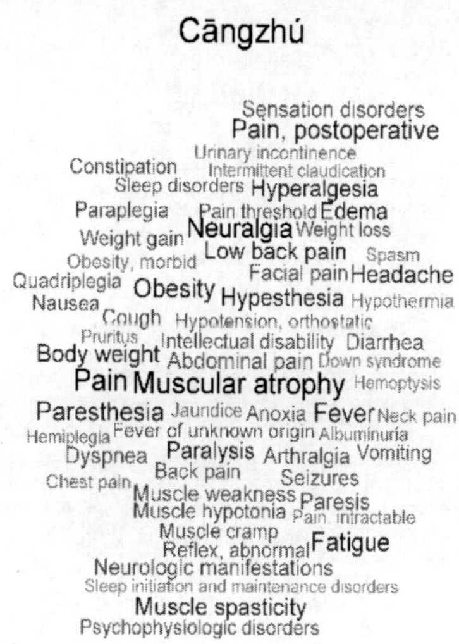

Figure 18.120. Cāngzhú symptom cloud.

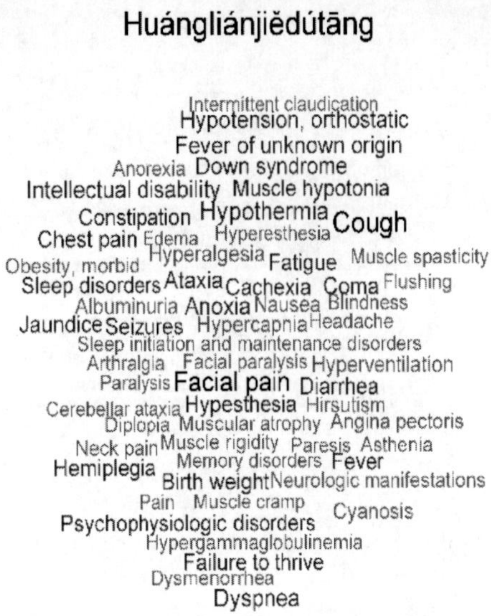

Figure 18.121. Huángliánjiědútāng symptom cloud.

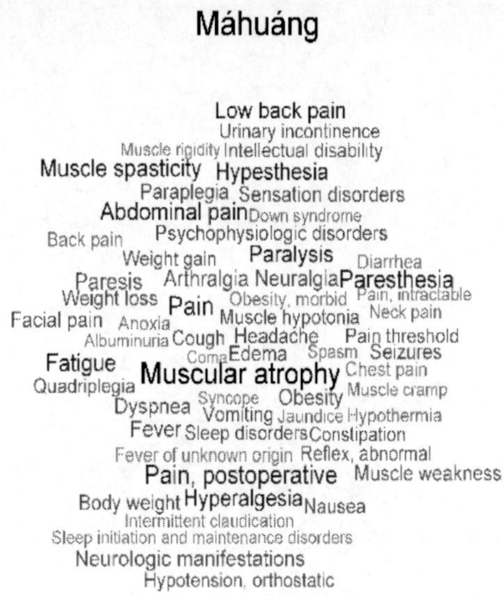

Figure 18.122. Máhuáng symptom cloud.

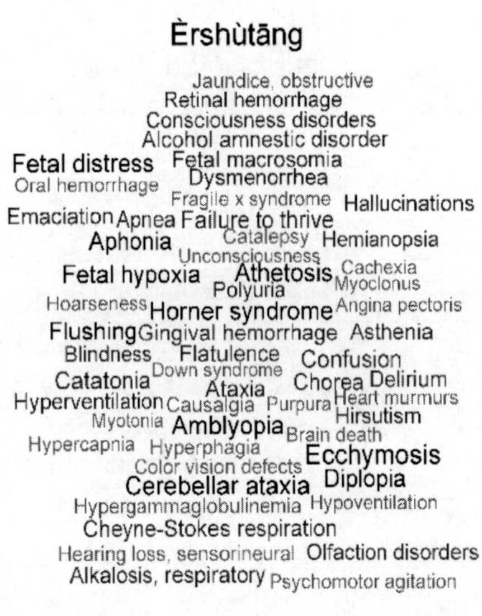

Figure 18.123. Èrshùtāng symptom cloud.

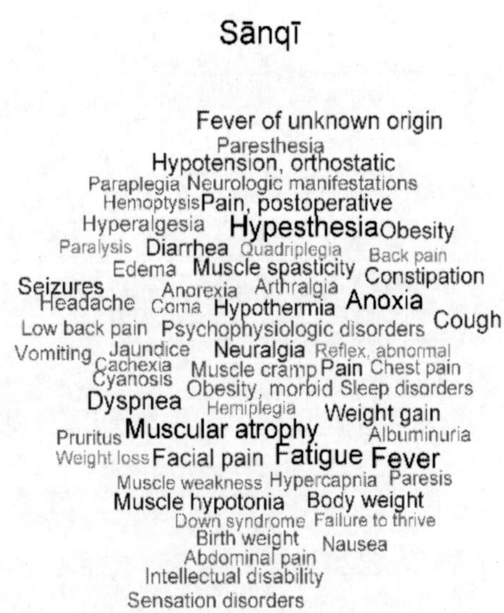

Figure 18.124. Sānqī symptom cloud.

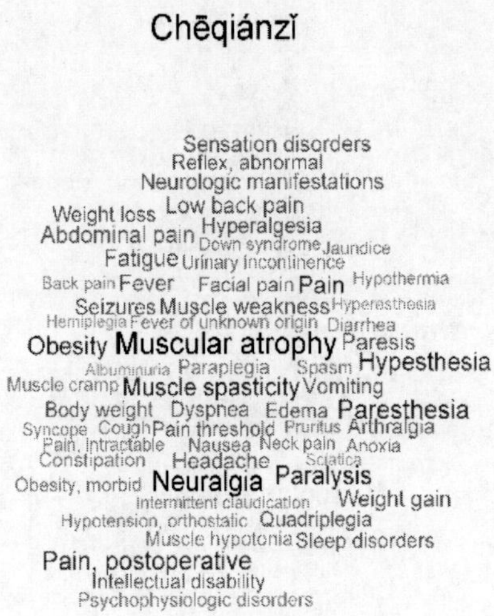

Figure 18.125. Chēqiánzǐ symptom cloud.

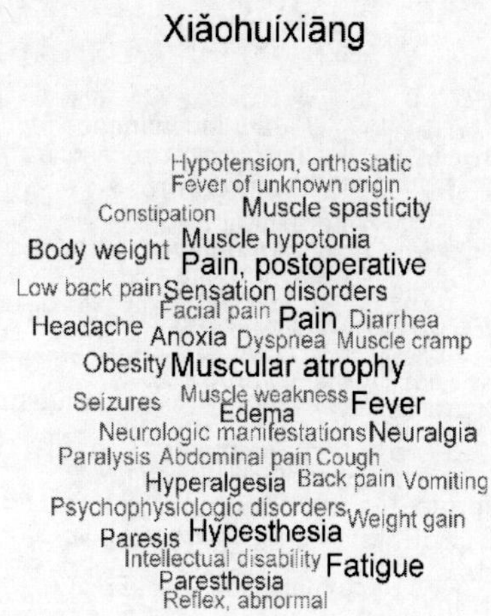

Figure 18.126. Xiǎohuíxiāng symptom cloud.

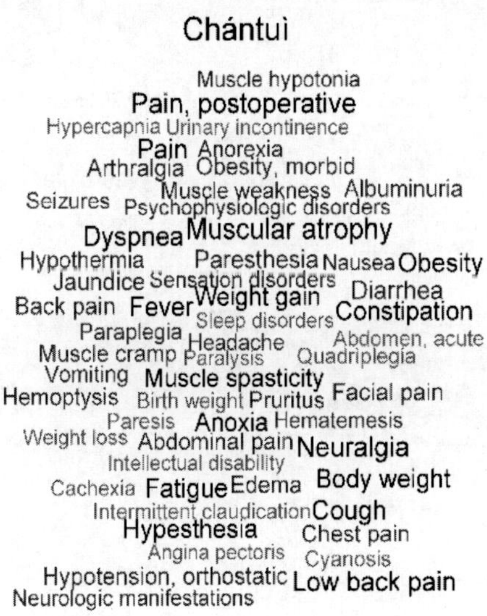

Figure 18.127. Chántuì symptom cloud.

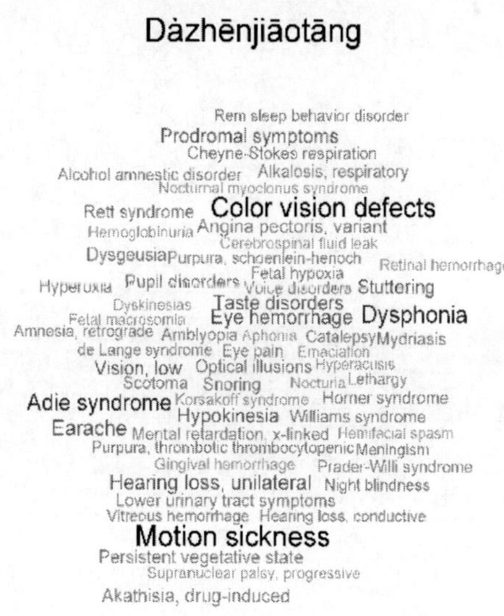

Figure 18.128. Dàzhēnjiāotāng symptom cloud.

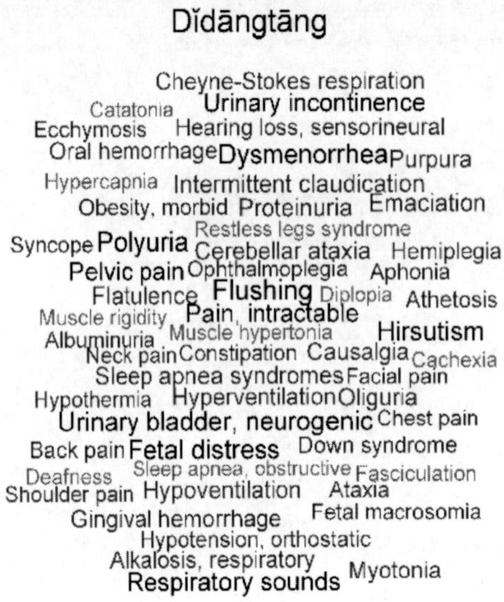

Figure 18.129. Dĭdāngtāng symptom cloud.

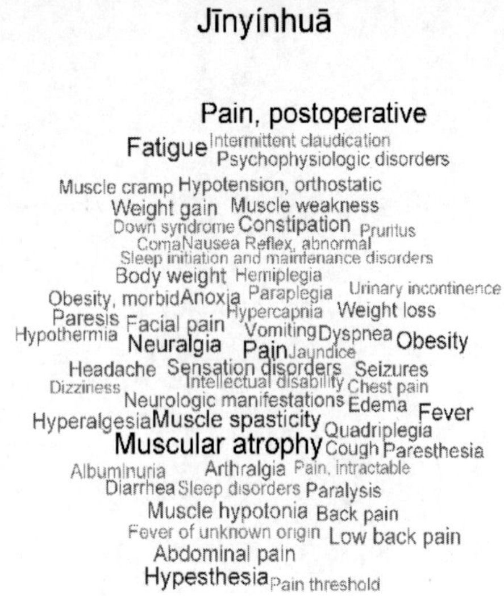

Figure 18.130. Jīnyínhuā symptom cloud.

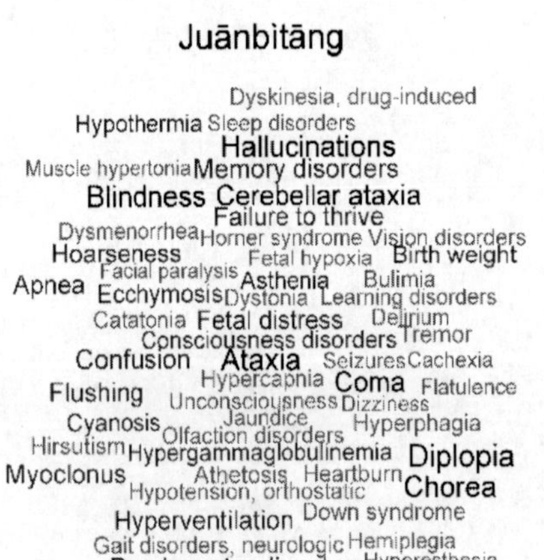

Figure 18.131. Juānbìtāng symptom cloud.

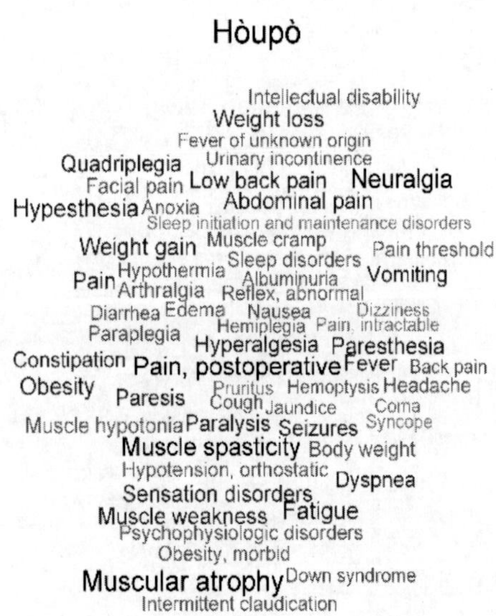

Figure 18.132. Hòupò symptom cloud.

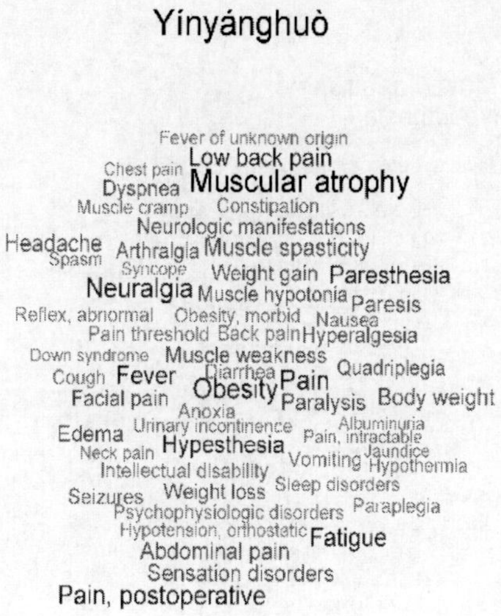

Figure 18.133. Yínyánghuò symptom cloud.

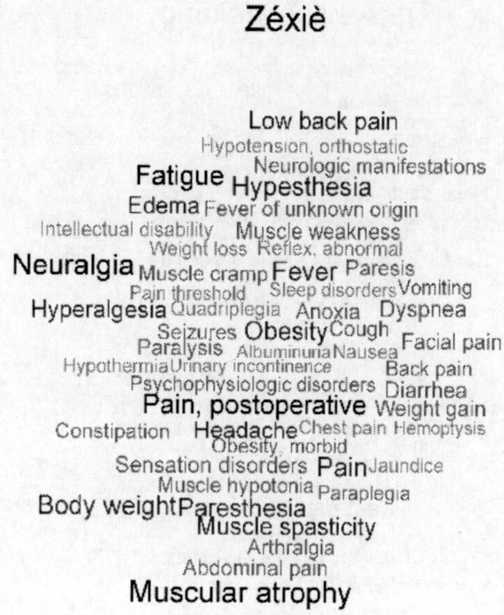

Figure 18.134. Zéxiè symptom cloud.

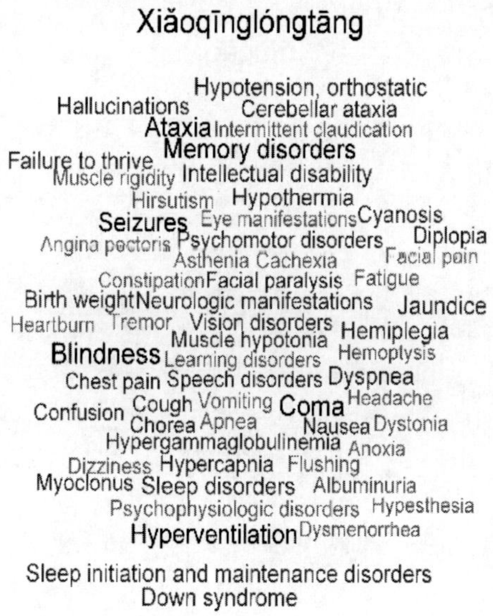

Figure 18.135. Xiǎoqīnglóngtāng symptom cloud.

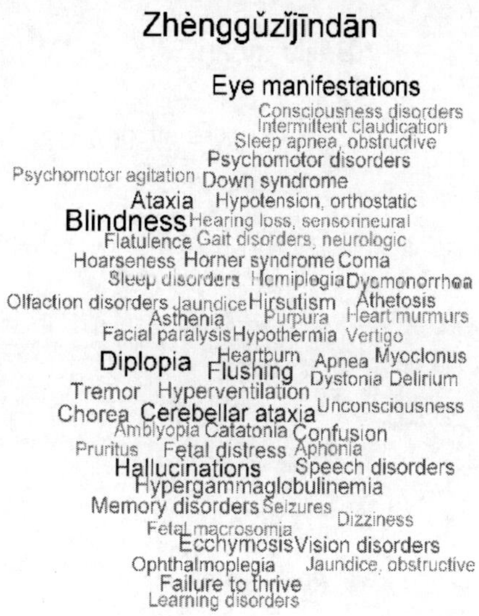

Figure 18.136. Zhènggǔzǐjīndān symptom cloud.

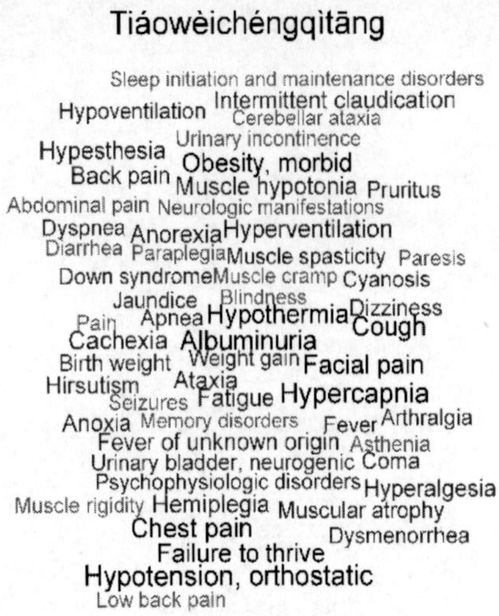

Figure 18.137. Tiáowèichéngqìtāng symptom cloud.

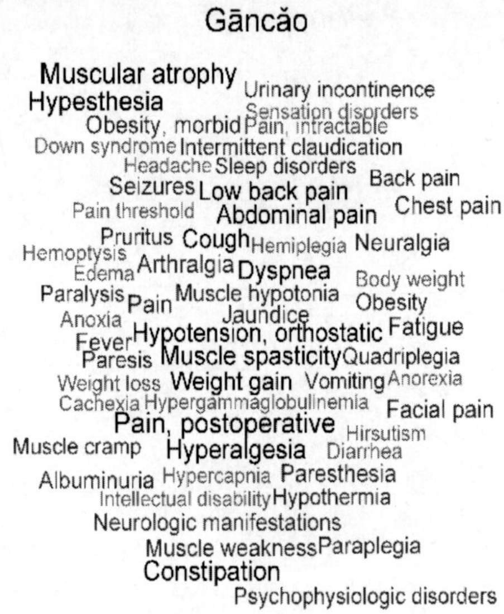

Figure 18.138. Gāncǎo symptom cloud.

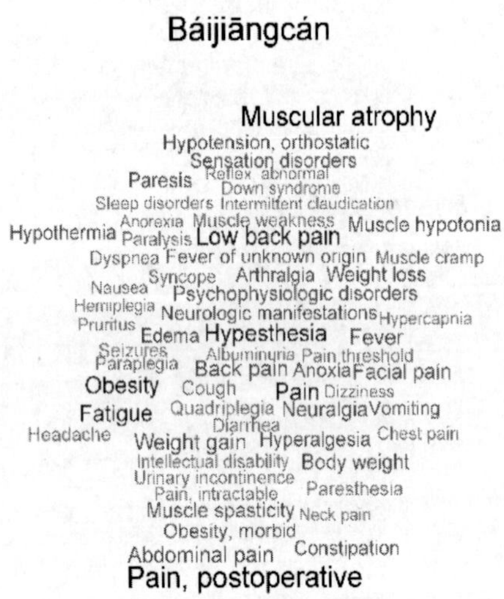

Figure 18.139. Báijiāngcán symptom cloud.

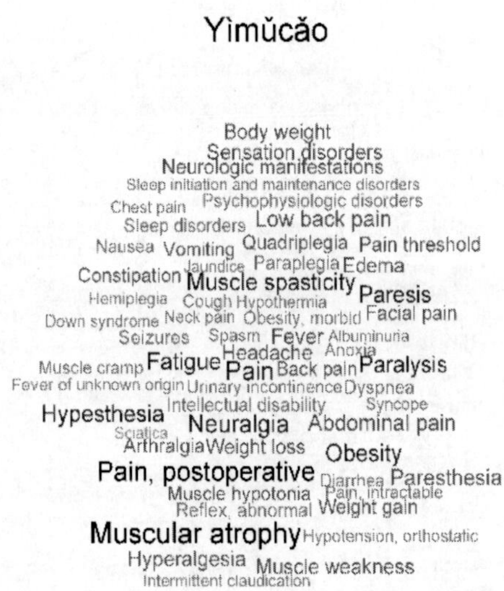

Figure 18.140. Yìmǔcǎo symptom cloud.

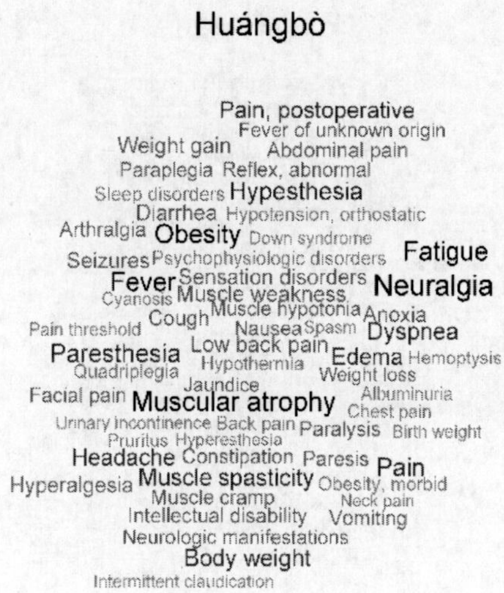

Figure 18.141. Huángbò symptom cloud.

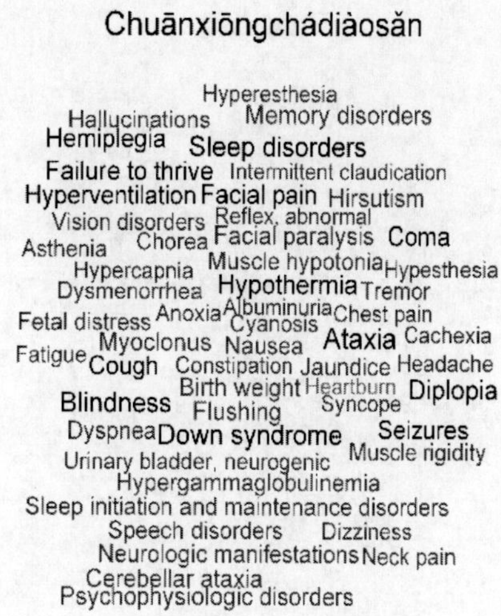

Figure 18.142. Chuānxiōngchádiàosǎn symptom cloud.

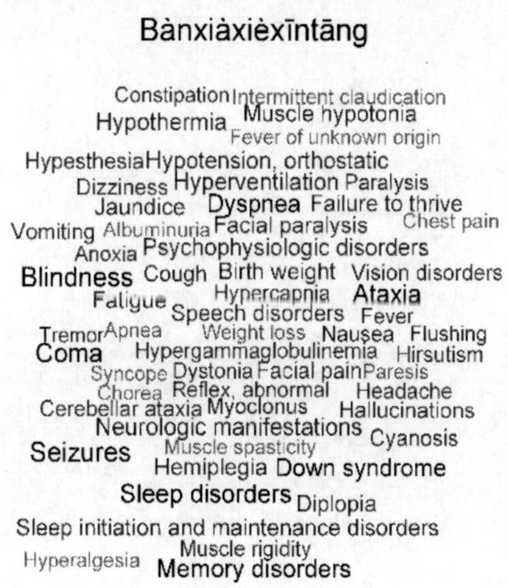

Figure 18.143. Bànxiàxièxīntāng symptom cloud.

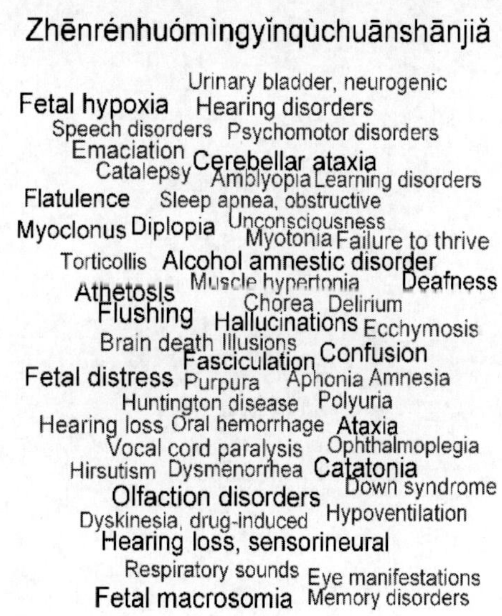

Figure 18.144. Zhēnrénhuómìngyǐnqùchuānshānjiǎ symptom cloud.

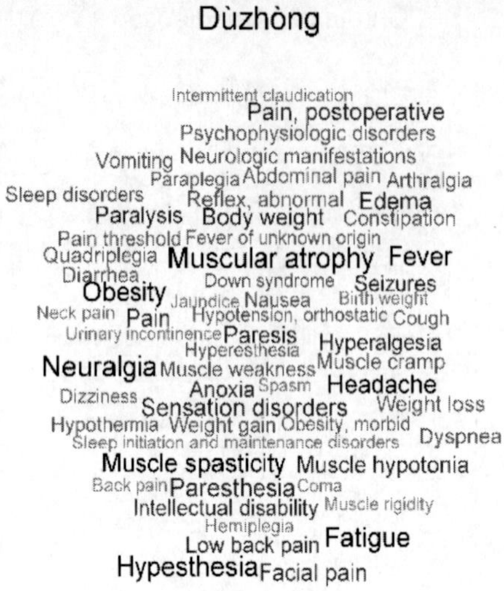

Figure 18.145. Dùzhòng symptom cloud.

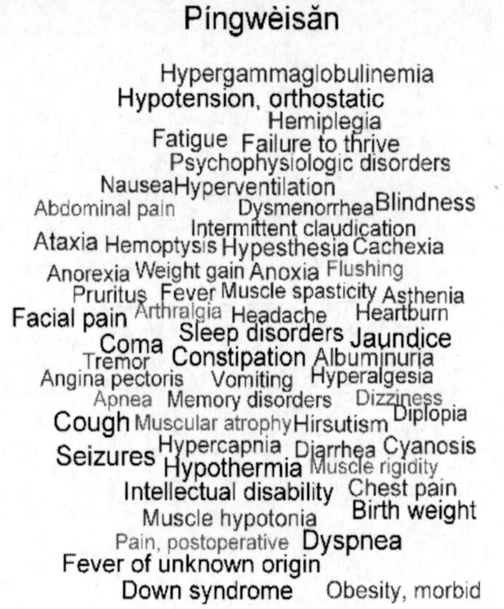

Figure 18.146. Píngwèisǎn symptom cloud.

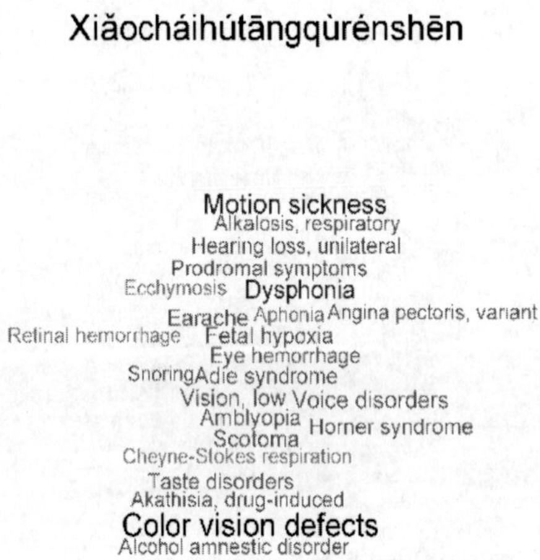

Figure 18.147. Xiǎocháihútāngqùrénshēn symptom cloud.

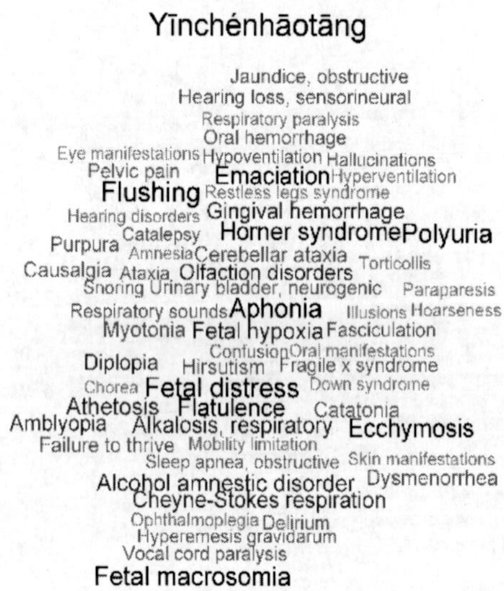

Figure 18.148. Yīnchénhāotāng symptom cloud.

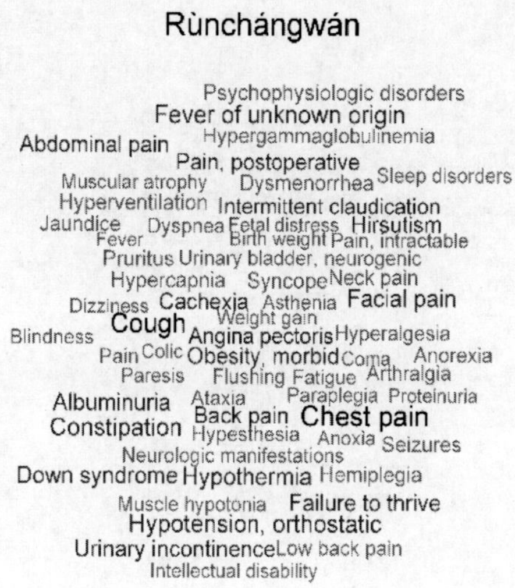

Figure 18.149. Rùnchángwán symptom cloud.

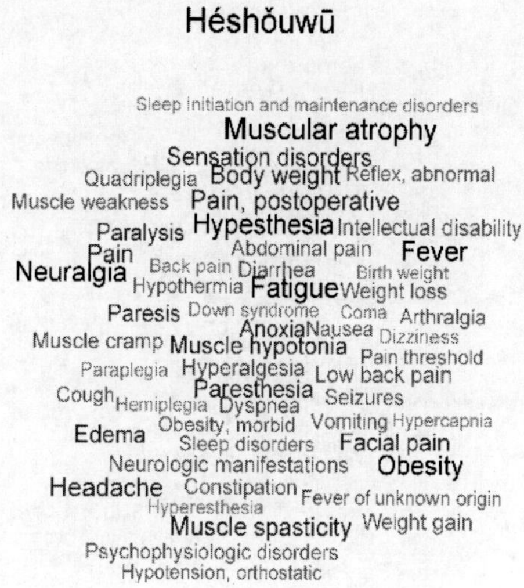

Figure 18.150. Héshǒuwū symptom cloud.

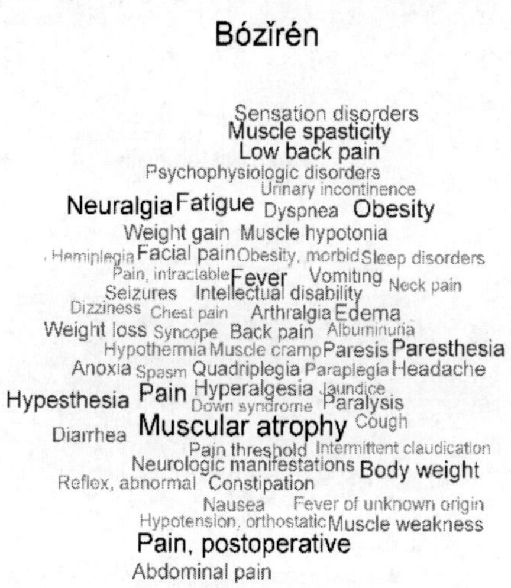

Figure 18.151. Bózǐrén symptom cloud.

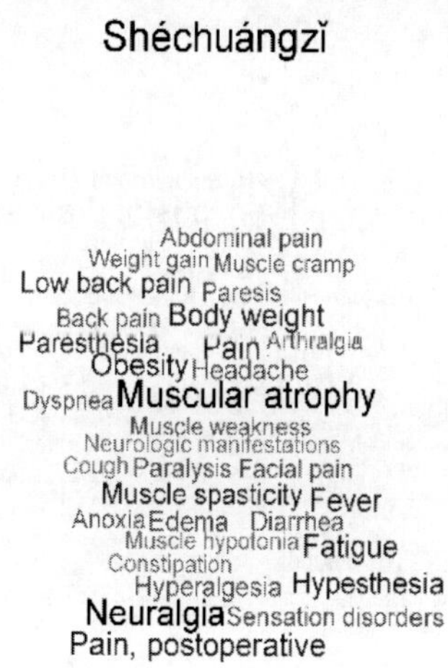

Figure 18.152. Shéchuángzǐ symptom cloud.

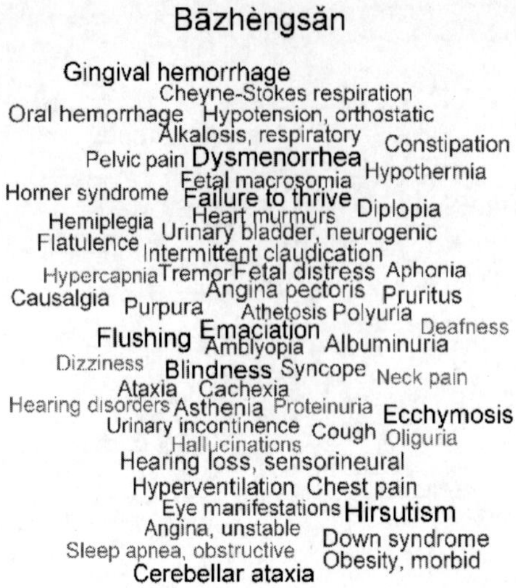

Figure 18.153. Bāzhèngsǎn symptom cloud.

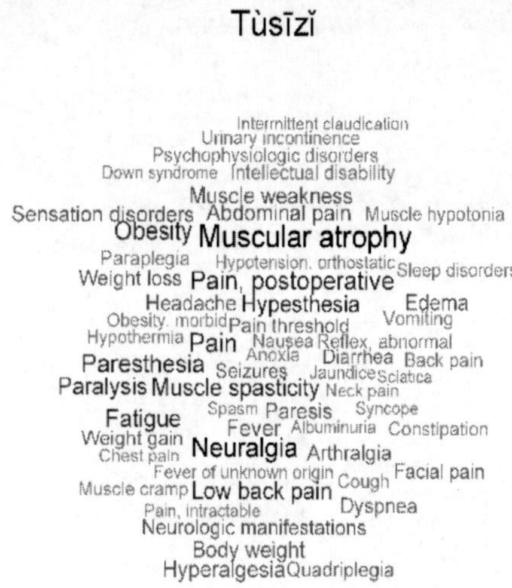

Figure 18.154. Tùsīzǐ symptom cloud.

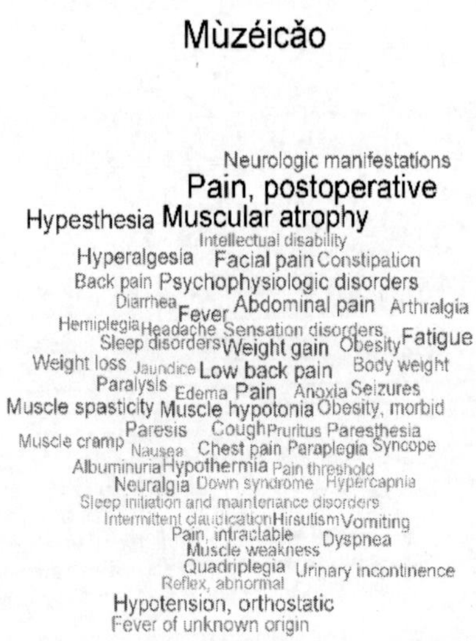

Figure 18.155. Mùzéicǎo symptom cloud.

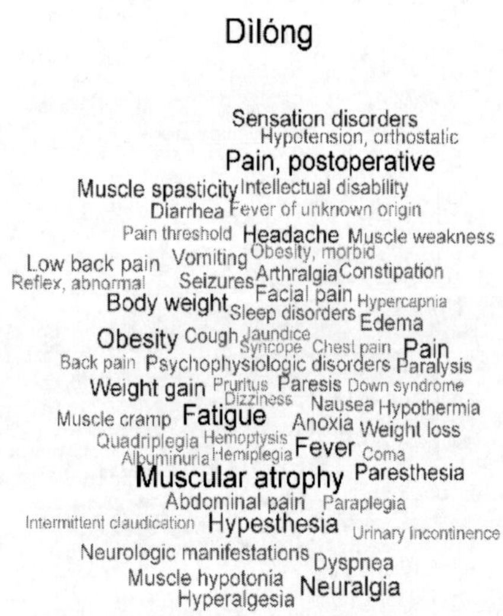

Figure 18.156. Dìlóng symptom cloud.

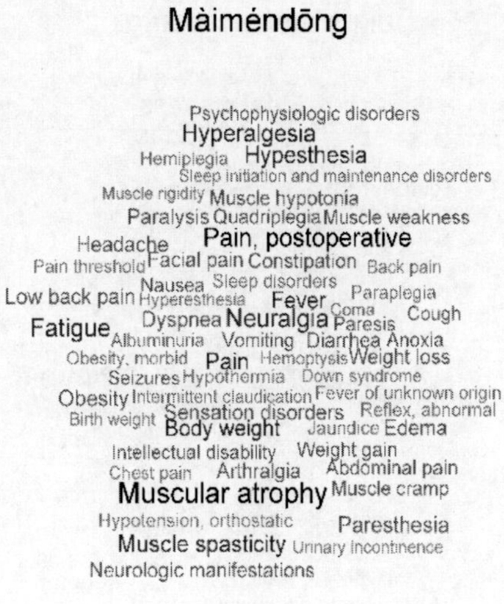

Figure 18.157. Màiméndōng symptom cloud.

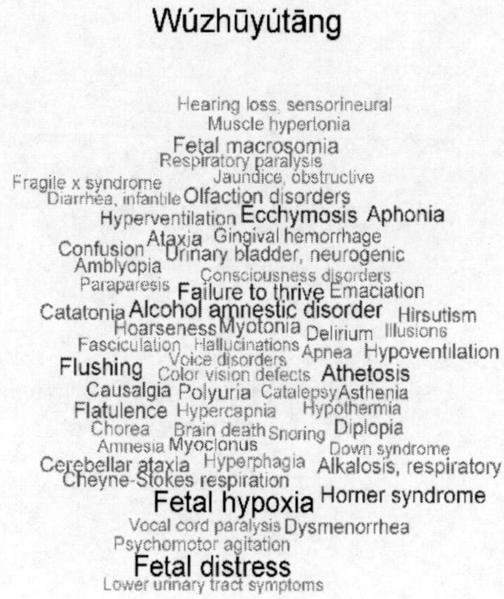

Figure 18.158. Wúzhūyútāng symptom cloud.

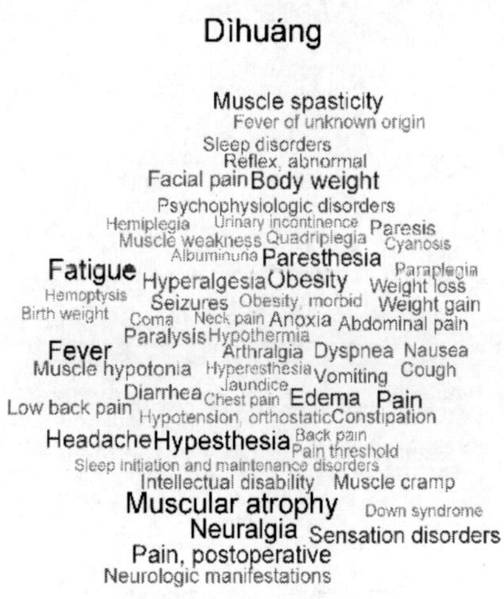

Figure 18.159. Dìhuáng symptom cloud.

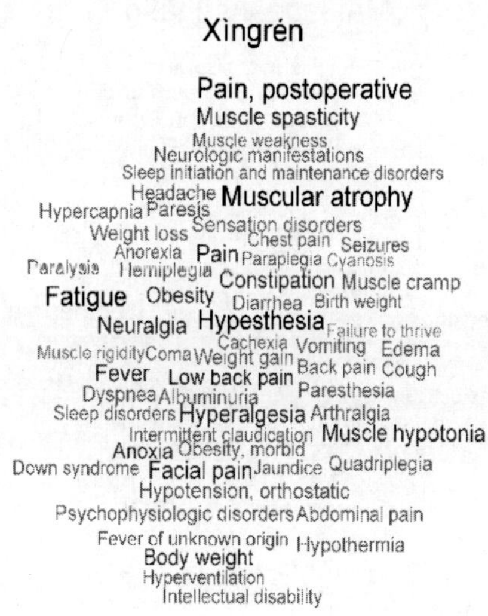

Figure 18.160. Xìngrén symptom cloud.

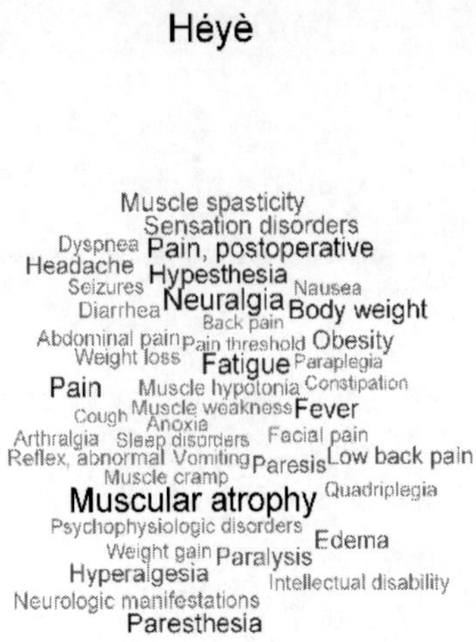

Figure 18.161. Héyè symptom cloud.

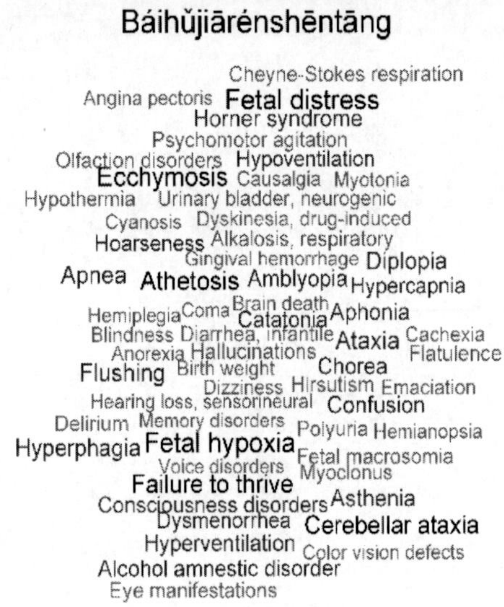

Figure 18.162. Báihǔjiārénshēntāng symptom cloud.

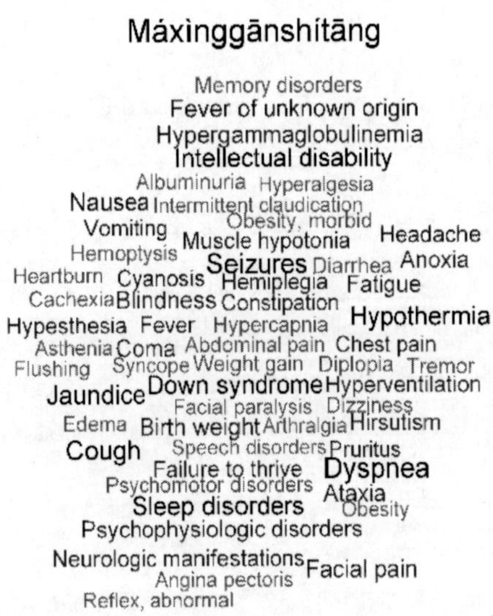

Figure 18.163. Máxìnggānshítāng symptom cloud.

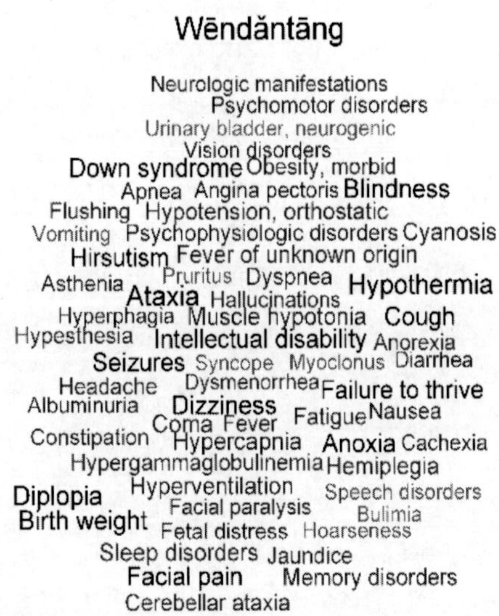

Figure 18.164. Wēndǎntāng symptom cloud.

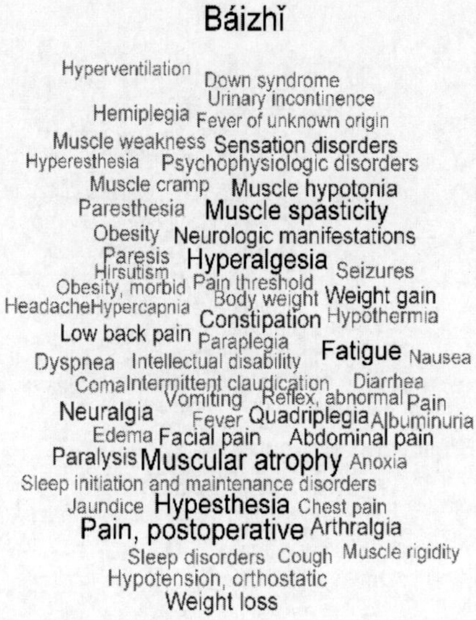

Figure 18.165. Báizhǐ symptom cloud.

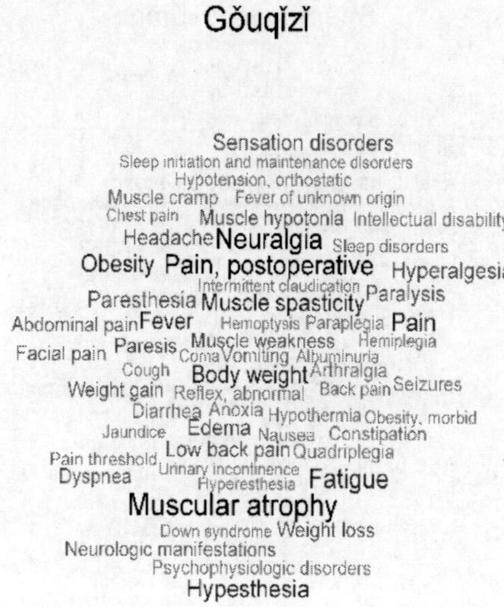

Figure 18.166. Gǒuqǐzǐ symptom cloud.

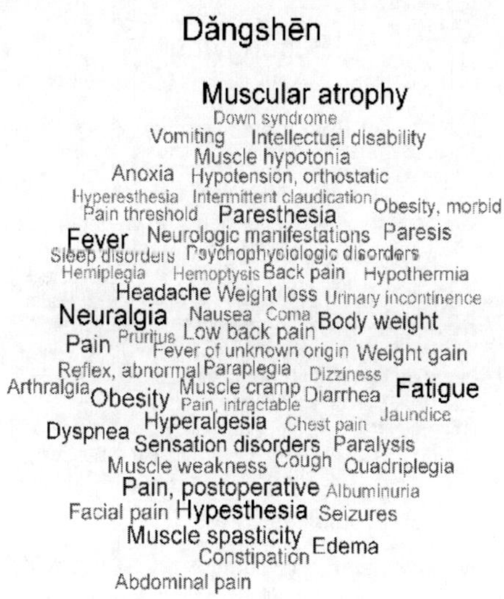

Figure 18.167. Dǎngshēn symptom cloud.

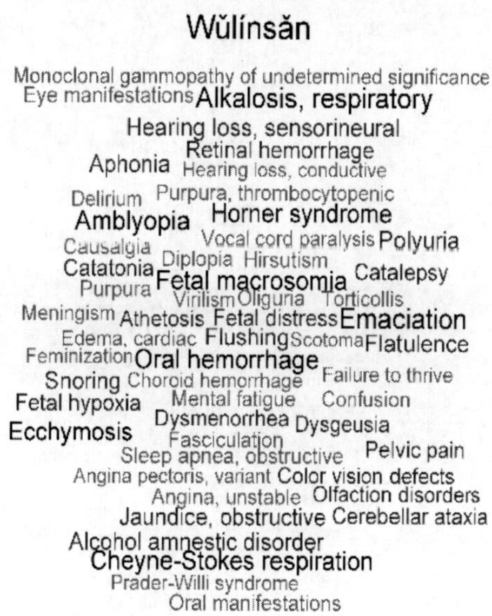

Figure 18.168. Wǔlínsǎn symptom cloud.

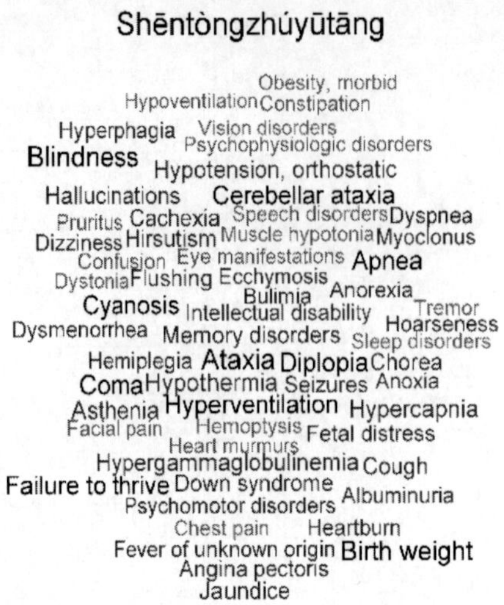

Figure 18.169. Shēntòngzhúyūtāng symptom cloud.

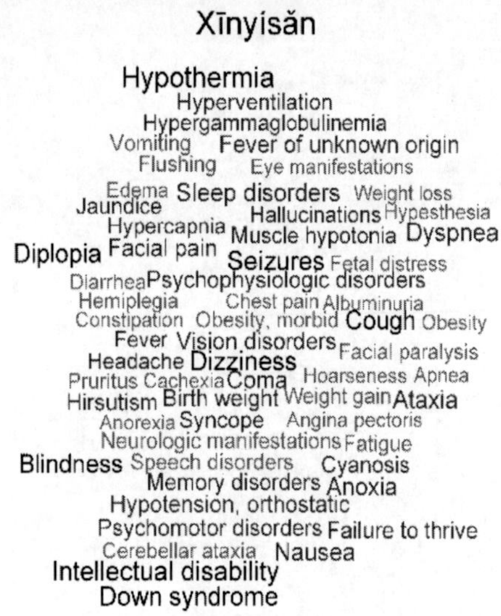

Figure 18.170. Xīnyísǎn symptom cloud.

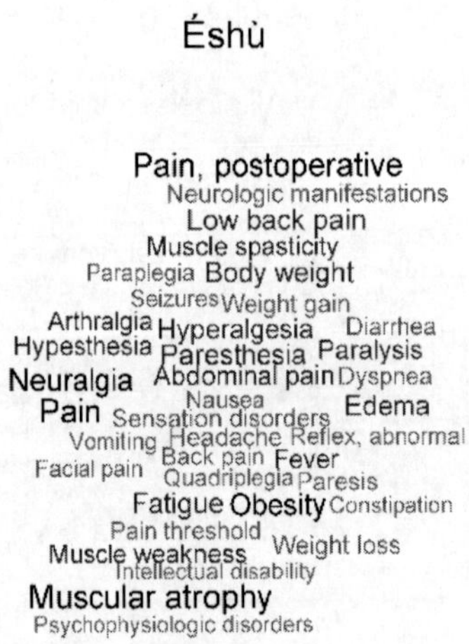

Figure 18.171. Éshù symptom cloud.

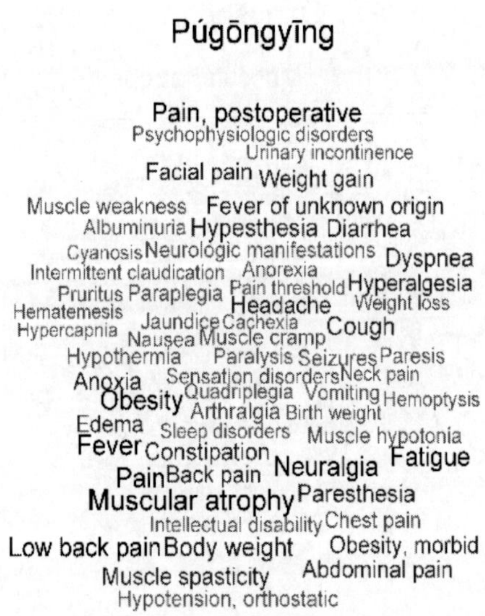

Figure 18.172. Púgōngyīng symptom cloud.

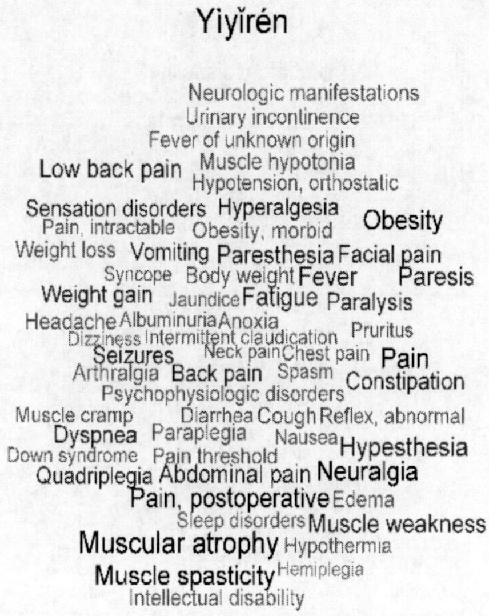

Figure 18.173. Yìyǐrén symptom cloud.

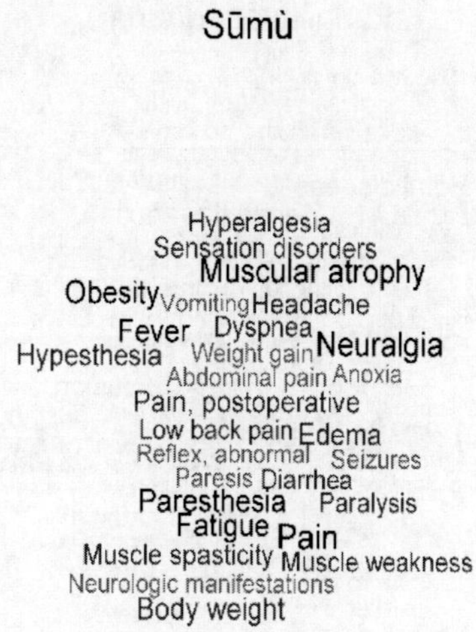

Figure 18.174. Sūmù symptom cloud.

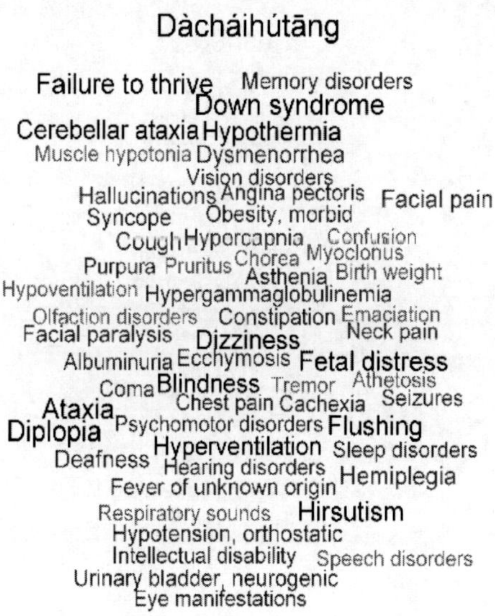

Figure 18.175. Dàcháihútāng symptom cloud.

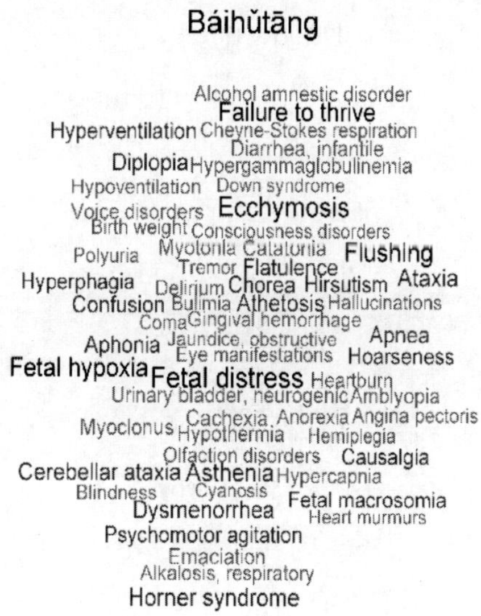

Figure 18.176. Báihǔtāng symptom cloud.

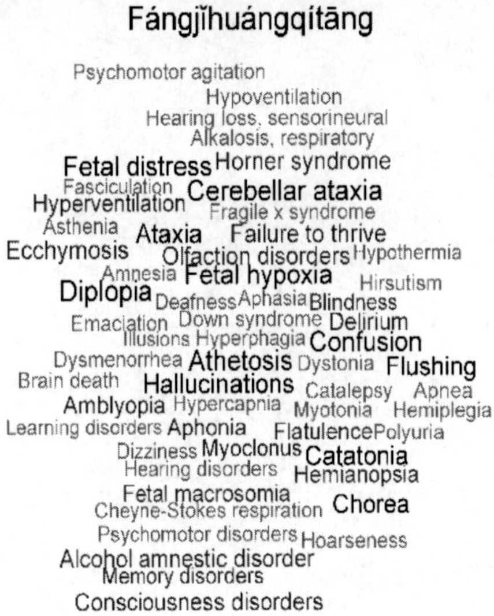

Figure 18.177. Fángjǐhuángqítāng symptom cloud.

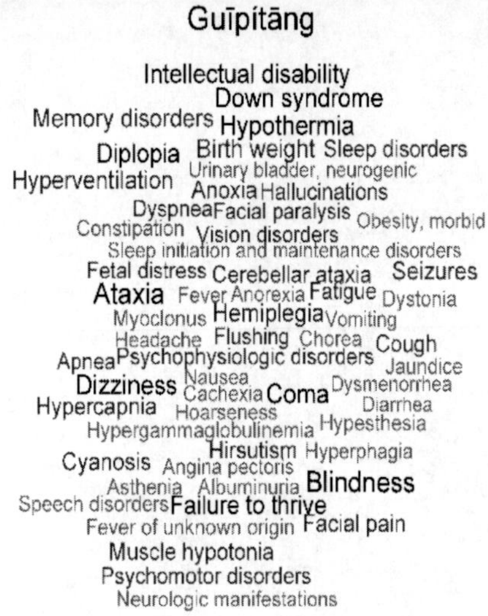

Figure 18.178. Guīpítāng symptom cloud.

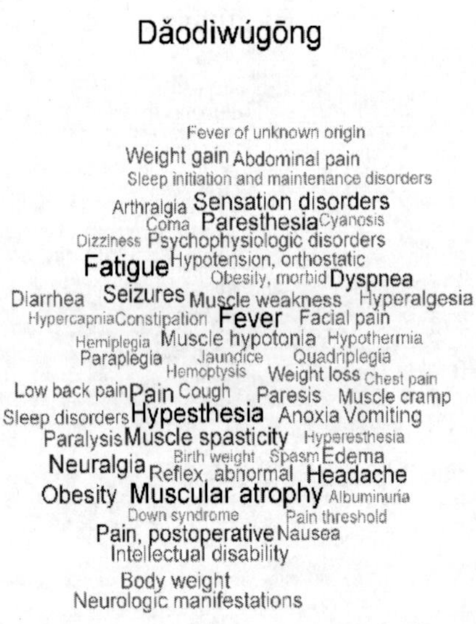

Figure 18.179. Dǎodìwúgōng symptom cloud.

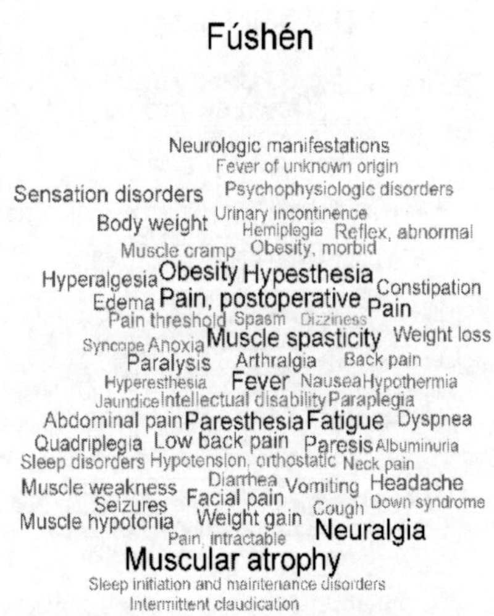

Figure 18.180. Fúshén symptom cloud.

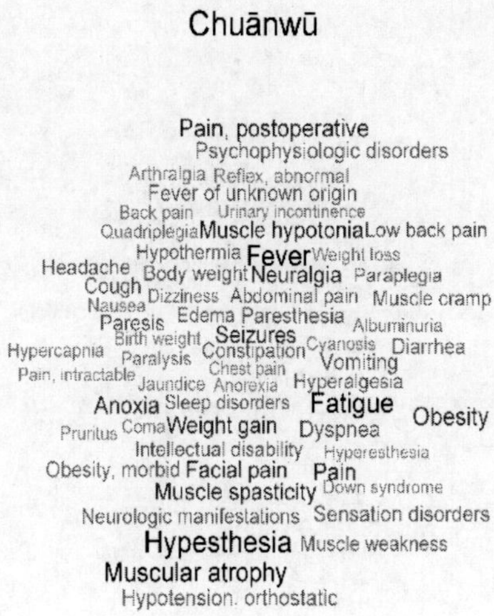

Figure 18.181. Chuānwū symptom cloud.

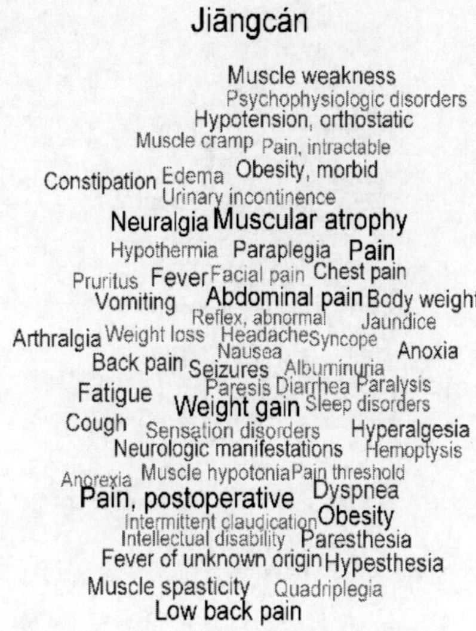

Figure 18.182. Jiāngcán symptom cloud.

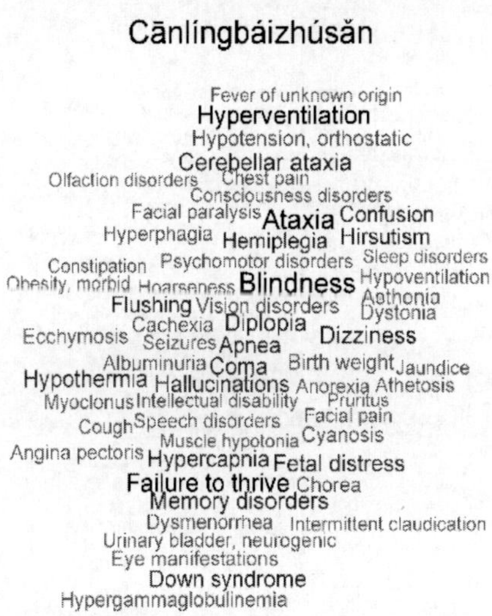

Figure 18.183. Cānlíngbáizhúsǎn symptom cloud.

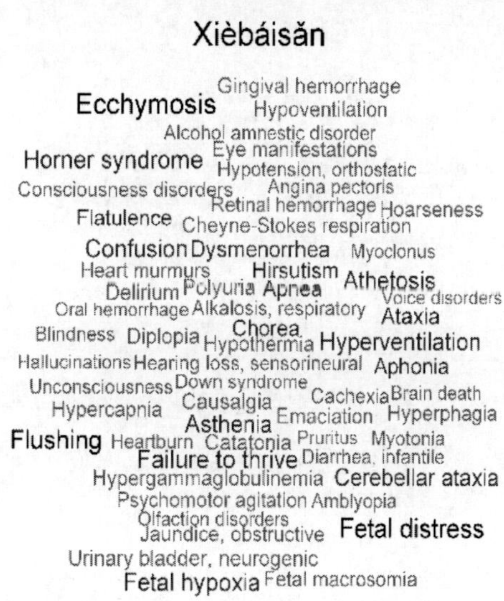

Figure 18.184. Xièbáisǎn symptom cloud.

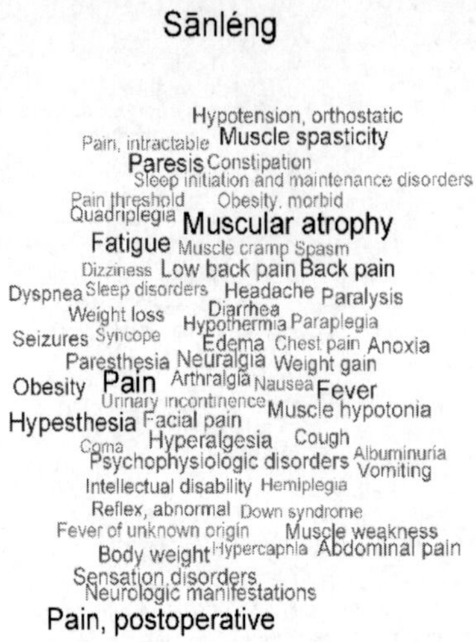

Figure 18.185. Sānléng symptom cloud.

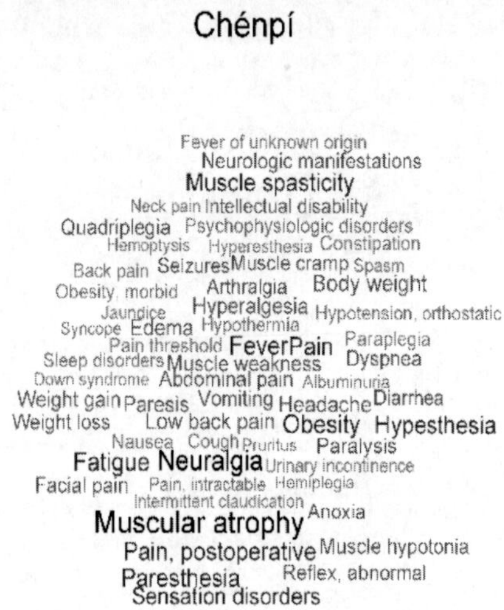

Figure 18.186. Chénpí symptom cloud.

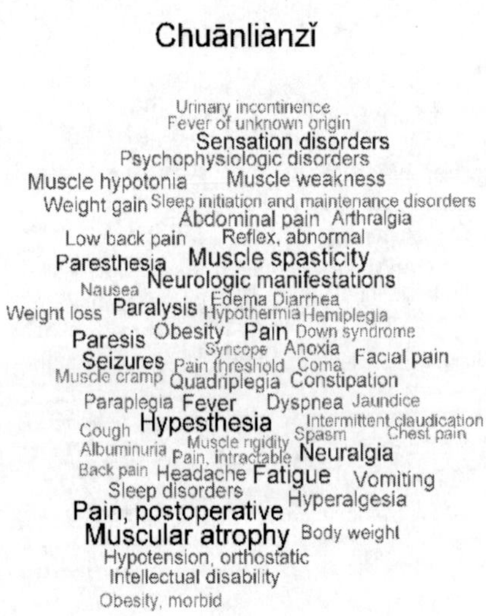

Figure 18.187. Chuānliànzǐ symptom cloud.

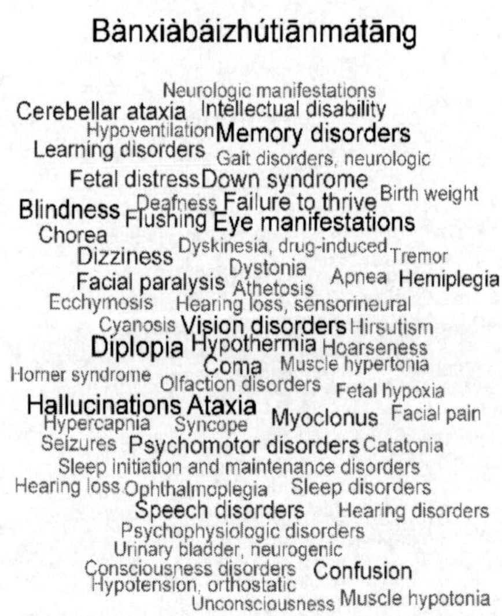

Figure 18.188. Bànxiàbáizhútiānmátāng symptom cloud.

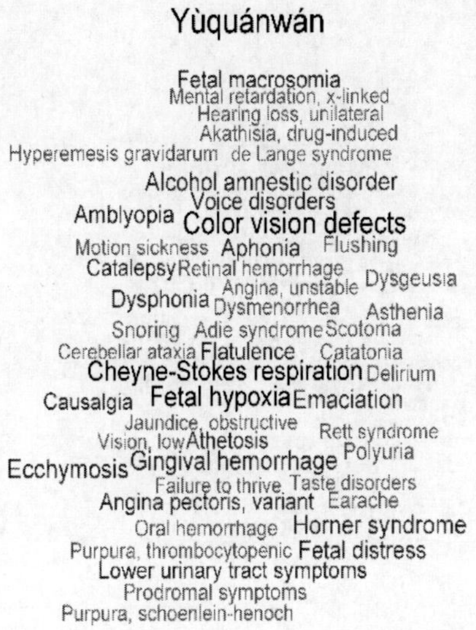

Figure 18.189. Yùquánwán symptom cloud.

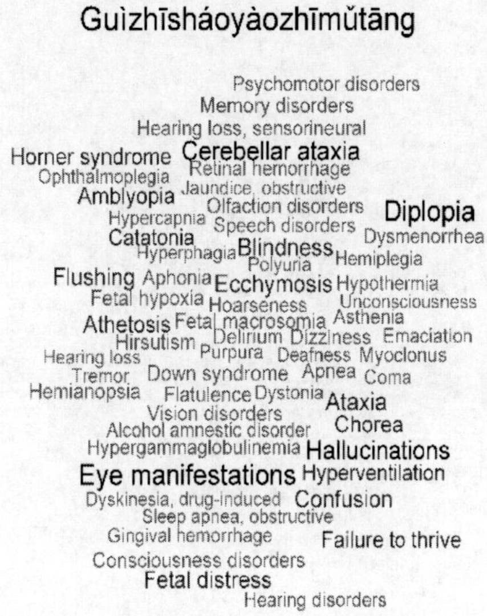

Figure 18.190. Guìzhīsháoyàozhīmǔtāng symptom cloud.

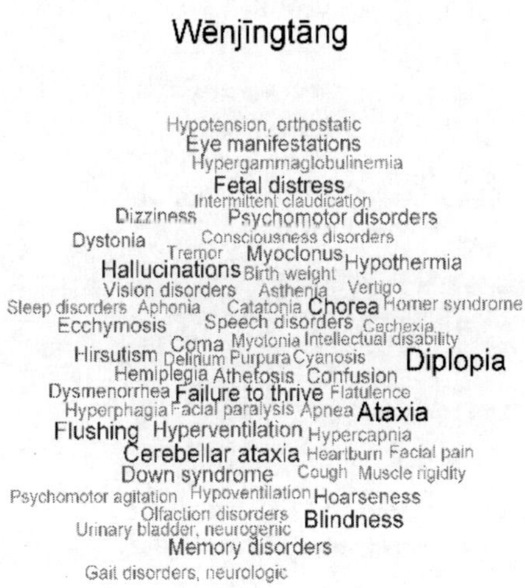

Figure 18.191. Wēnjīngtāng symptom cloud.

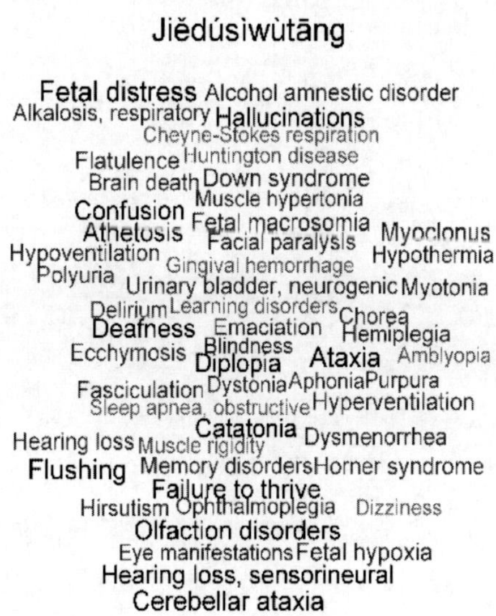

Figure 18.192. Jiědúsìwùtāng symptom cloud.

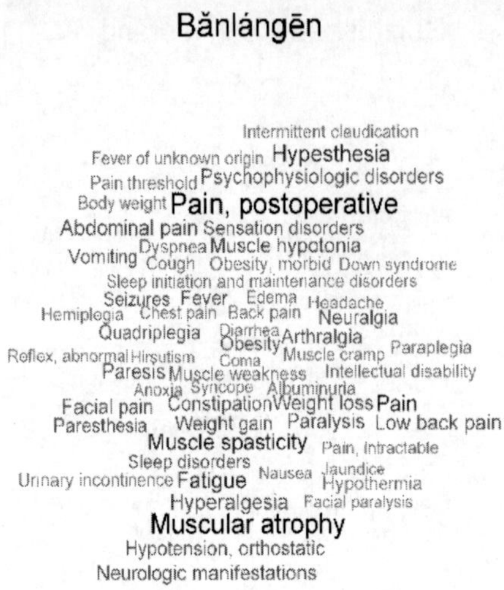

Figure 18.193. Bănlángēn symptom cloud.

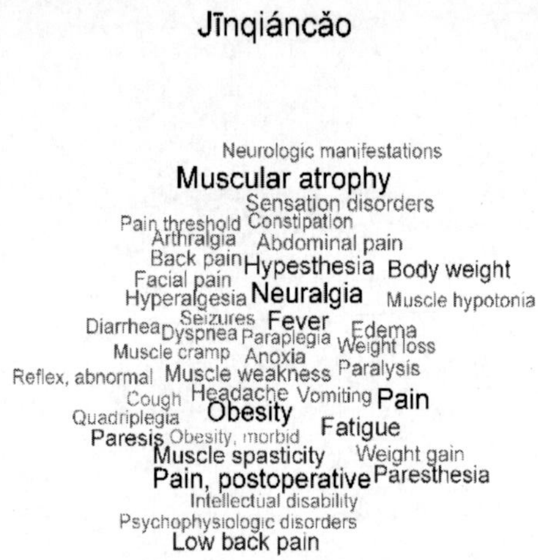

Figure 18.194. Jīnqiáncǎo symptom cloud.

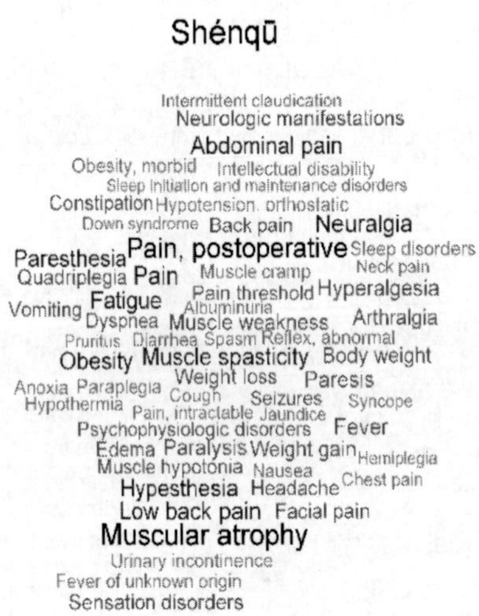

Figure 18.195. Shénqū symptom cloud.

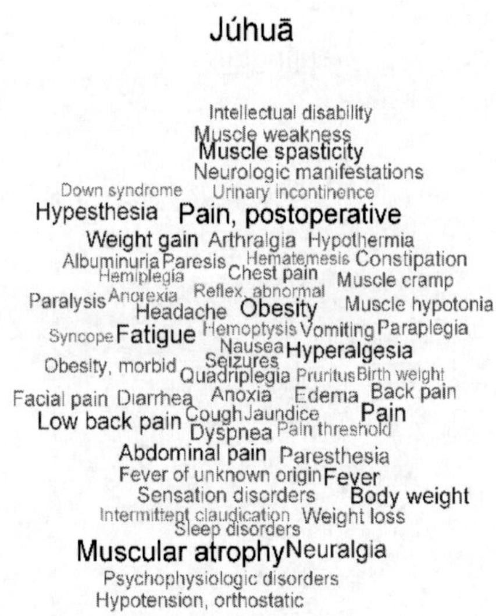

Figure 18.196. Júhuā symptom cloud.

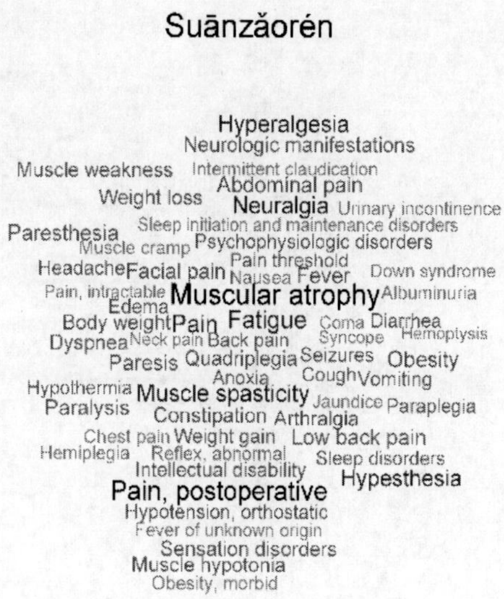

Figure 18.197. Suānzǎorén symptom cloud.

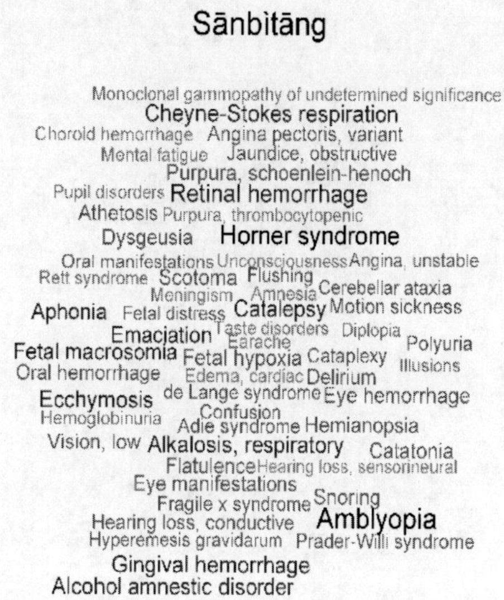

Figure 18.198. Sānbìtāng symptom cloud.

Appendix: Herbal Prescriptions by Multilingual Neural Machine Translation

Deep learning applications and performances have astonished the world since around 2016 (LeCun et al., 2015). The success of deep learning can be attributed to at least three concurrent developments: innovations in computational algorithms, availability of big data, and advances in computer hardware. Specifically, mathematic models, called artificial neural networks, are arranged into feedforward layers so that a layer in the model is able to abstractly represent the output of the preceding layer in the model (Wang, 2003, Chapter 5). Big data should be of high quality and diverse in the sense that images of a class, such as dog, should contain as many dog breeds, hair colors, body postures, camera angles and backgrounds as possible. Training of the model iteratively using a batch of dataset in a graphical processing unit can speed up the learning by up to a hundredfold. The "deep" in deep learning can therefore mean feeding data through so many layers in the artificial neural network model or training the model with so many batches in the data.

Besides the best-known achievement of deep learning in object recognition and computer vision, the other deep learning success is in machine translation and natural language processing. Different from the input pixel intensities in image classification, the input data in natural language processing are sequences of words. The state-of-the-art deep learning models for natural language processing tasks are the so-called Transformer (Vaswani et al., 2017), which, in addition to being multilayered, contains so-called self-attention layers to attend to individual positions in the sequence in order to better represent the sequence during language modeling or sentence translating tasks. As there exist so many natural languages in the world, if a Transformer model is trained to translate between a pair of languages, then so many models will need to be trained. It turned out that by pooling the vocabularies of individual languages into a single set of vocabulary supplemented with so-called language tags, a single Transformer model can be trained to translate between any language pairs, even between pairs that have no parallel sentences in the training data, achieving what is called zero-shot translation (Johnson et al., 2017; Zhang et al., 2020). This way of machine translation method is called multilingual neural machine translation (MNMT). A relevant development that uses Transformer encoder and accomplishes zero- or few-shot learning is the GPT-3 language model (Brown et al., 2020), which is the predecessor of ChatGPT that becomes well known today.

Encouraged by the success, we would like to harness the prowess of MNMT to the task of generating herbal prescriptions for signs and symptoms given that we have no pairs of herbal prescription and sign/symptom data, although we do have a large quantity, i.e., 42 million, of disease diagnoses and associated herbal prescriptions data (Wang, 2017). If we can manage to obtain disease and symptom pair data, then the issue is similar to the situation where we have only English to/from French sentences and English to/from German sentences, and we would like the MNMT to translate between French and German sentences utilizing MNMT's zero-shot translation capability. If the components of an herbal prescription are ordered according to their proportional weights in the prescription into a sequence like a sentence in a language, say French, then we have French sentences. And if the herbal prescription's matching disease diagnoses are ordered according to the primary disease diagnosis, secondary disease diagnosis, if any, and tertiary disease diagnosis, if any, of the patient in his medical insurance claim into a sequence like a sentence in a language, say English, then we have French-English sentence pairs (Wang, 2017). The next step is to get disease-symptom, i.e., English-German sentence, pairs. Note that, for convenience, we may neglect sign in sign and symptom.

To get diseases and their associated signs and symptoms, we searched all the articles in the PubMed server (https://pubmed.ncbi.nlm.nih.gov) for their disease and symptom MeSH terms (Zhou et al., 2014). MeSH stands for Medical Subject Headings and is the U.S. National Library of Medicine controlled vocabulary thesaurus for indexing articles in PubMed. The number of PubMed articles annotated with the MeSH terms of our interest is 1.49 million, as of February 2021. Each such article may contain multiple diseases and multiple signs/symptoms. The goal is to generate a disease-symptom sentence pair from each of such PubMed articles. Recall that a sentence is an ordered sequence of words. We ordered the disease MeSH terms in an article by disease prevalence in the population, which is available from our previous study (Wang, 2019). We ordered the sign and symptom MeSH terms into a sequence according to the tf-idf scores of individual sign and symptom MeSH terms calculated from the collection of 1.49 million records of sign and symptom MeSH terms. Tf-idf is a numeric statistic measuring how relevant a term is to a record in a collection of records. The rationale for the ordering is to give some rules for generating MeSH term sequences just like we use grammar while we write and speak a language. If we did not preprocess the data this way, a MeSH term could appear in any random position in a MeSH sentence and the Transformer model would be frustrated learning the random order. Finally, we have the desired disease-symptom sequence pairs or, in our analogy, the English-German sentence pairs for MNMT training. With the zero-shot translation capability of the MNMT method, the trained Transformer model is able to output herbal prescription given a sign or symptom and vice versa.

The other advantage of MNMT using a single transformer model is that we can mix English and German words, or disease and sign and symptom MeSH terms, into the input sentence and ask the trained model to output its French translation, or herbal prescription. This advantage results from the use of a single pooled vocabulary in the input and output layers of the transformer during MNMT training and cannot be achieved if we train two separately, i.e., German-English and English-French, bilingual models and use English as pivot to bridge between German and French translation. An example of exploiting this advantage in our context is that the trained transformer model is asked to output herbal prescriptions for a patient who has a diabetes diagnosis and at the same time presents with such signs and symptoms as overweight and fatigue.

The first layer in a transformer model is called embedding layer, whose functionality is to map individual words in the input sentence into points in a space whose dimension is usually very high, as high as e.g., 512. Every discrete word in the vocabulary then becomes represented by an array of 512 real numbers, called embedding vector. Before training, a word is initialized to 512 random values in the embedding space. As training begins, it can be imagined that the points in the embedding space start to move. In the end of the training when the discrepancy between model output sentences and the associated ground truth sentences does not improve anymore, we stop the training. It turns out that the embedding vectors in the trained model cluster in such a way that words of similar meaning cluster together, realizing what John Rupert Firth, an English Linguist, proposed in 1957 that "a word is characterized by the company it keeps." Furthermore, the other word embedding regularity is that the answer to "man is to king as woman is to ...?" can be obtained by searching for the words in the neighborhood of the resulting word embedding arithmetic: *king – man + woman* (Mikolov et al., 2013), where we italicize the word to indicate its word embedding vector. We exploited this property as a sanity check for the adequacy of our trained models and found the following example results:

Hyperplasia of prostate – Male + Female = Uterine leiomyoma
Angina Pectoris – Dānshēn + Bèimǔ = Cough
Morbid Obesity – Fángfēngtōngshèngsǎn + Jīngfángbàidúsǎn = Pruritus

In the embedding space neighborhood of the first arithmetic were also found "*Other disorders of cervical region*" and "*Female infertility*," which are female reproductive system disorders. In that of the second arithmetic was found "*Fever of Unknown Origin*," which, besides "*Cough*," is an indication of Bèimǔ. Note that the first word analogy concerns words from a single language, i.e., the disease diagnosis language, while the second and third analogies involve words from two different languages, i.e., the sign and symptom language and the prescription language. In other words, our MNMT training extends monolingual word analogy to multilingual word analogy, that is from *king – man + woman = queen* (man is to king as woman is to queen) to *roi – man + woman = reine* (man is to roi as woman is to reine).

Since diseases are coded in ICD-9-CM (International Classification of Diseases, 9th Revision, Clinical Modification https://www.cdc.gov/nchs/icd/icd9cm.htm) in the medical insurance claim data, the number of disease diagnoses is close to ten thousand (Wang, 2017). When preparing for the disease vocabulary, we created subwords so that the ten thousand different ICD-9-CM codes were represented by combinations of the subwords whose number was much smaller (Sennrich et al., 2016). With ordering of the MeSH terms, the number of unique pairs of disease sentences and their associated sign and symptom sentences dropped from 1.49 million to 0.37 million. We oversampled them so that the model did not bias its learning capacity against low resource language pairs (Arivazhagan et al., 2019). Other strategies in the MNMT that we found to improve the zero-shot performance include the random online backtranslation (Zhang et al., 2020) in fine tuning the model, top k random sampling, instead of beam search, to generate diverse outputs (Fan et al., 2018; Ippolito, et al., 2019) for backtranslation, and insertion of language tags in each target sentence in the training data (Li and Luo, 2021).

References

Arivazhagan, N., Bapna, A., Firat, O., Lepikhin, D., Johnson, M., Krikun, M., Chen, M. X., Cao, Y., Foster, G., Cherry, C., Macherey, W., Chen, Z., & Wu, Y. (2019). *Massively Multilingual Neural Machine Translation in the Wild: Findings and Challenges*. arXiv: https://doi.org/10.48550/arXiv.1907.05019.

Brown, T., Mann, B., Ryder, N., Subbiah, M., Kaplan, J. D., Dhariwal, P., Neelakantan, A., Shyam, P., Sastry, G., Askell, A., Agarwal, S., Herbert-Voss, A., Krueger, G., Henighan, T., Child, R., Ramesh, A., Ziegler, D., Wu, J., Winter, C., Hesse, C., Chen, M., Sigler, E., Litwin, M., Gray, S., Chess, B., Clark, J., Berner, C., McCandlish, S., Radford, A., Sutskever, I., & Amodei, D. (2020). Language models are few-shot learners. *NIPS'20: Proceedings of the 34th International Conference on Neural Information Processing Systems*, 1877–1901. https://dl.acm.org/doi/abs/10.5555/3495724.3495883.

Fan, A., Lewis, M., & Dauphin, Y. (2018). Hierarchical Neural Story Generation. *Proceedings of the 56th Annual Meeting of the Association for Computational Linguistics (Volume 1: Long Papers)*, 889–898. https://doi.org/10.18653/v1/p18-1082.

Ippolito, D., Kriz, R., Sedoc, J., Kustikova, M., & Callison-Burch, C. (2019). Comparison of Diverse Decoding Methods from Conditional Language Models. *Proceedings of the 57th Annual Meeting of the Association for Computational Linguistics*, 3752–3762. https://doi.org/10.18653/v1/p19-1365.

Johnson, M., Schuster, M., Le, Q. V., Krikun, M., Wu, Y., Chen, Z., Thorat, N., Viégas, F., Wattenberg, M., Corrado, G., Hughes, M., & Dean, J. (2017). Google's Multilingual Neural Machine Translation System: Enabling Zero-Shot Translation. *Transactions of the Association for Computational Linguistics*, *5*, 339–351. https://doi.org/10.1162/tacl_a_00065.

LeCun, Y., Bengio, Y., & Hinton, G. (2015). Deep Learning. *Nature*, *521*(7553), 436–444. https://doi.org/10.1038/nature14539.

Li, C., & Luo G. (2021). *Improving Zero-shot Multilingual Neural Machine Translation for Low-Resource Languages*. arXiv: https://doi.org/10.48550/arXiv.2110.00712.

Mikolov, T., Sutskever, I., Chen, K., Corrado, G., & Dean, J. (2013). Distributed representations of words and phrases and their compositionality. *NIPS'13: Proceedings of the 26th International Conference on Neural Information Processing Systems, 2*, 3111–3119. https://dl.acm.org/doi/10.5555/2999792.2999959.

Sennrich, R., Haddow, B., & Birch, A. (2016). Neural Machine Translation of Rare Words with Subword Units. *Proceedings of the 54th Annual Meeting of the Association for Computational Linguistics (Volume 1: Long Papers)*, 1715–1725. https://doi.org/10.18653/v1/p16-1162.

Vaswani, A., Shazeer, N., Parmar, N., Uszkoreit, J., Jones, L., Gomez, A. N., Kaiser, Ł., Polosukhin, I. (2017). Attention is all you need. *NIPS'17: Proceedings of the 31st International Conference on Neural Information Processing Systems*, 6000–6010. https://dl.acm.org/doi/10.5555/3295222.3295349.

Wang, S. C. (2003). *Interdisciplinary computing in Java programming language*. Kluwer Academic. https://doi.org/10.1007/978-1-4615-0377-4.

Wang, S. C. (2017). *Neural Machine Translation between Herbal Prescriptions and Diseases*. arXiv: https://doi.org/10.48550/arXiv.1707.02575.

Wang, S. C. (2019). *Clinical Herbal Prescriptions: Principles and Practices of Herbal Formulations from Deep Learning Health Insurance Herbal Prescription Big Data*. WSPC. https://doi.org/10.1142/11211.

Zhang, B., Williams, P., Titov, I., & Sennrich, R. (2020). Improving Massively Multilingual Neural Machine Translation and Zero-Shot Translation. *Proceedings of the 58th Annual Meeting of the Association for Computational Linguistics*, 1628–1639. https://doi.org/10.18653/v1/2020.acl-main.148.

Zhou, X., Menche, J., Barabási, A.-L., & Sharma, A. (2014). Human symptoms–disease network. *Nature Communications*, *5*, 4212. https://doi.org/10.1038/ncomms5212.

Index

B

D

E

F

G

H

I

N

Q

R

S

T

U

V

W

X

Author's Contact Information

Sun-Chong Wang
Department of Biomedical Sciences and Engineering
National Central University
Chungli, Taoyuan, Taiwan
sunchong.wang@gmail.com